AF688047

Handbook of Neuroprotection

Handbook of Neuroprotection

Editor: Craig Smith

MURPHY & MOORE
www.murphy-moorepublishing.com

www.murphy-moorepublishing.com

MURPHY & MOORE

Cataloging-in-Publication Data

Handbook of neuroprotection / edited by Craig Smith.
p. cm.
Includes bibliographical references and index.
ISBN 978-1-63987-773-7
1. Neurosciences. 2. Neurology. 3. Neuroprotective agents. I. Smith, Craig.
RC3434 .H36 2023
616.89--dc23

© Murphy & Moore Publishing, 2023

Murphy & Moore Publishing
1 Rockefeller Plaza,
New York City,
NY 10020, USA

ISBN 978-1-63987-773-7

This book contains information obtained from authentic and highly regarded sources. Copyright for all individual chapters remain with the respective authors as indicated. All chapters are published with permission under the Creative Commons Attribution License or equivalent. A wide variety of references are listed. Permission and sources are indicated; for detailed attributions, please refer to the permissions page and list of contributors. Reasonable efforts have been made to publish reliable data and information, but the authors, editors and publisher cannot assume any responsibility for the validity of all materials or the consequences of their use.

Trademark Notice: Registered trademark of products or corporate names are used only for explanation and identification without intent to infringe.

Contents

Preface

Neuroprotection refers to the preservation of neuronal structure and function. It is a well-researched therapy option for a variety of central nervous system (CNS) disorders comprising spinal cord injury, neurodegenerative diseases, traumatic brain injury, stroke and acute control of neurotoxin ingestion. Neuroprotection is focused on stopping or slowing down the loss of neurons in order to avoid or limit disease progression and consequent damage. Some of the mechanisms associated with neuronal injury are increased levels in oxidative stress, energy failure, decreased delivery of oxygen and glucose to the brain, and iron accumulation. Antioxidants and glutamate antagonists are two common neuroprotective therapies that aim to reduce oxidative stress and excitotoxicity, which are related with neuronal death. Neurotrophic factors, bioactive substances, cell engineering, and dietary nutrients may facilitate neuroprotection by improving pathogenic processes associated with neuronal death or degeneration. This book unravels the recent studies on neuroprotection. The readers would gain knowledge that would broaden their perspective about this area of neurology. It will serve as a valuable source of reference for graduate and post graduate students.

After months of intensive research and writing, this book is the end result of all who devoted their time and efforts in the initiation and progress of this book. It will surely be a source of reference in enhancing the required knowledge of the new developments in the area. During the course of developing this book, certain measures such as accuracy, authenticity and research focused analytical studies were given preference in order to produce a comprehensive book in the area of study.

This book would not have been possible without the efforts of the authors and the publisher. I extend my sincere thanks to them. Secondly, I express my gratitude to my family and well-wishers. And most importantly, I thank my students for constantly expressing their willingness and curiosity in enhancing their knowledge in the field, which encourages me to take up further research projects for the advancement of the area.

Editor

1

Neuroprotective Effect of Antioxidants in the Brain

Kyung Hee Lee [1], Myeounghoon Cha [2] and Bae Hwan Lee [2,3,*]

1 Department of Dental Hygiene, Division of Health Science, Dongseo University, Busan 47011, Korea; kyhee@dongseo.ac.kr
2 Department of Physiology, Yonsei University College of Medicine, Seoul 03722, Korea; mhcha@yuhs.ac
3 Brain Korea 21 PLUS Project for Medical Science, Yonsei University College of Medicine, Seoul 03722, Korea
* Correspondence: bhlee@yuhs.ac

Abstract: The brain is vulnerable to excessive oxidative insults because of its abundant lipid content, high energy requirements, and weak antioxidant capacity. Reactive oxygen species (ROS) increase susceptibility to neuronal damage and functional deficits, via oxidative changes in the brain in neurodegenerative diseases. Overabundance and abnormal levels of ROS and/or overload of metals are regulated by cellular defense mechanisms, intracellular signaling, and physiological functions of antioxidants in the brain. Single and/or complex antioxidant compounds targeting oxidative stress, redox metals, and neuronal cell death have been evaluated in multiple preclinical and clinical trials as a complementary therapeutic strategy for combating oxidative stress associated with neurodegenerative diseases. Herein, we present a general analysis and overview of various antioxidants and suggest potential courses of antioxidant treatments for the neuroprotection of the brain from oxidative injury. This review focuses on enzymatic and non-enzymatic antioxidant mechanisms in the brain and examines the relative advantages and methodological concerns when assessing antioxidant compounds for the treatment of neurodegenerative disorders.

Keywords: neuroprotection; antioxidant; brain; neurodegenerative disease; oxidative stress

1. Introduction

Oxidative stress is considered as a detrimental condition for normal brain functioning. Since the brain uses chemically diverse reactive species for signal transmission, it is susceptible to oxidative stress [1]. The human brain consists of more than 86 billion neurons and over 250–300 billion glial +cells, which consume over 20% of the total basal oxygen [2,3]. The mitochondria in the brain use the inspired basal oxygen to reduce O_2 to H_2O to support adenosine triphosphate (ATP) synthesis [4]. The electron transport chain in the mitochondria is not efficient and leakage of reactive oxygen species (ROS) from the mitochondria occurs when there is excess of oxygen [5]. Redox signaling in the brain functions as an intrinsic sensor to oxidative stress, when signals go awry during pathological conditions. Brain tissue has a high rate of oxidative metabolic activity, intense production of reactive oxygen metabolites, relatively low levels of antioxidants, low repair capacity, non-replicating neuronal cells, and a high membrane surface to cytoplasm ratio [6]. The cellular antioxidant system that prevents tissue damage is composed of endogenous and exogenous antioxidants that have the ability to reduce different chemicals. In biological antioxidant defense systems, both endogenous and exogenous antioxidants are classified into enzymatic antioxidants and non-enzymatic antioxidants, including oxidative enzyme inhibitors, antioxidant enzyme cofactors, ROS/RNS scavengers, and transition metal chelators [7,8]. These two main antioxidant systems play an important role in maintaining the balance between pro-oxidant and antioxidant agents in the brain and in mitigating oxidative stress [9]. The present review focuses on enzymatic and non-enzymatic antioxidant mechanisms in the brain and examines the relative advantages of antioxidant compounds for the treatment of various brain diseases. Therefore, this review will describe selective antioxidants shown to have neuroprotective effects that limit neurodegenerative disease.

2. Factors That Contribute to Vulnerability of the Brain to Oxidative Stress

Free radicals or other reactive molecules disturb cellular energy metabolism and cause oxidative stress. Endogenous redox imbalance by pro-oxidant and antioxidant agents occurs as a result of free radicals, which play an important role in oxidative stress, cell death, and tissue damage. Increased free radical production due to excess pro-oxidant mechanisms can react with lipids, proteins, nucleic acids, and other biomolecules which can alter their structure and function. A high concentration of polyunsaturated fatty acids exists in membrane lipids in the brain [10]. These are sources of decomposition reaction in the form of lipid peroxidation, in which a single initiating free radical can precipitate the destruction of adjacent molecules. Polyunsaturated fatty acids especially serve as major biological targets for oxidative damage induced by ROS. Other candidate molecules that serve as biological targets of free radicals are nucleic acids. Breaks in DNA or modified bases can result in aberrant gene expression and cell death [11]. Moreover, free radicals can also oxidize the backbone and side chains of proteins, thereby disrupting the function of enzymes, receptors, neurotransmitters, and structural proteins by oxidative modification [12]. Highly reactive oxygen radicals are produced in the brain as a result of interactions between various transition metals and their reducing equivalents. Transition metals including iron, copper, zinc, and manganese, are associated with increased free radical production by the Fenton reaction [13,14]. Since the brain has abundant lipid content, high energy requirements, and weak antioxidant capacity, it is an easy target for excessive oxidative insults. Specifically, ROS increase susceptibility to neuronal damage and functional decline via brain oxidation in Alzheimer's disease (AD), Parkinson's disease (PD), amyotrophic lateral sclerosis (ALS), cerebrovascular disorders, psychiatric disorders, and other neurodegenerative diseases [6,13,15] (Figure 1).

Considering a detailed perspective on signaling, the rationale underlying the vulnerability of the neurons in the brain to oxidative stress are as follows: In redox signaling, O_2^-/H_2O_2 generation by the reduced form of nicotinamide adenine dinucleotide phosphate (NADPH) oxidase 2 induces the activation of signaling proteins via sulfenic acid formation [16,17]. The brain is dependent on Ca^{2+} signaling for synaptic plasticity, a fundamental brain function, and it expends considerable amounts of ATP to maintain intracellular Ca^{2+} homeostasis. Synaptic terminal glutamate-induced Ca^{2+} transients activate neuronal nitric oxide synthase (nNOS)-mediated $NO^{\cdot}$ generation, and additionally, Ca^{2+} overloaded in the mitochondria induces O_2^-/H_2O_2 generation which can lead to $ONOO^{\cdot}$ production and excitotoxicity [18–20]. Particularly, the mitochondria generate O_2^- in complex I and complex III and the monoamine oxidase enzyme isoform catalyzes H_2O_2 generation during metabolism [21–23]. The human brain consumes over 25% circulating glucose to support neuronal function; however, protein inactivation by the formation of advanced end glycation products (AGE) due to decreased glycolytic rates can cause glucose-induced oxidative stress [24,25]. Neurotransmitters with a catechol group render the brain sensitive to oxidative stress. Redox-active transition metals catalyze the auto-oxidation of dopamine to a semiquinone radical during neurotransmitter oxidation [26–28]. The mature neurons of the brain have abundant and multiple mechanisms that promote long-term neuronal survival and prevent cell death; however, the brain has a comparatively weak endogenous antioxidant defense system relative to other tissues and is susceptible to imbalance in redox homeostasis. For instance, neurons with 50 times lower catalase content than hepatocytes have constrained glutathione peroxidase 4 (GPX4) activity (owing to low glutathione [GSH] content) and a modest antioxidant defense mechanism [29–31]. Microglia monitor neuronal activity for removal of unhealthy cells, neuronal wiring during development, and activity dependent synaptic plasticity. They generate O_2^- via NADPH oxidase 2 (NOX2) within an end-foot process, thus influencing brain oxidation [32,33]. Redox-active transition metals, such as Fe^{2+} and Cu^+, are enriched in the brain and therefore contribute to ferroptosis by catalyzing peroxyl ($ROO^{\cdot}$) and alkoxyl ($RO^{\cdot}$) radical generation [34,35]. Lipid peroxidation, which involves initiation, oxygenation, propagation, and termination, occurs within the neuronal cell membrane [36]. The brain uses nNOS and NOX isoforms to maintain essential functions. However, nNOS/NOX expression is associated with NO˙ generation, which can be spatially co-generated while producing ONOO˙ [37,38]. In summary, these interconnected, myriad factors render the brain vulnerable to oxidative stress. Furthermore, excessive production of reactive species and insufficient activity of antioxidant defense systems have been implicated in the pathogenesis of neurodegeneration.

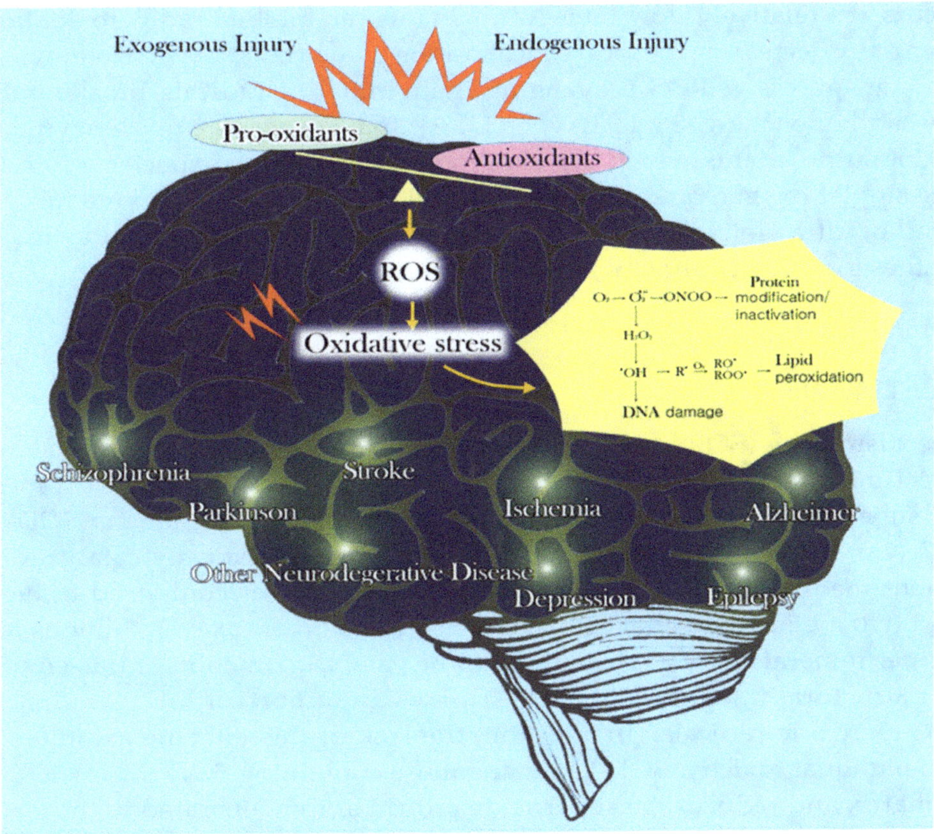

Figure 1. Development of various diseases by the pathophysiology of oxidative stress in the brain. Balance and imbalance between pro-oxidants and antioxidants against reactive oxygen species production induce oxidative stress and are consequently involved in neuronal damage resulting in the neurodegenerative diseases.

3. Role of Antioxidants in the Brain

Antioxidants act in two ways: First, the antioxidant defense systems, which are initiated against oxidative damage, prevent generation of ROS, and block and capture the generated radicals [39]. These systems are present in the aqueous and membrane compartments of cells; they can be enzymatic or non-enzymatic. The first line of defense has been identified as an enzymatic antioxidant system that includes superoxide dismutase, catalase, and glutathione peroxidase. The second line of defense is represented by reduced thiol and non-enzymatic antioxidants, including hydro- and lipo-soluble or metabolic compounds [7]. Second, during the antioxidant repair process, the removal of damaged biomolecules before their aggregation causes alterations in cell metabolism. The intervention by the repair systems consists of repairing oxidatively damaged nucleic acids by specific enzymes, removing oxidized proteins by the proteolytic systems, and repairing oxidized lipids by phospholipases, peroxidases, or acryl transferases [8,39,40].

Antioxidants act to directly scavenge oxidizing radicals and regenerate oxidized biomolecules in organisms. Neuronal cells possess several factors that minimize oxidative damage and a complex antioxidant system consisting of various antioxidant enzymes and non-enzymes. With regard to the mechanism of action of antioxidants, antioxidants respond to different steps of oxidative radical processing and can be considered by taking into account the different steps of lipid peroxidation in cell membranes such as: initiation, propagation, and chain termination [36]. The first step of initiation of lipid peroxidation can be promoted by diverse exogenous factors, endogenous enzyme systems, and the electron transport chain in the mitochondria. The propagation step of peroxidation is initiated by the addition of oxygen to carbon-centered radicals, which are generated at, or near, the diffusion-controlled rate. Propagation is represented by the transfer of a hydrogen atom to the chain carrying peroxyl radicals and occurs at a relatively slow rate. Antioxidants can inhibit lipid peroxidation by removing molecular oxygen or by decreasing the local concentration of molecular oxygen, removing pro-oxidative metal ions, trapping aggressive ROS, scavenging chain initiating radicals, breaking the chain of free radical reactions, and quenching singlet oxygen [7,41]. In its protective role, enzymatic antioxidants are chain-breaking antioxidants which are able to scavenge radical species while non-enzymatic antioxidants are singlet oxygen quenchers, metal chelators, oxidative enzyme inhibitors, peroxide decomposers, and/or ultra violet (UV) radiation absorbers [7]. Additionally, antioxidant enzymes can catalyze the synthesis or regeneration of non-enzymatic antioxidants.

3.1. Enzymatic Antioxidants

3.1.1. Superoxide Dismutase

Superoxide dismutase (SOD), which belongs to the enzymatic defense system, changes the superoxide radical anion to H_2O_2 by oxidative decay. Another function of SOD is to protect dehydratase from free radical superoxide inactivation. There are three forms of SOD in humans. SOD-1, a copper-zinc containing SOD (Cu, Zn-SOD), is present in the cytosol and specifically catalyzes dismutation in a pH-independent medium [42]. SOD-1 protein is a homodimer composed of eight antiparallel beta strands and two metal atoms that catalyze the conversion of toxic O_2^- anions to H_2O_2 and O_2. Specifically, copper minerals play a crucial role in the catalytic function of this enzyme, while zinc is important for structural integrity [43]. SOD-1 plays an important role as a first line of defense by detoxifying superoxide radicals. In addition, the lack of this enzyme exhibited a pronounced susceptibility to paraquat toxicity. SOD-2, a manganese containing SOD (Mn-SOD), is found in the mitochondrial matrix and reduces the superoxide radical anion generated in the electron transport chain [44]. A detailed analysis revealed that the SOD-2 subunit needs one metal atom and that it is functionally disabled in the absence of Mn atoms in the active site. SOD-2 attracts O_2^- and turns positive on the active side. The active metal provides electrons directly to O_2^- then reduces one molecule of O_2^- and one proton to be converted to form H_2O_2 (Figure 2). The amount of SOD-2 is different in each cell type, depending on the number of mitochondria. Specifically, the presence of SOD-2 is essential for the survival of aerobic cells and the development of cellular resistance to oxidative stress. SOD-3, an extracellular SOD (EC-SOD), also contains copper and zinc in its structure, is synthesized inside the cell and secreted into the extracellular matrix [45]. SOD-3 enzyme is not induced by its substrate or other oxidants and is regulated to coordinate with cytokines, rather than as a response of individual cells to oxidants [46].

In neurodegenerative diseases, SOD-1 and SOD-2 genes appear to be disrupted and/or mutated. SOD-1 gene mutations produce diverse cellular changes such as alteration of gene expression, unusual protein interactions, caspase activation, mitochondrial dysfunction, and cytoskeletal abnormalities in familial ALS [47]. Overexpression of SOD-1 protects neurons against the neurotoxic effects of amyloid beta (Aβ), and loss of SOD-1 accelerates aging-related pathologies and reduces lifespan in mice [48–50]. SOD-1 deficiency in an AD model showed that it was associated with augmented Aβ oligomerization and memory impairment mediated by oxidative stress [51]. Overexpression of SOD-2 by treatment with sodium orthovanadate could rescue synaptic failure and neuronal cell death in the hippocampus after kainic acid (KA)-induced oxidative stress; moreover, an increase in SOD-2 protected the neuronal death from oxidative injury [52]. Impaired SOD-2 is a common potential pathogenesis related to oxidative stress in PD and AD [6]. In human amyloid precursor protein (hAPP) transgenic mice with over 50% reduced SOD-2 activity, increased SOD-2 protects the age-related brain against hAPP/Aβ-induced impairments [53]. Extracellularly administered SOD was effective in inhibiting cell death and restoring healthy mitochondrial morphology in a monosodium glutamate-induced excitotoxicity disease model [54]. An increase in SOD-2 can be expected to assist or improve neuronal function and vascular pathology in AD as a therapeutic effect.

3.1.2. Catalase

Catalase (CAT), a heme-containing tetrameric protein is a common antioxidant enzyme naturally produced by the body when exposed to oxygen. H_2O_2 generated inside the cell is enzymatically catabolized in aerobic organisms by catalase and the activity of several peroxidases. CAT is one of the most efficient enzymes that cannot be saturated by H_2O_2 at any concentration. It reacts with H_2O_2 to form water/alcohol and oxygen using Fe as a cofactor [55,56]. CAT protects cells by detoxification of the generated H_2O_2 and plays an important role in the acquisition of tolerance to oxidative stress as an adaptive response [57]. CAT can maintain the concentration of O_2 either for repeated rounds of chemical reduction or for direct interaction with the toxin [58] (Figure 2). Furthermore, inhibition of CAT activity results in enhanced cytotoxicity and increased ROS, indicating an important role of CAT in maintaining the oxidative balance [59]. Specifically, mislocalized CAT is associated with accumulation of H_2O_2 [60] and other ROS in the cells leading to compromised neurological function [61]. Thus, deficiency or malfunction of CAT is postulated to be related to the pathogenesis of many age-associated degenerative diseases.

CAT treatment reduces H_2O_2 levels and improves neuronal survival following Aβ-induced toxicity in neuronal culture [62]. In Aβ toxicity, CAT–SKL (serine-lysine-leucine) treatment reduced the pathology of microglial activation, and rat brains did not show long-term memory impairments via the reduction of H_2O_2 levels [63]. In the PD model, mutant α-synuclein inhibited the expression and activity of CAT and induced low catalase activity and high H_2O_2 production [64]. This antioxidant enzyme plays an important role in maintaining oxidative balance.

3.1.3. Glutathione Peroxidase

Glutathione peroxidase (GPx) catalyzes the reduction of a variety of hydroperoxides (ROOH and H_2O_2) to water or the corresponding alcohols using GSH to protect mammalian cells against oxidative damage [65] (Figure 2). GPx has four identical subunits containing one selenocysteine in each residue for essential enzyme activity, which are classified as selenium-containing GPxs (GPx1–4 and 6) and their non-selenium congeners (GPx5, 7, and 8) [30]. The glutathione redox cycle is mostly active during low levels of oxidant stress, while CAT is more significant in protecting against severe oxidant stress. GPx isoenzymes appear to have antioxidant functions at different locations and cellular compartments, and the levels of expression of each isoform vary depending on the type of tissue, even though their expression is omnipresent. Furthermore, GPx is responsible for the conversion of GSH to oxidized glutathione disulfide (GSSG) and glutathione reductase (GR) reduces GSSG back to GSH [66]. GPx1 and GPx4 are found in most tissues and the predominant forms of GPx are found in brain tissue. GPx1 reduces H_2O_2 and organic hydroperoxides and is expressed both in neurons and astrocytes [67]. GPx4, the phospholipid hydroperoxide glutathione peroxidase, is located in the cytosol and a membrane fraction that can directly reduce phospholipid hydroperoxides, fatty acid hydroperoxides, and cholesterol hydroperoxides [68]. In the brain, mitochondrial and cytosolic GPx4 isoforms have been detected in neurons of the cerebral cortex, hippocampus, and cerebellum. In contrast, GPx4 in glial cells is barely activated under normal physiological conditions, whereas reactive astrocytes upregulate the expression of GPx4 following selective brain injury [31]. Recently, GPx4 has become well known as a key regulatory factor in ferroptosis which is a non-apoptotic and iron-dependent programmed cell death pathway that causes a rapid elevation of oxidative stress [69].

As the function of GPx is related to normal development and cellular metabolism via the regulation of oxidative stress, GPx4 function is potentially the key for cell survival.

GPx activity decreased significantly in PC12 cells during oxygen-glucose deprivation [70], and a two-fold increase in GPx and a three-fold increase in CAT activities were observed during a time course that reflected the temporal increase in nerve growth factor (NGF) in a brain contusion model [71]. The ferroptotic potential of neurons in the forebrain regions of the hippocampus and cerebral cortex is severely affected in AD patients, with increased vulnerability to ferroptosis. The role of GPx4 as a key regulator of ferroptosis was observed in Gpx4BIKO transgenic mice, a mouse model with a conditional deletion of GPx4 in forebrain neurons. Gpx4BIKO transgenic mice showed significant deficits in spatial learning and memory function and exhibited hippocampal neurodegeneration compared to control mice [72]. In human PD tissue biopsies, GPx4 expression was upregulated and ferroptosis-related events were observed [73].

3.1.4. Thioredoxin

The thioredoxin (Trx) system consists of two types of antioxidant oxidoreductase proteins, Trx and thioredoxin reductase (TrxRs) with NADPH as an electron donor. Trx has a conserved active site such as Cys-Pro-Gly-Cys, that has an important function of acting as an active oxidoreductase and electron donor of some peroxiredoxins (Prx) which are crucial for the reduction of peroxides [74]. Trx is an important regulator of cellular function that can respond to redox balance by modulating signaling pathways, transcription factors, and immunological responses for cell survival in many conditions, including neurodegenerative diseases [75]. There are three isoforms in the Trx family such as Trx1 in the cytosol, Trx2 in the mitochondria, and a testis-specific Trx3 in mammalian cells. Trx1 exists in cell compartments such as the nucleus and the plasma membrane or as a secreted protein, depending on its localization and function in different cell types [76]. Trx1 is coupled with Prx 1/2 and methionine sulfoxide reductase and is essential role in the control of growth and apoptosis. TrxR 1 and Trx 1 are observed in neuronal synaptic vesicles. In addition, Trx 1 and 2 expressions are also present mainly in rat brain neurons. Neurons with mitochondrial dysfunction by complex IV inhibition show low levels of Trx and are thus, more vulnerable to H_2O_2. Reduced Trx is a powerful reductase that acts through a disulfide–dithiol exchange mechanism to catalyze the conversion of disulfide bonds into thiols with high efficiency [77]. The disulfides in the oxidized Trx are converted to thiols by the consumption of NADPH [78] (Figure 2). TrxR, a homodimer, catalyzes the reduction of the disulfide at the Trx active site and is encoded by three distinct genes: the cytosolic TrxR (*TrxR1*), mitochondrial TrxR (*TrxR2*), and thioredoxin-glutaredoxin reductase (*TrxR3*). TrxR can directly reduce substrates such as peroxides, including lipid hydroperoxides, H_2O_2, and protein disulfide isomerase [76,79]. TrxR is also involved in the regeneration of other antioxidant molecules such as dehydroascorbate, lipoic acid, and ubiquinone [80–82]. TrxR is very important when other selenoproteins including GPx lose most of their activity and it effectively donates electrons during DNA synthesis [83]. TrxR activation in the rat brain can be maintained at a certain level under severe selenium (Se)-deficient conditions. Both Trx and TrxR are widely expressed in tissues and organs, including the brain. In a central nervous system (CNS) study, it has been suggested that increased expression of Trx and TrxR is closely associated with cell damage due to oxidative stress [84,85]. In addition, NADPH and human TrxR are efficient electron donors to human plasma peroxidase and reduce hyperoxides, even with low GSH capacity [86].

The upregulation of Trx was observed as a neuroprotective effect on retinal ganglion cells against oxidative stress-induced neurodegeneration [87]. Overexpression of Trx1 attenuated endoplasmic reticulum stress by regulating the activation of the molecular mechanism for neuroprotection in an in vitro and in vivo model of PD [88]. In AD brains, TrxR activity was increased in the cerebellum and amygdala [89]. It has been implied that TrxR activation increases a compensatory mechanism during increased oxidative stress that is limited by the substrate Trx and the subsequent neurodegeneration seen in AD. Another evidence for the peripheral response to oxidative stress during neurodegeneration is the reduction of Trx1 and TrxR1 in the plasma and erythrocytes in blood samples from patients with Huntington's disease (HD) [90]. Exogenously administered human recombinant Trx attenuates the generation of ROS involved in cytotoxic mechanisms, ameliorates neuronal damage, and augments neurogenesis following brain ischemia/reperfusion injury in rats [91]. In the ischemic brain, administration of Prx3 and Trx2 shows substantial neuroprotective effects by reducing oxidative stress [92].

Important enzymatic antioxidants such as SOD, CAT, GPx, and Trx remove superoxide and peroxides before they react with metal catalysts to form more reactive species (Figure 2). Peroxidative chain reactions initiated by reactive species that escape enzymatic degradation are terminated via chain-breaking antioxidants, including water-soluble ascorbate, lipid-soluble vitamin E, and ubiquinone. To enhance the antioxidative effect, oxidative stress should be controlled by supplying all the antioxidant nutrients and by minimizing the effect of substances that stimulate reactive oxygen metabolites (ROM) [93].

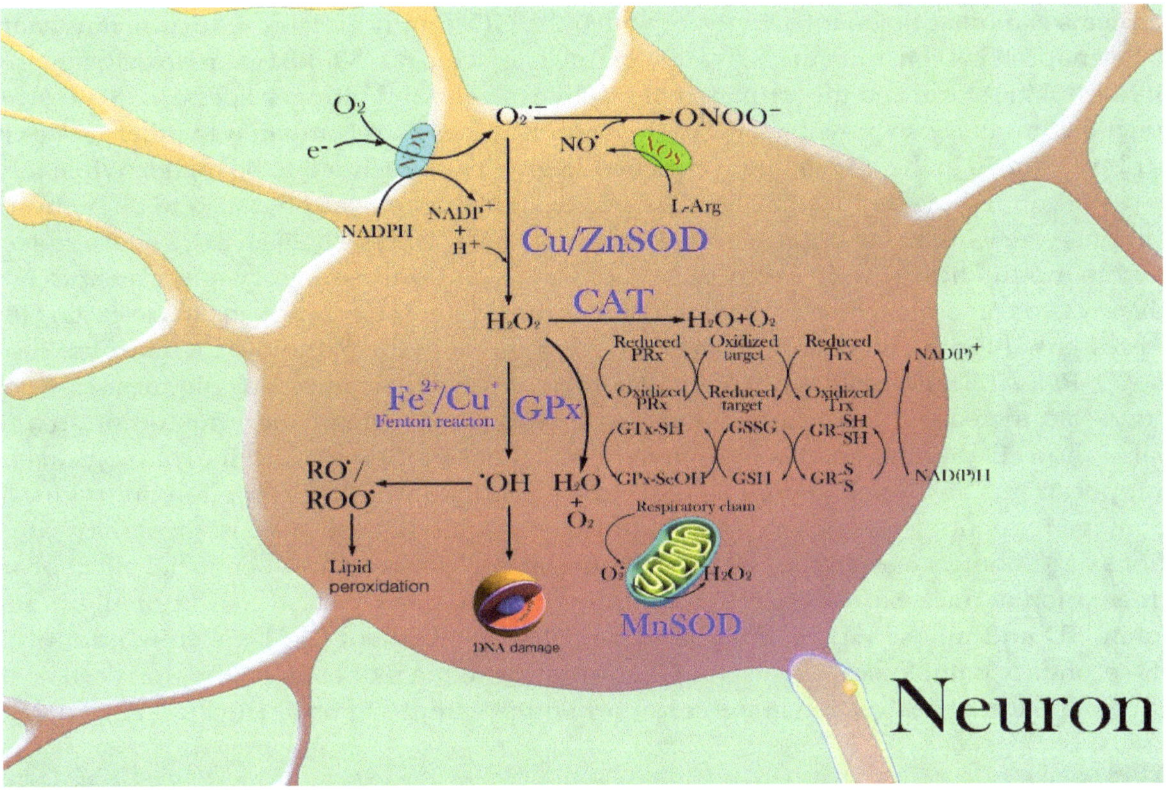

Figure 2. Enzymatic antioxidant defense system against the production of reactive oxygen species (ROS). Various pathways of cell death caused by ROS and its transformation are observed in brain injury. NADPH oxidase and mitochondrial respiratory transport chain are known as major cellular sources of the superoxide radical anion (O_2^-). The superoxide radical anion reacts with nitric oxide (NO) to form the peroxynitrite anion ($ONOO^-$) which mediates oxidative modification of protein residues via an interaction with NO. The superoxide radical is dismuted by the superoxide dismutase enzyme (SOD) to form hydrogen peroxide. In addition, manganese containing superoxide dismutase (Mn-SOD) reduces the superoxide radical anion generated during the electron transport chain in the mitochondrial matrix. Catalase (CAT) and/or glutathione peroxidase (GPx) decomposes hydrogen peroxide to water and oxygen by enzymatic reactions. Hydrogen peroxide is decomposed into reactive hydroxyl radicals by reaction with catalytically active redox metals such as (copper and iron). Hydroxyl radicals can react with oxygen to form peroxyl or alkoxyl radicals which can lead to lipid peroxidation and react with DNA and primarily cause damage to DNA. Peroxiredoxins (Prx) and thioredoxin (Trx) act as redox-regulated proteins to additional redox relay bases.

3.2. Non-Enzymatic Antioxidants

3.2.1. Antioxidant Enzyme Cofactors (Selenium, Coenzyme Q10, Zinc)

Selenium

Selenium (Se) is an enzymatic cofactor and an essential component of selenoaminoacids and selenoproteins. Se has numerous biological functions related to redox signaling, antioxidant defense systems, thyroid hormone metabolism, and humoral and cell-mediated immune responses [94]. Se reacts with redox signals involving one- or two-electron transitions; however, it is less reactive and prefers higher oxidation states. The biological activity of Se varies depending on its concentration: normal growth and development at low concentrations, homeostatic function at moderate concentrations, and induced toxicity at high concentrations [95]. The complex biological functions of Se are found in general body proteins that mainly and effectively act through 25 selenoproteins that have selenocysteine at their active center in humans [96]. Over half of the selenoproteins exhibit antioxidant activity, of which the GPx family and Trx reductase family are well known. Selenoproteins constrain the activation of nuclear factor-κB (NF-κB) via redox signaling, which prohibits a cytokine storm and the formation of reactive oxygen and nitrogen species. Se is essential for brain function, but the Se expression level in the brain is rather poor compared to other tissues [97,98]. The distribution of Se in the human brain enriched in gray matter tended to be higher, while the white matter was found to have reduced Se levels. Specifically, Se level was observed to be highest in the hippocampus, cerebellum, and brainstem in the rat brain [99]. The mechanism of Se neuroprotection is attributed to modulation of Ca^{2+} influx via ion channels, anti-inflammatory effect by abrogation of microglia invasion, and biosynthesis stimulation of antioxidative selenoproteins in the brain [100,101].

Se is essential for the brain and plays an important role in the pathology of neuronal disorders such as AD, PD, ALS, and epilepsy [96]. In Se-deficient transgenic mice, Aβ plaques showed more than a two-fold increase compared to Se-adequate ones [102]. Selenite administration in a rat AD model also showed attenuation of cognitive deficits, oxidative damage and morphological changes in the hippocampus and cerebral cortex [103]. In a paraquat induced PD model, bradykinesia and DNA damage reduction were observed by supplementing Se with selenite in drinking water [104]. Alterations of Se homeostasis in the HD model have been observed and a beneficial effect of selenite supplementation in mice expressing mutant huntingtin has been reported. Additionally, autopsy of the human HD and mouse HD brain showed decreased Se content [105]. Selenite administration prevents secondary pathological events, thus, contributing to the reduction of apoptotic cell death and prevention of neuronal destruction in the cortex and hippocampus of traumatic brain injury [106,107]

Coenzyme Q

Coenzyme Q (CoQ) is a remarkable liposoluble ubiquinone with a long isoprenoid side chain and a main component of the internal mitochondria membrane, Golgi complex membrane, and lysosomal membrane. CoQ is an endogenous free radical scavenger and enzyme cofactor produced by most human cells and is abundant in the brain and intestine in mitochondria, the site of oxidative phosphorylation [108]. It is biosynthesized by all membranes and a component of the mitochondrial respiratory chain, which participates in electron transport [109]. CoQ in either reduced form, hydroquinone or ubiquinol, is a potent lipophilic antioxidant and is also involved in the regeneration and recycling of other antioxidants such as tocopherol and ascorbate [110]. CoQ is an important antioxidant that protects cellular membranes and lipoproteins against the toxic effects of free radicals that are generated during general metabolism [111]. The redox functions of CoQ mainly occur in the mitochondria as electrons shuttle between complexes I and II of the respiratory chain. Dehydrogenases oxidize NADH, NADPH, and dihydroflavine-adenine dinucleotide (FADH2) and transfer protons and electrons to ubiquinone, which is converted to ubiquinol. Finally, the protons transfer to the mitochondrial matrix and the electrons move to the cytochromes. Thus, cytochromes reduce the superoxide radical anion to water with electrons and protons from the matrix. These processes are required to produce ATP [108]. TrxRs within the cytosol induce the reduction of CoQ to ubiquinol and maintain the extra-mitochondrial antioxidant defense [112]. CoQ is synthesized by at least 12 proteins that form a multiprotein complex in the mitochondria, and the pathogenesis of CoQ10 deficiency involves deficient ATP production and excessive ROS formation in humans. However, CoQ10 deficiency is unique among mitochondrial disorders because an effective treatment is available by oral CoQ10 supplementation, to which many patients respond well [113,114]. However, dietary supplementation is still challenging due to the low bioavailability of the compound. Because CoQ10 levels decline with age, it has been studied in a variety of neurodegenerative disorders and aging but with disparate results [115].

In KA-induced oxidative injury in vitro [116], an increased number of surviving CA3 neurons was observed at 0.1 and 1 μM concentrations in CoQ10-treated groups using cresyl violet staining. CoQ10 (0.01, 0.1, and 1 μM) treatment significantly decreased 2,7-dichlorofluorescein fluorescence, and the expression of NQO1 in the CoQ10-treated groups was significantly lower than that in controls, indicating the protective role of CoQ10 in hippocampal neurons against oxidative stress. Rats exposed to intrastriatal CoQ10 showed a larger number of dopaminergic neurons, higher expression of neurogenetic and angiogenetic factors, and less inflammation, and these effects were more prominent than the orally administered CoQ10. Thus, continuous intrastriatal administration of low doses of CoQ10 showed a more effective strategy to prevent dopaminergic neuronal degeneration in a PD rat model induced by 6-hydroxydopamine [117]. In patients with acute ischemic stroke, a significant increase in CoQ10 level was observed with the administration of CoQ10 (300 mg/day group) compared with the placebo group. CoQ10 supplementation attenuated oxidative stress and neuroinflammatory marker levels and improved the neurological outcome scale and antioxidant enzyme activity [118]. In PD patients, the total Unified Parkinson's Disease Rating Scale (UPDRS) scores decreased in the CoQ10-treated group, indicating amelioration of the symptoms and significant improvement in wearing-off in PD [119]. CoQ10 increased a reduced glutathione and SOD levels in patients with pregabalin-treated fibromyalgia. The supplementation of CoQ10 effectively reduced pain sensation, anxiety and brain activity, mitochondrial oxidative stress, and inflammation [120].

Zinc and Essential Metals

Zinc, a redox inactive metal, does not directly interact with ROS but has a crucial role in maintaining redox balance for the antioxidant defense system in various ways in the cell. Zinc increases the activation of antioxidant enzymes such as SOD, GPx, and CAT. It also acts as a direct cofactor of SOD-1 and SOD-3 and as an indirect cofactor for GPx [121]. Zinc inhibits important pro-oxidant enzymes such as NADPH oxidase, inducible nitric oxide synthetase (iNOS), and the reduced form of nicotinamide adenine dinucleotide (NMDA) and regulates oxidant production and metal-induced oxidative damage. Zinc is dynamically associated with sulfur in protein cysteine clusters. It mediates the induction of the zinc-binding protein metallothionein which releases the metal under oxidative conditions and acts as an Se scavenging oxidant. Zinc is involved in the regulation of glutathione metabolism and the overall protein thiol redox status [122]. Zinc competes with redox-active transition metals, iron and copper, for certain binding sites. When zinc binds to these sites, copper and iron are forced to undergo hydrolytic polymerization into unreactive structures, thereby prohibiting the catalysis of free radical formation and the initiation of lipid peroxidation [121–123]. Zinc is mainly expressed in the hippocampus, amygdala, cerebral cortex, thalamus, and olfactory cortex in the brain [124] and is stored as free zinc ions (Zn^{2+}) in the presynaptic glutamatergic neurons. Zinc in synaptic vesicles is released with glutamate and acts as a potent extracellular modulator by interacting with many synaptic receptors during synaptic activity [123].

Co-treatment with zinc and Se significantly decreased mitochondrial dysfunction, ROS levels, and lipid peroxidation levels, while significantly increasing cognitive performance, SOD, glutathione peroxidase, and catalase activity in the mitochondria of the brain in an AD rat model [125]. In a double-blind, placebo-controlled trial of zinc supplementation for premenstrual syndrome, sixty women (18–30 years) were randomly assigned to receive either 30 mg of zinc gluconate and/or placebo for 12 weeks. The zinc-administered group showed beneficial effects on physical and psychological symptoms of premenstrual syndrome, total antioxidant capacity, and brain-derived neurotrophic factor [126].

Other essential metals, such as copper, iron, and magnesium, play an important role in the maintenance of cell homeostasis and preservation of life. They display important structural, regulatory, and catalytic functions in different types of proteins, such as enzymes, receptors, and transporters. Cu^{+} and magnesium are the cofactors for enzymes such as COX and/or supper zinc, SOD, and neuronal Cu enrichment predispose to Cu^{2+}-catalyzed Fenton chemistry and H_2O_2-assisted protein oxidation. In particularly, iron continuously shifts between ferrous ion (Fe^{2+}) and ferric ion (Fe^{3+}) states in a redox reaction in the presence of O_2. The constitution of iron in the body is in the form of 65% (Fe^{2+}) ions bound to hemoglobin; less than 10% of ions are expressed with myoglobin (Fe^{2+}), cytochromes (Fe^{2+} or Fe^{3+}), and iron-containing enzymes, and 25% of the ions are bound to iron-storage proteins such as transferrin, ferritin, and hemosiderin [127]. Iron present in the cells in the reduced (Fe^{2+}) and oxidized (Fe^{3+}) states can serve both as an electron donor and electron acceptor. Particularly, the ferrous form of iron can act as a catalyst in the potentiation of oxygen toxicity by generating a wide range of free radical species, including hydroxyl radicals. In addition, an excessive amount of this essential metal induces toxicity, leading to pathological conditions generated by oxidative stress and neurodegeneration [128]. Although homeostasis of iron is essential for physiological functions in the brain, less than 2% of total body iron is present in the brain. Iron contributes to the activity of various enzymes involved in neurotransmitter synthesis and myelination of axons of motor neurons in the brain. Iron accumulation induces features of neurodegenerative disorders including AD, PD, HD, ALS, and neurodegeneration with brain iron accumulation (NBIA). The pathogenesis of neurodegenerative diseases shows a relationship with a dramatic increase in iron content in the brain, which is correlated with the production of ROS [127].

3.2.2. ROS/RNS Scavengers (Vitamin C, E, and A)

Vitamin C

Ascorbate (ascorbic acid, AA), a ubiquitous water-soluble antioxidant and a cofactor for several enzymes, can inhibit the generation of ROS, directly scavenge ROS/RNS, and repair other oxidized scavengers [129]. ROS generation is limited by ascorbate through the inhibition of NOX and nNOS. It also helps in the regeneration of alpha-tocopherol from alpha-tocopheroxyl radical and repair of glutathione. The highest concentration of ascorbate is expressed in the brain and is involved in CNS homeostasis. Endogenous ascorbate exists in two biological forms, the deprotonated ascorbate anion and dehydroascorbate (DHA), which is the product of the two-electron reversible oxidation of ascorbate [129]. The mechanism of ascorbate uptake involves absorption of dietary ascorbate in the intestine by sodium-dependent transporter-1 (SVCT-1) and dissolution in the blood. Ascorbate enters the CNS by slow transport from the plasma to the cerebrospinal fluid across the choroid plexus epithelium. Ascorbate can easily enter the brain through the glucose transporter (GLUT1) when a considerable amount of DHA is present in the blood. Ascorbate or DHA in the cerebrospinal fluid enters the neuron via sodium-dependent transporter-2 (SVCT-2) or GLUT1 transporters [130,131]. Once they enter the neuron, DHA can be reduced to ascorbate or released by GLUT1. Ascorbate produces ascorbate free radicals as one electron donor, which is reduced back to ascorbate within the cells by NADH- and NADPH-dependent reductase. Glial cells obtain ascorbate by reduction of DHA through GLUT1, and ascorbate uptake does not involve SVCT-2, which is different from neurons [131]. DHA goes through GLUT1 slowly to enter the choroid plexus and astrocytes [132–134]. The rapid entry of ascorbate is driven by SVCT-2 through the blood-brain-barrier (BBB) to neurons, and ascorbate modulates SVCT-2 translocation to the plasma membrane, ensuring optimal ascorbate uptake in the neurons [135,136] (Figure 3). The oxidizing and free radical scavenging activity of ascorbate inside the cell is not limited to the aqueous phase, but also includes protection of membranes and other hydrophobic compartments through interaction with vitamin E [137]. Aging decreases the extracellular concentration and the uptake of ascorbate in the brain, which is consistent with an increase in oxidative stress. The neurobiological role of ascorbate in the brain is seen in neuromodulation and neuroprotection [129]. In the role of a neuromodulator, ascorbate release is involved in the uptake or clearance of glutamate from the synapse after its release from the axon terminals. Specifically, L-glutamate promotes ascorbate release as a consequence of removing glutamate from the synapse [138]. Although ascorbate does not act as a classical neurotransmitter, extracellular ascorbate may influence neurotransmission. In particular, ascorbate directly modulates neural excitability through inhibition of T-type Ca^{2+} channels [139], participates in the reduction of extracellular oxidants, which effects the redox status of catecholamines [140], and influences the release of biogenic amines in striatum [141] and pituitary neuropeptides [142]. Another neuroprotective role of ascorbate is the attenuation of neurotoxicity, which results from the scavenging activity [143]. Ascorbate inhibits the oxidative stress triggered by various neurotoxins and protects against ethanol-induced apoptotic neurodegeneration in prenatal rat hippocampal neurons [144]. Oxidative stress in stroke, hypoxia, ischemia, and seizure activity leads to massive glutamate release and subsequent excitotoxicity, a result of over-activation of glutamate receptors [145]. Therefore, ascorbate can protect against glutamate-induced excitotoxicity and neurodegeneration.

Many researchers have reported that neurodegeneration can be reversed or lessened by ascorbate treatment [146–148]. From the viewpoint of the effect of aging, the extracellular concentration and uptake of ascorbate is decreased in the brain, which is consistent with an increase in oxidative stress [149]. Moreover, excess ascorbate intake or deficiency may influence brain aging [150]. Thus, careful maintenance of ascorbate levels in the brain may be important during the life span. There have been extensive reviews on the role of ascorbate in the brain with a focus on neurodegenerative disease [130,131]. Even though ascorbate has a complicated interaction with the neurotransmitter system, ascorbate is considered relevant for use as an antioxidant therapy because neurons are sensitive to ascorbate deficiency and excess oxidant stress. In our previous work [151], we studied the protective effects of AA and DHA on KA-induced oxidative stress using organotypic hippocampal slice cultures. After 12 h of KA treatment, significant delayed neuronal death was detected in the CA3, but not in the CA1 region. Pretreatment with intermediate doses of AA and DHA significantly prevented cell death and reduced ROS levels, as well as mitochondrial dysfunction in the CA3 region. However, pretreatment with high doses of AA or DHA was not effective. Attempting to elevate the brain ascorbate by the systemic administration of high doses of ascorbate is very difficult. The level of AA in the extracellular fluid of the striatum was decreased in a transgenic mouse model of HD; hence, restoring striatal extracellular AA levels with high doses of ascorbate improved behavior [152,153].

Vitamin E

Vitamin E is a major group of lipid-soluble antioxidants called tocopherols and tocotrienols, of which the most biologically active isoform is α-tocopherol [154]. It is a major chain-breaking antioxidant and exists in a low molar ratio compared to unsaturated phospholipids. The most important function of vitamin E is its antioxidant activity, which protects the integrity of cellular membranes from polyunsaturated fatty acid-generated oxygen free radicals and to act as a direct scavenger of superoxide and hydroxyl radicals [154,155]. Based on studies of brain capillary endothelial cells, the mechanism of entry of α-tocopherol into the CNS correlated to α-tocopherol and scavenger receptor class B type 1 (SRB1) levels. α-Tocopherol uptake occurs via a selective high-density lipoprotein (HDL) pathway, which modulates the expression of SRB1 receptor [156–158]. Once α-tocopherol passes through the BBB, it may be directly delivered to specialized astrocytes. Astrocyte-synthesized apolipoprotein E (ApoE) moves through the cerebral spinal fluid transporting α-tocopherol between various cell types in the CNS cell [154,159]. ApoE lipoprotein particles in astrocytes are secreted through membrane proteins and interact with low-density lipoprotein receptor-related protein (LRP) on the neurons [160].

The neurons take up these ApoE particles and distribute them throughout the body, axon, and dendrites to preserve the membrane from lipid peroxidation (Figure 3). The expression of α-tocopherol transfer protein is enhanced by an increase in ROS, and it is useful for combating neuronal damage.

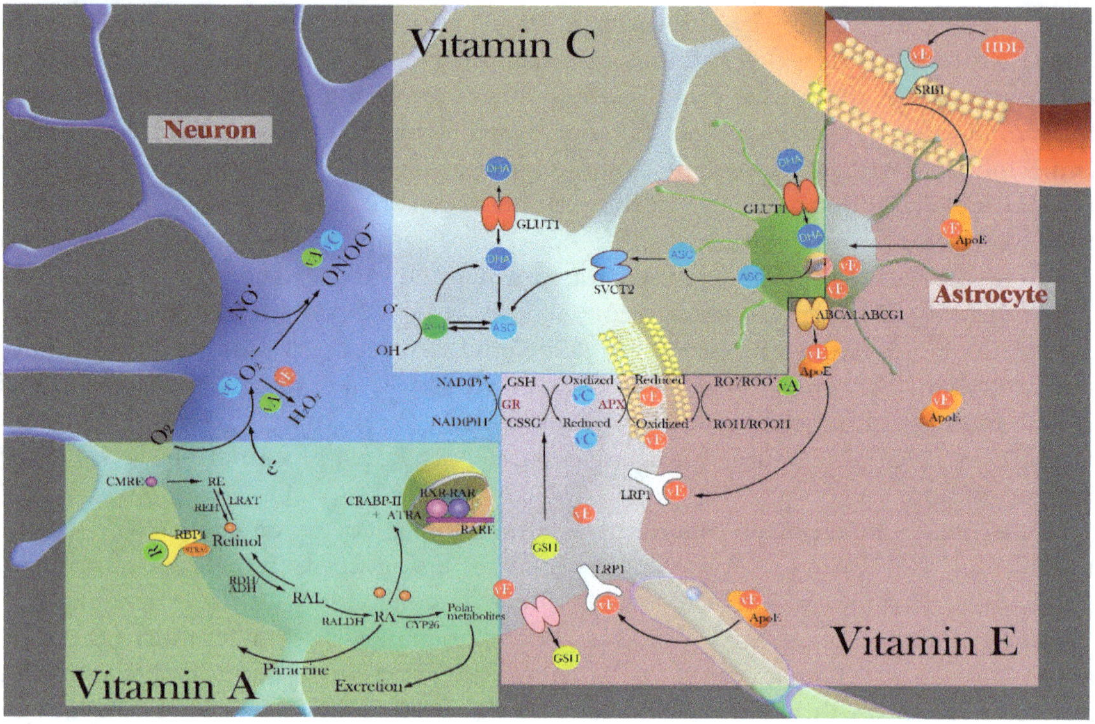

Figure 3. Schematic representation of vitamin uptake and protective mechanisms by exogenous vitamins as antioxidants. **Vitamin C:** During uptake in the CNS, ascorbate passes through the BBB to enter directly through the SVCT-2 and/or possibly DHA through GLUT1s. Moreover, the neuronal uptake of ascorbate occurs through SVCT-2 and DHA via the GLUT1s. In the neuron, DHA can be reduced to ascorbate or released back into the extracellular space by GLUT1. Ascorbate free radicals convert to form DHA and ascorbate. Ascorbate recycles both the ascorbate free radical and DHA by cellular metabolism. Astrocytes contain ascorbate from recycling of DHA which is taken up through GLUT1s. Neurons directly acquire ascorbate via SVCT-2. **Vitamin E:** With respect to vitamin E uptake, HDL particles can pass through SRB1 receptors expressed on endothelial cells. Astrocytes that exist adjacent to the BBB take up vitamin E into the inner cell membrane. Synthesized ApoE lipoproteins take up vitamin E that is left out of an ABC transporter, for transport into neurons through LRP1 requiring vitamin E for maintenance or during conditions of oxidative stress. **Vitamin A:** In cellular retinoid signaling pathways, retinol is metabolized to all-trans-retinoic acid (ATRA). Vitamin A (retinol, ROL) binds to plasma retinol binding protein (RBP4) and circulates; RBP4 protein binds to the membrane receptor STAR6 to promote cellular absorption of retinol from the cells. A chylomicron remnant (CMRE), as a form of circulating vitamin A, can serve as a source of vitamin A for the cells and retinol is esterified and stored by lecithin: retinol acyltransferase (LRAT) and is reversibly oxidized to retinaldehyde (RAL) by retinol dehydrogenase (RDH/ADH). In addition, retinol is further oxidized to RA in an irreversible manner by retinaldehyde dehydrogenase (RALDH). ATRA regulates gene transcription through retinoic acid receptors (RAR) and/or retinoid X receptors (RXRs) which are bound to retinoic acid response elements (RARE) in the nucleus. These representative schematics are modified from [130,154,161]. Abbreviations: VC, vitamin C; VE, vitamin E; VA, vitamin A; ASC, ascorbate; ASF, ascorbate free radical; DHA, dehydroascorbic acid; GLUT1, glucose transports; SVTC-2, sodium-dependent transporters; LRP, lipoprotein receptor-related protein; GSH, glutathione; ApoE, apolipoprotein E; HDL, density lipoprotein; CMRE, chylomicron remnant; CRABP, cellular retinoic acid-binding protein; LRAT, lethicin: retinol acyltransferase; RBP, retinol binding protein; RAL, retinaldehyde; RDH/ADH, retinol dehydrogenase; RALDH, retinaldehyde dehydrogenase; RXR, retinoid X receptors; RAR, retinoic acid receptors; ATRA, all-trans-retinoic acid; BBB, blood–brain barrier.

The antioxidant ability of vitamin E is continuously restored via vitamin E recycling by other antioxidants such as vitamin C, ubiquinols, and thiols. The half-life of vitamin E in the brain tissue is slower than that of other vitamins, and it is also actively retained and protected from auto-oxidation in the brain [162]. The distribution of α-tocopherol is significantly different in the brain. These CNS-regional disparities are suggestive of the specific protective antioxidant effect of α-tocopherol. Specifically, the concentrations of α-tocopherol were relatively higher in the nuclear membranes than in the other membranes of the brain. It has been suggested that α-tocopherol may play a role in nuclear-associated functions in the cerebellum and striatum, wherein preferential accumulation of α-tocopherol in the membrane was most apparent [163]. Vitamin E, similar to other radical scavengers/trappers, influences the flux of lipid hydroperoxide (LOOH), which is derived from both spontaneous and enzymatic formation of lipid peroxyl radicals ($LOO^{\bullet}$) on the cellular membrane [164]. The effects of vitamin E on peroxidation activity appear to involve both the radical scavenging mechanism such as the H atom donor activity and a physical interaction with the polyunsaturated lipid substrate. Tocotrienols, another form of vitamin E that are highly metabolized, show more potent inhibition of the phospholipase A2/lipoxygenases pathway as compared to tocopherols, and have different cellular bioavailability, distribution, and protein interaction in the saturated and unsaturated form of vitamin E in the brain [165]. Deficiency of vitamin E showed increased biochemical and histological markers of oxidative stress, including total glutathione and lipid peroxidation in the CNS.

Therapeutic effects of α-tocopherol by application of vitamin E in neurological lesions caused by neuronal excitotoxicity and the conditional activation of neuroglial cells have also been reported. In KA treatment-induced oxidative stress [166], delayed neuronal death was detected in the hippocampal CA3 region and ROS formation and lipid peroxidation were also increased. Both co-treatment and post-treatment with α-tocopherol (100 μM) or α-tocotrienol (100 μM) significantly increased cell survival and reduced the number of TUNEL-positive cells in the CA3 region. Increased dichlorofluorescein (DCF) fluorescence and thiobarbiturate reactive substance (TBARS) levels were decreased by drug treatment (Figure 4). In AD patients, long-term administration of vitamin D and E alone or in combination could inhibit morphological changes of neurons and improve learning and memory [167]. Vitamin E prevented the memory impairment associated with post-traumatic stress disorder (PTSD)-like behavior in rats. Significant decreases in oxidative stress biomarkers were detected with reduced glutathione/oxidized glutathione (GSH/GSSG) ratio [168]. In PD patients, omega-3 fatty acid and vitamin E co-supplementation had favorable effects on the UPDRS score and increased the total antioxidant capacity (TAC) and GSH concentration compared to placebo [169].

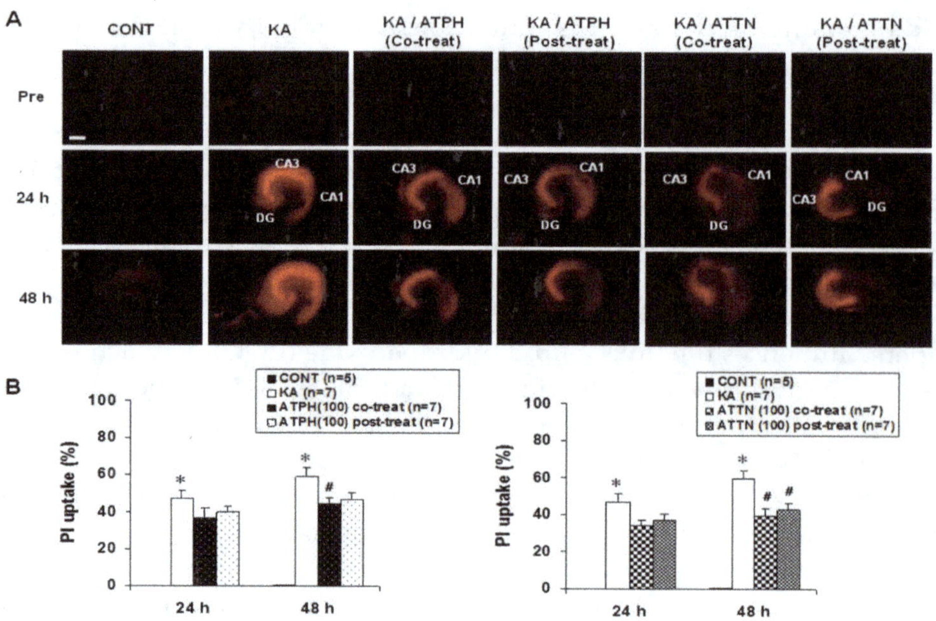

Figure 4. Neuroprotective effect of vitamin E. (**A**): Representative propidium iodide (PI) images. When hippocampal slices were exposed to 5 μM KA for 15 h, PI uptake in the CA3 region was significantly higher than the CA1 region. Co-treatment using ATPH (100 μM) or ATTN (100 μM) with KA significantly reduced PI uptake in the CA3 region compared with KA treatment alone. (**B**): Quantification of PI intensity. * $p < 0.05$, # $p < 0.05$; one-way ANOVA followed by Dunnett's post hoc comparison (* $p < 0.05$ vs. normal, # $p < 0.05$ vs. KA-treated cultures). This present data is a part of our previous research showing neuronal rescue after oxidative stress by alpha-tocopherol and tocotrienol treatment [166]. Abbreviations: ATPH, alpha-tocopherol; ATTN, alpha-tocotrienol; OHSC, organotypic hippocampal slice culture; KA, kainic acid; PI, propidium iodide; DCF, dichlorofluorescein.

Vitamin A

Vitamin A, carotenoids including retinol and beta-carotene, are fat-soluble chemicals synthesized by plants and some microorganisms and have many functions in human growth, development, and health [170,171]. Vitamin A is available in the human diet as pro-vitamin A carotenoids and preformed vitamin A (retinol-alcohol form, retinal-aldehyde form, retinoic acid-carboxylic acid form, and retinyl ester-ester form). The preformed vitamin A from animal-derived food and pro-vitamin A carotenoids from plant-derived foods are converted to all-trans-retinol as vitamin A alcohol by a series of reactions in the intestine. Carotenoids, mainly via dietary intake, can function directly as antioxidants by quenching ROS through energy transfer [172]. Vitamin A deprivation was investigated in the deficiency of cognitive function in adult mice and rats, which highlights the importance of adequate vitamin A status by the retinoid signaling pathways [161]. Carotenoids are classified into pro-vitamin A carotenoids such as β-carotene and β-cryptoxanthin, which are capable of converting to retinal, and non-pro-vitamin A carotenoids such as lycopene and lutein, which cannot be converted to retinal [173]. Carotenoids act through several pathways and interact with free radicals in the plasma, mitochondria, and nuclear membranes of cells via electron transfer, hydrogen abstraction, and physical quenching [174]. Carotenoids indirectly react with cell signaling cascades, including the nuclear factor elytroid 2 (NF-E2)-related factor 2 (Nrf2), NF-κB, or mitogen-activated protein kinase (MAPK) [175,176]. The antioxidant action of carotenoids involves singlet oxygen quenching and trapping of peroxyl radicals. Retinol-binding proteins observed in the BBB regulate the access of retinol into the brain [177]. High concentrations of retinol and carotenoids have been observed in the postmortem human frontal lobe cortex [178]. β-carotene, a precursor of retinol and retinoic acid, is reported to be a potent free radical quencher, singlet oxygen scavenger, and lipid antioxidant in tissues and plasma. Therefore, β-carotene acts in a hydrophobic environment such as the lipid core of the membranes and is used faster than α-tocopherol, implying that β-carotene is more favorable than α-tocopherol to quench lipophilic radicals in the membrane. The most efficient synergistic inhibition during oxidative stress was observed with a combination treatment of α-tocopherol and ascorbic acid [179].

Retinoids, compounds structurally related to vitamin A, are considered vitamin A derivatives that contribute to regular cellular morphogenesis, proliferation, and differentiation. Retinoids are involved in normal signaling cascades in modulating brain functions [180]. Retinoids modulate the availability of glucocorticosteroids in the brain, an important biological mechanism that can be explored in many stress-related pathologies to prevent alterations in the plasticity of the hippocampus [181]. Retinol metabolic pathways have shown that retinol can be stored intracellularly as retinyl esters and metabolized into all-trans-retinoic acid (ATRA) as a bioactive derivative. ATRA induces cellular differentiation and growth by reacting to retinoic acid receptors (RARs). Cellular retinol-binding proteins (CRBP-I and II) and cellular retinoic acid-binding proteins (CRABP-I, II) are distributed in the adult CNS. Furthermore, CRBP-I distribution parallels that of ATRA with expression in the meninges, hippocampus, amygdala, and olfactory bulb [182] (Figure 3). Under oxidative stress conditions such as metal exposure and production and accumulation of ROS, retinoids protect the cells against this imbalance through multiple mechanisms, including interference with ROS production, scavenging free radicals directly, upregulation of antioxidant enzymes, and signaling pathways involved in defense system such as Nrf2 signaling [183]. It has also been observed that retinoic acid has a protective effect on neuronal apoptosis and oxidative damage by reducing glutathione [184] and restoring SOD-1 and SOD-2 in the hippocampal cells [185]. The role of retinoid signal transduction in the control of dopaminergic neurotransmission was observed in the presence of high levels of retinoic acid-synthesizing enzymes [186] and RAR, which may play a critical role in controlling the survival, adaptation, and homeostatic regulation of the dopaminergic system [187]. Retinoid signaling play a physiological role in synaptic plasticity and learning and memory behaviors [188].

Retinoic acid supplementation upregulated μ-type opioid receptor 1 (MOR1) and its signaling and alleviated dyskinetic movements, which is a known consequence of prolonged administration of L-DOPA, in Pitx3$^{ak/ak}$ mice [189]. Moreover, RA triggered the neuroprotective effect on DA neurons in MPTP-treated mice model of PD. Administration of RA-loaded polymeric nanoparticle significantly reduced the loss of DA neuron in the substantia nigra as well as their neuronal fiber/axonal innervations in the striatum [190]. Moreover, oral administration of lycopene (5–20 mg/kg), a carotenoid with unique pharmacological properties, attenuated oxidative stress in mice with PD, which was induced with intraperitoneal injection of 1-methyl-4-phenyl-1,2,3,6-tetrahydropyridine (MPTP). Lycopene supplementation also inhibits apoptosis in PD mice by decreasing Bax and caspases, and contrarily increasing Bcl-2 [191]. Dietary supplementation with astaxanthin, another carotenoid family member, significantly decreased intracellular ROS accumulation in a hippocampal neuronal cell line after exposure to glutamate and induced antioxidant mediators, such as heme oxygenase-1 (HO-1) and nuclear Nrf2 expression in vitro [192]. In multiple sclerosis (MS) patients, vitamin A supplementation had a significant effect in the treatment group for fatigue and depression. In addition, when a synthetic retinoid was tested, it showed reduction in inflammation, Aβ burden, and tau phosphorylation with associated cognitive benefits in AD patients [193,194].

Aside from elucidating the efficiency of endogenous antioxidants, several studies have increasingly accredited the role of various exogenous antioxidants. Limited clinical studies are reported herein and are illustrated in Table 1. Table 1 also shows several examples of previously mentioned exogenous antioxidant reactions that have worked in clinical settings. Although the administration of exogenous antioxidants showed positive effects, there are some inconsistencies in clinical trials. The clinical trials performed multivariable analyses with various factors, such as sample size, replication or validation studies using the same agent and outcome measures, assessment of vitamins, different conditions of endogenous antioxidants, long-term monitoring, etc., which caused variability because of inconsistencies. In general, several common antioxidants and their clinical effects are described in Table 1.

Table 1. Clinical trials of antioxidant in neurodegenerative diseases.

Antioxidant	Number of Patients	Follow up Period	Dosage	Route	Effects	Disease	Reference
CoQ10	609 40	60 month 96 week	2400 mg/day 300 mg/day	Oral Oral	No Y	Huntington Parkinson	[119,195]
Selenium	7540	7 year 6 month	200 μg/day 1000 μg/day	Oral I.V.	No Y	Alzheimer Traumatic brain injury	[107,196]
Zinc	43	12 week	20 mg/day	Oral	Y	Depression with multiple sclerosis	[197]
Vitamin A	50 101	28 day 6 month	30 mg/day 25,000 UI/day	Oral Oral	Y Y	Alzheimer Multiple sclerosis	[191,198]
Vitamin C	12 60	6 day 3 month	2 g/day 500 mg/day	Oral Oral	Y Y	Hyperoxia Trauma surgery	[147,199]
Vitamin E	7540 60 50	7 year 3 month 12 month	400 UI/day 400 UI/day 45 UI/day	Oral Oral Oral	No Y Y	Alzheimer Parkinson Parkinson	[168,196,200]

3.2.3. Nrf2 Antioxidant System

The transcription factor Nrf2 is characterized as a regulator of redox homeostasis and antioxidant defense mechanisms. This protective pathway also encompasses the activation of a detoxification network such as oxidation/reduction factors (Phase I), metabolizing enzymes (Phase II), efflux transporters (Phase III), and free radical scavengers [201]. Oxidation/reduction factors consisting of nearly 500 genes encoding proteins, including redox balancing factors, stress response proteins, detoxifying enzymes, and metabolic enzymes such as NAD(P)H quinone oxidoreductase (NQO1), HO-1, SOD, GST, GSR, GSH-Px, carbonyl reductase (CR), and glutamate-cysteine ligase (GCL) play important roles in antioxidant and pro-survival effects and detoxification of xenobiotics. Nrf2 is generally targeted for ubiquitin-mediated degradation by its endogenous inhibitor Keap1, but oxidative modification of Keap1 inhibits the Nrf2 degradation process during conditions of redox imbalance [202]. To maintain cellular redox homeostasis, basal Nrf2 accumulation increases to mediate the normal expression of antioxidant response element (ARE)-dependent genes in the nucleus. The mitochondrial membrane directly interacts with Nrf2 which can respond to mitochondrial oxidative stressors that can collapse cellular bioenergetics leading to cell apoptosis [203]. Thus, the Keap1/Nrf2 system is another good homeostatic regulator of intrinsic cellular antioxidant defense and mitochondrial health. The suppression of Nrf2 activity increases the susceptibility of the brain to the damaging effects of oxidative stress and inflammatory stimuli [204]. Nrf2 activation promotes neuroprotective effects in both in vitro and in vivo neurodegenerative models. Nrf2 activity diminishes with age, and consequently, the effect of antioxidant enzyme activity decreases. Nrf2/ARE system impairment leads to higher susceptibility to oxidative injury, abnormal protein aggregation and neurodegeneration in the brain. Many studies have demonstrated the importance of the Nrf2/ARE pathway in the pathogenesis and control of neurological disorders, including PD, AD, ischemia, and other neurodegenerative diseases.

After middle cerebral artery occlusion (MCAO) in rats, Keap1 levels are decreased and this loss is correlated with an increase in Nrf2 and its downstream proteins, such as thioredoxins, GSH synthases, and HO-1 [205]. Stroke models of Nrf2-deficient mice exhibit higher levels of ROS than the wild-type littermates, which supports the natural compensatory mechanism of Nrf2 [206]. In AD transgenic mice, Nrf2-deficiency brains presented increased marker of oxidative stress and exhibited deficits in spatial learning and memory [204]. Nrf2 knockout and wild-type mice can be administered MPTP with doses ranging from 20 to 60 mg/kg for an animal model of PD. Nrf2$^{-/-}$ mice exhibited increased sensitivity to the dopaminergic toxins MPTP and 6-OHDA [207]. Nrf2 deficiency increased the MPTP sensitivity by 30 mg/kg administration of MPTP, but astrocytic Nrf2 overexpression showed the amelioration of MPTP toxicity in ARE-hPAP mice [208]. Astrocytic Nrf2 reduced the MPTP neurotoxicity by β-lapachone treatment in PD models [209].

4. Conclusions

Brains are metabolically active and have a high demand for large amounts of ATP to maintain their physiological function. Additionally, the brain has a relatively low level of antioxidants, low repair capacity, non-replicating nature of neuronal cells, and a high ratio of membrane surface to cytoplasm. ROS production is largely through oxidative phosphorylation and increased free radicals play a central role in neurological disorders by the imbalance of pro-oxidant and antioxidant agents in the brain. This underpins the importance of targeting antioxidant systems to counteract the oxidative stress and associated brain diseases. Indeed, the antioxidant system is important for the rescue of neuronal cells from oxidative stress and preservation of the right redox balance in the brain tissue by promoting antioxidative defenses for neutralizing ROS and by blocking transcription. Currently, there is growing research interest in the development of new/combination exogenous supplementation of antioxidants, retention of the functional integrity of intrinsic antioxidant systems for preventing harmful CNS disorders, and identification of novel approaches to therapy to prevent and/or reduce brain injury. Thus, high levels and variable metabolites in the brain indicate an increased requirement for antioxidant defense systems as enzymatic and non-enzymatic molecules. Redox biology fulfills important physiological functions that extend beyond its role on oxidative stress, such as cell signaling [210,211]. Perhaps, ROS generation may be necessary for cell function. Although their role is still ill-defined, the antioxidant systems may contribute to the controlled release of ROS for normal brain function.

Author Contributions: All authors contributed substantially to the preparation of this study. K.H.L. designed the study and drafted the manuscript. M.C. assisted with drafting of the manuscript and preparation of the figures. B.H.L. supervised the entire project and prepared the manuscript draft. All authors have read and agreed to the published version of the manuscript.

Abbreviations

AD	Alzheimer disease
ALS	amyotrophic lateral sclerosis
ApoE	apolipoprotein E
ARE	antioxidant response element
ATP	adenosine triphosphate
ATPH	alpha-tocopherol
ATRA	all-trans-retinoic acid
ATTN	alpha-tocotrienol
Aβ	beta-amyloid
CA3	cornu ammonis 3
CAT	catalase
CNS	central nervous system
CoQ	coenzyme Q
COX	cyclooxygenase
CR	carbonyl reductase
CRABP	cellular retinoic acid-binding proteins
CRBP	cellular retinol binding proteins
DCF	dichlorofluorescein
DHA	dehydroascorbate
EC-SOD	extracellular superoxide dismutase
FADH2	dihydroflavine-adenine dinucleotide
Fe^{2+}	ferrous ion
Fe^{3+}	ferric ion

GCL	glutamate-cysteine ligase
GLUT1	glucose transports
GPx	glutathione peroxidase
GR	glutathione reductase
GSH	glutathione
GSSG	glutathione disulfide
hAPP	human amyloid precursor protein
HD	Huntington's disease
HDL	high density lipoprotein
HO-1	heme oxygenase-1
iNOS	inducible nitric oxide synthase
KA	kainic acid
LRP	lipoprotein receptor-related protein
MAPK	mitogen-activated protein kinase
MCAO	middle cerebral artery occlusion
Mn-SOD	manganese containing superoxide dismutase
MOR	μ-type opioid receptor
MPTP	1-methyl-4-phenyl-1,2,3,6-tetrahydropyridine
NADH	reduced form of nicotinamide adenine dinucleotide
NADPH	reduced form of nicotinamide adenine dinucleotide phosphate
NBIA	neurodegeneration brain iron accumulation
NF-κB	nuclear factor-κB
nNOS	neuronal nitric oxide synthase
NOX	NADPH oxidase
NQO1	NADPH quinone oxidoreductase
Nrf2	nuclear factor elytroid 2-related factor 2
6-OHDA	6-hydroxydopamine
OHSC	organotypic hippocampal slice culture
PD	Parkinson disease
PI	propidium iodide
PTSD	post-traumatic stress disorder
RAR	retinoic acid receptors
RNS	reactive nitrogen species
ROS	reactive oxygen species
Se	selenium
SOD	superoxide dismutase
SRB1	scavenger receptor class B type 1
SVCT	sodium-vitamin C co-transporters
TAC	total antioxidant capacity
TBARS	thiobarbiturate reactive substance
Trx	thioredoxin
TrxR	thioredoxin reductase
UV	ultra violet

References

1. Cobley, J.N.; Fiorello, M.L.; Bailey, D.M. 13 reasons why the brain is susceptible to oxidative stress. *Redox Biol.* **2018**, *15*, 490–503. [CrossRef] [PubMed]
2. Magistretti, P.J.; Allaman, I. A cellular perspective on brain energy metabolism and functional imaging. *Neuron* **2015**, *86*, 883–901. [CrossRef] [PubMed]
3. Nedergaard, M.; Ransom, B.; Goldman, S.A. New roles for astrocytes: Redefining the functional architecture of the brain. *Trends Neurosci.* **2003**, *26*, 523–530. [CrossRef] [PubMed]
4. Bailey, D.M.; Bärtsch, P.; Knauth, M.; Baumgartner, R.W. Emerging concepts in acute mountain sickness and high-altitude cerebral edema: From the molecular to the morphological. *Cell. Mol. Life Sci.* **2009**, *66*, 3583–3594. [CrossRef] [PubMed]

5. Turrens, J.F. Mitochondrial formation of reactive oxygen species. *J. Physiol.* **2003**, *552*, 335–344. [CrossRef] [PubMed]
6. Niedzielska, E.; Smaga, I.; Gawlik, M.; Moniczewski, A.; Stankowicz, P.; Pera, J.; Filip, M. Oxidative stress in neurodegenerative diseases. *Mol. Neurobiol.* **2016**, *53*, 4094–4125. [CrossRef] [PubMed]
7. Pisoschi, A.M.; Pop, A. The role of antioxidants in the chemistry of oxidative stress: A review. *Eur. J. Med. Chem.* **2015**, *97*, 55–74. [CrossRef] [PubMed]
8. Poljsak, B.; Šuput, D.; Milisav, I. Achieving the balance between ROS and antioxidants: When to use the synthetic antioxidants. *Oxid. Med. Cell. Longev.* **2013**, *2013*, 956792. [CrossRef]
9. Jiang, T.; Sun, Q.; Chen, S. Oxidative stress: A major pathogenesis and potential therapeutic target of antioxidative agents in Parkinson's disease and Alzheimer's disease. *Prog. Neurobiol.* **2016**, *147*, 1–19. [CrossRef]
10. Watson, B.D. Evaluation of the concomitance of lipid peroxidation in experimental models of cerebral ischemia and stroke. In *Progress in Brain Research*; Elsevier: Amsterdam, The Netherlands, 1993; Volume 96, pp. 69–95.
11. Choi, B.H. Oxygen, antioxidants and brain dysfunction. *Yonsei Med. J.* **1993**, *34*, 1–10. [CrossRef]
12. Poon, H.F.; Calabrese, V.; Scapagnini, G.; Butterfield, D.A. Free radicals: Key to brain aging and heme oxygenase as a cellular response to oxidative stress. *J. Gerontol. A Biol. Sci. Med. Sci.* **2004**, *59*, M478–M493. [CrossRef] [PubMed]
13. Rao, A.; Balachandran, B. Role of oxidative stress and antioxidants in neurodegenerative diseases. *Nutr. Neurosci.* **2002**, *5*, 291–309. [CrossRef] [PubMed]
14. Packer, L. Oxidative stress, Antioxidants, Aging and Disease. In *Oxidative Stress and Aging*; Springer: Berlin/Heidelberg, Germany, 1995; pp. 1–14.
15. Li, J.; Li, W.; Jiang, Z.G.; Ghanbari, H.A. Oxidative stress and neurodegenerative disorders. *Int. J. Mol. Sci.* **2013**, *14*, 24438–24475. [CrossRef] [PubMed]
16. Conway, M.E.; Lee, C. The redox switch that regulates molecular chaperones. *Biomol. Concepts* **2015**, *6*, 269–284. [CrossRef]
17. Dickinson, B.C.; Peltier, J.; Stone, D.; Schaffer, D.V.; Chang, C.J. Nox2 redox signaling maintains essential cell populations in the brain. *Nat. Chem. Biol.* **2011**, *7*, 106–112. [CrossRef]
18. Brown, G.C. Nitric oxide and mitochondrial respiration. *Biochim. Biophys. Acta* **1999**, *1411*, 351–369. [CrossRef]
19. Carballal, S.; Bartesaghi, S.; Radi, R. Kinetic and mechanistic considerations to assess the biological fate of peroxynitrite. *Biochim. Biophys. Acta* **2014**, *1840*, 768–780. [CrossRef]
20. Lipton, S.A.; Choi, Y.B.; Pan, Z.H.; Lei, S.Z.; Chen, H.S.; Sucher, N.J.; Loscalzo, J.; Singel, D.J.; Stamler, J.S. A redox-based mechanism for the neuroprotective and neurodestructive effects of nitric oxide and related nitroso-compounds. *Nature* **1993**, *364*, 626–632. [CrossRef]
21. Sena, L.A.; Chandel, N.S. Physiological roles of mitochondrial reactive oxygen species. *Mol. Cell* **2012**, *48*, 158–167. [CrossRef]
22. Brand, M.D.; Goncalves, R.L.; Orr, A.L.; Vargas, L.; Gerencser, A.A.; Jensen, M.B.; Wang, Y.T.; Melov, S.; Turk, C.N.; Matzen, J.T. Suppressors of superoxide-H_2O_2 production at site IQ of mitochondrial complex I protect against stem cell hyperplasia and ischemia-reperfusion injury. *Cell Metab.* **2016**, *24*, 582–592. [CrossRef]
23. Goncalves, R.L.; Rothschild, D.E.; Quinlan, C.L.; Scott, G.K.; Benz, C.C.; Brand, M.D. Sources of superoxide/H_2O_2 during mitochondrial proline oxidation. *Redox Biol.* **2014**, *2*, 901–909. [CrossRef]
24. Bélanger, M.; Allaman, I.; Magistretti, P.J. Brain energy metabolism: Focus on astrocyte-neuron metabolic cooperation. *Cell Metab.* **2011**, *14*, 724–738. [CrossRef] [PubMed]
25. Pun, P.B.L.; Logan, A.; Darley-Usmar, V.; Chacko, B.; Johnson, M.S.; Huang, G.W.; Rogatti, S.; Prime, T.A.; Methner, C.; Krieg, T. A mitochondria-targeted mass spectrometry probe to detect glyoxals: Implications for diabetes. *Free Radic. Biol. Med.* **2014**, *67*, 437–450. [CrossRef] [PubMed]
26. Przedborski, S. The two-century journey of Parkinson disease research. *Nat. Rev. Neurosci.* **2017**, *18*, 251. [CrossRef] [PubMed]
27. Cohen, G.; Heikkila, R.E. The generation of hydrogen peroxide, superoxide radical, and hydroxyl radical by 6-hydroxydopamine, dialuric acid, and related cytotoxic agents. *J. Biol. Chem.* **1974**, *249*, 2447–2452.

28. Miller, D.M.; Buettner, G.R.; Aust, S.D. Transition metals as catalysts of "autoxidation" reactions. *Free Radic. Biol. Med.* **1990**, *8*, 95–108. [CrossRef]
29. Patra, R.; Swarup, D.; Dwivedi, S. Antioxidant effects of α tocopherol, ascorbic acid and L-methionine on lead induced oxidative stress to the liver, kidney and brain in rats. *Toxicology* **2001**, *162*, 81–88. [CrossRef]
30. Brigelius-Flohé, R.; Maiorino, M. Glutathione peroxidases. *Biochim. Biophys. Acta* **2013**, *1830*, 3289–3303. [CrossRef]
31. Savaskan, N.E.; Borchert, A.; Bräuer, A.U.; Kuhn, H. Role for glutathione peroxidase-4 in brain development and neuronal apoptosis: Specific induction of enzyme expression in reactive astrocytes following brain injury. *Free Radic. Biol. Med.* **2007**, *43*, 191–201. [CrossRef]
32. Hong, S.; Dissing-Olesen, L.; Stevens, B. New insights on the role of microglia in synaptic pruning in health and disease. *Curr. Opin. Neurobiol.* **2016**, *36*, 128–134. [CrossRef]
33. Bedard, K.; Krause, K.-H. The NOX family of ROS-generating NADPH oxidases: Physiology and pathophysiology. *Physiol. Rev.* **2007**, *87*, 245–313. [CrossRef] [PubMed]
34. Cheng, Z.; Li, Y. What is responsible for the initiating chemistry of iron-mediated lipid peroxidation: An update. *Chem. Rev.* **2007**, *107*, 748–766. [CrossRef] [PubMed]
35. Halliwell, B. Oxidative stress and neurodegeneration: Where are we now? *J. Neurochem.* **2006**, *97*, 1634–1658. [CrossRef] [PubMed]
36. Yin, H.; Xu, L.; Porter, N.A. Free Radical Lipid Peroxidation: Mechanisms and Analysis. *Chem. Rev.* **2011**, *111*, 5944–5972. [CrossRef] [PubMed]
37. Ferrer-Sueta, G.; Radi, R. Chemical biology of peroxynitrite: Kinetics, diffusion, and radicals. *ACS Chem. Biol.* **2009**, *4*, 161–177. [CrossRef]
38. Thomas, D.D. Breathing new life into nitric oxide signaling: A brief overview of the interplay between oxygen and nitric oxide. *Redox Biol.* **2015**, *5*, 225–233. [CrossRef]
39. Lobo, V.; Patil, A.; Phatak, A.; Chandra, N. Free radicals, antioxidants and functional foods: Impact on human health. *Pharmacogn. Rev.* **2010**, *4*, 118. [CrossRef]
40. Cadet, J.; Davies, K.J. Oxidative DNA damage & repair: An introduction. *Free Radic. Biol. Med.* **2017**, *107*, 2–12.
41. Gutteridge, J. Biological origin of free radicals, and mechanisms of antioxidant protection. *Chem. Biol. Interact.* **1994**, *91*, 133–140. [CrossRef]
42. Ellerby, L.M.; Cabelli, D.E.; Graden, J.A.; Valentine, J.S. Copper−zinc superoxide dismutase: Why not pH-dependent? *J. Am. Chem. Soc.* **1996**, *118*, 6556–6561. [CrossRef]
43. Banci, L.; Benedetto, M.; Bertini, I.; Del Conte, R.; Piccioli, M.; Viezzoli, M.S. Solution structure of reduced monomeric Q133M2 copper, zinc superoxide dismutase (SOD). Why is SOD a dimeric enzyme? *Biochemistry* **1998**, *37*, 11780–11791. [CrossRef] [PubMed]
44. Guan, Y.; Hickey, M.J.; Borgstahl, G.E.; Hallewell, R.A.; Lepock, J.R.; O'Connor, D.; Hsieh, Y.; Nick, H.S.; Silverman, D.N.; Tainer, J.A. Crystal structure of Y34F mutant human mitochondrial manganese superoxide dismutase and the functional role of tyrosine 34. *Biochemistry* **1998**, *37*, 4722–4730. [CrossRef] [PubMed]
45. Adachi, T.; Wang, X.L. Association of extracellular-superoxide dismutase phenotype with the endothelial constitutive nitric oxide synthase polymorphism. *FEBS Lett.* **1998**, *433*, 166–168. [CrossRef]
46. Matés, J.M.; Sánchez-Jiménez, F. Antioxidant enzymes and their implications in pathophysiologic processes. *Front. Biosci.* **1999**, *4*, D339–D345. [CrossRef] [PubMed]
47. Liu, J.; Lillo, C.; Jonsson, P.A.; Velde, C.V.; Ward, C.M.; Miller, T.M.; Subramaniam, J.R.; Rothstein, J.D.; Marklund, S.; Andersen, P.M. Toxicity of familial ALS-linked SOD1 mutants from selective recruitment to spinal mitochondria. *Neuron* **2004**, *43*, 5–17. [CrossRef]
48. Li, Q.X.; Mok, S.S.; Laughton, K.M.; McLean, C.A.; Volitakis, I.; Cherny, R.A.; Cheung, N.S.; White, A.R.; Masters, C.L. Overexpression of Aβ is associated with acceleration of onset of motor impairment and superoxide dismutase 1 aggregation in an amyotrophic lateral sclerosis mouse model. *Aging Cell* **2006**, *5*, 153–165. [CrossRef]
49. Iadecola, C.; Zhang, F.; Niwa, K.; Eckman, C.; Turner, S.K.; Fischer, E.; Younkin, S.; Borchelt, D.R.; Hsiao, K.K.; Carlson, G.A. SOD1 rescues cerebral endothelial dysfunction in mice overexpressing amyloid precursor protein. *Nat. Neurosci.* **1999**, *2*, 157–161. [CrossRef]

50. De Haan, J.B.; Newman, J.D.; Kola, I. Cu/Zn superoxide dismutase mRNA and enzyme activity, and susceptibility to lipid peroxidation, increases with aging in murine brains. *Brain Res. Mol. Brain Res.* **1992**, *13*, 179–187. [CrossRef]
51. Murakami, K.; Murata, N.; Noda, Y.; Tahara, S.; Kaneko, T.; Kinoshita, N.; Hatsuta, H.; Murayama, S.; Barnham, K.J.; Irie, K. SOD1 (copper/zinc superoxide dismutase) deficiency drives amyloid β protein oligomerization and memory loss in mouse model of Alzheimer disease. *J. Biol. Chem.* **2011**, *286*, 44557–44568. [CrossRef]
52. Kim, U.J.; Lee, B.H.; Lee, K.H. Neuroprotective effects of a protein tyrosine phosphatase inhibitor against hippocampal excitotoxic injury. *Brain Res.* **2019**, *1719*, 133–139. [CrossRef]
53. Esposito, L.; Raber, J.; Kekonius, L.; Yan, F.; Yu, G.-Q.; Bien-Ly, N.; Puoliväli, J.; Scearce-Levie, K.; Masliah, E.; Mucke, L. Reduction in mitochondrial superoxide dismutase modulates Alzheimer's disease-like pathology and accelerates the onset of behavioral changes in human amyloid precursor protein transgenic mice. *J. Neurosci.* **2006**, *26*, 5167–5179. [CrossRef] [PubMed]
54. Liao, R.; Wood, T.R.; Nance, E. Superoxide dismutase reduces monosodium glutamate-induced injury in an organotypic whole hemisphere brain slice model of excitotoxicity. *J. Biol. Eng.* **2020**, *14*, 1–12.
55. Hunt, C.R.; Sim, J.E.; Sullivan, S.J.; Featherstone, T.; Golden, W.; Von Kapp-Herr, C.; Hock, R.A.; Gomez, R.A.; Parsian, A.J.; Spitz, D.R. Genomic instability and catalase gene amplification induced by chronic exposure to oxidative stress. *Cancer Res.* **1998**, *58*, 3986–3992. [PubMed]
56. Fita, I.; Rossmann, M.G. The active center of catalase. *J. Mol. Biol.* **1985**, *185*, 21–37. [CrossRef]
57. Usui, S.; Komeima, K.; Lee, S.Y.; Jo, Y.-J.; Ueno, S.; Rogers, B.S.; Wu, Z.; Shen, J.; Lu, L.; Oveson, B.C. Increased expression of catalase and superoxide dismutase 2 reduces cone cell death in retinitis pigmentosa. *Mol. Ther.* **2009**, *17*, 778–786. [CrossRef]
58. Speranza, M.J.; Bagley, A.; Lynch, R. Cells enriched for catalase are sensitized to the toxicities of bleomycin, adriamycin, and paraquat. *J. Biol. Chem.* **1993**, *268*, 19039–19043.
59. Terlecky, S.R.; Koepke, J.I.; Walton, P.A. Peroxisomes and aging. *Biochim. Biophy. Acta* **2006**, *1763*, 1749–1754. [CrossRef]
60. Sheikh, F.G.; Pahan, K.; Khan, M.; Barbosa, E.; Singh, I. Abnormality in catalase import into peroxisomes leads to severe neurological disorder. *Proc. Natl. Acad. Sci. USA* **1998**, *95*, 2961–2966. [CrossRef]
61. Baxter, P.S.; Bell, K.F.; Hasel, P.; Kaindl, A.M.; Fricker, M.; Thomson, D.; Cregan, S.P.; Gillingwater, T.H.; Hardingham, G.E. Synaptic NMDA receptor activity is coupled to the transcriptional control of the glutathione system. *Nat. Commun.* **2015**, *6*, 1–13. [CrossRef]
62. Zhang, Z.; Rydel, R.E.; Drzewiecki, G.J.; Fuson, K.; Wright, S.; Wogulis, M.; Audia, J.E.; May, P.C.; Hyslop, P.A. Amyloid β-mediated oxidative and metabolic stress in rat cortical neurons: No direct evidence for a role for H_2O_2 generation. *J. Neurochem.* **1996**, *67*, 1595–1606. [CrossRef]
63. Nell, H.J.; Au, J.L.; Giordano, C.R.; Terlecky, S.R.; Walton, P.A.; Whitehead, S.N.; Cechetto, D.F. Targeted antioxidant, catalase–SKL, reduces beta-amyloid toxicity in the rat brain. *Brain Pathol.* **2017**, *27*, 86–94. [CrossRef] [PubMed]
64. Yakunin, E.; Kisos, H.; Kulik, W.; Grigoletto, J.; Wanders, R.J.; Sharon, R. The regulation of catalase activity by PPAR γ is affected by α-synuclein. *Ann. Clin. Transl. Neurol.* **2014**, *1*, 145–159. [CrossRef] [PubMed]
65. Ursini, F.; Maiorino, M.; Brigelius-Flohé, R.; Aumann, K.D.; Roveri, A.; Schomburg, D.; Flohé, L. Diversity of glutathione peroxidases. *Methods Enzymol.* **1995**, *252*, 38–53. [PubMed]
66. Kemp, M.; Go, Y.M.; Jones, D.P. Nonequilibrium thermodynamics of thiol/disulfide redox systems: A perspective on redox systems biology. *Free Radic. Biol. Med.* **2008**, *44*, 921–937. [CrossRef] [PubMed]
67. Taylor, J.M.; Ali, U.; Iannello, R.C.; Hertzog, P.; Crack, P.J. Diminished Akt phosphorylation in neurons lacking glutathione peroxidase-1 (Gpx1) leads to increased susceptibility to oxidative stress-induced cell death. *J. Neurochem.* **2005**, *92*, 283–293. [CrossRef] [PubMed]
68. Cardoso, B.R.; Hare, D.J.; Bush, A.I.; Roberts, B.R. Glutathione peroxidase 4: A new player in neurodegeneration? *Mol. Psychiatry* **2017**, *22*, 328–335. [CrossRef]
69. Dixon, S.J.; Lemberg, K.M.; Lamprecht, M.R.; Skouta, R.; Zaitsev, E.M.; Gleason, C.E.; Patel, D.N.; Bauer, A.J.; Cantley, A.M.; Yang, W.S. Ferroptosis: An iron-dependent form of nonapoptotic cell death. *Cell* **2012**, *149*, 1060–1072. [CrossRef]
70. Chen, Z.H.; Yoshida, Y.; Saito, Y.; Niki, E. Adaptation to hydrogen peroxide enhances PC12 cell tolerance against oxidative damage. *Neurosci. Lett.* **2005**, *383*, 256–259. [CrossRef]

71. Goss, J.R.; Taffe, K.M.; Kochanek, P.M.; DeKosky, S.T. The antioxidant enzymes glutathione peroxidase and catalase increase following traumatic brain injury in the rat. *Exp. Neurol.* **1997**, *146*, 291–294. [CrossRef]
72. Hambright, W.S.; Fonseca, R.S.; Chen, L.; Na, R.; Ran, Q. Ablation of ferroptosis regulator glutathione peroxidase 4 in forebrain neurons promotes cognitive impairment and neurodegeneration. *Redox Biol.* **2017**, *12*, 8–17. [CrossRef]
73. Do Van, B.; Gouel, F.; Jonneaux, A.; Timmerman, K.; Gelé, P.; Pétrault, M.; Bastide, M.; Laloux, C.; Moreau, C.; Bordet, R. Ferroptosis, a newly characterized form of cell death in Parkinson's disease that is regulated by PKC. *Neurobiol. Dis.* **2016**, *94*, 169–178. [CrossRef] [PubMed]
74. Chae, H.Z.; Kim, H.J.; Kang, S.W.; Rhee, S.G. Characterization of three isoforms of mammalian peroxiredoxin that reduce peroxides in the presence of thioredoxin. *Diabetes Res. Clin. Pract.* **1999**, *45*, 101–112. [CrossRef]
75. Burke-Gaffney, A.; Callister, M.E.; Nakamura, H. Thioredoxin: Friend or foe in human disease? *Trends Pharmacol. Sci.* **2005**, *26*, 398–404. [CrossRef] [PubMed]
76. Silva-Adaya, D.; Gonsebatt, M.E.; Guevara, J. Thioredoxin system regulation in the central nervous system: Experimental models and clinical evidence. *Oxid. Med. Cell. Longev.* **2014**, *2014*, 590808. [CrossRef]
77. Ren, X.; Zou, L.; Zhang, X.; Branco, V.; Wang, J.; Carvalho, C.; Holmgren, A.; Lu, J. Redox signaling mediated by thioredoxin and glutathione systems in the central nervous system. *Antioxid. Redox Signal.* **2017**, *27*, 989–1010. [CrossRef]
78. Lundström, J.; Holmgren, A. Protein disulfide-isomerase is a substrate for thioredoxin reductase and has thioredoxin-like activity. *J. Biol. Chem.* **1990**, *265*, 9114–9120.
79. Soerensen, J.; Jakupoglu, C.; Beck, H.; Förster, H.; Schmidt, J.; Schmahl, W.; Schweizer, U.; Conrad, M.; Brielmeier, M. The role of thioredoxin reductases in brain development. *PLoS ONE* **2008**, *3*, e1813. [CrossRef]
80. May, J.M.; Cobb, C.E.; Mendiratta, S.; Hill, K.E.; Burk, R.F. Reduction of the ascorbyl free radical to ascorbate by thioredoxin reductase. *J. Biol. Chem.* **1998**, *273*, 23039–23045. [CrossRef]
81. Arnér, E.S.; Nordberg, J.; Holmgren, A. Efficient reduction of lipoamide and lipoic acid by mammalian thioredoxin reductase. *Biochem. Biophys. Res. Commun.* **1996**, *225*, 268–274. [CrossRef]
82. Xia, L.; Björnstedt, M.; Nordman, T.; Eriksson, L.C.; Olsson, J.M. Reduction of ubiquinone by lipoamide dehydrogenase: An antioxidant regenerating pathway. *Eur. J. Biochem.* **2001**, *268*, 1486–1490. [CrossRef]
83. Lu, J.; Zhong, L.; Lönn, M.E.; Burk, R.F.; Hill, K.E.; Holmgren, A. Penultimate selenocysteine residue replaced by cysteine in thioredoxin reductase from selenium-deficient rat liver. *FASEB J.* **2009**, *23*, 2394–2402. [CrossRef] [PubMed]
84. Takagi, Y.; Hattori, I.; Nozaki, K.; Mitsui, A.; Ishikawa, M.; Hashimoto, N.; Yodoi, J. Excitotoxic hippocampal injury is attenuated in thioredoxin transgenic mice. *J. Cereb. Blood Flow Metab.* **2000**, *20*, 829–833. [CrossRef] [PubMed]
85. Takagi, Y.; Mitsui, A.; Nishiyama, A.; Nozaki, K.; Sono, H.; Gon, Y.; Hashimoto, N.; Yodoi, J. Overexpression of thioredoxin in transgenic mice attenuates focal ischemic brain damage. *Proc. Natl. Acad. Sci. USA* **1999**, *96*, 4131–4136. [CrossRef]
86. Björnstedt, M.; Xue, J.; Huang, W.; Akesson, B.; Holmgren, A. The thioredoxin and glutaredoxin systems are efficient electron donors to human plasma glutathione peroxidase. *J. Biol. Chem.* **1994**, *269*, 29382–29384. [PubMed]
87. Munemasa, Y.; Kim, S.H.; Ahn, J.H.; Kwong, J.M.; Caprioli, J.; Piri, N. Protective effect of thioredoxins 1 and 2 in retinal ganglion cells after optic nerve transection and oxidative stress. *Investig. Ophthalmol. Vis. Sci.* **2008**, *49*, 3535–3543. [CrossRef] [PubMed]
88. Zeng, X.S.; Jia, J.J.; Kwon, Y.; Wang, S.D.; Bai, J. The role of thioredoxin-1 in suppression of endoplasmic reticulum stress in Parkinson disease. *Free Radic. Biol. Med.* **2014**, *67*, 10–18. [CrossRef]
89. Lovell, M.A.; Xie, C.; Gabbita, S.P.; Markesbery, W.R. Decreased thioredoxin and increased thioredoxin reductase levels in Alzheimer's disease brain. *Free Radic. Biol. Med.* **2000**, *28*, 418–427. [CrossRef]
90. Sánchez-López, F.; Tasset, I.; Agüera, E.; Feijóo, M.; Fernández-Bolaños, R.; Sánchez, F.M.; Ruiz, M.C.; Cruz, A.H.; Gascón, F.; Túnez, I. Oxidative stress and inflammation biomarkers in the blood of patients with Huntington's disease. *Neurol. Res.* **2012**, *34*, 721–724. [CrossRef]
91. Zhou, F.; Liu, P.P.; Ying, G.Y.; Zhu, X.D.; Shen, H.; Chen, G. Effects of thioredoxin-1 on neurogenesis after brain ischemia/reperfusion injury. *CNS Neurosci. Ther.* **2013**, *19*, 204. [CrossRef]

92. Hwang, I.K.; Yoo, K.-Y.; Kim, D.W.; Lee, C.H.; Choi, J.H.; Kwon, Y.-G.; Kim, Y.-M.; Choi, S.Y.; Won, M.-H. Changes in the expression of mitochondrial peroxiredoxin and thioredoxin in neurons and glia and their protective effects in experimental cerebral ischemic damage. *Free Radic. Biol. Med.* **2010**, *48*, 1242–1251. [CrossRef]
93. Miller, J.; Brzezinska-Slebodzinska, E.; Madsen, F. Oxidative stress, antioxidants, and animal function. *J. Dairy Sci.* **1993**, *76*, 2812–2823. [CrossRef]
94. Hardy, G.; Hardy, I.; Manzanares, W. Selenium supplementation in the critically ill. *Nutr. Clin. Pract.* **2012**, *27*, 21–33. [CrossRef] [PubMed]
95. Hamilton, S.J. Review of selenium toxicity in the aquatic food chain. *Sci. Total Environ.* **2004**, *326*, 1–31. [CrossRef] [PubMed]
96. Solovyev, N.D. Importance of selenium and selenoprotein for brain function: From antioxidant protection to neuronal signalling. *J. Inorg. Biochem.* **2015**, *153*, 1–12. [CrossRef]
97. Santamaría, A.; Vázquez-Román, B.; La cruz, V.P.D.; González-Cortés, C.; Trejo-Solís, M.C.; Galván-Arzate, S.; Jara-Prado, A.; Guevara-Fonseca, J.; Ali, S.F. Selenium reduces the proapoptotic signaling associated to NF-κB pathway and stimulates glutathione peroxidase activity during excitotoxic damage produced by quinolinate in rat corpus striatum. *Synapse* **2005**, *58*, 258–266. [CrossRef] [PubMed]
98. Zachara, B.A.; Pawluk, H.; Bloch-Boguslawska, E.; Śliwka, K.M.; Korenkiewicz, J.; Skok, Ź.; Ryć, K. Tissue level, distribution and total body selenium content in healthy and diseased humans in Poland. *Arch. Environ. Health* **2001**, *56*, 461–466. [CrossRef]
99. Kühbacher, M.; Bartel, J.; Hoppe, B.; Alber, D.; Bukalis, G.; Bräuer, A.U.; Behne, D.; Kyriakopoulos, A. The brain selenoproteome: Priorities in the hierarchy and different levels of selenium homeostasis in the brain of selenium-deficient rats. *J. Neurochem.* **2009**, *110*, 133–142. [CrossRef]
100. Dalla Puppa, L.; Savaskan, N.E.; Braeuer, A.U.; Behne, D.; Kyriakopoulos, A. The role of selenite on microglial migration. *Ann. N. Y. Acad. Sci.* **2007**, *1096*, 179–183. [CrossRef]
101. Uğuz, A.C.; Nazıroğlu, M. Effects of selenium on calcium signaling and apoptosis in rat dorsal root ganglion neurons induced by oxidative stress. *Neurochem. Res.* **2012**, *37*, 1631–1638. [CrossRef]
102. Haratake, M.; Yoshida, S.; Mandai, M.; Fuchigami, T.; Nakayama, M. Elevated amyloid-β plaque deposition in dietary selenium-deficient Tg2576 transgenic mice. *Metallomics* **2013**, *5*, 479–483. [CrossRef]
103. Ishrat, T.; Parveen, K.; Khan, M.M.; Khuwaja, G.; Khan, M.B.; Yousuf, S.; Ahmad, A.; Shrivastav, P.; Islam, F. Selenium prevents cognitive decline and oxidative damage in rat model of streptozotocin-induced experimental dementia of Alzheimer's type. *Brain Res.* **2009**, *1281*, 117–127. [CrossRef] [PubMed]
104. Ellwanger, J.H.; Molz, P.; Dallemole, D.R.; dos Santos, A.P.; Müller, T.E.; Cappelletti, L.; da Silva, M.G.; Franke, S.I.R.; Prá, D.; Henriques, J.A.P. Selenium reduces bradykinesia and DNA damage in a rat model of Parkinson's disease. *Nutrition* **2015**, *31*, 359–365. [CrossRef] [PubMed]
105. Lu, Z.; Marks, E.; Chen, J.; Moline, J.; Barrows, L.; Raisbeck, M.; Volitakis, I.; Cherny, R.A.; Chopra, V.; Bush, A.I. Altered selenium status in Huntington's disease: Neuroprotection by selenite in the N171-82Q mouse model. *Neurobiol. Dis.* **2014**, *71*, 34–42. [CrossRef] [PubMed]
106. Yeo, J.E.; Kang, S.K. Selenium effectively inhibits ROS-mediated apoptotic neural precursor cell death in vitro and in vivo in traumatic brain injury. *Biochim. Biophys. Acta* **2007**, *1772*, 1199–1210. [CrossRef]
107. Khalili, H.; Ahl, R.; Cao, Y.; Paydar, S.; Sjölin, G.; Niakan, A.; Dabiri, G.; Mohseni, S. Early selenium treatment for traumatic brain injury: Does it improve survival and functional outcome? *Injury* **2017**, *48*, 1922–1926. [CrossRef] [PubMed]
108. Nohl, H.; Kozlov, A.V.; Staniek, K.; Gille, L. The multiple functions of coenzyme Q. *Bioorg. Chem.* **2001**, *29*, 1–13. [CrossRef] [PubMed]
109. Ernster, L.; Dallner, G. Biochemical, physiological and medical aspects of ubiquinone function. *Biochim. Biophys. Acta* **1995**, *1271*, 195–204. [CrossRef]
110. Bhagavan, H.N.; Chopra, R.K. Coenzyme Q10: Absorption, tissue uptake, metabolism and pharmacokinetics. *Free Radic. Res.* **2006**, *40*, 445–453. [CrossRef]
111. Hargreaves, I.P. Ubiquinone: Cholesterol's reclusive cousin. *Ann. Clin. Biochem.* **2003**, *40*, 207–218. [CrossRef]
112. Xia, L.; Nordman, T.; Olsson, J.M.; Damdimopoulos, A.; Björkhem-Bergman, L.; Nalvarte, I.; Eriksson, L.C.; Arnér, E.S.; Spyrou, G.; Björnstedt, M. The mammalian cytosolic selenoenzyme thioredoxin reductase reduces ubiquinone a novel mechanism for defense against oxidative stress. *J. Biol. Chem.* **2003**, *278*, 2141–2146. [CrossRef]

113. Montini, G.; Malaventura, C.; Salviati, L. Early coenzyme Q10 supplementation in primary coenzyme Q10 deficiency. *N. Engl. J. Med.* **2008**, *358*, 2849–2850. [CrossRef] [PubMed]

114. Salviati, L.; Sacconi, S.; Murer, L.; Zacchello, G.; Franceschini, L.; Laverda, A.M.; Basso, G.; Quinzii, C.; Angelini, C.; Hirano, M.; et al. Infantile encephalomyopathy and nephropathy with CoQ10 deficiency: A CoQ10-responsive condition. *Neurology* **2005**, *65*, 606–608. [CrossRef]

115. Hargreaves, I.; Mantle, D. Supplementation with selenium and coenzyme Q10 in critically ill patients. *Br. J. Hosp. Med.* **2019**, *80*, 589–593. [CrossRef] [PubMed]

116. Won, R.; Lee, K.H.; Lee, B.H. Coenzyme Q10 protects neurons against neurotoxicity in hippocampal slice culture. *Neuroreport* **2011**, *22*, 721–726. [CrossRef] [PubMed]

117. Park, H.W.; Park, C.G.; Park, M.; Lee, S.H.; Park, H.R.; Lim, J.; Paek, S.H.; Choy, Y.B. Intrastriatal administration of coenzyme Q10 enhances neuroprotection in a Parkinson's disease rat model. *Sci. Rep.* **2020**, *10*, 1–12. [CrossRef] [PubMed]

118. Ramezani, M.; Sahraei, Z.; Simani, L.; Heydari, K.; Shahidi, F. Coenzyme Q10 supplementation in acute ischemic stroke: Is it beneficial in short-term administration? *Nutr. Neurosci.* **2020**, *23*, 640–645. [CrossRef] [PubMed]

119. Yoritaka, A.; Kawajiri, S.; Yamamoto, Y.; Nakahara, T.; Ando, M.; Hashimoto, K.; Nagase, M.; Saito, Y.; Hattori, N. Randomized, double-blind, placebo-controlled pilot trial of reduced coenzyme Q10 for Parkinson's disease. *Parkinsonism Relat. Disord.* **2015**, *21*, 911–916. [CrossRef] [PubMed]

120. Sawaddiruk, P.; Apaijai, N.; Paiboonworachat, S.; Kaewchur, T.; Kasitanon, N.; Jaiwongkam, T.; Kerdphoo, S.; Chattipakorn, N.; Chattipakorn, S.C. Coenzyme Q10 supplementation alleviates pain in pregabalin-treated fibromyalgia patients via reducing brain activity and mitochondrial dysfunction. *Free Radic. Res.* **2019**, *53*, 901–909. [CrossRef] [PubMed]

121. Kloubert, V.; Rink, L. Zinc as a micronutrient and its preventive role of oxidative damage in cells. *Food Funct.* **2015**, *6*, 3195–3204. [CrossRef] [PubMed]

122. Oteiza, P.I. Zinc and the modulation of redox homeostasis. *Free Radic. Biol. Med.* **2012**, *53*, 1748–1759. [CrossRef] [PubMed]

123. Kawahara, M.; Tanaka, K.-i.; Kato-Negishi, M. Zinc, carnosine, and neurodegenerative diseases. *Nutrients* **2018**, *10*, 147. [CrossRef]

124. Frederickson, C.J.; Suh, S.W.; Silva, D.; Frederickson, C.J.; Thompson, R.B. Importance of zinc in the central nervous system: The zinc-containing neuron. *J. Nutr.* **2000**, *130*, 1471S–1483S. [CrossRef] [PubMed]

125. Farbood, Y.; Sarkaki, A.; Mahdavinia, M.; Ghadiri, A.; Teimoori, A.; Seif, F.; Dehghani, M.A.; Navabi, S.P. Protective effects of co-administration of zinc and selenium against streptozotocin-induced Alzheimer's disease: Behavioral, mitochondrial oxidative stress, and GPR39 expression alterations in rats. *Neurotox. Res.* **2020**, *38*, 398–407. [CrossRef] [PubMed]

126. Jafari, F.; Amani, R.; Tarrahi, M.J. Effect of zinc supplementation on physical and psychological symptoms, biomarkers of inflammation, oxidative stress, and brain-derived neurotrophic factor in young women with premenstrual syndrome: A randomized, double-blind, placebo-controlled trial. *Biol. Trace Elem. Res.* **2020**, *194*, 89–95. [CrossRef] [PubMed]

127. Carocci, A.; Catalano, A.; Sinicropi, M.S.; Genchi, G. Oxidative stress and neurodegeneration: The involvement of iron. *Biometals* **2018**, *31*, 715–735. [CrossRef] [PubMed]

128. Farina, M.; Avila, D.S.; Da Rocha, J.B.T.; Aschner, M. Metals, oxidative stress and neurodegeneration: A focus on iron, manganese and mercury. *Neurochem. Int.* **2013**, *62*, 575–594. [CrossRef] [PubMed]

129. Ballaz, S.J.; Rebec, G.V. Neurobiology of vitamin C: Expanding the focus from antioxidant to endogenous neuromodulator. *Pharmacol. Res.* **2019**, *146*, 104321. [CrossRef]

130. Moretti, M.; Fraga, D.B.; Rodrigues, A.L.S. Preventive and therapeutic potential of ascorbic acid in neurodegenerative diseases. *CNS Neurosci. Ther.* **2017**, *23*, 921–929. [CrossRef]

131. Harrison, F.E.; May, J.M. Vitamin C function in the brain: Vital role of the ascorbate transporter SVCT2. *Free Radic. Biol. Med.* **2009**, *46*, 719–730. [CrossRef]

132. García-Krauss, A.; Ferrada, L.; Astuya, A.; Salazar, K.; Cisternas, P.; Martínez, F.; Ramírez, E.; Nualart, F. Dehydroascorbic acid promotes cell death in neurons under oxidative stress: A protective role for astrocytes. *Mol. Neurobiol.* **2016**, *53*, 5847–5863. [CrossRef]

133. Astuya, A.; Caprile, T.; Castro, M.; Salazar, K.; García, M.d.l.A.; Reinicke, K.; Rodríguez, F.; Vera, J.C.; Millán, C.; Ulloa, V. Vitamin C uptake and recycling among normal and tumor cells from the central nervous system. *J. Neurosci. Res.* **2005**, *79*, 146–156. [CrossRef]
134. Ulloa, V.; García-Robles, M.; Martínez, F.; Salazar, K.; Reinicke, K.; Pérez, F.; Godoy, D.F.; Godoy, A.S.; Nualart, F. Human choroid plexus papilloma cells efficiently transport glucose and vitamin C. *J. Neurochem.* **2013**, *127*, 403–414. [CrossRef] [PubMed]
135. Ziylan, Y.Z.; Diler, A.S.; Lefauconnier, J.-M.; Bourre, J.-M. Evidence for ascorbic acid transport system in rat brain capillaries. *Int. J. Neurosci.* **2006**, *116*, 25–38. [CrossRef]
136. Covarrubias-Pinto, A.; Acuna, A.; Boncompain, G.; Papic, E.; Burgos, P.; Perez, F.; Castro, M. Ascorbic acid increases SVCT2 localization at the plasma membrane by accelerating its trafficking from early secretory compartments and through the endocytic-recycling pathway. *Free Radic. Biol. Med.* **2018**, *120*, 181–191. [CrossRef] [PubMed]
137. Getoff, N. Vitamin C: Electron emission, free radicals and biological versatility. *In Vivo* **2013**, *27*, 565–570. [PubMed]
138. Lane, D.J.; Lawen, A. Ascorbate and plasma membrane electron transport—Enzymes vs efflux. *Free Radic. Biol. Med.* **2009**, *47*, 485–495. [CrossRef] [PubMed]
139. Nelson, M.T.; Joksovic, P.M.; Su, P.; Kang, H.-W.; Van Deusen, A.; Baumgart, J.P.; David, L.S.; Snutch, T.P.; Barrett, P.Q.; Lee, J.-H. Molecular mechanisms of subtype-specific inhibition of neuronal T-type calcium channels by ascorbate. *J. Neurosci.* **2007**, *27*, 12577–12583. [CrossRef]
140. Smythies, J. Redox aspects of signaling by catecholamines and their metabolites. *Antioxid. Redox Signal.* **2000**, *2*, 575–583. [CrossRef]
141. Sandstrom, M.I.; Rebec, G.V. Extracellular ascorbate modulates glutamate dynamics: Role of behavioral activation. *BMC Neurosci.* **2007**, *8*, 1–6. [CrossRef]
142. Karanth, S.; Wen, H.Y.; Walczewska, A.; Mastronardi, C.A.; McCann, S.M. Ascorbic acid stimulates gonadotropin release by autocrine action by means of NO. *Proc. Natl. Acad. Sci. USA* **2001**, *98*, 11783–11788. [CrossRef]
143. Harrison, F.; Dawes, S.; Meredith, M.; Babaev, V.; Li, L.; May, J. Low vitamin C and increased oxidative stress and cell death in mice that lack the sodium-dependent vitamin C transporter SVCT2. *Free Radic. Biol. Med.* **2010**, *49*, 821–829. [CrossRef] [PubMed]
144. Naseer, M.; Ullah, N.; Ullah, I.; Koh, P.; Lee, H.; Park, M.; Kim, M. Vitamin C protects against ethanol and PTZ-induced apoptotic neurodegeneration in prenatal rat hippocampal neurons. *Synapse* **2011**, *65*, 562–571. [CrossRef] [PubMed]
145. Choi, D.W. Excitotoxic cell death. *J. Neurobiol.* **1992**, *23*, 1261–1276. [CrossRef] [PubMed]
146. Barak, O.F.; Caljkusic, K.; Hoiland, R.L.; Ainslie, P.N.; Thom, S.R.; Yang, M.; Jovanov, P.; Dujic, Z. Differential influence of vitamin C on the peripheral and cerebral circulation after diving and exposure to hyperoxia. *Am. J. Physiol. Regul. Integr. Comp. Physiol.* **2018**, *315*, R759–R767. [CrossRef]
147. Jain, S.K.; Dar, M.Y.; Kumar, S.; Yadav, A.; Kearns, S.R. Role of anti-oxidant (Vitamin-C) in post-operative pain relief in foot and ankle trauma surgery: A prospective randomized trial. *Foot Ankle Surg.* **2019**, *25*, 542–545. [CrossRef]
148. Kim, E.J.; Park, Y.G.; Baik, E.J.; Jung, S.J.; Won, R.; Nahm, T.S.; Lee, B.H. Dehydroascorbic acid prevents oxidative cell death through a glutathione pathway in primary astrocytes. *J. Neurosci. Res.* **2005**, *79*, 670–679. [CrossRef]
149. Siqueira, I.R.; Elsner, V.R.; Leite, M.C.; Vanzella, C.; dos Santos Moysés, F.; Spindler, C.; Godinho, G.; Battú, C.; Wofchuk, S.; Souza, D.O. Ascorbate uptake is decreased in the hippocampus of ageing rats. *Neurochem. Int.* **2011**, *58*, 527–532. [CrossRef]
150. Naziroglu, M.; Butterworth, P.J.; Sonmez, T.T. Dietary vitamin C and E modulates antioxidant levels in blood, brain, liver, muscle, and testes in diabetic aged rats. *Int. J. Vitam Nutr. Res.* **2011**, *81*, 347. [CrossRef]
151. Kim, E.J.; Won, R.; Sohn, J.-H.; Chung, M.-A.; Nam, T.S.; Lee, H.-J.; Lee, B.H. Anti-oxidant effect of ascorbic and dehydroascorbic acids in hippocampal slice culture. *Biochem. Biophys. Res. Commun.* **2008**, *366*, 8–14. [CrossRef]

152. Rebec, G.V.; Barton, S.J.; Ennis, M.D. Dysregulation of ascorbate release in the striatum of behaving mice expressing the Huntington's disease gene. *J. Neurosci.* **2002**, *22*, RC202. [CrossRef]
153. Rebec, G.V.; Barton, S.J.; Marseilles, A.M.; Collins, K. Ascorbate treatment attenuates the Huntington behavioral phenotype in mice. *Neuroreport* **2003**, *14*, 1263–1265. [CrossRef] [PubMed]
154. Lee, P.; Ulatowski, L.M. Vitamin E: Mechanism of transport and regulation in the CNS. *IUBMB Life* **2019**, *71*, 424–429. [CrossRef] [PubMed]
155. Atkinson, J.; Epand, R.F.; Epand, R.M. Tocopherols and tocotrienols in membranes: A critical review. *Free Radic. Biol. Med.* **2008**, *44*, 739–764. [CrossRef] [PubMed]
156. Goti, D.; Hrzenjak, A.; Levak-Frank, S.; Frank, S.; Van Der Westhuyzen, D.R.; Malle, E.; Sattler, W. Scavenger receptor class B, type I is expressed in porcine brain capillary endothelial cells and contributes to selective uptake of HDL-associated vitamin E. *J. Neurochem.* **2001**, *76*, 498–508. [CrossRef] [PubMed]
157. Balazs, Z.; Panzenboeck, U.; Hammer, A.; Sovic, A.; Quehenberger, O.; Malle, E.; Sattler, W. Uptake and transport of high-density lipoprotein (HDL) and HDL-associated α-tocopherol by an in vitro blood–brain barrier model. *J. Neurochem.* **2004**, *89*, 939–950. [CrossRef]
158. Acton, S.; Rigotti, A.; Landschulz, K.T.; Xu, S.; Hobbs, H.H.; Krieger, M. Identification of scavenger receptor SR-BI as a high density lipoprotein receptor. *Science* **1996**, *271*, 518–520. [CrossRef]
159. Vance, J.E.; Hayashi, H. Formation and function of apolipoprotein E-containing lipoproteins in the nervous system. *Biochim. Biophys. Acta* **2010**, *1801*, 806–818. [CrossRef]
160. Hayashi, H.; Campenot, R.B.; Vance, D.E.; Vance, J.E. Apolipoprotein E-containing lipoproteins protect neurons from apoptosis via a signaling pathway involving low-density lipoprotein receptor-related protein-1. *J. Neurosci.* **2007**, *27*, 1933–1941. [CrossRef]
161. Lane, M.A.; Bailey, S.J. Role of retinoid signalling in the adult brain. *Prog. Neurobiol.* **2005**, *75*, 275–293. [CrossRef]
162. Ambrogini, P.; Torquato, P.; Bartolini, D.; Albertini, M.C.; Lattanzi, D.; Di Palma, M.; Marinelli, R.; Betti, M.; Minelli, A.; Cuppini, R. Excitotoxicity, neuroinflammation and oxidant stress as molecular bases of epileptogenesis and epilepsy-derived neurodegeneration: The role of vitamin E. *Biochim. Biophys. Acta* **2019**, *1865*, 1098–1112. [CrossRef]
163. Mohn, E.S.; Kuchan, M.J.; Erdman, J.W.; Neuringer, M.; Matthan, N.R.; Chen, C.-Y.O.; Johnson, E.J. The subcellular distribution of alpha-tocopherol in the adult primate brain and its relationship with membrane arachidonic acid and its oxidation products. *Antioxidants* **2017**, *6*, 97. [CrossRef] [PubMed]
164. Shah, R.; Shchepinov, M.S.; Pratt, D.A. Resolving the role of lipoxygenases in the initiation and execution of ferroptosis. *ACS Cent. Sci.* **2018**, *4*, 387–396. [CrossRef] [PubMed]
165. Sen, C.K.; Khanna, S.; Rink, C.; Roy, S. Tocotrienols: The Emerging Face of Natural Vitamin E. In *Vitam. Horm*; Academic Press: Cambridge, MA, USA, 2007; Volume 76, pp. 203–261.
166. Jung, N.Y.; Lee, K.H.; Won, R.; Lee, B.H. Neuroprotective effects of α-tocotrienol on kainic acid-induced neurotoxicity in organotypic hippocampal slice cultures. *Int. J. Mol. Sci.* **2013**, *14*, 18256–18268. [CrossRef]
167. Mehrabadi, S.; Sadr, S.S. Administration of Vitamin D3 and E supplements reduces neuronal loss and oxidative stress in a model of rats with Alzheimer's disease. *Neurol. Res.* **2020**, *38*, 1–7. [CrossRef] [PubMed]
168. Ahmed, M.; Alzoubi, K.H.; Khabour, O.F. Vitamin E prevents the cognitive impairments in post-traumatic stress disorder rat model: Behavioral and molecular study. *Psychopharmacology (Berlin)* **2020**, *237*, 599–607. [CrossRef]
169. Taghizadeh, M.; Tamtaji, O.R.; Dadgostar, E.; Kakhaki, R.D.; Bahmani, F.; Abolhassani, J.; Aarabi, M.H.; Kouchaki, E.; Memarzadeh, M.R.; Asemi, Z. The effects of omega-3 fatty acids and vitamin E co-supplementation on clinical and metabolic status in patients with Parkinson's disease: A randomized, double-blind, placebo-controlled trial. *Neurochem. Int.* **2017**, *108*, 183–189. [CrossRef]
170. Shannon, S.R.; Moise, A.R.; Trainor, P.A. New insights and changing paradigms in the regulation of vitamin A metabolism in development. *Wiley Interdiscip. Rev. Dev. Biol.* **2017**, *6*, e264. [CrossRef]
171. Duester, G. Retinoic acid synthesis and signaling during early organogenesis. *Cell* **2008**, *134*, 921–931. [CrossRef]
172. Mueller, L.; Boehm, V. Antioxidant activity of β-carotene compounds in different in vitro assays. *Molecules* **2011**, *16*, 1055–1069. [CrossRef]

173. Honarvar, N.M.; Saedisomeolia, A.; Abdolahi, M.; Shayeganrad, A.; Sangsari, G.T.; Rad, B.H.; Muench, G. Molecular anti-inflammatory mechanisms of retinoids and carotenoids in Alzheimer's disease: A review of current evidence. *J. Mol. Neurosci.* **2017**, *61*, 289–304. [CrossRef]

174. Woodall, A.A.; Lee, S.W.-M.; Weesie, R.J.; Jackson, M.J.; Britton, G. Oxidation of carotenoids by free radicals: Relationship between structure and reactivity. *Biochim. Biophys. Acta* **1997**, *1336*, 33–42. [CrossRef]

175. Ben-Dor, A.; Steiner, M.; Gheber, L.; Danilenko, M.; Dubi, N.; Linnewiel, K.; Zick, A.; Sharoni, Y.; Levy, J. Carotenoids activate the antioxidant response element transcription system. *Mol. Cancer Ther.* **2005**, *4*, 177–186. [PubMed]

176. Palozza, P.; Serini, S.; Torsello, A.; Nicuolo, F.D.; Piccioni, E.; Ubaldi, V.; Pioli, C.; Wolf, F.I.; Calviello, G. Nutrient-gene interactions-b-carotene regulates NF-kB DNA-binding activity by a redox mechanism in human leukemia and colon adenocarcinoma cells. *J. Nutr.* **2003**, *133*, 381–388. [CrossRef] [PubMed]

177. MacDonald, P.N.; Bok, D.; Ong, D.E. Localization of cellular retinol-binding protein and retinol-binding protein in cells comprising the blood-brain barrier of rat and human. *Proc. Natl. Acad. Sci. USA* **1990**, *87*, 4265–4269. [CrossRef]

178. Craft, N.; Haitema, T.; Garnett, K.; Fitch, K.; Dorey, C. Carotenoid, tocopherol, and retinol concentrations in elderly human brain. *Exp. Anim.* **2004**, *21*, 22.

179. de Oliveira, B.F.; Veloso, C.A.; Nogueira-Machado, J.A.; de Moraes, E.N.; dos Santos, R.R.; Cintra, M.T.G.; Chaves, M.M. Ascorbic acid, alpha-tocopherol, and beta-carotene reduce oxidative stress and proinflammatory cytokines in mononuclear cells of Alzheimer's disease patients. *Nutr. Neurosci.* **2012**, *15*, 244–251. [CrossRef]

180. Shudo, K.; Fukasawa, H.; Nakagomi, M.; Yamagata, N. Towards retinoid therapy for Alzheimer's disease. *Curr. Alzheimer Res.* **2009**, *6*, 302–311. [CrossRef]

181. Bonhomme, D.; Minni, A.M.; Alfos, S.; Roux, P.; Richard, E.; Higueret, P.; Moisan, M.-P.; Pallet, V.; Touyarot, K. Vitamin A status regulates glucocorticoid availability in Wistar rats: Consequences on cognitive functions and hippocampal neurogenesis? *Front. Behav. Neurosci.* **2014**, *8*, 20. [CrossRef]

182. Zetterström, R.H.; Lindqvist, E.; De Urquiza, A.M.; Tomac, A.; Eriksson, U.; Perlmann, T.; Olson, L. Role of retinoids in the CNS: Differential expression of retinoid binding proteins and receptors and evidence for presence of retinoic acid. *Eur. J. Neurosci.* **1999**, *11*, 407–416. [CrossRef]

183. Sodhi, R.K.; Singh, N. Retinoids as potential targets for Alzheimer's disease. *Pharmacol. Biochem. Behav.* **2014**, *120*, 117–123. [CrossRef]

184. Ahlemeyer, B.; Krieglstein, J. Inhibition of glutathione depletion by retinoic acid and tocopherol protects cultured neurons from staurosporine-induced oxidative stress and apoptosis. *Neurochem. Int.* **2000**, *36*, 1–5. [CrossRef]

185. Ahlemeyer, B.; Bauerbach, E.; Plath, M.; Steuber, M.; Heers, C.; Tegtmeier, F.; Krieglstein, J. Retinoic acid reduces apoptosis and oxidative stress by preservation of SOD protein level. *Free Radic. Biol. Med.* **2001**, *30*, 1067–1077. [CrossRef]

186. McCaffery, P.; Dräger, U.C. High levels of a retinoic acid-generating dehydrogenase in the meso-telencephalic dopamine system. *Proc. Natl. Acad. Sci. USA* **1994**, *91*, 7772–7776. [CrossRef] [PubMed]

187. Lévesque, D.; Rouillard, C. Nur77 and retinoid X receptors: Crucial factors in dopamine-related neuroadaptation. *Trends Neurosci.* **2007**, *30*, 22–30. [CrossRef]

188. Crandall, J.; Sakai, Y.; Zhang, J.; Koul, O.; Mineur, Y.; Crusio, W.E.; McCaffery, P. 13-cis-retinoic acid suppresses hippocampal cell division and hippocampal-dependent learning in mice. *Proc. Natl. Acad. Sci. USA* **2004**, *101*, 5111–5116. [CrossRef]

189. Pan, J.; Yu, J.; Sun, L.; Xie, C.; Chang, L.; Wu, J.; Hawes, S.; Saez–Atienzar, S.; Zheng, W.; Kung, J. ALDH1A1 regulates postsynaptic μ–opioid receptor expression in dorsal striatal projection neurons and mitigates dyskinesia through transsynaptic retinoic acid signaling. *Sci. Rep.* **2019**, *9*, 1–14. [CrossRef]

190. Esteves, M.; Cristóvão, A.C.; Saraiva, T.; Rocha, S.M.; Baltazar, G.; Ferreira, L.; Bernardino, L. Retinoic acid-loaded polymeric nanoparticles induce neuroprotection in a mouse model for Parkinson's disease. *Front. Aging Neurosci.* **2015**, *7*, 20. [CrossRef]

191. Prema, A.; Janakiraman, U.; Manivasagam, T.; Thenmozhi, A.J. Neuroprotective effect of lycopene against MPTP induced experimental Parkinson's disease in mice. *Neurosci. Lett.* **2015**, *599*, 12–19. [CrossRef]

192. Wen, X.; Huang, A.; Hu, J.; Zhong, Z.; Liu, Y.; Li, Z.; Pan, X.; Liu, Z. Neuroprotective effect of astaxanthin against glutamate-induced cytotoxicity in HT22 cells: Involvement of the Akt/GSK-3β pathway. *Neuroscience* **2015**, *303*, 558–568. [CrossRef]
193. Bitarafan, S.; Saboor-Yaraghi, A.; Sahraian, M.-A.; Soltani, D.; Nafissi, S.; Togha, M.; Moghadam, N.B.; Roostaei, T.; Honarvar, N.M.; Harirchian, M.-H. Effect of vitamin A supplementation on fatigue and depression in multiple sclerosis patients: A double-blind placebo-controlled clinical trial. *Iran. J. Allergy Asthma Immunol.* **2016**, *15*, 13–19.
194. Corbett, A.; Pickett, J.; Burns, A.; Corcoran, J.; Dunnett, S.B.; Edison, P.; Hagan, J.J.; Holmes, C.; Jones, E.; Katona, C. Drug repositioning for Alzheimer's disease. *Nat. Rev. Drug Discov.* **2012**, *11*, 833–846. [CrossRef] [PubMed]
195. McGarry, A.; McDermott, M.; Kieburtz, K.; de Blieck, E.A.; Beal, F.; Marder, K.; Ross, C.; Shoulson, I.; Gilbert, P.; Mallonee, W.M. A randomized, double-blind, placebo-controlled trial of coenzyme Q10 in Huntington disease. *Neurology* **2017**, *88*, 152–159. [CrossRef] [PubMed]
196. Kryscio, R.J.; Abner, E.L.; Caban-Holt, A.; Lovell, M.; Goodman, P.; Darke, A.K.; Yee, M.; Crowley, J.; Schmitt, F.A. Association of antioxidant supplement use and dementia in the prevention of Alzheimer's disease by vitamin E and selenium trial (PREADViSE). *JAMA Neurol.* **2017**, *74*, 567–573. [CrossRef] [PubMed]
197. Salari, S.; Khomand, P.; Arasteh, M.; Yousefzamani, B.; Hassanzadeh, K. Zinc sulphate: A reasonable choice for depression management in patients with multiple sclerosis: A randomized, double-blind, placebo-controlled clinical trial. *Pharmacol. Rep.* **2015**, *67*, 606–609. [CrossRef]
198. Endres, K.; Fahrenholz, F.; Lotz, J.; Hiemke, C.; Teipel, S.; Lieb, K.; Tüscher, O.; Fellgiebel, A. Increased CSF APPs-α levels in patients with Alzheimer disease treated with acitretin. *Neurology* **2014**, *83*, 1930–1935. [CrossRef]
199. Thorsen, E.; Haave, H.; Hofsø, D.; Ulvik, R.J. Exposure to hyperoxia in diving and hyperbaric medicine–effects on blood cell counts and serum ferritin. *Undersea Hyperb. Med.* **2001**, *28*, 57–62.
200. Group, P.S. Effects of tocopherol and deprenyl on the progression of disability in early Parkinson's disease. *N. Engl. J. Med.* **1993**, *328*, 176–183.
201. Zhang, D.; Hannink, D.D. Distinct Cysteine residues in keap1 are required for keap1-dependent ubiquitination of Nrf2 and for stabilization of Nrf2 by chemopreventive agents and oxidative stress. *Mol. Cell. Biol.* **2003**, *23*, 8137–8151. [CrossRef]
202. Suzuki, T.; Motohashi, H.; Yamamoto, M. Toward clinical application of the Keap1–Nrf2 pathway. *Trends Pharmacol. Sci.* **2013**, *34*, 340–346. [CrossRef]
203. Strom, J.; Xu, B.; Tian, X.; Chen, Q.M. Nrf2 protects mitochondrial decay by oxidative stress. *FASEB J.* **2016**, *30*, 66–80. [CrossRef]
204. Rojo, A.I.; Pajares, M.; Rada, P.; Nuñez, A.; Nevado-Holgado, A.J.; Killik, R.; Van Leuven, F.; Ribe, E.; Lovestone, S.; Yamamoto, M.; et al. NRF_2 deficiency replicates transcriptomic changes in Alzheimer's patients and worsens APP and TAU pathology. *Redox Biol.* **2017**, *13*, 444–451. [CrossRef] [PubMed]
205. Tanaka, N.; Ikeda, Y.; Ohta, Y.; Deguchi, K.; Tian, F.; Shang, J.; Matsuura, T.; Abe, K. Expression of Keap1–Nrf2 system and antioxidative proteins in mouse brain after transient middle cerebral artery occlusion. *Brain Res.* **2011**, *1370*, 246–253. [CrossRef]
206. Zhao, X.; Sun, G.; Zhang, J.; Strong, R.; Dash, P.K.; Kan, Y.W.; Grotta, J.C.; Aronowski, J. Transcription factor Nrf2 protects the brain from damage produced by intracerebral hemorrhage. *Stroke* **2007**, *38*, 3280–3286. [CrossRef] [PubMed]
207. Burton, N.C.; Kensler, T.W.; Guilarte, T.R. In vivo modulation of the Parkinsonian phenotype by Nrf2. *Neurotoxicology* **2006**, *27*, 1094–1100. [CrossRef] [PubMed]
208. Chen, P.C.; Vargas, M.R.; Pani, A.K.; Smeyne, R.J.; Johnson, D.A.; Kan, Y.W.; Johnson, J.A. Nrf2-mediated neuroprotection in the MPTP mouse model of Parkinson's disease: Critical role for the astrocyte. *Proc. Natl. Acad. Sci. USA* **2009**, *106*, 2933–2938. [CrossRef] [PubMed]
209. Park, J.S.; Leem, Y.H.; Park, J.E.; Kim, D.Y.; Kim, H.S. Neuroprotective effect of β-lapachone in MPTP-induced Parkinson's disease mouse model: Involvement of astroglial p-AMPK/Nrf2/HO-1 signaling pathways. *Biomol. Ther.* **2019**, *27*, 178. [CrossRef] [PubMed]
210. Rhee, S.G. Cell signaling. H2O2, a necessary evil for cell signaling. *Science* **2006**, *312*, 1882–1883. [CrossRef]
211. Schieber, M.; Chandel, N.S. ROS function in redox signaling and oxidative stress. *Curr. Biol.* **2014**, *24*, R453–R462. [CrossRef]

2

Preventive Triple Gene Therapy Reduces the Negative Consequences of Ischemia-Induced Brain Injury after Modelling Stroke in a Rat

Vage Markosyan [1], Zufar Safiullov [1], Andrei Izmailov [1], Filip Fadeev [1], Mikhail Sokolov [1], Maksim Kuznetsov [1], Dmitry Trofimov [1], Evgeny Kim [1], Grayr Kundakchyan [2], Airat Gibadullin [1], Ilnur Salafutdinov [2], Leniz Nurullin [3], Farid Bashirov [1] and Rustem Islamov [1,*]

1 Department of Medical Biology and Genetics, Kazan State Medical University, 420012 Kazan, Russia; vage.markosyan@gmail.com (V.M.); redblackwhite@mail.ru (Z.S.); gostev.andrei@gmail.com (A.I.); philip.fadeyev@gmail.com (F.F.); supermihon@yandex.ru (M.S.); qmaxksmu@yandex.ru (M.K.); t.dima19961996@gmail.com (D.T.); profzh@yandex.ru (E.K.); halsoulo@gmail.com (A.G.); faridbashirov@yandex.ru (F.B.)

2 Institute of Fundamental Medicine and Biology, Kazan [Volga Region] Federal University, 420008 Kazan, Russia; grayr23@gmail.com (G.K.); sal.ilnur@gmail.com (I.S.)

3 Kazan Institute of Biochemistry and Biophysics, Federal Research Center of Kazan Scientific Center of Russian Academy of Sciences, 119991 Kazan, Russia; leniz2001@mail.ru

* Correspondence: rustem.islamov@gmail.com

Abstract: Currently, the main fundamental and clinical interest for stroke therapy is focused on developing a neuroprotective treatment of a penumbra region within the therapeutic window. The development of treatments for ischemic stroke in at-risk patients is of particular interest. Preventive gene therapy may significantly reduce the negative consequences of ischemia-induced brain injury. In the present study, we suggest the approach of preventive gene therapy for stroke. Adenoviral vectors carrying genes encoding vascular endothelial growth factor (VEGF), glial cell-derived neurotrophic factor (GDNF) and neural cell adhesion molecule (NCAM) or gene engineered umbilical cord blood mononuclear cells (UCB-MC) overexpressing recombinant VEGF, GDNF, and NCAM were intrathecally injected before distal occlusion of the middle cerebral artery in rats. Post-ischemic brain recovery was investigated 21 days after stroke modelling. Morphometric and immunofluorescent analysis revealed a reduction of infarction volume accompanied with a lower number of apoptotic cells and decreased expression of Hsp70 in the peri-infarct region in gene-treated animals. The lower immunopositive areas for astrocytes and microglial cells markers, higher number of oligodendrocytes and increased expression of synaptic proteins suggest the inhibition of astrogliosis, supporting the corresponding myelination and functional recovery of neurons in animals receiving preventive gene therapy. In this study, for the first time, we provide evidence of the beneficial effects of preventive triple gene therapy by an adenoviral- or UCB-MC-mediated intrathecal simultaneous delivery combination of *vegf165*, *gdnf*, and *ncam1* on the preservation and recovery of the brain in rats with subsequent modelling of stroke.

Keywords: stroke; preventive gene therapy; adenoviral vector; VEGF; GDNF; NCAM; human umbilical cord blood mononuclear cells

---

1. Introduction

The current options for ischemic stroke treatment are extremely limited and are aimed at restoring blood flow in the ischemic area by intravenous infusion of recombinant tissue plasminogen activator and/or physical removal of the clots [1]. To date, the main fundamental and clinical interest is focused on developing a neuroprotective treatment of the penumbra region within the therapeutic window. The strategy of cell-, gene-, and gene-cell therapy for neuroprotection in stroke treatment has been proven by numerous experiments in animal models [2–4]. Besides brain-specific cell types, umbilical cord blood (UCB) is widely used for neuroprotection in the central nervous system (CNS) for different pathological conditions [5]. UCB cells are considered a valuable source of stem cells, growth and neurotrophic factors for cell therapy. The mononuclear fraction of UCB contains populations of different immature cells that are capable of differentiating into many cell types [6] and, thus, represent an alternative to embryonic stem cells for transplantation to patients with post-ischemic, post-traumatic and degenerative diseases [7,8]. To date, the following have been discovered in UCB: Hematopoietic stem cells (HSCs), endothelial progenitor cells, mesenchymal stem cells (MSCs), unrestricted somatic stem cells (USSCs), and side population cells (SP) [9–12].

Due to the immaturity of the immune system of a new-born, the use of UCB cells for cell therapy does not require matching of genes relating to HLA (Human Leucocyte Antigens) human tissue compatibility, as evidenced by the absence of an acute or chronic form of the disease "graft-versus-host" (graft versus host disease) [13,14]. In addition, with UCB cell transplantation, tumor transformation of cells in the recipient's body is practically prevented [15].

Another attractive reason for using UCB cells for cell therapy is their ability to produce various biologically active molecules, such as proteins which are antioxidant, angiogenic, neurotrophic, and growth factors [16–20]. Thus, transplantation of UCB cells can be aimed at replacing dead cells and at preventing the further death of surviving cells due to secreted biologically active molecules. Enhancement of the positive effects of UCB cells on tissue regeneration after their genetic modification is a relatively new and promising gene-cell approach in cell therapy to stimulate post-traumatic or post-ischemic brain injury [21,22]. Gene-modified UCB cells may provide addressed delivery of therapeutic genes and supply the expression of the recombinant molecules at the site of regeneration.

In our previous studies, we showed the positive effect of gene-modified umbilical cord blood mononuclear cells (UCB-MC), simultaneously producing three recombinant molecules—vascular endothelial growth factor (VEGF), glial cell-derived neurotrophic factor (GDNF) and neural cell adhesion molecule (NCAM)—in animal models of amyotrophic lateral sclerosis [23], spinal cord injury [24], and stroke [25]. The rationale of using a combination of two neurotrophic factors with cell adhesion molecules is based on the well-known neuroprotective effects of VEGF and GDNF [26,27], with the expression of NCAM increasing the homing and survivability of UCB-MC at the brain injury site [28] supporting local production of the therapeutic molecules. In the model of middle cerebral artery occlusion (MCAO) in rats, we demonstrated that intrathecal injection of genetically-engineered UCB-MC over-expressing VEGF, GDNF, and NCAM, four hours after MCAO results in a reduction of infarct volume, the positive reaction of neuroglial cells and an increase in synaptic protein expression. Thus, ex vivo gene modification may enhance the naïve neuroprotective properties of UCB-MC.

The development of treatment under the threat of stroke is of particular interest. Preventive therapy may highly reduce the consequences of a stroke-induced brain injury. In the present study, we suggest the approach of preventive cell-mediated gene therapy for stroke. The efficacy of gene-engineered UCB-MC overexpressing recombinant molecules-stimulants of neuroregeneration VEGF, GDNF, and NCAM, administered intrathecally 3 days before MCAO in rats, was investigated using morphometric and immunofluorescent methods.

2. Results

2.1. Molecular Analysis of Gene-Modified UCBC

The efficiency of UCB-MC transduction by Ad5-GFP adenoviral vector was confirmed after 72 h of UCB-MC+Ad5-GFP cultivation using fluorescent microscopy. In the cytoplasm of UCB-MC+Ad5-GFP, a specific green glow was detected (Figure 1A). By the flow cytometry method, it was established that the percentage of GFP-positive human UCB-MC at multiplicity of infection (MOI) equal to 10 reaches 29.5% (Figure 1B).

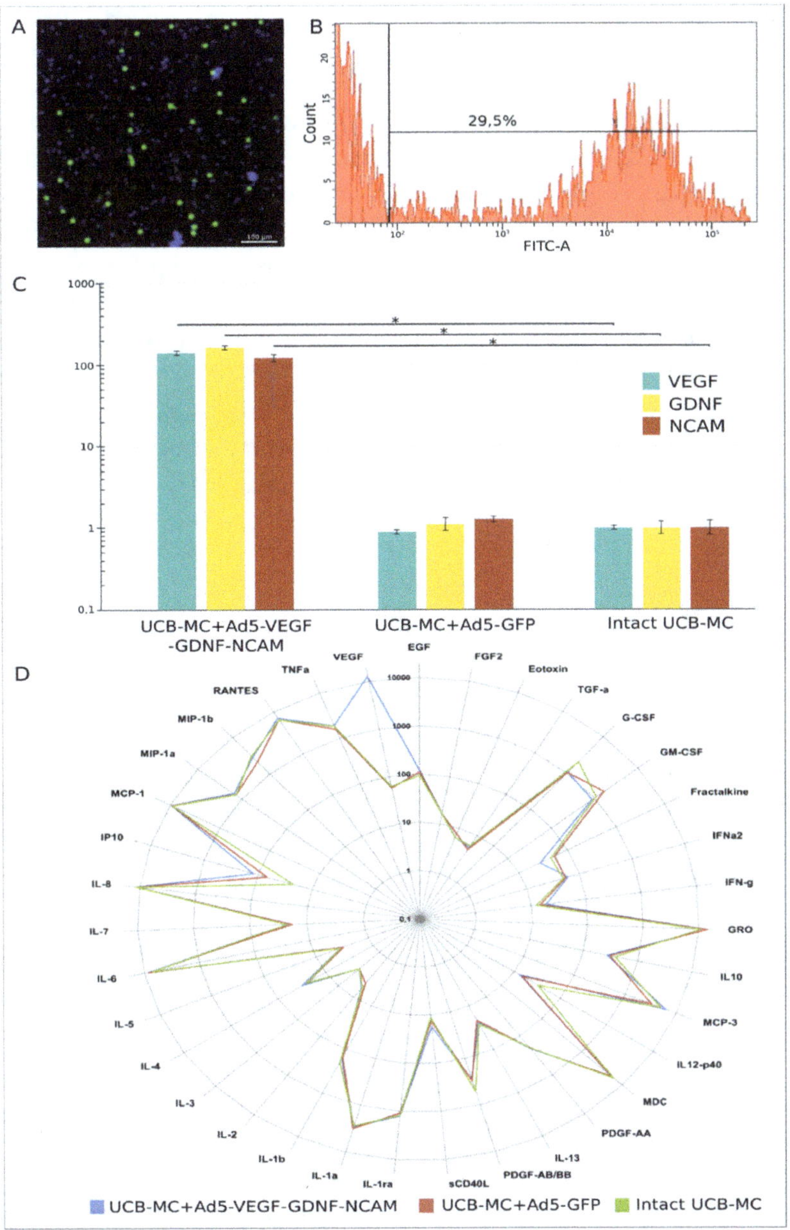

Figure 1. Molecular analysis of gene modified umbilical cord blood mononuclear cells (UCB-MC). (**A**,**B**)—Production of green fluorescent protein (GFP) in UCB-MC, 72 h after transduction with Ad5-GFP (MOI = 10). (**A**)—fluorescent microscopy shows a specific green glow in UCB-MC+Ad5-GFP. Cell nuclei are stained with Hoechst 33342 (blue glow). Scale bar = 200 μm. (**B**)—flow cytometry analysis demonstrates that 29.5% of UCB-MC effectively produce reporter GFP. (**C**)—Quantitative analysis of mRNA *vegf165*, *gdnf*, and *ncam1* levels in intact (naïve) UCB-MC and genetically-modified UCB-MC, 72 h after transduction with three adenoviral vectors simultaneously carrying the therapeutic genes (Ad5-VEGF, Ad5-GDNF, and Ad5-NCAM) or with Ad5-GFP (UCBC + Ad5-GFP), with a MOI = 10. Data from two independent experiments are represented as an average value of ± SE, *—$p < 0.05$. (**D**)—Radial comparative diagram of cytokine, chemokines and growth factors in supernatant obtained 72 h after incubation of gene modified UCB-MC (UCB-MC+Ad5- vascular endothelial growth factor (VEGF)- glial cell-derived neurotrophic factor (GDNF)- neural cell adhesion molecule (NCAM) and UCB-MC+Ad5-GFP) and intact UCB-MC.

Evaluation of mRNA levels of transgenes (*vegf165*, *gdnf*, and *ncam1*) in genetically-modified UCB-MC was performed by RT-PCR, 72 h after incubation of UCB-MC+Ad5-VEGF-GDNF-NCAM. The molecular analysis revealed that the content of mRNA *vegf165* increased 141.8 ± 8.24 times, *gdnf* mRNA 167.51 ± 6.85 times and *ncam1* mRNA 122.9 ± 13.5 times compared with intact (naïve) UCB-MC (Figure 1C).

Multiplex analysis of cytokines, chemokines and growth factors in supernatants harvested after the cultivation of naïve UCB-MC identified a wide range of pro- and anti-inflammatory cytokines, chemokines and growth factors (Figure 1D). However, the concentrations of Flt-3L, IL12-p70, IL-15, IL-17a, IL-9, and TNFb were lower than the detection level. Genetic modification of human UCB-MC by recombinant adenovirus Ad5-GFP does not affect the secretory profile of modified cells in relation to the investigated factors when compared to the naïve cells. UCB-MC simultaneously transduced with Ad5-VEGF, Ad5-GDNF, and Ad5-NCAM also preserves the qualitative and quantitative profile of expression of the investigated factors. However, as expected, in comparison with the naïve and UCB-MC+Ad5-GFP, we observed a 200-fold increase of VEGF level. The presented results correlate with PCR-RT data above and confirm the efficiency of UCB-MC transduction and its ability to synthesize and secrete recombinant molecules, as with the example of VEGF. In addition, the results support that adenoviral vector does not affect the production of the studied biologically active molecules by human UCB-MC.

2.2. *Morphometric Analysis of Infarct Area*

Three weeks after ischemic stroke modelling, cerebral infarction volume analysis revealed an infarct zone located in the parietal lobe (parietal cortex, area 1 (Par1), which corresponds to the site of MCAO (Figure 2A,B). Morphometric analysis of the brain cortex infarct cavities volume showed the differences between therapeutic and control groups (Figure 2C,D). The infarct cavities volume was significantly less in the Ad5-VEGF-GDNF-NCAM (0.177 [0.155; 0.197]) and UCB-MC+Ad5-VEGF-GDNF-NCAM (0.070 [0.014; 0.245]) groups when compared with the control saline (0.607 [0.568; 0.759]) and Ad5-GFP (0.817 [0.754; 0.865]) groups ($p < 0.05$). In the UCB-MC+Ad5-GFP (0.249 [0.119; 0.305]) group, the infarction volume did not differ from the gene-treated groups and was lower when compared with the saline group ($p < 0.05$) (Figure 2E).

2.3. *Immunofluorescent Study of Brain*

Comparative analysis of the molecular and cellular changes in the peri-infarct zone (Figure 2C) of experimental rats' brains revealed different patterns in the expression of cellular stress, apoptosis, and synaptic proteins and in the reorganization of neuroglial cells in relation to data obtained from intact animals.

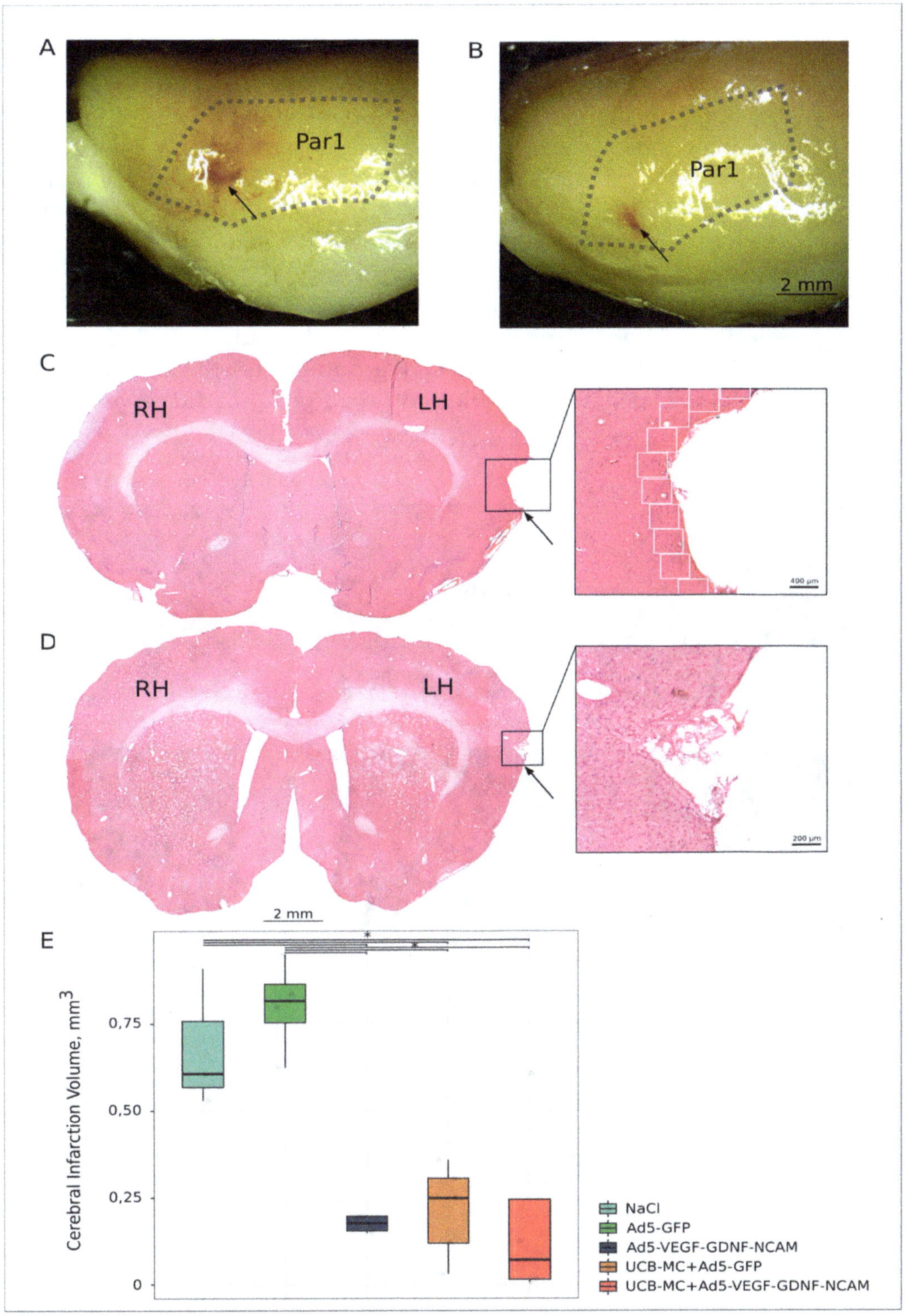

Figure 2. Ischemic stroke in rats 3 weeks after the distal middle cerebral artery occlusion. (**A**,**C**)—The brain from the control (NaCl) group. (**B**,**D**)—The brain from the therapeutic (UCB-MC+Ad5-VEGF-GDNF-NCAM) group. In (**A**) and (**B**) the stroke area in the parietal lobe of the brain is shown with the arrow. Par1—cortex parietals, area 1 is marked by a dotted line. In (**C**) and (**D**)—frontal sections of the brain in the stroke area stained with hematoxylin and eosin. RH—right hemisphere; LH—left hemisphere. Inserts with arrows show the stroke area with the maximum depth and the maximum radius of the infarct cavities at higher magnification. White boxes in the insert in (**C**) panel indicate areas with S = 0.05 mm^2 in the peri-infarct zone used for immunofluorescent analysis. (**E**)—comparative morphometric analysis of the infarct cavities volume in experimental groups; *—$p < 0.05$.

2.3.1. Cellular Stress and Apoptosis Proteins

The expression of heat shock protein 70 kDa (Hsp70) in neural and glial brain cells has constitutional and inductive options. Thus, Hsp70 expression is significantly upregulated in ischemic conditions [29]. In this study, analysis of the intensity of immunofluorescent brain cortex staining with antibodies against Hsp70 revealed a different response of brain cells in the area of ischemic damage in experimental animals when compared with intact animals (Figure 3A,G). The Hsp70 expression level in control (NaCl) (Figure 3B,G) and Ad5-GFP (Figure 3C,G) groups was 27.375 [24.940; 28.649] and 34.361 [31.315; 35.612], respectively, and was significantly higher than that of intact animals (18.422 [17.786; 19.510]). In the therapeutic groups with preventive gene therapy with Ad5-VEGF-GDNF-NCAM (20.419 [18.510; 22.950]) (Figure 3E,G) and UCB-MC+Ad5-VEGF-GDNF-NCAM (18.169 [17.462; 18.964]) (Figure 3F,G), Hsp70 immunoexpression was lower compared to the control groups ($p < 0.05$) and did not differ from intact group ($p < 0.05$). In the UCB-MC+Ad5-GFP group (Figure 3D,G), the expression level of Hsp70 (17.651 [17.648; 20.832]) was lower than the control groups and did not differ from the intact and therapeutic groups.

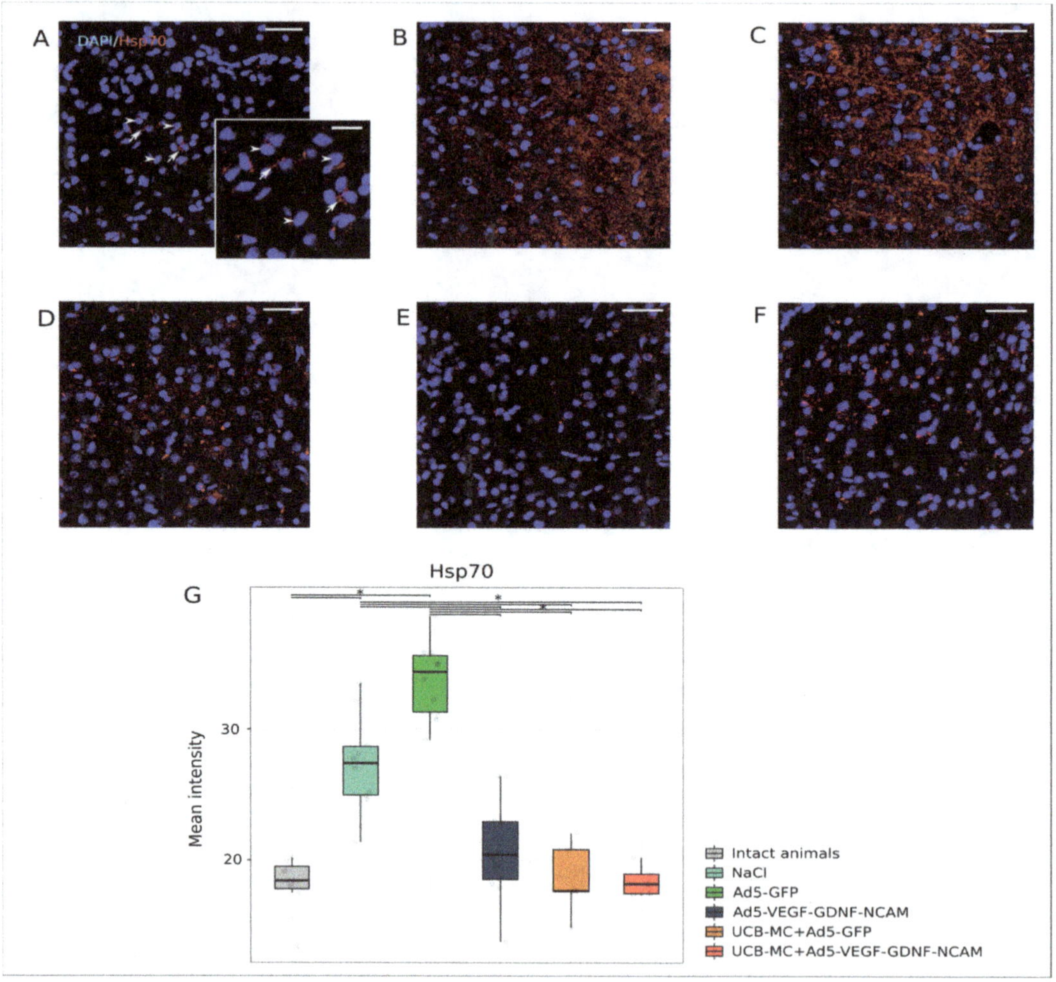

Figure 3. Immunoexpression of Hsp70 in the rat brain cortex, 21 days after the middle cerebral artery occlusion. Immunofluorescent staining with antibody to heat shock protein 70 kDa in intact (**A**), control NaCl (**B**) and Ad5-GFP (**C**), and therapeutic UCB-MC+Ad5-GFP (**D**), Ad5-VEGF-GDNF-NCAM (**E**) and UCB-MC+Ad5-VEGF-GDNF-NCAM (**F**) groups. Arrows indicate cytoplasmic localization of Hsp70 (red glow) in brain cells. Arrowheads point to cell nuclei visualized using DAPI (blue glow). Scale bar in (**A–F**) = 50 μm; scale bar in the insert = 20 μm. (**G**)—comparative analysis of fluorescence intensity level of Hsp70 in experimental groups; *—$p < 0.05$.

Activation of Caspase3 enzyme characterizes the irreversible phase of nuclear DNA degradation and subsequent cell death. In the present study, the activity of the pro-apoptotic protein Caspase3 was studied in the ischemic brain cortex in experimental rats (Figure 4A–F). It was found that the therapeutic groups Ad5-VEGF-GDNF-NCAM (12.00 [9.00; 13.00]) (Figure 4D,F) and UCB-MC+Ad5-VEGF-GDNF-NCAM (9.00 [7.50; 9.00]) (Figure 4E,F) had significantly less Caspase3-positive cells than the control NaCl (25.00 [22.00; 27.00]) group (Figure 4A,F). The number of apoptotic cells in the UCB-MC+Ad5-VEGF-GDNF-NCAM group was also lower than the Ad5-GFP control group (15.50 [11.75; 19.00]) (Figure 4B,F) ($p < 0.05$). In the UCBC+Ad5-GFP group (6.00 [3.25; 9.75]) (Figure 4C,F), the content of Caspase3-positive cells was lower than in the control groups ($p < 0.05$) and did not differ from other therapeutic groups.

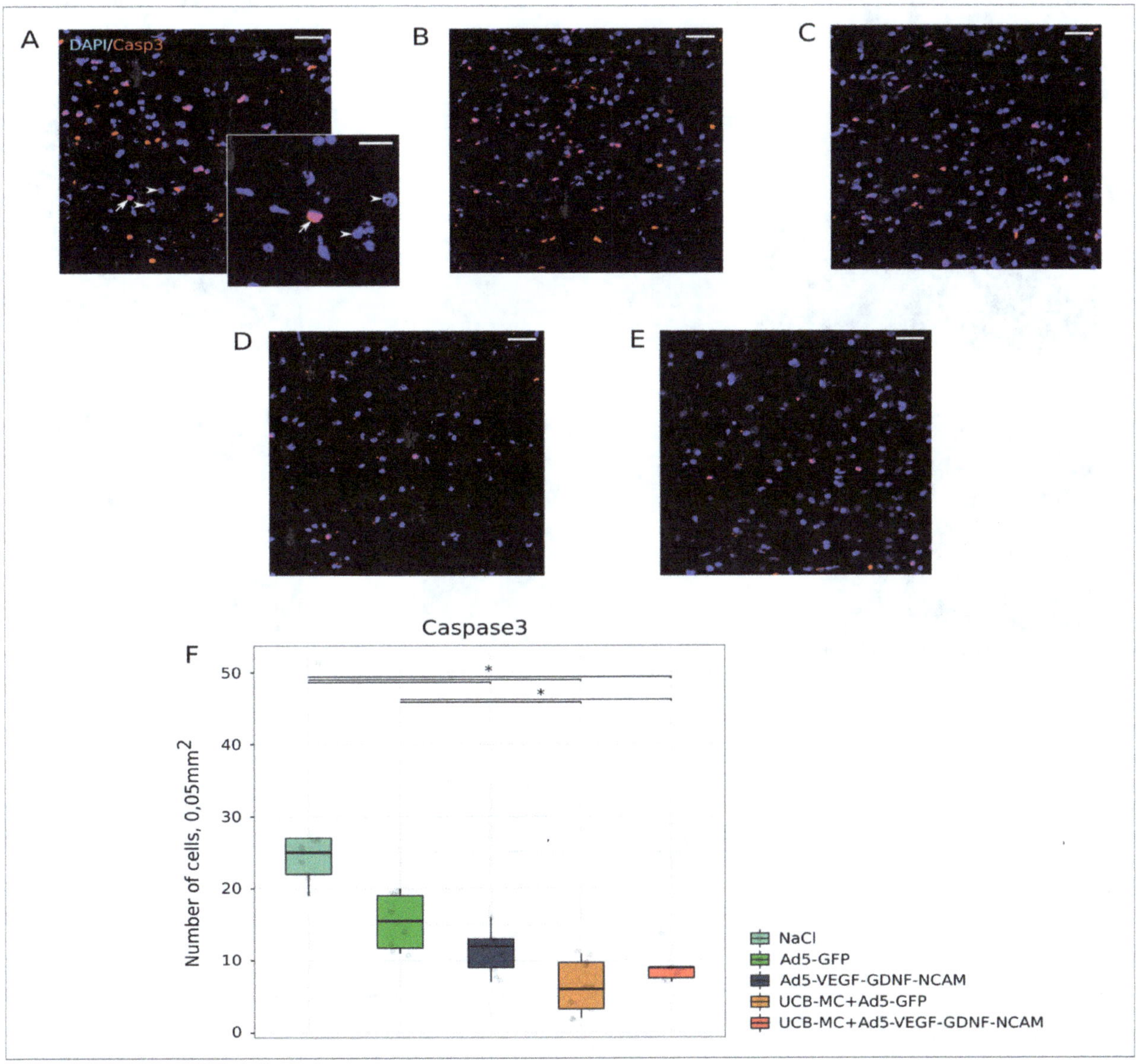

Figure 4. Count of Caspase3-positive cells in the rat brain cortex, 21 days after the middle cerebral artery occlusion. Immunofluorescent staining with antibody to Caspase3 in control NaCl (**A**) and Ad5-GFP (**B**), and therapeutic UCB-MC+Ad5-GFP (**C**), Ad5-VEGF-GDNF-NCAM (**D**) and UCB-MC+Ad5-VEGF-GDNF-NCAM (**E**) groups. Arrow indicates nuclear localization of Caspase3 (red glow) in brain cells. Arrowheads point to cell nuclei visualized using DAPI (blue glow). Scale bar in (**A–E**) = 50 μm; scale bar in the insert = 20 μm. (**F**)—comparative analysis of Caspase3-positive cells number in experimental groups; *—$p < 0.05$.

2.3.2. Neuroglia Cells

Analysis of GFAP-positive cells (astrocytes), Olig2-positive cells (oligodendrocytes), and Iba1-positive cells (microglia) revealed different reactions of neuroglia cells in the ischemic area of the brain in experimental animals.

Microglial cells are the dominant cell type involved in post-stroke neuroinflammation and the organization of the glial scar. In the intact group, the immunopositive area for microglia cells detected with Iba1 marker was lower (5.42 [4.96; 5.98]) (Figure 5A,G) than in the control NaCl (12.57 [10.31; 16.82]) (Figure 5B,G) and Ad5-GFP (14.43 [12.93; 16.01]) (Figure 5C,G) groups and in the therapeutic UCB-MC+Ad5-GFP (10.07 [7.67; 10.52]]) group (Figure 5D,G) ($p < 0.05$). The Iba1-positive area in the therapeutic Ad5-VEGF-GDNF-NCAM (5.60 [4.89; 6.69]) (Figure 5E,G) and UCBC+Ad5-VEGF-GDNF-NCAM (8.80 [6.37; 9.99]) (Figure 5F,G) groups was lower when compared with the control groups and did not differ from the intact group ($p < 0.05$).

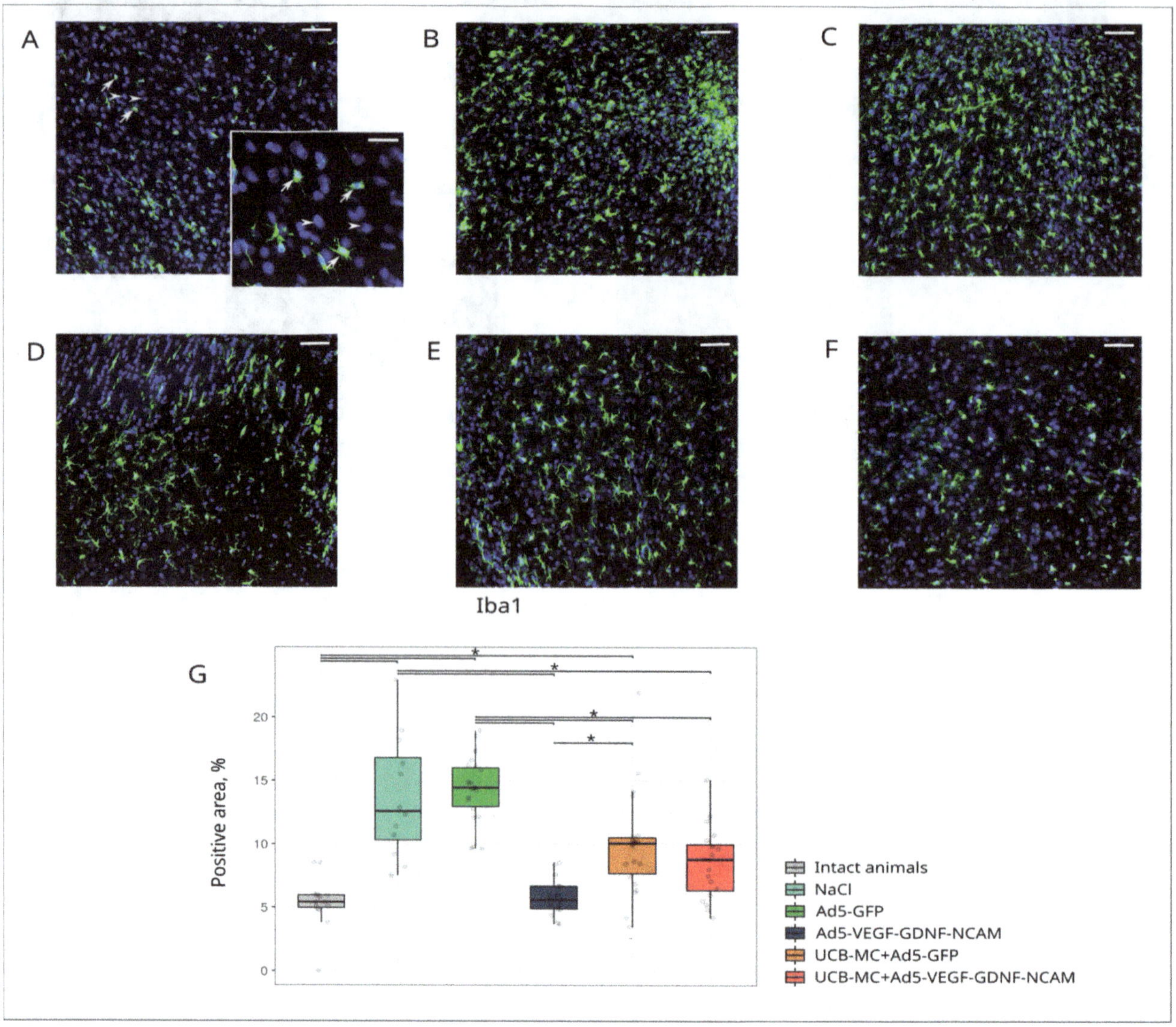

Figure 5. Immunoexpression of Iba1 in the rat brain cortex, 21 days after the middle cerebral artery occlusion. Immunofluorescent staining with antibody to microglia specific calcium-binding protein Iba1 in intact (**A**), control NaCl (**B**) and Ad5-GFP (**C**), and therapeutic UCB-MC+Ad5-GFP (**D**), Ad5-VEGF-GDNF-NCAM (**E**), and UCB-MC+Ad5-VEGF-GDNF-NCAM (**F**) groups. Arrows indicate cytoplasmic localization of Iba1 (green glow) in microglial cells. Arrowheads point to cell nuclei visualized using DAPI (blue glow). Scale bar in (**A**–**F**) = 50 μm; scale bar in the insert = 20 μm. (**G**)—comparative analysis of Iba1-positive areas in experimental groups; *—$p < 0.05$.

Astrocytes in the post-ischemic brain, in association with microglial cells, are involved in the formation of the glial scar, with physical and chemical properties inhibitory for brain recovery. Decreased astrogliosis often correlates with reduced volume of ischemic infarct [30]. The GFAP-positive areas in the brains of the intact group was lower (4.12 [3.36; 4.85]) (Figure 6A,G) than in the control NaCl (9.34 [8.08; 10.15]) (Figure 6B,G) and Ad5-GFP (8.92 [6.25; 12.42]]) (Figure 6C,G) groups ($p < 0.05$). In the therapeutic groups Ad5-VEGF-GDNF-NCAM (4.22 [3.36; 5.19]) (Figure 5E,G) and UCBC+Ad5-VEGF-GDNF-NCAM (3.43 [2.81; 4.19]) (Figure 5F,G), the GFAP-positive areas were lower than in the control (NaCl and Ad5-GFP) groups and did not differ from intact group ($p < 0.05$). In the UCBC+Ad5-GFP (Figure 5D,G) group, the GFAP-positive area did not differ in comparison with all experimental groups ($p < 0.05$).

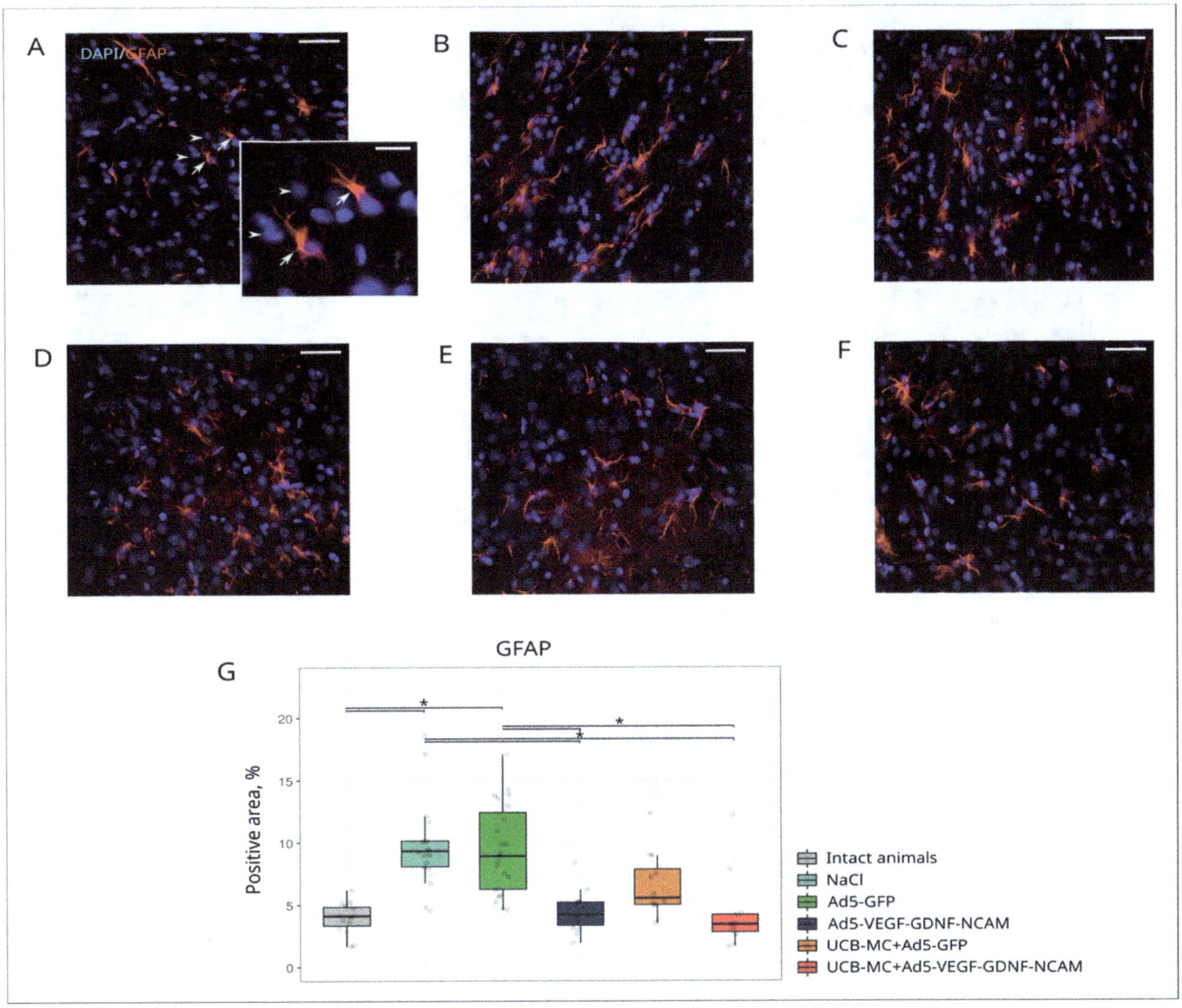

Figure 6. Immunoexpression of GFAP in the rat brain cortex, 21 days after the middle cerebral artery occlusion. Immunofluorescent staining with antibody to astrocyte specific cytoskeletal glial fibrillary acidic protein GFAP in intact (**A**), control NaCl (**B**) and Ad5-GFP (**C**), and therapeutic UCB-MC+Ad5-GFP (**D**), Ad5-VEGF-GDNF-NCAM (**E**) and UCB-MC+Ad5-VEGF-GDNF-NCAM (**F**) groups. Arrows indicate cytoplasmic localization of GFAP (red glow) in astrocytes. Arrowheads point to cell nuclei visualized using DAPI (blue glow). Scale bar in (**A**–**F**) = 50 μm; scale bar in the insert = 20 μm. (**G**)—comparative analysis of GFAP-positive areas in experimental groups; *—$p < 0.05$.

Postischemic brain damage is accompanied by the destruction of oligodendrocytes and the subsequent demyelination of neural processes [31]. The number of Olig2-positive cells was significantly reduced in the control NaCl (10.00 [9.00; 11.00]) (Figure 7B,G) and Ad5-GFP (10.00 [9.00; 11.00]) (Figure 7C,G) groups and in the UCBC+Ad5-GFP group (9.00 [9.00; 11.00]) (Figure 7D,G) relative to the intact group (14 [13; 19]) (Figure 7A,G) ($p < 0.05$). The number of Olig2-positive cells in the intact group did not differ from the therapeutic Ad5-VEGF-GDNF-NCAM (12.00 [9.00; 18.00]) (Figure 7E,G) and UCBC+Ad5-VEGF-GDNF-NCAM (14.00 [12.00; 16.00]) (Figure 7F,G) groups. It is important to note that there were more oligodendrocytes in the UCBC+Ad5-VEGF-GDNF-NCAM group than in the control groups and in the UCBC+Ad5-GFP group ($p < 0.05$), but the number did not differ from the Ad5-VEGF-GDNF-NCAM group.

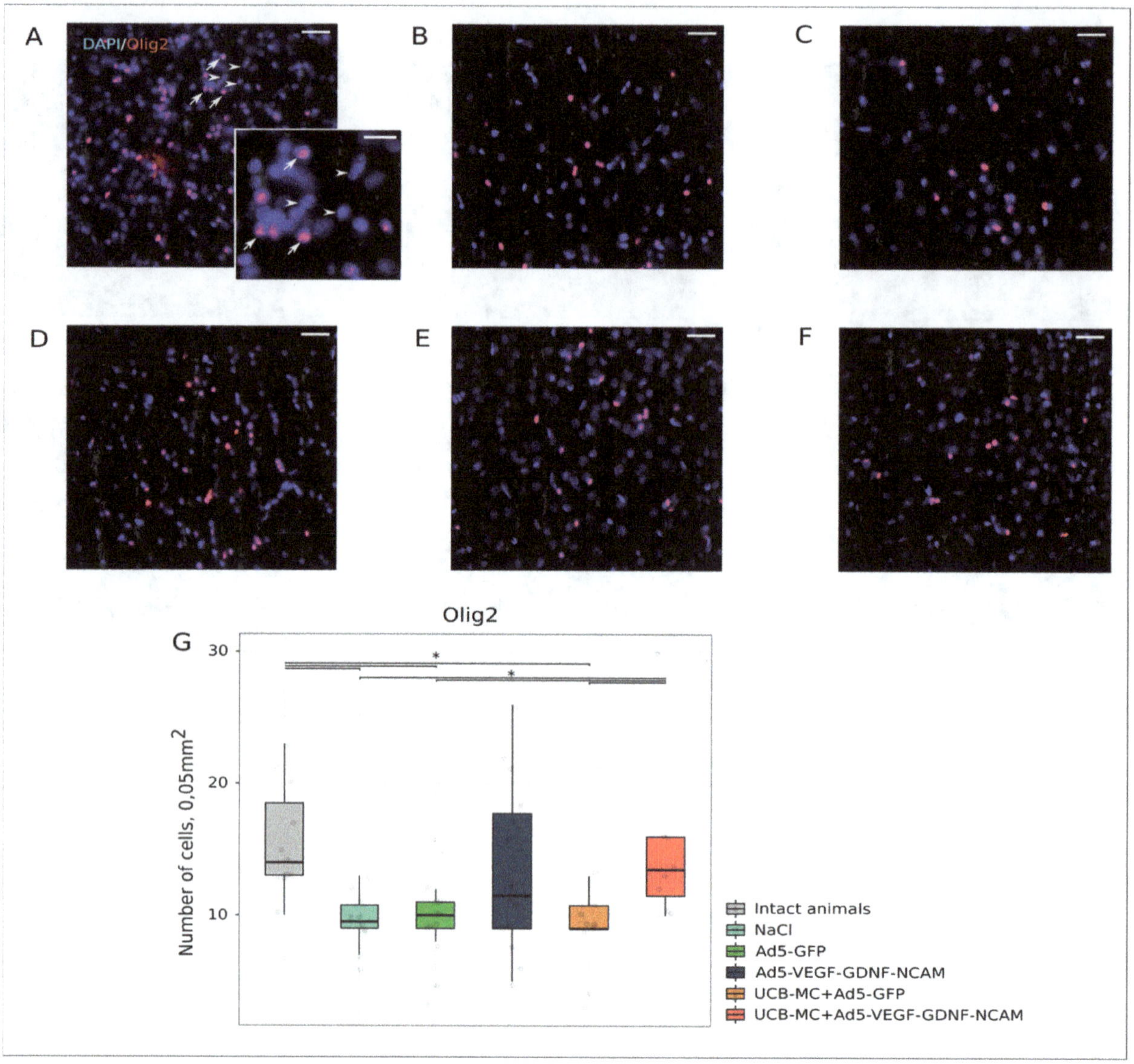

Figure 7. Count of Olig2-positive oligodendrocytes in the rat brain cortex, 21 days after the middle cerebral artery occlusion. Immunofluorescent staining with antibody to oligodendrocyte transcription factor Olig2 (red glow) in intact (**A**), control NaCl (**B**), and Ad5-GFP (**C**), and therapeutic UCB-MC+Ad5-GFP (**D**), Ad5-VEGF-GDNF-NCAM (**E**), and UCB-MC+Ad5-VEGF-GDNF-NCAM (**F**) groups. Arrows indicate nuclear localization of Olig2 (red glow) in oligodendrocytes. Arrowheads point to cell nuclei visualized using DAPI (blue glow). Scale bar in (**A**–**F**) = 50 µm; scale bar in the insert = 20 µm. (**G**)—comparative analysis of Olig2-positive cells number in experimental groups; *—$p < 0.05$.

2.3.3. Synaptic Proteins

Synaptothysin is associated with synaptic vesicles involved in nerve impulse transmission, and its content in the presynaptic area reflects the functional activity of neurons. The synaptophysin level of fluorescence was reduced in the control NaCl (55.00 [53.00; 61.00]) (Figure 8B,G) and Ad5-GFP (56.00 [48.00; 59.00]) (Figure 8C,G) groups when compared with the intact group (78.00 [61.00; 87.00]) (Figure 8A,G) ($p < 0.05$). Immunoexpression of synaptophysin in the therapeutic Ad5-VEGF-GDNF-NCAM (64.00 [61.00; 72.00]) (Figure 8E,G), UCBC+Ad5-VEGF-GDNF-NCAM (62.00 [61.00; 65.00]) (Figure 8F,G) and UCBC+Ad5-GFP groups (79.00 [76.00; 81.00]) (Figure 8D,G) was higher than in the control groups and did not differ from the intact group ($p < 0.05$).

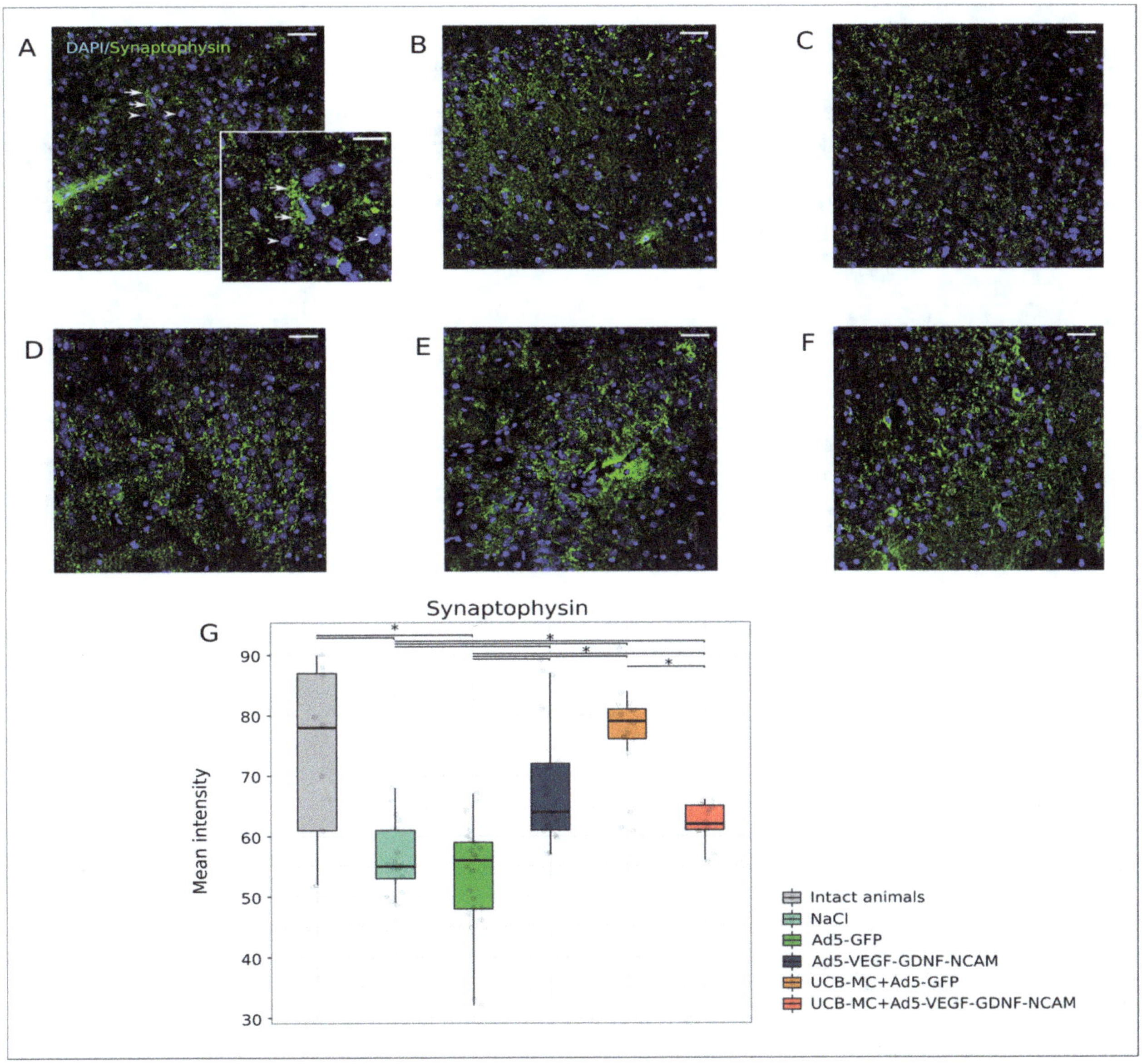

Figure 8. Immunoexpression of Synaptophysin in the rat brain cortex, 21 days after the middle cerebral artery occlusion. Immunofluorescent staining with antibody to synaptic vesicle membrane protein Synaptophysin in intact (**A**), control NaCl (**B**) and Ad5-GFP (**C**), and therapeutic UCB-MC+Ad5-GFP (**D**), Ad5-VEGF-GDNF-NCAM (**E**) and UCB-MC+Ad5-VEGF-GDNF-NCAM (**F**) groups. Arrows indicate Synaptophysin (green glow) in neurons. Arrowheads point to cell nuclei visualized using DAPI (blue glow). Scale bar in (**A**—**F**) = 50 μm; scale bar in the insert = 20 μm. (**G**)—comparative analysis of fluorescence intensity level of Synaptophysin in experimental groups; *—$p < 0.05$.

Postsynaptic density protein 95 kDa (PSD95) is associated with the functional activity of the postsynaptic membrane, providing its stability and plasticity in interactions with neurotransmitters. As for the intact group, the immune expression of PSD95 (65.0 [62.00; 69.00]) (Figure 9A,G) was reduced in all experimental groups except for the group UCBC+Ad5-VEGF-GDNF-NCAM (55.00 [50.00; 57.00]) ($p < 0.05$) (Figure 9F,G). However, the level of PSD95 fluorescence was significantly higher in the therapeutic Ad5-VEGF-GDNF-NCAM (62.50 [57.75; 67.00]) (Figure 9E,G), UCBC+Ad5-VEGF-GDNF-NCAM and UCBC+Ad5-GFP (50.00 [48.50; 57.50]) (Figure 9D,G) groups, in comparison with the control group NaCl (43.00 [38.50; 46.00]) (Figure 9B,G), which did not differ from the Ad5-GFP group (49.00 [46.00; 51.00]) (Figure 9C,G) ($p < 0.05$).

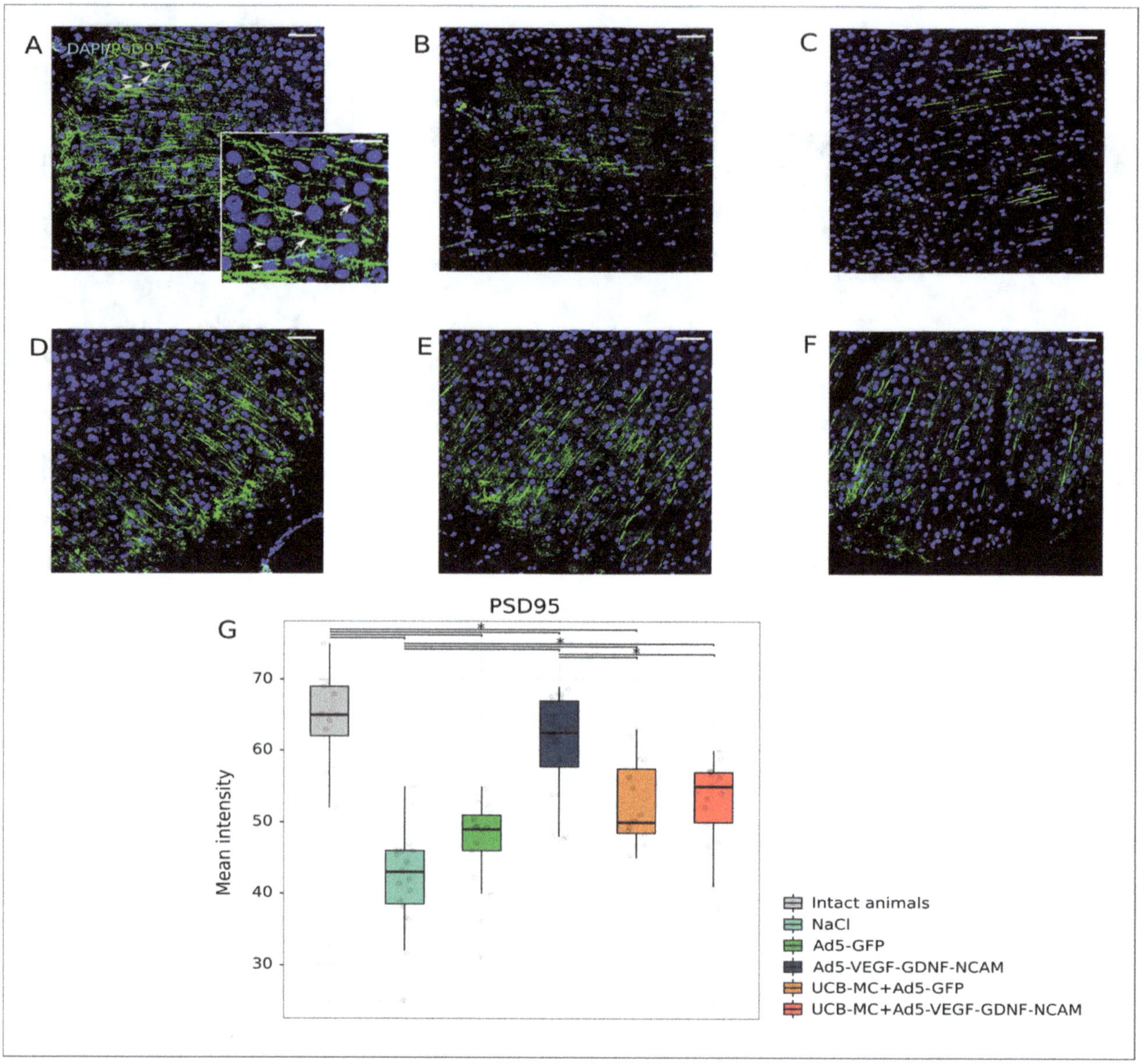

Figure 9. Immunoexpression of PSD95 in the rat brain cortex 21 days after the middle cerebral artery occlusion. Immunofluorescent staining with antibody to postsynaptic membrane protein PSD95 in intact (**A**), control NaCl (**B**) and Ad5-GFP (**C**), and therapeutic UCB-MC+Ad5-GFP (**D**), Ad5-VEGF-GDNF-NCAM (**E**) and UCB-MC+Ad5-VEGF-GDNF-NCAM (**F**) groups. Arrows indicate PSD95 (green glow) in neurons. Arrowheads point to cell nuclei visualized using DAPI (blue glow). Scale bar in (**A**–**F**) = 50 μm; scale bar in the insert = 20 μm. (**G**)—Comparative analysis of fluorescence intensity level of PSD95 in experimental groups; *—$p < 0.05$.

2.4. Expression of Recombinant Molecules in the Rat Brain after Intrathecal Adenoviral-Mediated Delivery of Transgenes

The expression of the reporter *gfp* and therapeutic *vegf165, gdnf* and *ncam1* genes was studied in the stroke area of rat brains, 25 days after an intrathecal injection of Ad5-GFP or Ad5-VEGF-GDNF-NCAM. Green fluorescent protein was detected in brain cells by laser microscopy (Figure 10A). Immunofluorescent analysis using specific antibodies to VEGF, GDNF, and NCAM also revealed target molecules in the brain cells (Figure 10B–D). In the peri-infarct zone, we observed an approximately equal distribution of the cells producing reporter GFP or recombinant VEGF, GDNF, and NCAM molecules.

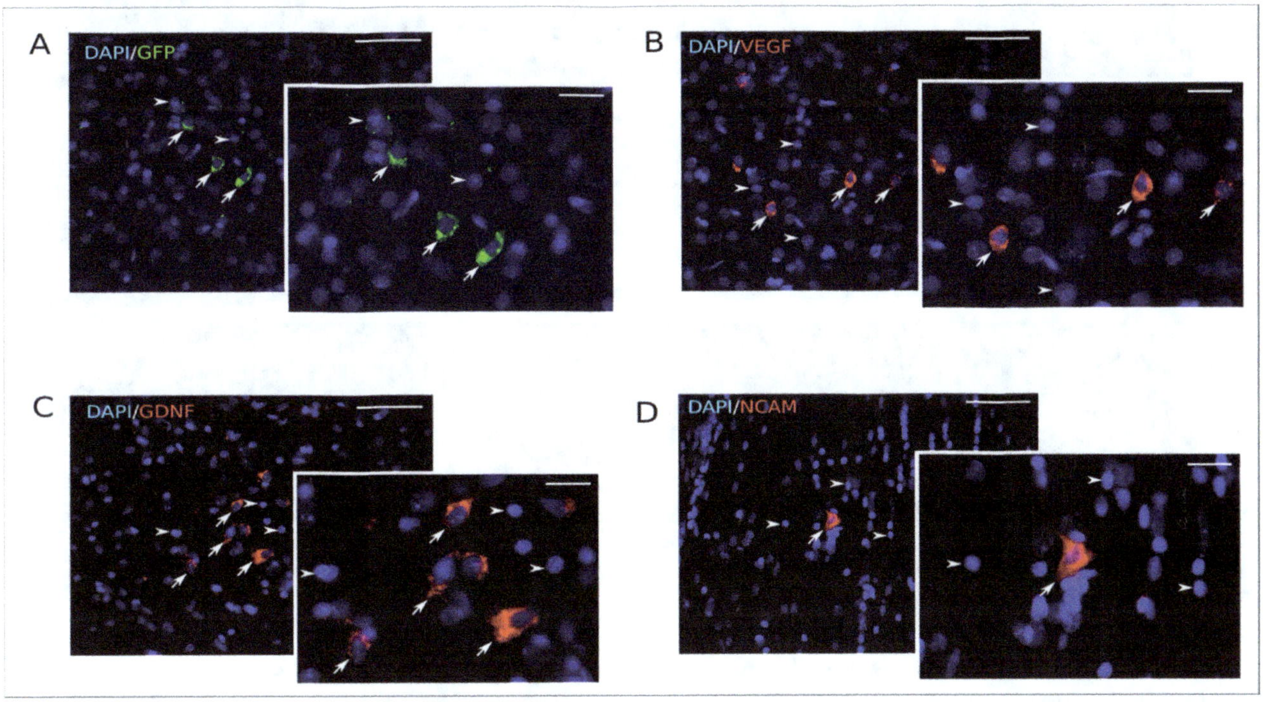

Figure 10. Expression of recombinant molecules in rat brain on 25th day after intrathecal injection of Ad5-GFP and Ad5-VEGF-GDNF-NCAM. (**A**)—Specific green glow of GFP in the transduced brain cells. (**B**)—Immune reaction with antibody to vascular endothelial growth factor (VEGF) in brain cells (red glow). (**C**)—Immune reaction with antibody to glial-derived neurotrophic factor (GDNF) (red glow). (**D**)—Immune reaction with antibody to neuronal cell adhesion molecule (NCAM) (red glow). Arrows point to the transduced brain cells. Arrowheads indicate cell nuclei visualized using DAPI (blue glow). Scale bar in (**A–D**) = 50 μm; scale bar in the inserts = 20 μm.

2.5. Expression of Recombinant Molecules in Rat Brain after Intrathecal UCB-MC-Mediated Delivery of Transgenes

The synthesis of the reporter GFP in UCB-MC in vivo was studied on day 24 after intrathecal injection of UCB-MC transduced with Ad-GFP. Antibody to human nuclear antigen (HNA) was used for the identification of UCB-MC in the rat brain cortex. HNA-positive cells producing GFP were revealed in the peri-infarct zone (Figure 11A). The production of therapeutic molecules (VEGF, GDNF, and NCAM) in transplanted, genetically-modified UCB-MC was studied using a double immunofluorescent staining method with antibodies against HNA and to one of the recombinant molecules. HNA-positive cells producing recombinant human molecules VEGF (Figure 11B), GDNF (Figure 11C), and NCAM (Figure 11D) were detected in the left hemisphere, 24 days after the intrathecal injection of UCB-MC+Ad5-VEGF-GDNF-NCAM.

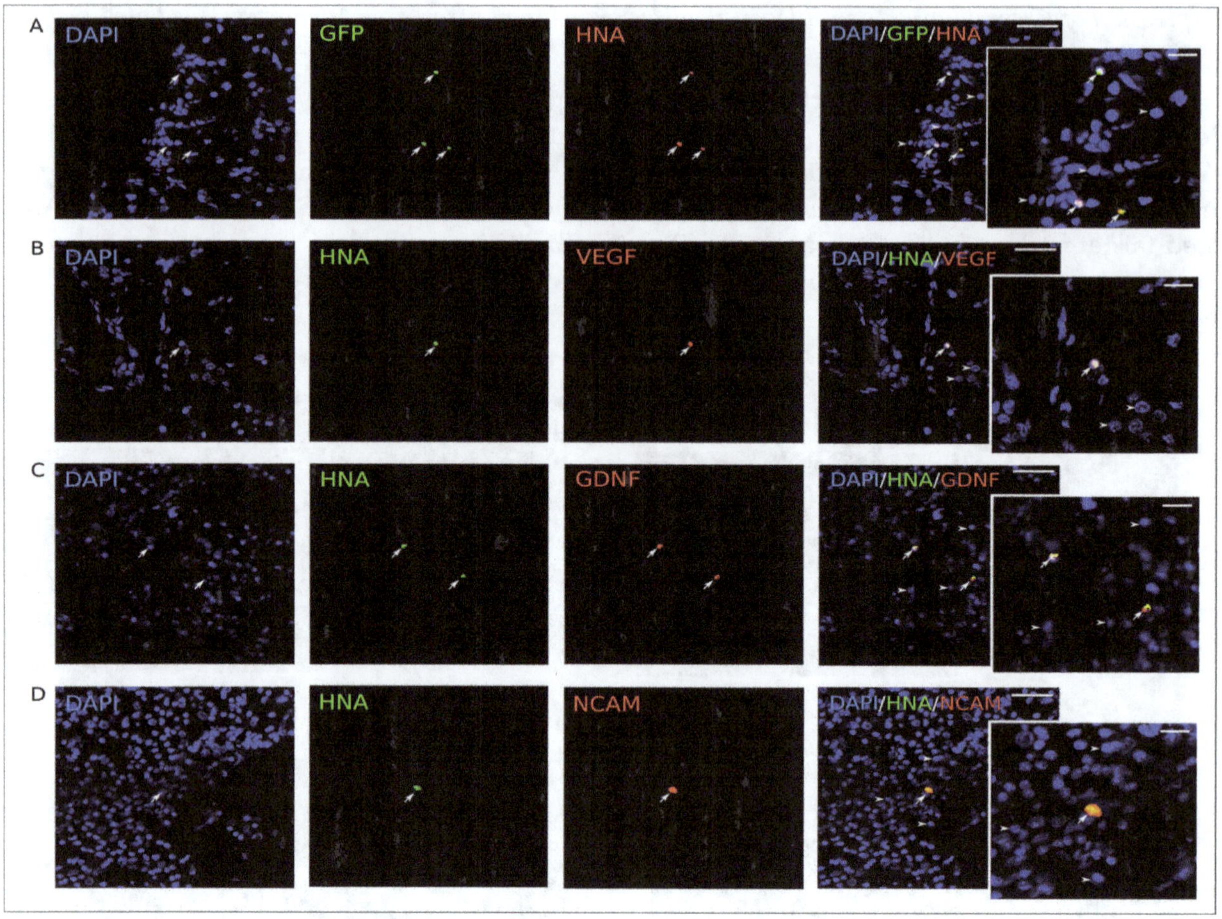

Figure 11. Expression of recombinant molecules in rat brain on the 24th day after intrathecal injection of UCB-MC+Ad5-GFP and UCB-MC+Ad-VEGF-GDNF-NCAM. UCB-MC+Ad-VEGF-GDNF-NCAM are visualized with antibody against the human nuclear antigen (HNA). Cell nuclei are counterstained with DAPI (blue glow). (**A**)—Specific green glow in UCB-MC+Ad5-GFP. (**B**)—Immune reaction with antibody against vascular endothelial growth factor (VEGF) (red glow). (**C**)—Immune response with antibody against glial-derived neurotrophic factor (GDNF) (red glow). (**D**)—Immune response with antibody against neuronal cell adhesion molecule (NCAM) (red glow). Arrows point to the UCB-MC. Arrowheads indicate cell nuclei visualized using DAPI (blue glow). Scale bar in (**A–D**) = 50 µm; scale bar in the inserts = 20 µm.

2.6. Multiplex Analysis of Cytokines, Chemokines and Growth Factors in Blood (Serum) and Cerebrospinal Fluid (Liquor) Samples of Experimental and Intact Animals

Granulocyte colony-stimulating factor (G-CSF), granulocyte and monocyte colony-stimulating factor (GM-CSF), interferon-γ (IFN-γ), interleukin-4 (IL-4), interleukin-10 (IL-10), interleukin-12 (IL-12), and VEGF are considered cytokines with neuroprotective action, while interleukin-1 (IL-1), interleukin-6 (IL-6), interleukin-17 (IL-17), and tumor necrosis factor-α (TNF-α) can cause secondary death of nerve cells. In the present study, preliminary analysis of endogenous cytokines, chemokines and growth factors in cerebrospinal fluid in animals from the control group NaCl showed no significant differences in comparison with intact rats, which probably indicates the cessation of inflammatory response 21 days after modelling a stroke. In addition, intrathecal injection of a combination of adenoviral vectors carrying cDNA encoding VEGF, GDNF, and NCAM, or genetically-modified UCB-MC+Ad5-VEGF-GDNF-NCAM on day 21 of the experiment does not reliably affect the cytokine levels in liquor samples when compared with intact rats.

3. Discussion

It is known that ischemic stroke leads to massive loss of neurons and glial cells immediately after acute arterial occlusion. Neuron death caused by necrosis and apoptosis is the result of blood flow impairment, oxidative stress, mitochondrial dysfunction, and excitotoxicity. Unfortunately, these irreversible changes rapidly spread beyond the epicenter of the ischemic damage, resulting in progressive neurodegeneration on the following days, and even over the following week [32]. However, during the first hours, an ischemic penumbra with blood supply below a normal level is formed around the ischemic core with irreversible changes. The viability of cells in the penumbra is limited to a 3–6-h period of the therapeutic window, during which it is possible to restrain the entry into apoptosis of neurons and glial cells and thus prevent the increase of infarction volume.

Despite the improved efficiency of modern therapy for ischemic brain stroke, recovery of patients is not satisfactory. Today, specific therapy for acute stroke is aimed at restoring blood circulation in the ischemic area and maintaining the metabolism of brain cells. However, the drugs used in practical medicine are not effective in controlling the death of nerve cells in the ischemic penumbra, which results in an extensive increase in brain infarction. It is known that there are natural limitations neuroregeneration in the CNS; therefore, there is a need to develop new effective approaches to maintain the viability of nerve cells in the ischemic penumbra in the 3–6-h therapeutic window.

It is known that neuroontogenesis (addressed migration of brain cells, directed axon growth and establishment of intercellular contacts) involves an information exchange between neurons, which is realized through neurotrophic factors produced in some neurons or in non-neural cells that affect other neurons. In postnatal ontogenesis, there is no formation of new cortical neurons. Therefore, dying neurons are not restored. This does not mean that there is no regeneration in brain cortex; however, as regeneration is carried out due to intracellular regeneration of damaged neurons, growth of their neuritis and restoration of synaptic connections between regenerating and intact neurons. During neuroregeneration, neurotrophic factors support neuronal survival, stimulate axonal growth, and establish lost synaptic contacts.

At present, the most promising of the actively developed strategies to prevent brain cell death in penumbra is the development of gene and cellular technologies. Gene therapy is mainly aimed at the delivery of therapeutic genes encoding neurotrophic factors. Among them, the most promising are genes encoding neurotrophic factors (BDNF, CNTF, GDNF, VEGF), anti-apoptotic proteins (Bcl-2, Bcl-XL), heat shock proteins (Hsp25, Hsp70), and anti-inflammatory molecules (IL-1RA). The neuroprotective effect of these factors has been experimentally proven, but there is no unequivocal, let alone exhaustive, answer to the question of which of these factors may be recommended as neuroprotective factors in practical medicine. It has been established that combinations of several neurotrophic factors may have a more pronounced effect on nerve cell survival [25,28].

Other equally important issues in the strategy for the gene therapy of stroke include the development of technology to deliver transgenes to the brain. Difficulties in the delivery of therapeutic genes to the cerebral infarction area are one of the main reasons for the unavailability of effective gene therapy in treating post-ischemic negative consequences in the brain. Direct (in vivo) gene therapy provides for the delivery of transgenes into the recipient brain plasmid or viral genetic vectors [33]. Cell-mediated (ex vivo) gene therapy is based on the delivery of therapeutic genes using cells that serve as carriers of transgenes, as well as producers of recombinant protein molecules.

For the treatment of stroke, various methods of gene therapy are known, the effectiveness of which has been proven in numerous experiments on animals [2,4,34]. Injections of viral vectors carrying transgenes into the ventricles or the infarction area are mainly used to deliver the therapeutic genes to the brain. Genetic vectors based on Sendai virus vectors containing *gdnf* or *ngf* genes were injected 30 min after stroke simulation [35]. The adeno-associated viral vector carrying *gdnf* was injected 2 days after the stroke modelling [36]. In other studies, viral vectors carrying therapeutic genes were delivered before modelling the stroke. The positive effect was shown after local delivery to the brain of *gdnf* or *cntf* genes—7 days [37], *bdnf*—2 weeks [38], *gdnf*—4 weeks [39], or *ngf* and *bdnf*—4 to 5 weeks [40] before stroke modelling.

The list of genes employed in gene therapy for stroke is quite long. Of these, we find *vegf, gdnf,* and *ncam* to be the most promising.

In addition to angiogenic action, VEGF exhibits the properties of a typical neurotrophic factor. It supports survival of sensitive [41] and motor neurons [42] and stimulates proliferation of astrocytes [43], neural stem cells [44], and Schwann's cells [41]. GDNF has a pronounced neuroprotective effect on dopaminergic brain neurons and cholinergic spinal cord motoneurons [45] and stimulates the growth of nerve processes [46]. NCAM (CD56) is expressed on the surface of neurons and glial cells. Intercellular interactions mediated by NCAM in neuro-ontogenesis and posttraumatic regeneration provide survival and migration of neurons, directed neurite growth and synaptogenesis.

The efficiency of cell therapy for stroke treatment in experiments using neural precursors derived from embryonic stem cells [47], induced pluripotent cells [48], MSCs isolated from red bone marrow [49] or UCB [50] suggests the use of these cells as carriers of therapeutic genes for delivery to the brain. Thus, MSCs were used for delivery of *bdnf* [51], *pigf* [52], and *vegf165* [53] to the brain. Of particular interest is the transduction of cell carriers by two or more expression vectors [28]. This approach allows simultaneous overexpression of several molecules/stimulants of neuroregeneration to be obtained. In our studies, in addition to the gene encoding neurotrophic factors, a gene encoding NCAM was delivered into UCB-MC, which, according to the obtained data, promoted the addressed migration of transplanted cells into the CNS after intravenous injection, increased their survival in the recipient's tissues and supported prolonged production of recombinant therapeutic molecules [28]. In clinical investigations, autologous cells isolated from the red bone marrow (mononuclear and MSCs) or peripheral blood (CD34+) are predominantly used in the cell therapy of patients after stroke [54,55].

The most promising cell carriers of therapeutic genes are UCB-MC [56–58]. The basis for their application is the suitability for both allografting and autotransplantation in humans, availability, and the ease of obtaining and storage. An important factor is the absence of legal, ethical, and religious prohibitions related to blood cell transplantation. In our previous study, we showed that intrathecal injection of adenoviral vectors carrying *vegf, gdnf,* and *ncam*, or genetically-modified UCB-MC+Ad5-VEGF-GDNF-NCAM, 4 h after stroke modelling in rats, had a positive effect on the morpho-functional recovery of the post-ischemic brain [25]. Adenoviral vectors and genetically-modified UCB-MC with cerebrospinal fluid reached the ischemic area and delivered the production of recombinant VEGF, GDNF, and NCAM, lasting up to 21 days in the experiment.

Other important issues in the strategy for the treatment of ischemic stroke include the development of approaches to enhance the viability of neurons with the threat of a stroke. Patients with transient ischemic attacks, arterial hypertension, atrial fibrillation, disorders of lipid metabolism with high cholesterol and diabetes are at high risk of ischemic stroke. Preventive therapy aimed at increasing the survivability of neurons in at-risk patients may prevent severe post-ischemic consequences in the brain, or improve the outcome of the disease. Currently, in medical practice, measures to prevent stroke are based on the use of anticoagulants and prosthetics of blood vessels. At the same time, the preventive methods that are able to considerably decrease the death of neurons in the "ischemic penumbra" during the 3–6-h "therapeutic window" are unknown. Enhancement of the viability of nerve cells at risk of stroke is also associated with the delivery of therapeutic genes that encode molecules to the brain, which inhibit neuronal death and stimulate neuroregeneration. In this study, for the first time, we propose the approach of preventive gene therapy to improve the viability of brain neurons under threat of ischemic stroke to contain neuronal death in the first hours of a stroke. The use of leucocytes for delivery of therapeutic genes (*vegf165, gdnf,* and *ncam1*) in the brain was based on their biological properties. Leucocytes are cells with high secretory and migration potentials, which suggest their exclusive role as cell carriers for addressed delivery and effective expression of transgenes. The results obtained in the study demonstrate that preventive intrathecal adenoviral- or UCB-MC-mediated delivery of *vegf165, gdnf,* and *ncam1* results in a reduction of apoptosis and, consequently, the infraction volume.

In addition to the decrease in expression of proteins of cellular stress and restraining neuronal death in the area of ischemic damage, we found evidence of the restoration of functional activity of neurons (increase in expression of synaptic proteins), maintenance of myelinization (increase in the number of oligodendrocytes) and an obstacle to astrogliosis development (decrease in the immunopositive areas for astrocytes and microglial cells markers). Importantly, transplantation of gene-modified UCB-MC is safer and more efficacious compared with direct gene therapy. These data are in line with our results using the same gene and gene-cell constructs for ischemic stroke treatment in rats and allow us to conclude that preventive gene therapy may be effective in overcoming the negative consequences of ischemic stroke in the rehabilitation period.

Recently, for personalized ex vivo gene therapy, we suggested the use of gene-modified leucoconcentrate (GML) prepared from patient's peripheral blood and chimeric adenoviral vectors (Ad5/35F) carrying one or a combination of therapeutic genes [59]. Taken together with the concept of GML-therapy and the data of this study, we propose the use of GML carrying *vegf165*, *gdnf*, and *ncam1* for personalized preventive gene therapy in the threat of stroke.

4. Materials and Methods

4.1. Preparation and Molecular Analysis of Gene-Modified UCB-MC

Human (*vegf165, gdnf, ncam1*) and reporter (*gfp*) genes were inserted into recombinant replication-defective adenovirus serotype 5 (Ad5) in the Gamaleya Research Institute of Epidemiology and Microbiology (Moscow, Russia), as described previously [25]. Viral vectors were grown in HEK-293 cell culture, purified by exclusion chromatography and the titres of Ad5-VEGF (2.6×10^9 PFU/mL), Ad5-GDNF (1.7×10^{10} PFU/mL), Ad5-NCAM (2.4×10^{10} PFU/mL) and Ad5-GFP (1.2×10^{10} PFU/mL) were determined in the HEK-293 cell culture using the plaque formation technique.

The fraction of mononuclear cells from UCB was isolated onto a density barrier by the standard technique of sedimentation, seeded in 10 cm culture dishes and simultaneously transduced with three adenoviral vectors at an equal ratio: Ad5-VEGF (1/3)+Ad5-GDNF (1/3)+Ad5-NCAM (1/3) or with Ad5-GFP with MOI of 10, as described previously [25]. To confirm the efficacy of UCB-MC transduction, the gene-modified cells were cultured for 96 h. Transduction with therapeutic genes (*vegf165, gdnf, ncam1*) was confirmed by a real-time polymerase chain reaction (RT-PCR) and with reporter green fluorescent protein (*gfp*) using fluorescent microscopy, as described previously [57].

For direct (in vivo) preventive gene therapy, a mixture of 2×10^7 virus particles in an equal ratio of Ad5-VEGF (1/3)+Ad5-GDNF (1/3)+Ad5-NCAM (1/3) in 20 μL of saline and Ad5-GFP in 20 μL of saline were prepared. For cell-mediated (ex vivo) preventive gene therapy, 2×10^6 UCB-MC+Ad5-VEGF+Ad5-GDNF+Ad5-NCAM in 20 μL of saline and 2×10^6 UCB-MC+Ad5-GFP in 20 μL of saline were prepared.

The efficiency of UCB-MC genetic modification by adenoviral vector, bearing green fluorescent protein reporter gene, was analyzed 72 h after cell transduction. The production of green fluorescent protein UCB-MC+Ad5-GFP was examined with the Axio Oberver Z1 inverted fluorescence microscope (Carl Zeiss, Germany). The number of transduced UCBC was estimated using a BD FACSAria III flow cytomography fluorimeter (BD Bioscience, New York, NY, USA) and BD FACS Diva7 software (BD Bioscience, New York, NY, USA).

mRNA levels of *vegf165, gdnf,* and *ncam1* transgenes in the UCB-MC, simultaneously transduced by a combination of three adenoviral vectors Ad5-VEGF, Ad5-GDNF and Ad5-NCAM, were analyzed with PCR-RT. Extraction of common RNA from UCB-MC+Ad5-VEGF-GDNF-NCAM and UCB-MC+Ad5-GFP, 72 h after cell incubation, was carried out using a set Yellow Solve (Silex), according to the manufacturer's instructions. Reference samples of common RNA were derived from non-transduced UCBC. The cDNA synthesis was performed using six nucleotide random primers and reverse transcriptase RevertAid Reverse Transcriptase (Thermo Fisher Scientific). Quantitative level analysis mRNA of the target cDNA was performed using a CFX 96 Real-Time PCR System thermocirculator (BioRad, Hercules, CA, USA), using the TaqMan system. Sequences of primers and probes of the reaction mixture are presented in Table 1. Received data was normalized by the 18S rRNA reference gene. For each target gene, the results were obtained in two independent experiments and presented as a mean value ± SE, $p < 0.05$.

Table 1. Experimental groups of animals.

Groups	Preparation for Animals Treatment	Number of Animals
Control	20 μL 0.9% NaCl intrathecally injected 4 days before ischemic stroke modelling	5
Ad5-GFP	Ad5 carrying *gfp* in 20 μL of saline intrathecally injected 4 days before ischemic stroke modelling	6
Ad5-VEGF+Ad5-GDNF+Ad5-NCAM	Mixture of the three Ad5 carrying *vegf165*, *gdnf* and *ncam1* in 20 μL of saline intrathecally injected 4 days before ischemic stroke modelling	6
UCBC+Ad5-GFP	2 × 10^6 UCBC transduced with Ad5 carrying *gfp* in 20 μL of saline intrathecally injected 3 days before ischemic stroke modelling	6
UCBC+Ad5-VEGF-GDNF-NCAM	2 × 10^6 UCBC simultaneously transduced with three Ad5 carrying *vegf165*, *gdnf* and *ncam1* in 20 μL of saline intrathecally injected 3 days before ischemic stroke modelling	6

Supernatant obtained 72 h after incubation of gene-modified UCB-MC (UCB-MC+Ad5-VEGF -GDNF-NCAM and UCB-MC+Ad5-GFP) and intact UCB-MC were used for multiplex profiling. In this work, commercially available panels, Human Cytokine/Chemokine Magnetic Bead Panel (HCYTMAG-60K-PX41), were applied, containing the following analytes: EGF, FGF2, Eotoxin, TGF-a, G-CSF, Flt-3L, GM-CSF, Fractalkine, IFNa2, IFN-g, GRO, IL10, MCP-3, IL12-p40, MDC, IL12-p70, PDGF-AA, IL-13, PDGF-AB/BB, IL-15, sCD40L, IL-17a, IL-1ra, IL-1a, IL-9, IL-1bIL-2, IL-3, IL-4, IL-5, IL-6, IL-7, IL-8, IP10, MCP-1, MIP-1a, MIP-1b, RANTES, TNFa, TNFb, and VEGF (Millipore). The quantitative analysis of target molecules was performed on a Bio-Plex200 System (BioRad, USA) according to the protocol recommended by the manufacturer and using Bio-Plex Manager 4.1 software (Bio-RadLaboratories). The results were statistically processed using the following methods, using linear models implemented in the limma package. Fold Change was used as an estimate for the effect size, obtained for pairwise comparison.

4.2. Animals and Treatments

The animal protocols were conducted in strict compliance with the guidelines established by the Kazan State Medical University Animal Care and Use Committee (approval No. 10, 2017). Experiments were performed on adult female Wistar rats (weight of 200–250 g) obtained from Pushchino Laboratory (Pushchino, Russia). Animals were housed one per cage according to approved procedures for the use of animals in laboratory experiments.

For preventive gene therapy, rats were deeply anesthetized intraperitoneally with Zolitil 100 (Virbac Laboratoires, France) 3 mg/kg and Xyla (Interchemie werken "De Adelaar" B.V., Netherlands) 4.8 mg/kg. A laminectomy was made over the L4–L5 vertebral level and gene-modified UCBC or adenoviral vectors were infused intrathecally. The rats were divided into five experimental groups according to the injected substances (Table 1).

Ischemic stroke in the rats was induced 3 days after intrathecal injection of UCB-MC+Ad5-GFP and UCB-MC+Ad5-VEGF-GDNF-NCAM or 4 days after intrathecal injection of 0.9% NaCl, Ad5-GFP and Ad5-VEGF-GDNF-NCAM. The ischemic stroke was induced by permanent MCAO, as described previously [25]. In brief, to reduce blood flow in the circle of Willis, the right common carotid artery was ligated with surgical silk. In the left side, a 4–5 mm hole was drilled in the temporal bone and MCAO was performed by thermocoagulation using an operating microscope.

To reduce suffering and distress, post-operative care included analgesic therapy with Ketamine (Dr. Reddy's Laboratories, Ltd., Hyderabad, Andhra Pradesh, India) intramuscularly (2.5 mg/kg) once-a-day and antibacterial therapy with Ceftriaxone (Sandoz, Austria) intramuscularly (50 mg/kg) once-a-day for 5 days. Based on our previous study [25] for evaluation of preventive gene therapy, experimental animals were sacrificed three weeks after MCAO.

4.3. Morphometric and Immunofluorescent Analysis of the Brain

For histological analysis, rats were deeply anesthetized by intraperitoneal injection of sodium pentobarbital (60 mg/kg) and intracardially perfused with 4% paraformaldehyde (PFA, Sigma) in phosphate-buffered saline (PBS, pH 7.4). The brains of the rats were isolated from the skull, post-fixed in 4% paraformaldehyde and cryoprotected in 30% sucrose. Frozen frontal sections of the brain were obtained through the epicenter of ischemic injury using a cryostat (Microm HM 560, Thermo Scientific, Waltham, MA, USA).

Morphometric analysis of the volume of the cerebral infarction included macroscopic evaluation of the infarct area of the whole brain by capturing digital images and microscopic study every 10 frontal brain sections (with 200 μm interval) through the ischemic injury area, after staining with hematoxylin and eosin. To calculate the infarction volume, maximal depth and maximal diameter of the infarct cavities were estimated using ImageJ software (NIH). The calculation was carried out as $V = 1/3 \times \text{maximal depth} \times \pi \times (\text{maximal diameter}/2)^2$.

Immunofluorescent staining was performed on 20 μm sections of frontal brain using primary antibodies (Ab) reacting with cell specific markers (Table 2). The viability of neural cells was evaluated using Ab to pro-apoptotic protein (Caspase3) and heat shock protein 70 kDa (Hsp70). Synaptic function of preserved neurons was assessed with Ab against synaptophysin and postsynaptic density protein 95 kDa (PSD95). Responses of glial cells were assessed with Ab to GFAP for astrocytes, Ab to Olig2 for oligodendrocytes and Ab to Iba1 for microglia. Anti-human nuclear antigen (HNA) antibodies were used for identification of human UCBC in the rat brain. Double immunofluorescent staining with Ab to HNA and Ab to human VEGF, GDNF, and NCAM were employed to analyze the expression of those recombinant molecules in UCB-MC. For immunofluorescent labelling, sections were incubated with secondary antibodies (Table 2). Appropriate secondary Alexa Fluor 647 and 488 conjugated Abs were used for immunofluorescent labelling of the target molecules. Cell nuclear counterstaining was performed with DAPI (10 μg/mL in PBS, Sigma), sections were embedded in glycerol (GalenoPharm, Saint Petersburg, Russia) and observed under a LEICA TCS SP5 MP microscope (Leica Microsystems, Wetzlar, Germany).

Digital images were captured using identical confocal settings in areas of 0.05 mm^2 and analyzed with ImageJ software (NIH) in 10 captured fields in the peri-infarct zone (Figure 2C) in each section, as described previously [25]. The number of immunopositive cells for apoptosis protein Caspase3 and oligodendroglial cells transcription factor Olig2 were counted in regard to nuclear counterstaining with DAPI. Neuroglial markers for astrocytes (GFAP) and microglia (Iba1) were evaluated as the immunopositive areas and presented in percentages. The level of synaptic proteins (synaptophysin and PSD95) and Hsp70 immunoexpression in brain sections was evaluated as mean pixel intensities.

Table 2. Antibodies used in immunofluorescent analysis.

Antibody against:	Host	Dilution	Source
Caspase3	Rabbit	1:200	Abcam
Glial cell-derived neurotrophic factor (GDNF)	Rabbit	1:100	Santa Cruz
Glial fibrillary acidic protein (GFAP)	Mouse	1:200	Santa Cruz
Ionized calcium binding adaptor molecule 1 (Iba1)	Rabbit	1:150	Biocare Medical
Human Nuclear Antigen (HNA)	Mouse	1:150	Millipore
Heat shock protein 70 kDa (Hsp70)	Rabbit	1:200	Abcam
Oligodendrocyte transcription factor 2 (Olig2)	Rabbit	1:100	Santa Cruz
Neural cell adhesion molecule (NCAM)	Rabbit	1:100	Santa Cruz
Postsynaptic density protein 95 kDa (PSD95)	Rabbit	1:200	Abcam
Synaptophysin Vascular endothelial growth factor (VEGF)	Rabbit Goat	1:100 1:300	Abcam Sigma
Rabbit IgG conjugated with Alexa 647	Donkey	1:200	Invitrogen
Mouse IgG conjugated with Alexa 488	Donkey	1:200	Invitrogen

4.4. Multiplex Cytokine Analysis of the Cerebrospinal Fluid

Multiplex profiling was performed in cerebrospinal fluid (liquor) of experimental and intact animals using the commercially available Bio-Plex Pro™ Rat Cytokine 23-Plex Assay panel, containing the following analytes: G-SCF, GM-CSF, GRO/KC, IFN-g, IL-10, IL-12p70, IL-13, IL-18, IL-1a, IL-1b, IL-2, IL-4, IL-5, IL-6, IL-7, IL17A, M-CSF, MCP-1, MIP1a, MIP3a, RANTES, TNFa, and VEGF. Quantitative analysis of target molecules was performed on a Bio-Plex200 System analyzer (BioRad, USA), as recommended by the manufacturer, using Bio-Plex Manager 4.1 software (Bio-RadLaboratories). The statistical processing of obtained results was carried out using linear models implemented in the limma package.

4.5. Statistics

Statistical data analysis and visualizations were performed using R version 3.5.3 (R Foundation for Statistical Computing, Vienna, Austria). Sample distributions of quantitative values were visualized using box plots, and descriptive statistics are presented as: (Median [1st quartile; 3rd quartile]). The Kruskal–Wallis test was used to compare morphometric and immunofluorescent staining data between experimental groups when a null hypothesis was rejected; we used Dunn's-test as the post hoc method. Differences were considered statistically significant where $p < 0.05$.

5. Conclusions

Methods of preventive gene therapy of ischemic stroke in at-risk patients are currently unknown. In this study, for the first time, we provide evidence of the beneficial effects of preventive triple gene therapy by an adenoviral- or UCB-MC-mediated intrathecal simultaneous delivery combination of *vegf165*, *gdnf*, and *ncam1* on the preservation and recovery of the brain in rats with subsequent modelling of stroke. The obtained data represent a novel and potentially successful approach for ischemic stroke treatment in patients.

Author Contributions: Conceptualization, R.I.; Data curation, V.M. and M.K.; Formal analysis, M.K.; Investigation, V.M., F.F., M.S., D.T., E.K., G.K., A.G. and I.S.; Methodology, Z.S., A.I. and F.F.; Project administration, V.M., Z.S., A.I., F.F. and M.S.; Supervision, F.B. and R.I.; Visualization, A.I. and L.N.; Writing—original draft and review & editing, R.I. All authors have read and agreed to the published version of the manuscript.

Acknowledgments: Some experiments were carried out as part of the state assignment of the Federal Research Center "Kazan Scientific Center of the Russian Academy of Sciences".

References

1. Karlupia, N.; Manley, N.C.; Prasad, K.; Schäfer, R.; Steinberg, G.K. Intraarterial transplantation of human umbilical cord blood mononuclear cells is more efficacious and safer compared with umbilical cord mesenchymal stromal cells in a rodent stroke model. *Stem Cell Res. Ther.* **2014**, *5*, 45. [CrossRef] [PubMed]
2. Rhim, T.; Lee, M. Targeted delivery of growth factors in ischemic stroke animal models. *Expert Opin. Drug Deliv.* **2016**, *13*, 709–723. [CrossRef] [PubMed]
3. Yamashita, T.; Deguchi, K.; Nagotani, S.; Kamiya, T.; Abe, K. Gene and Stem Cell Therapy in Ischemic Stroke. *Cell Transplant.* **2009**, *18*, 999–1002. [CrossRef] [PubMed]
4. Ooboshi, H. Gene Therapy as a Novel Pharmaceutical Intervention for Stroke. *Curr. Pharm. Des.* **2011**, *17*, 424–433. [CrossRef] [PubMed]
5. Yang, W.Z.; Zhang, Y.; Wu, F.; Min, W.P.; Minev, B.; Zhang, M.; Luo, X.L.; Ramos, F.; Ichim, T.E.; Riordan, N.H.; et al. Safety evaluation of allogeneic umbilical cord blood mononuclear cell therapy for degenerative conditions. *J. Transl. Med.* **2010**, *8*, 75. [CrossRef]
6. Harris, D.T.; Rogers, I. Umbilical cord blood: A unique source of pluripotent stem cells for regenerative medicine. *Curr. Stem Cell Res. Ther.* **2007**, *2*, 301–309. [CrossRef]
7. Arien-Zakay, H.; Lazarovici, P.; Nagler, A. Tissue regeneration potential in human umbilical cord blood. *Best Pract. Res. Clin. Haematol.* **2010**, *23*, 291–303. [CrossRef]
8. Arien-Zakay, H.; Lecht, S.; Nagler, A.; Lazarovici, P. Human umbilical cord blood stem cells: Rational for use as a neuroprotectant in ischemic brain disease. *Int. J. Mol. Sci.* **2010**, *11*, 3513–3528. [CrossRef]
9. Erices, A.; Conget, P.; Minguell, J.J. Mesenchymal progenitor cells in human umbilical cord blood. *Br. J. Haematol.* **2000**, *109*, 235–242. [CrossRef]
10. Kögler, G.; Sensken, S.; Airey, J.A.; Trapp, T.; Müschen, M.; Feldhahn, N.; Liedtke, S.; Sorg, R.V.; Fischer, J.; Rosenbaum, C.; et al. A new human somatic stem cell from placental cord blood with intrinsic pluripotent differentiation potential. *J. Exp. Med.* **2004**, *200*, 123–135. [CrossRef]
11. Gluckman, E. Ten years of cord blood transplantation: From bench to bedside. *Br. J. Haematol.* **2009**, *147*, 192–199. [CrossRef] [PubMed]
12. Pimentel-Coelho, P.M.; Rosado-de-Castro, P.H.; Barbosa da Fonseca, L.M.; Mendez-Otero, R. Umbilical cord blood mononuclear cell transplantation for neonatal hypoxic–ischemic encephalopathy. *Pediatr. Res.* **2012**, *71*, 464–473. [CrossRef] [PubMed]
13. Goldstein, G.; Toren, A.; Nagler, A. Transplantation and Other Uses of Human Umbilical Cord Blood and Stem Cells. *Curr. Pharm. Des.* **2007**, *13*, 1363–1373. [CrossRef] [PubMed]
14. Rocha, V.; Labopin, M.; Sanz, G.; Arcese, W.; Schwerdtfeger, R.; Bosi, A.; Jacobsen, N.; Ruutu, T.; De Lima, M.; Finke, J.; et al. Transplants of umbilical-cord blood or bone marrow from unrelated donors in adults with acute leukemia. *N. Engl. J. Med.* **2004**, *351*, 2276–2285. [CrossRef]
15. Balassa, K.; Rocha, V. Anticancer cellular immunotherapies derived from umbilical cord blood. *Expert Opin. Biol. Ther.* **2018**, *18*, 121–134. [CrossRef]
16. Arien-Zakay, H.; Lecht, S.; Bercu, M.M.; Tabakman, R.; Kohen, R.; Galski, H.; Nagler, A.; Lazarovici, P. Neuroprotection by cord blood neural progenitors involves antioxidants, neurotrophic and angiogenic factors. *Exp. Neurol.* **2009**, *216*, 83–94. [CrossRef]
17. Bachstetter, A.D.; Pabon, M.M.; Cole, M.J.; Hudson, C.E.; Sanberg, P.R.; Willing, A.E.; Bickford, P.C.; Gemma, C. Peripheral injection of human umbilical cord blood stimulates neurogenesis in the aged rat brain. *BMC Neurosci.* **2008**, *9*, 22. [CrossRef]
18. Dasari, V.R.; Spomar, D.G.; Li, L.; Gujrati, M.; Rao, J.S.; Dinh, D.H. Umbilical cord blood stem cell mediated downregulation of Fas improves functional recovery of rats after spinal cord injury. *Neurochem. Res.* **2008**, *33*, 134–149. [CrossRef]
19. Schira, J.; Gasis, M.; Estrada, V.; Hendricks, M.; Schmitz, C.; Trapp, T.; Kruse, F.; Kögler, G.; Wernet, P.; Hartung, H.P.; et al. Significant clinical, neuropathological and behavioural recovery from acute spinal cord trauma by transplantation of a well-defined somatic stem cell from human umbilical cord blood. *Brain* **2012**, *135*, 431–446. [CrossRef]

20. Xiao, J.; Nan, Z.; Motooka, Y.; Low, W.C. Transplantation of a novel cell line population of umbilical cord blood stem cells ameliorates neurological deficits associated with ischemic brain injury. *Stem Cells Dev.* **2005**, *14*, 722–733. [CrossRef]
21. Ikeda, Y.; Fukuda, N.; Wada, M.; Matsumoto, T.; Satomi, A.; Yokoyama, S.-I.; Saito, S.; Matsumoto, K.; Kanmatsuse, K.; Mugishima, H. Development of angiogenic cell and gene therapy by transplantation of umbilical cord blood with vascular endothelial growth factor gene. *Hypertens. Res.* **2004**, *27*, 119–128. [CrossRef] [PubMed]
22. Chen, H.K.; Hung, H.F.; Shyu, K.G.; Wang, B.W.; Sheu, J.R.; Liang, Y.J.; Chang, C.C.; Kuan, P. Combined cord blood stem cells and gene therapy enhances angiogenesis and improves cardiac performance in mouse after acute myocardial infarction. *Eur. J. Clin. Investig.* **2005**, *35*, 677–686. [CrossRef]
23. Islamov, R.R.; Sokolov, M.E.; Bashirov, F.V.; Fadeev, F.O.; Shmarov, M.M.; Naroditskiy, B.S.; Povysheva, T.V.; Shaymardanova, G.F.; Yakupov, R.A.; Chelyshev, Y.A.; et al. A pilot study of cell-mediated gene therapy for spinal cord injury in mini pigs. *Neurosci. Lett.* **2017**, *644*, 67–75. [CrossRef] [PubMed]
24. Izmailov, A.A.; Povysheva, T.V.; Bashirov, F.V.; Sokolov, M.E.; Fadeev, F.O.; Garifulin, R.R.; Naroditsky, B.S.; Logunov, D.Y.; Salafutdinov, I.I.; Chelyshev, Y.A.; et al. Spinal Cord Molecular and Cellular Changes Induced by Adenoviral Vector- and Cell-Mediated Triple Gene Therapy after Severe Contusion. *Front. Pharmacol.* **2017**, *8*, 813. [CrossRef] [PubMed]
25. Sokolov, M.E.; Bashirov, F.V.; Markosyan, V.A.; Povysheva, T.V.; Fadeev, F.O.; Izmailov, A.A.; Kuztetsov, M.S.; Safiullov, Z.Z.; Shmarov, M.M.; Naroditskyi, B.S.; et al. Triple-Gene Therapy for Stroke: A Proof-of-Concept in Vivo Study in Rats. *Front. Pharmacol.* **2018**, *9*, 111. [CrossRef] [PubMed]
26. Mothe, A.J.; Tator, C.H. Review of transplantation of neural stem/progenitor cells for spinal cord injury. *Int. J. Dev. Neurosci.* **2013**, *31*, 701–713. [CrossRef]
27. Razavi, S.; Ghasemi, N.; Mardani, M.; Salehi, H. Remyelination improvement after neurotrophic factors secreting cells transplantation in rat spinal cord injury. *Iran. J. Basic Med. Sci.* **2017**, *20*, 392–398. [CrossRef] [PubMed]
28. Safiullov, Z.Z.; Garanina, E.E.; Izmailov, A.A.; Garifulin, R.R.; Fedotova, V.Y.; Salafutdinov, I.I.; Rizvanov, A.A.; Islamov, R.R. Homing and survivability of genetically modified mononuclear umbilical cord blood cells after transplantation into transgenic G93A mice with amyotrophic lateral sclerosis. *Genes Cells* **2015**, *X*, 1–4.
29. Franklin, T.B.; Krueger-Naug, A.M.; Clarke, D.B.; Arrigo, A.-P.; Currie, R.W. The role of heat shock proteins Hsp70 and Hsp27 in cellular protection of the central nervous system. *Int. J. Hyperth.* **2005**, *21*, 379–392. [CrossRef]
30. Barreto, G.E.; White, R.; Ouyang, Y.; Xu, L.G.; Giffard, R. Astrocytes: Targets for Neuroprotection in Stroke. *Cent. Nerv. Syst. Agents Med. Chem.* **2012**, *11*, 164–173. [CrossRef]
31. Dewar, D.; Underhill, S.M.; Goldberg, M.P. Oligodendrocytes and ischemic brain injury. *J. Cereb. Blood Flow Metab.* **2003**, *23*, 263–274. [CrossRef] [PubMed]
32. Du, C.; Hu, R.; Csernansky, C.A.; Hsu, C.Y.; Choi, D.W. Very delayed infarction after mild focal cerebral ischemia: A role for apoptosis? *J. Cereb. Blood Flow Metab.* **1996**, *16*, 195–201. [CrossRef] [PubMed]
33. Abdellatif, A.A.; Pelt, J.L.; Benton, R.L.; Howard, R.M.; Tsoulfas, P.; Ping, P.; Xu, X.-M.; Whittemore, S.R. Gene delivery to the spinal cord: Comparison between lentiviral, adenoviral, and retroviral vector delivery systems. *J. Neurosci. Res.* **2006**, *84*, 553–567. [CrossRef] [PubMed]
34. Craig, A.J.; Housley, G.D. Evaluation of Gene Therapy as an Intervention Strategy to Treat Brain Injury from Stroke. *Front. Mol. Neurosci.* **2016**, *9*, 34. [CrossRef] [PubMed]
35. Shirakura, M.; Inoue, M.; Fujikawa, S.; Washizawa, K.; Komaba, S.; Maeda, M.; Watabe, K.; Yoshikawa, Y.; Hasegawa, M. Postischemic administration of Sendai virus vector carrying neurotrophic factor genes prevents delayed neuronal death in gerbils. *Gene Ther.* **2004**, *11*, 784–790. [CrossRef] [PubMed]
36. Mätlik, K.; Abo-Ramadan, U.; Harvey, B.K.; Arumäe, U.; Airavaara, M. AAV-mediated targeting of gene expression to the peri-infarct region in rat cortical stroke model. *J. Neurosci. Methods* **2014**, *236*, 107–113. [CrossRef]
37. Hermann, D.M.; Kilic, E.; Kügler, S.; Isenmann, S.; Bähr, M. Adenovirus-mediated GDNF and CNTF pretreatment protects against striatal injury following transient middle cerebral artery occlusion in mice. *Neurobiol. Dis.* **2001**, *8*, 655–666. [CrossRef]

38. Zhang, J.; Yu, Z.; Yu, Z.; Yang, Z.; Zhao, H.; Liu, L.; Zhao, J. rAAV-mediated delivery of brain-derived neurotrophic factor promotes neurite outgrowth and protects neurodegeneration in focal ischemic model. *Int. J. Clin. Exp. Pathol.* **2011**, *4*, 496–504.
39. Arvidsson, A.; Kirik, D.; Lundberg, C.; Mandel, R.J.; Andsberg, G.; Kokaia, Z.; Lindvall, O. Elevated GDNF levels following viral vector-mediated gene transfer can increase neuronal death after stroke in rats. *Neurobiol. Dis.* **2003**, *14*, 542–556. [CrossRef]
40. Andsberg, G.; Kokaia, Z.; Klein, R.L.; Muzyczka, N.; Lindvall, O.; Mandel, R.J. Neuropathological and behavioral consequences of adeno-associated viral vector-mediated continuous intrastriatal neurotrophin delivery in a focal ischemia model in rats. *Neurobiol. Dis.* **2002**, *9*, 187–204. [CrossRef]
41. Sondell, M.; Lundborg, G.; Kanje, M. Vascular endothelial growth factor has neurotrophic activity and stimulates axonal outgrowth, enhancing cell survival and Schwann cell proliferation in the peripheral nervous system. *J. Neurosci.* **1999**, *19*, 5731–5740. [CrossRef] [PubMed]
42. Islamov, R.R.; Chintalgattu, V.; Pak, E.S.; Katwa, L.C.; Murashov, A.K. Induction of VEGF and its Flt-1 receptor after sciatic nerve crush injury. *Neuroreport* **2004**, *15*, 2117–2121. [CrossRef] [PubMed]
43. Rosenstein, J.M.; Mani, N.; Silverman, W.F.; Krum, J.M. Patterns of brain angiogenesis after vascular endothelial growth factor administration in vitro and in vivo. *Proc. Natl. Acad. Sci. USA* **1998**, *95*, 7086–7091. [CrossRef] [PubMed]
44. Jin, L.; Neff, T.; Blau, C.A. Marrow sensitization to 5-fluorouracil using the ligands for Flt-3 and c-Kit. *Exp. Hematol.* **1999**, *27*, 520–525. [CrossRef]
45. Cheng, H.; Wu, J.-P.; Tzeng, S.-F. Neuroprotection of glial cell line-derived neurotrophic factor in damaged spinal cords following contusive injury. *J. Neurosci. Res.* **2002**, *69*, 397–405. [CrossRef]
46. Iannotti, C.; Li, H.; Yan, P.; Lu, X.; Wirthlin, L.; Xu, X.M. Glial cell line-derived neurotrophic factor-enriched bridging transplants promote propriospinal axonal regeneration and enhance myelination after spinal cord injury. *Exp. Neurol.* **2003**, *183*, 379–393. [CrossRef]
47. Drury-Stewart, D.; Song, M.; Mohamad, O.; Guo, Y.; Gu, X.; Chen, D.; Wei, L. Highly efficient differentiation of neural precursors from human embryonic stem cells and benefits of transplantation after ischemic stroke in mice. *Stem Cell Res. Ther.* **2013**, *4*, 93. [CrossRef]
48. Yuan, T.; Liao, W.; Feng, N.-H.; Lou, Y.-L.; Niu, X.; Zhang, A.-J.; Wang, Y.; Deng, Z.-F. Human induced pluripotent stem cell-derived neural stem cells survive, migrate, differentiate, and improve neurologic function in a rat model of middle cerebral artery occlusion. *Stem Cell Res. Ther.* **2013**, *4*, 73. [CrossRef]
49. He, B.; Yao, Q.; Liang, Z.; Lin, J.; Xie, Y.; Li, S.; Wu, G.; Yang, Z.; Xu, P. The Dose of Intravenously Transplanted Bone Marrow Stromal Cells Determines the Therapeutic Effect on Vascular Remodeling in a Rat Model of Ischemic Stroke. *Cell Transplant.* **2016**, *25*, 2173–2185. [CrossRef]
50. Zhu, H.; Poon, W.; Liu, Y.; Leung, G.K.-K.; Wong, Y.; Feng, Y.; Ng, S.C.P.; Tsang, K.S.; Sun, D.T.F.; Yeung, D.K.; et al. Phase III Clinical Trial Assessing Safety and Efficacy of Umbilical Cord Blood Mononuclear Cell Transplant Therapy of Chronic Complete Spinal Cord Injury. *Cell Transplant.* **2016**, *25*, 1925–1943. [CrossRef]
51. Nomura, T.; Honmou, O.; Harada, K.; Houkin, K.; Hamada, H.; Kocsis, J.D. IV Infusion of brain-derived neurotrophic factor gene-modified human mesenchymal stem cells protects against injury in a cerebral ischemia model in adult rat. *Neuroscience* **2005**, *136*, 161–169. [CrossRef] [PubMed]
52. Liu, H.; Honmou, O.; Harada, K.; Nakamura, K.; Houkin, K.; Hamada, H.; Kocsis, J.D. Neuroprotection by PlGF gene-modified human mesenchymal stem cells after cerebral ischaemia. *Brain* **2006**, *129*, 2734–2745. [CrossRef] [PubMed]
53. Chen, Y.; Zhu, H.; Liao, J.; Yi, Y.; Wang, G.; Tong, L.; Ge, J. Regulation of naotai recipe on the expression of HIF-1α/VEGF signaling pathway in cerebral ischemia/reperfusion rats. *Zhongguo Zhong xi yi jie he za zhi Zhongguo Zhongxiyi jiehe zazhi = Chin. J. Integr. Tradit. West. Med.* **2014**, *34*, 1225–1230.
54. Wang, X.-L.; Zhao, Y.-S.; Hu, M.-Y.; Sun, Y.-Q.; Chen, Y.-X.; Bi, X.-H. Umbilical cord blood cells regulate endogenous neural stem cell proliferation via hedgehog signaling in hypoxic ischemic neonatal rats. *Brain Res.* **2013**, *1518*, 26–35. [CrossRef]
55. Chernykh, E.R.; Shevela, E.Y.; Starostina, N.M.; Morozov, S.A.; Davydova, M.N.; Menyaeva, E.V.; Ostanin, A.A. Safety and Therapeutic Potential of M2 Macrophages in Stroke Treatment. *Cell Transplant.* **2016**, *25*, 1461–1471. [CrossRef]
56. Hernández, J.; Torres-Espín, A.; Navarro, X. Adult stem cell transplants for spinal cord injury repair: Current state in preclinical research. *Curr. Stem Cell Res. Ther.* **2011**, *6*, 273–287. [CrossRef]

57. Islamov, R.R.; Rizvanov, A.A.; Mukhamedyarov, M.A.; Salafutdinov, I.I.; Garanina, E.E.; Fedotova, V.Y.; Solovyeva, V.V.; Mukhamedshina, Y.O.; Safiullov, Z.Z.; Izmailov, A.A.; et al. Symptomatic improvement, increased life-span and sustained cell homing in amyotrophic lateral sclerosis after transplantation of human umbilical cord blood cells genetically modified with adeno-viral vectors expressing a neuro-protective factor and a neur. *Curr. Gene Ther.* **2015**, *15*, 266–276. [CrossRef]
58. Park, D.-H.; Lee, J.-H.; Borlongan, C.V.; Sanberg, P.R.; Chung, Y.-G.; Cho, T.-H. Transplantation of Umbilical Cord Blood Stem Cells for Treating Spinal Cord Injury. *Stem Cell Rev. Rep.* **2011**, *7*, 181–194. [CrossRef]
59. Islamov, R.R.; Bashirov, F.V.; Sokolov, M.E.; Izmailov, A.A.; Fadeev, F.O.; Markosyan, V.A.; Davleeva, M.A.; Zubkova, O.V.; Smarov, M.M.; Logunov, D.Y.; et al. Gene-modified leucoconcentrate for personalized ex vivo gene therapy in a mini pig model of moderate spinal cord injury. *Neural Regen. Res.* **2020**, *16*, 357–361. [CrossRef]

3

An Inhibitor of the Sodium–Hydrogen Exchanger-1 (NHE-1), Amiloride, Reduced Zinc Accumulation and Hippocampal Neuronal Death after Ischemia

Beom Seok Kang [1], Bo Young Choi [1], A Ra Kho [1], Song Hee Lee [1], Dae Ki Hong [1], Jeong Hyun Jeong [1], Dong Hyeon Kang [2], Min Kyu Park [1] and Sang Won Suh [1,*]

1 Department of Physiology, College of Medicine, Hallym University, Chuncheon 24252, Korea; ttiger1993@gmail.com (B.S.K.); bychoi@hallym.ac.kr (B.Y.C.); rnlduadkfk136@hallym.ac.kr (A.R.K.); sshlee@hallym.ac.kr (S.H.L.); zxnm01220@gmail.com (D.K.H.); jd1422@hanmail.net (J.H.J.); bagmingyu50@gmail.com (M.K.P.)

2 Department of Medical Science, College of Medicine, Hallym University, Chuncheon 24252, Korea; ehdgus6312@gmail.com

* Correspondence: swsuh@hallym.ac.kr

Abstract: Acidosis in the brain plays an important role in neuronal injury and is a common feature of several neurological diseases. It has been reported that the sodium–hydrogen exchanger-1 (NHE-1) is a key mediator of acidosis-induced neuronal injury. It modulates the concentration of intra- and extra-cellular sodium and hydrogen ions. During the ischemic state, excessive sodium ions enter neurons and inappropriately activate the sodium–calcium exchanger (NCX). Zinc can also enter neurons through voltage-gated calcium channels and NCX. Here, we tested the hypothesis that zinc enters the intracellular space through NCX and the subsequent zinc accumulation induces neuronal cell death after global cerebral ischemia (GCI). Thus, we conducted the present study to confirm whether inhibition of NHE-1 by amiloride attenuates zinc accumulation and subsequent hippocampus neuronal death following GCI. Mice were subjected to GCI by bilateral common carotid artery (BCCA) occlusion for 30 min, followed by restoration of blood flow and resuscitation. Amiloride (10 mg/kg, intraperitoneally (*i.p.*)) was immediately injected, which reduced zinc accumulation and neuronal death after GCI. Therefore, the present study demonstrates that amiloride attenuates GCI-induced neuronal injury, likely via the prevention of intracellular zinc accumulation. Consequently, we suggest that amiloride may have a high therapeutic potential for the prevention of GCI-induced neuronal death.

Keywords: global cerebral ischemia; amiloride; sodium–hydrogen exchanger-1; zinc; neuronal death; neuroprotection

1. Introduction

Ischemic stroke is one of the most severe cerebral pathological conditions and can manifest via a number of clinical symptoms such as problems in cognition, dizziness, or loss of vision on one side of the visual field [1]. In particular, the development of ischemic conditions in the brain is very dangerous because only a momentary lack of adequate blood flow to the brain can lead to oxygen deprivation, insufficient nutrient provision, and potentially irreversible neural injury [2–4]. There are two basic types of ischemic injury: global and focal ischemia. Global ischemia impacts wide areas of brain tissue at once due to the blockage of blood flow to an entire region of the brain, while focal ischemia is limited to a specific region of the brain tissue and is due to the more local disruption of cerebral blood flow. Ischemia-induced brain damage can be recovered by early reperfusion, but this reperfusion process can also initiate independent cascades of cell death pathways such as zinc release, microglial activation, and blood–brain barrier (BBB) disruption [5]. If the interruption of blood circulation happens for an extended period prior to the restoration of circulation, brain damage can be permanent.

Furthermore, after a long period of ischemia, secondary brain damage occurs when blood flow is initiated, which is known as "reperfusion injury". The sudden recovery of blood supply leads to mitochondrial dysfunction, producing excessive reactive oxygen species (ROS) and, finally, cell death [6]. Under healthy conditions, superoxide production via neuronal nicotinamide adenine dinucleotide phosphate (NADPH) oxidase is thought to play a part in normal physiological processes such as long-term potentiation and intracellular signaling [7,8]. However, under ischemic conditions, mitochondrial dysfunction and excessive ROS generation predominate and promote pathological responses such as leukocyte invasion and the disruption of the BBB [9,10]. Also, tissue pH is typically reduced to 6.0–6.5 during ischemia, falling even lower during severe ischemic conditions [11–13]. As a result, this study suggests that the increase in NADPH activity after ischemia may also promote cell death by acidifying brain cells.

Zinc is one of the most essential transition metals in our body, especially in the brain. Furthermore, zinc regulates physiological functions that control DNA synthesis, cell division, and signal transduction. Most of the zinc is present in a protein-bound form in neuronal cytoplasm. Free or chelatable zinc is localized within the vesicles of synaptic terminals [14,15]. Taken together, these lines of circumstantial evidence suggest that zinc plays a key role in maintaining cellular homeostasis. However, previous studies have demonstrated that excessive neuronal zinc accumulation occurs after traumatic brain injury, ischemia, hyperglycemia, and epilepsy [16–19]. Under these various pathological conditions, ROS changes the protein-mediated sequestration of zinc and, thus, increases intracellular free zinc levels which increases ROS production. If this condition is maintained for long periods, it can lead to neuronal death [18]. Several neurological injuries, accelerate zinc release from synaptic vesicles, and zinc then moves into neurons via multiple classes of membrane-bound channels [20,21].

Sodium–hydrogen exchangers (NHEs) are membrane transporters that mediate hydrogen efflux into cells. Sodium–hydrogen exchanger-1 (NHE-1) is a ubiquitous and essential membrane ion transporter that mediates the electroneutral exchange of hydrogen and sodium to regulate intracellular pH [22]. Other NHEs, namely, NHE-2–5, indicate more distinct cell-type- and tissue-dependent expressions than NHE-1 and play key roles in regulating transcellular sodium and potassium ion absorption [23]. The NHE-6 expression is localized to early endosomes [24]. The NHE-7 and -8 isoforms have not been localized in the brain, and the NHE-9 isoform is localized to late recycling endosomes [25]. Here, we focused on NHE-1 which is expressed in high abundance in the brain.

Amiloride, also known as thiazide, is related to other loop diuretic agents and blocks sodium hydrogen exchanger-1 [26]. Amiloride, an inhibitor of NHE-1, has demonstrated neuroprotective effects in various neuropathological conditions involving brain injuries such as ischemia, dementia, and epilepsy [27,28]. Previous studies have suggested that injection of amiloride can reduce cerebral-hypoxia-induced neuronal death after seizure and spinal cord injury [29–31]. Under the acidic conditions found in the post-ischemic state, as NHE-1 becomes activated, hydrogen is released into the extracellular space and sodium moves into the intracellular compartment. Thus, intracellular sodium is increased and the sodium–calcium exchanger (NCX) becomes activated, so that sodium is released into the extracellular space driving calcium entry, leading to a calcium overload state and, ultimately, resulting in neuronal death. Considering this, we hypothesized that not only calcium, but also zinc may enter via NCX and that NHE-1 blockade by amiloride decreases zinc accumulation and neuronal death through reduced NCX activity. Therefore, we investigated whether the administration of amiloride (10 mg/kg, intraperitoneally (*i.p.*)) reduces zinc accumulation, neuronal degeneration, oxidative stress, and microtubule damage after global cerebral ischemia. As a result, the present study proved that the administration of amiloride reduces ischemia-induced neuronal degeneration.

2. Results

2.1. *Amiloride Reduced Global Cerebral Ischemia-Induced Hippocampus Neuronal Death after 24 Hour Post-Insult*

To investigate whether amiloride has neuroprotective effects after global cerebral ischemia (GCI)-induced hippocampus neuronal death, experimental mice were immediately intraperitoneally injected with amiloride (10 mg/kg) after GCI. The mice were sacrificed 24 h after GCI with or without amiloride treatment. After insult, a histological evaluation to detect degenerating neurons was conducted in the hippocampal subiculum (Sub), cornus ammonis 1 (CA1), CA2, and CA3 regions. Fluoro-Jade B (FJB) staining showed widespread neuronal degeneration in the Sub, CA1, CA2, and CA3 regions of the hippocampus ($p < 0.05$) (Figure 1A). This staining protocol is a sensitive and selective marker of degenerating neurons. The number of degenerating neurons was increased in the GCI-induced group compared with the sham-operated group. When compared with the GCI-vehicle-treated groups, the amiloride-injected groups showed a dramatically reduced number of degenerating hippocampal neurons. Figure 1B shows the quantified FJB (+) neurons in the Sub, CA1, CA2, and CA3 regions. Amiloride-administered groups displayed a reduction of FJB (+) neurons of approximately 64% in the Sub (GCI-vehicle, 76.9 ± 8.4; GCI-amiloride, 27.2 ± 10.5), 84% in the CA1 (GCI-vehicle, 126.2 ± 18.5; GCI-amiloride, 19.5 ± 17.6), 83% in the CA2 (GCI-vehicle, 125.3 ± 22; GCI-amiloride, 20.7 ± 17.9), and 50% in the CA3 (GCI-vehicle, 220.6 ± 30.3; GCI-amiloride, 109.5 ± 29) regions compared with the vehicle-treated groups.

2.2. *Amiloride Reduced Global Cerebral Ischemia-Induced Hippocampal Zinc Accumulation after 24 Hour Post-Insult*

To estimate GCI-induced zinc accumulation, brain sections were histologically evaluated by *N*-(6-methoxy-8-quinolyl)-para-toluenesulfonamide (TSQ) staining 24 h after GCI. Zinc accumulation is known to advance the neuronal NADPH oxidase activity and ROS responsible for neuronal death. Under normal conditions, zinc levels are controlled by zinc transporters and zinc-binding proteins [32]. However, under conditions such as ischemia, traumatic brain injury, and seizure, neuronal death occurs in part by the destruction of zinc homeostasis. Thus, we performed TSQ fluorescence staining to confirm whether amiloride can reduce zinc accumulation in the brain hippocampal CA1 region. The intensity of TSQ staining in the CA1 region was reduced in the amiloride-treated group compared with the GCI-induced group ($p < 0.05$) (Figure 1C,D). Amiloride-administered groups displayed an approximately 44% reduction of TSQ (+) neurons in the CA1 region (GCI-vehicle, 36.9 ± 5.9; GCI-amiloride, 20.6 ± 4.1) compared with the vehicle-treated groups.

2.3. *Amiloride Reduced Global Cerebral Ischemia-Induced Astrocyte and Microglial Activation 24 Hour Post-Insult*

Multiple studies have previously reported that ischemia induces astrocyte and microglial activation in the brain hippocampal region [3,18,33], and it is well known that inflammation contributes to the severity of astrocyte and microglial activation. In addition, activated astrocytes are potentially harmful, because they can produce nitric oxide synthase (NOS) and neurotoxic nitric oxide (NO). To test whether amiloride affects GCI-induced glial activation, we performed immunofluorescence staining using the marker glial fibrillary acidic protein (GFAP) and ionized calcium-binding adaptor molecule 1 (Iba-1). We confirmed an assessment of the microglia number, morphology, and intensity and astrocyte intensity [34]. Global cerebral ischemia triggers astroglia and microglial activation which is considered to have macrophage-like activity. However, activated astrocytes were reduced by approximately 45% in the GCI–amiloride groups compared with the GCI-vehicle groups in the CA1 region (GCI-vehicle, 33.2 ± 3.3; GCI–amiloride, 18.2 ± 1.8). Further, activated microglia were reduced by 32% in the GCI–amiloride groups in the CA1 region (GCI-vehicle, 5.8 ± 0.3; GCI–amiloride, 3.9 ± 0.3) (Figure 2B,D).

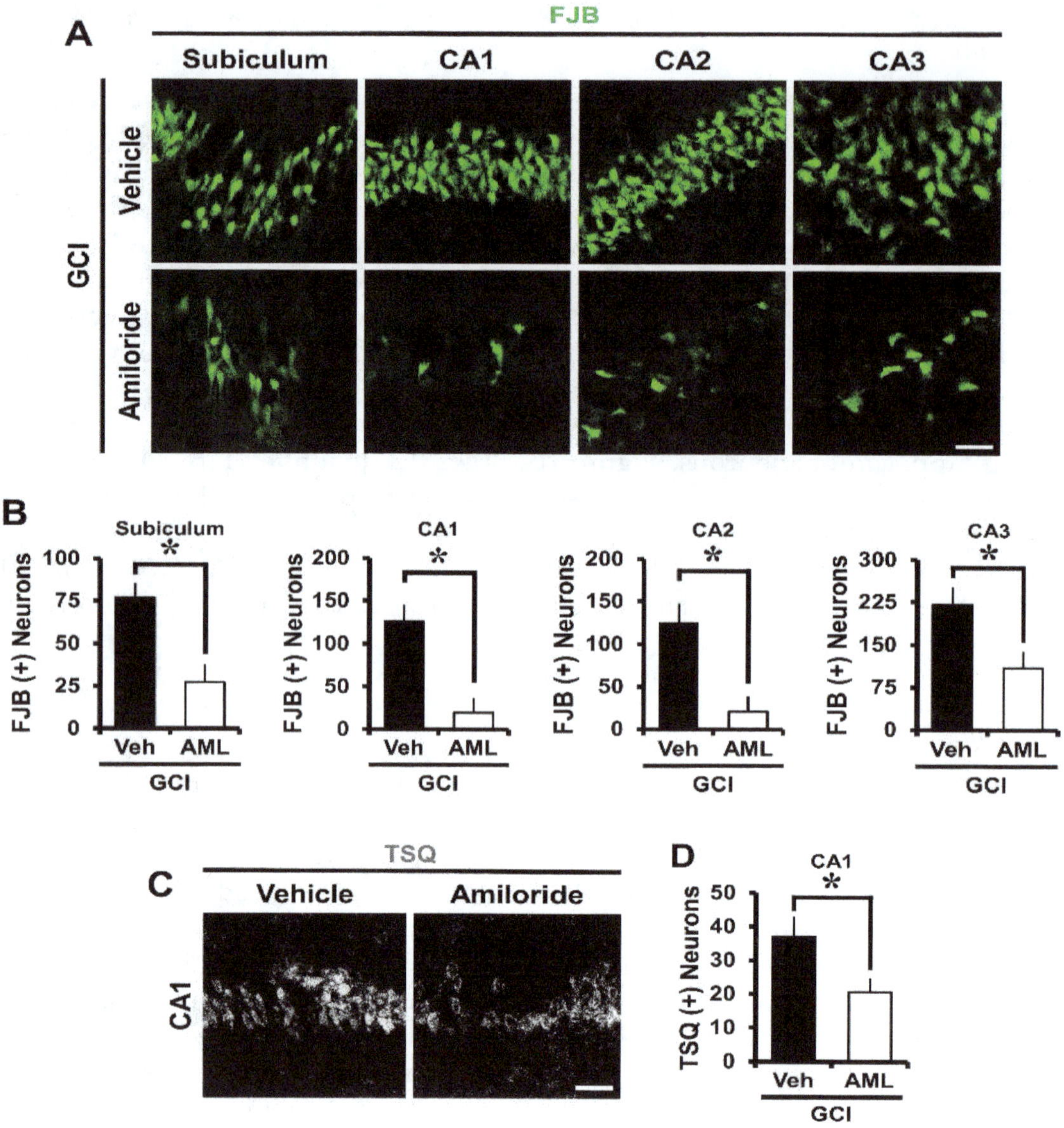

Figure 1. Amiloride treatment decreased the number of degenerating neurons and zinc accumulation after global cerebral ischemia (GCI). GCI-induced hippocampus neuronal death was confirmed in the subiculum (Sub), cornus ammonis 1 (CA1), CA2, and CA3 regions after ischemic insult. Zinc accumulation was confirmed in the CA1 region after ischemic insult. (**A**) Fluorescent images show degenerated neurons in the Sub, CA1, CA2, and CA3 regions. Intraperitoneal post-treatment with amiloride (10 mg/kg) reduced neuronal death in the Sub, CA1, CA2, and CA3 regions at 24 h after ischemia. Scale bar = 20 μm. (**B**) Bar graph displaying the quantification of degenerating neurons in the hippocampal regions. The number of FJB (+) neurons was decreased in the amiloride-injected (10 mg/kg) group in the Sub, CA1, CA2, and CA3 regions compared with the vehicle-treated group (GCI-vehicle, $n = 8$; GCI-amiloride, $n = 8$). (**C**) Representative images show *N*-(6-methoxy-8-quinolyl)-para-toluenesulfonamide (TSQ) (+) neurons in the CA1 region. Scale bar = 20 μm. (**D**) The bar graph indicates the TSQ (+) neurons in the hippocampal CA1 region (GCI-vehicle, $n = 8$; GCI-amiloride, $n = 10$). Data are mean ± S.E.M. * Considerably different from the vehicle-treated group, $p < 0.05$. (Mann–Whitney U test (B) Sub: z = 2.626, $p = 0.007$; CA1: z = 2.838, $p = 0.003$; CA2: z = 2.836, $p = 0.003$; CA3: z = 2.205, $p = 0.028$; (D) CA1: z = 2.134, $p = 0.034$).

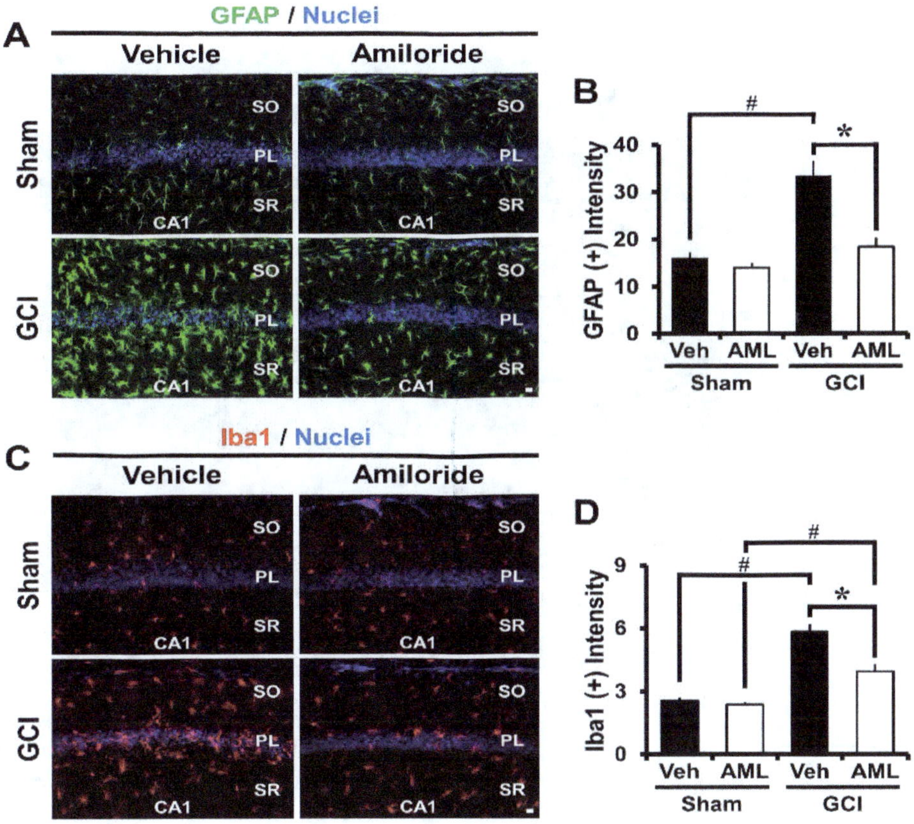

Figure 2. Amiloride treatment reduced astrocyte and microglial activation. GCI induces an inflammatory response by promoting astrocyte and microglia activation in the damaged brain. This figure shows astrocyte and microglia activation in the CA1 region 24 h after GCI. (**A**,**C**) show glial fibrillary acidic protein (GFAP) and Ionized calcium-binding adaptor molecule-1 (Iba-1) activation and (**B**,**D**) show GFAP and Iba-1 quantification in the CA1 region from sham-operated or GCI-induced mice. It was increased in the GCI-induced group compared with the sham-operated group. However, the amiloride-treated group showed reduced astrocyte and microglia activation after GCI. Scale bar = 20 μm. (Sham-vehicle, $n = 5$; sham-amiloride, $n = 5$; GCI-vehicle, $n = 6$; GCI-amiloride, $n = 8$). Data are mean ± SEM. * Considerably different from the vehicle-treated group, $p < 0.05$; # sham versus vehicle-operated group; sham versus vehicle-treated group, $p < 0.05$. (Kruskal–Wallis test (B) Chi square = 14.612, df = 3, $p = 0.002$; (D) Chi square = 18.606, df = 3, $p < 0.001$) (SO: stratum oriens; PL: pyramidal cell layer; SR: stratum lacunosum-moleculare).

2.4. Amiloride Reduces Global Cerebral Ischemia-Induced Oxidative Damage after 24 Hour Post-Insult

We estimated oxidative stress by using 4-hydroxynonenal (4HNE) staining. The brain was immunohistochemically stained with a 4HNE antibody 24 h after global cerebral ischemia induction to discover whether hippocampal neurons had experienced oxidative stress. The sham-vehicle and amiloride-injected groups showed no difference in 4HNE fluorescence signals. However, the 4HNE fluorescence signal of the GCI-vehicle groups increased in the hippocampal Sub, CA1, CA2, and CA3 regions. The amiloride-treated group showed a significant reduction of 4HNE intensity compared with the vehicle-treated groups (Figure 3A). Oxidative damage was reduced in the GCI-amiloride groups compared with the GCI-vehicle groups by approximately 42% in the Sub (GCI-vehicle, 21.8 ± 2.4; GCI-amiloride, 12.6 ± 0.5), 48% in the CA1 (GCI-vehicle, 23.5 ± 2.3; GCI-amiloride, 12.2 ± 1.5), 36% in the CA2 (GCI-vehicle, 21.5 ± 2.4; GCI-amiloride, 13.7 ± 1.4), and 48% in the CA3 (GCI-vehicle, 31.2 ± 3.3; GCI-amiloride, 16.1 ± 2.2) regions (Figure 3B).

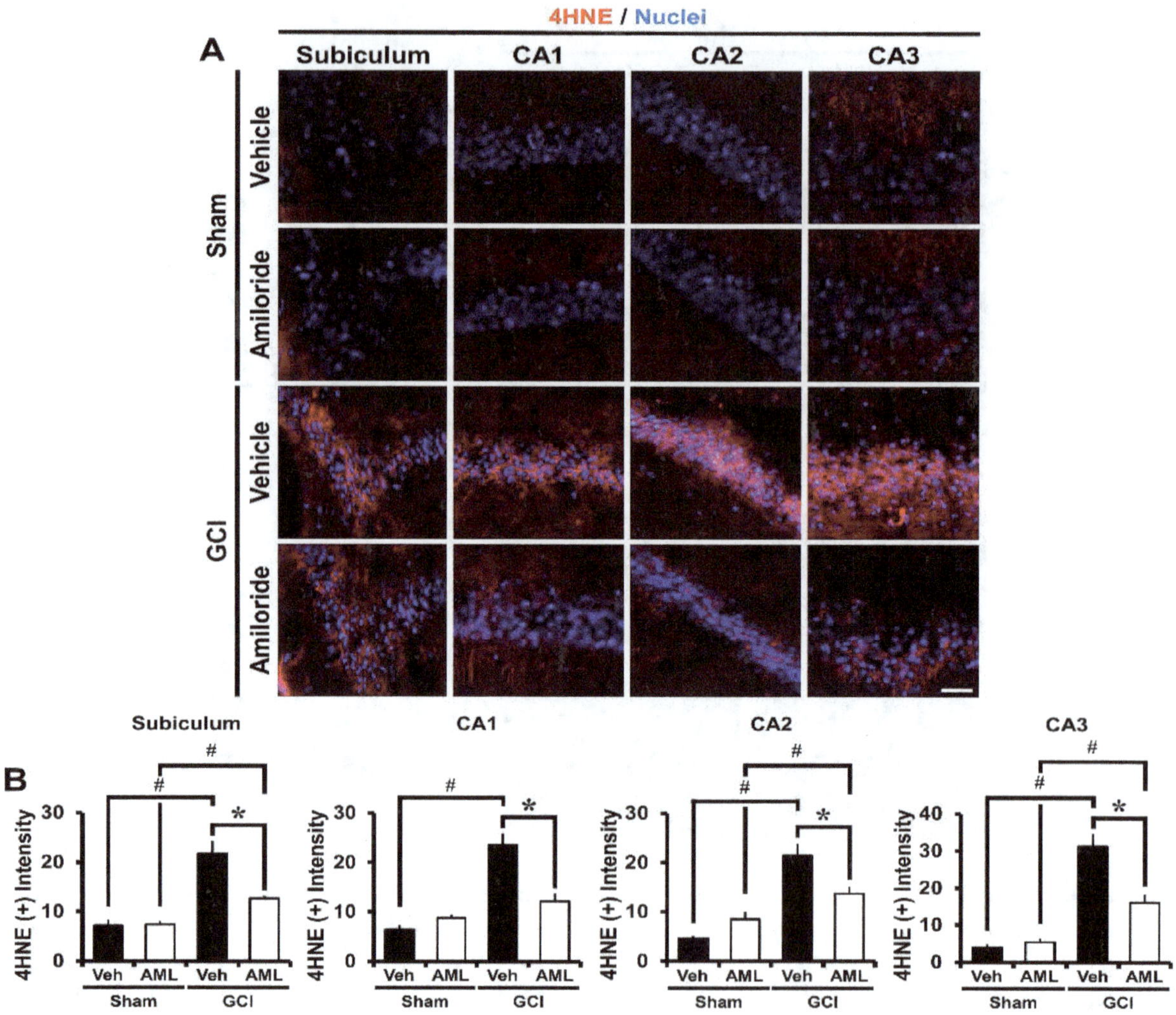

Figure 3. Amiloride reduced oxidative injury after GCI. Oxidative injury was detected by 4-hydroxynonenal (4HNE, red color) staining from the hippocampal Sub, CA1, CA2, and CA3 regions 24 h after GCI. (**A**) Sham-operated groups showed minimal 4HNE fluorescence signals in the hippocampus. Amiloride-treated groups showed reduced immunoreactive fluorescence intensity for 4HNE in the hippocampus compared with the vehicle-treated group after GCI. Scale bar = 20 μm. (**B**) The bar graph presents the 4HNE fluorescence intensity in the Sub, CA1, CA2, and CA3 regions. The fluorescence intensity showed a significant difference among groups (sham-vehicle, $n = 6$; sham-amiloride, $n = 5$; GCI-vehicle, $n = 8$; GCI-amiloride, $n = 8$). Data are mean ± S.E.M. * Considerably different from the vehicle-treated group, $p < 0.05$; # sham versus vehicle-operated group, sham versus vehicle-treated group, $p < 0.05$. (Kruskal–Wallis test (B) Sub: Chi square = 22.444, df = 3, $p < 0.001$; CA1: Chi square = 17.896, df = 3, $p < 0.001$; CA2: Chi square = 20.967, df = 3, $p < 0.001$; CA3: Chi square = 20.986, df = 3, $p < 0.001$).

2.5. Amiloride Reduced Global Cerebral Ischemia-Induced Microtubule Damage after 24 Hour Post-Insult

To evaluate whether GCI-induced microtubule damage occurred, brain sections were histologically processed with antibodies against microtubule-associated protein 2 (MAP2) 24 h after GCI. The GCI-vehicle groups showed a significant reduction in MAP2 immunoreactivity (IR) in the hippocampus and cortex compared with the GCI-amiloride group, indicating a loss of microtubules. Amiloride injection reduced GCI-induced microtubule damage compared with the vehicle-treated group (Figure 4A). Microtubule intensity was increased in the GCI-amiloride groups compared with the GCI-vehicle groups by approximately 42% in the Sub (GCI-vehicle, 41.9 ± 6.3; GCI-amiloride, 72.5 ± 7.2), 60% in the CA1 (GCI-vehicle, 43.3 ± 8.4; GCI-amiloride, 109.7 ± 12.5), 43% in the CA2

(GCI-vehicle, 56.2 ± 11; GCI-amiloride, 99.6 ± 10.1), and 59% in the CA3 (GCI-vehicle, 23.2 ± 5.9; GCI-amiloride, 57.2 ± 10.6) regions (Figure 4B).

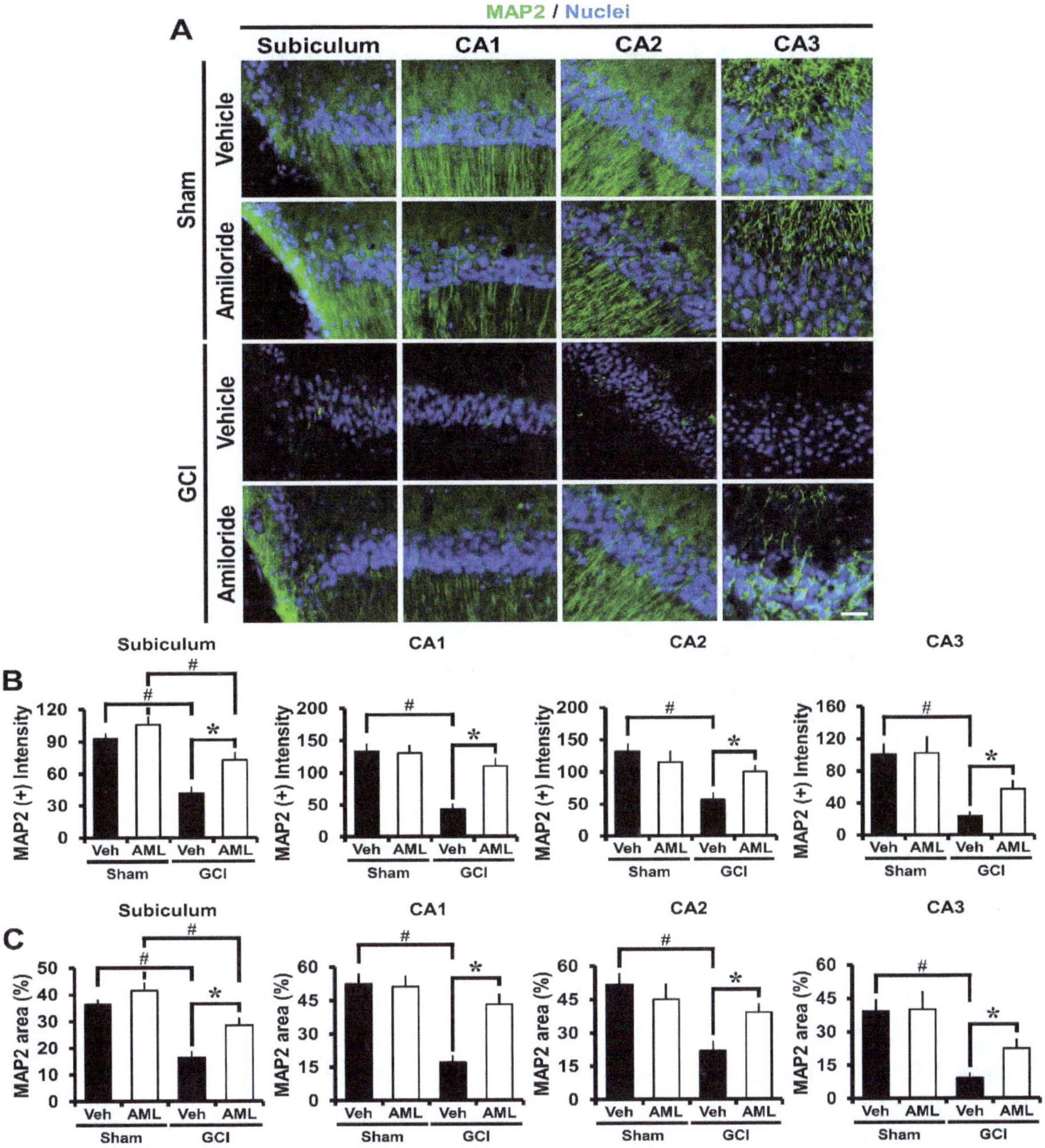

Figure 4. Microtubule damage was detected by microtubule-associated protein 2 (MAP2, green color) staining at the hippocampal Sub, CA1, CA2, and CA3 regions 24 h after GCI. (**A**) Sham-operated groups showed MAP2 fluorescence signals in the hippocampus. Amiloride-administered groups showed a reduced microtubule loss in the hippocampal regions compared with the vehicle-treated group. Scale bar = 20 μm. (**B**) The bar graph indicates the MAP2 fluorescence intensity in the hippocampus. (**C**) The bar graph indicates the MAP2 percent area in the hippocampus (sham-vehicle, $n = 6$; sham-amiloride, $n = 5$; GCI-vehicle, $n = 8$; GCI-amiloride, $n = 8$). Data are mean ± S.E.M. * Considerably different from the vehicle-treated group, $p < 0.05$; # sham versus vehicle-operated group, sham versus vehicle-treated group, $p < 0.05$. (Kruskal–Wallis test (B) Sub: Chi square = 18.901, df = 3, $p < 0.001$; CA1: Chi square = 15.166, df = 3, $p < 0.002$; CA2: Chi square = 15.054, df = 3, $p < 0.002$; CA3: Chi square = 17.137, df = 3, $p < 0.001$).

2.6. Amiloride Prevented Global Cerebral Ischemia-Induced Blood–Brain Barrier Disruption after 24 Hour Post-Insult

To verify the degree of blood–brain barrier (BBB) disruption, we stained brain sections to evaluate extravasation of serum immunoglobulin G (IgG) by using immunohistochemistry as described before [35,36]. In sham-operated brain sections, leakage of IgG was not detected. However, in ischemia-induced mice, we observed excessive extravascular IgG leakage in the hippocampus (Figure 5A). Figure 5B shows a bar graph of the scale of IgG extravasation from the damaged BBB in the hippocampus. IgG leakage was reduced by 24% in the GCI-amiloride group compared with the GCI-vehicle group (GCI-vehicle, 1.37 ± 0.09; GCI-amiloride, 1.04 ± 0.07) (Figure 5B).

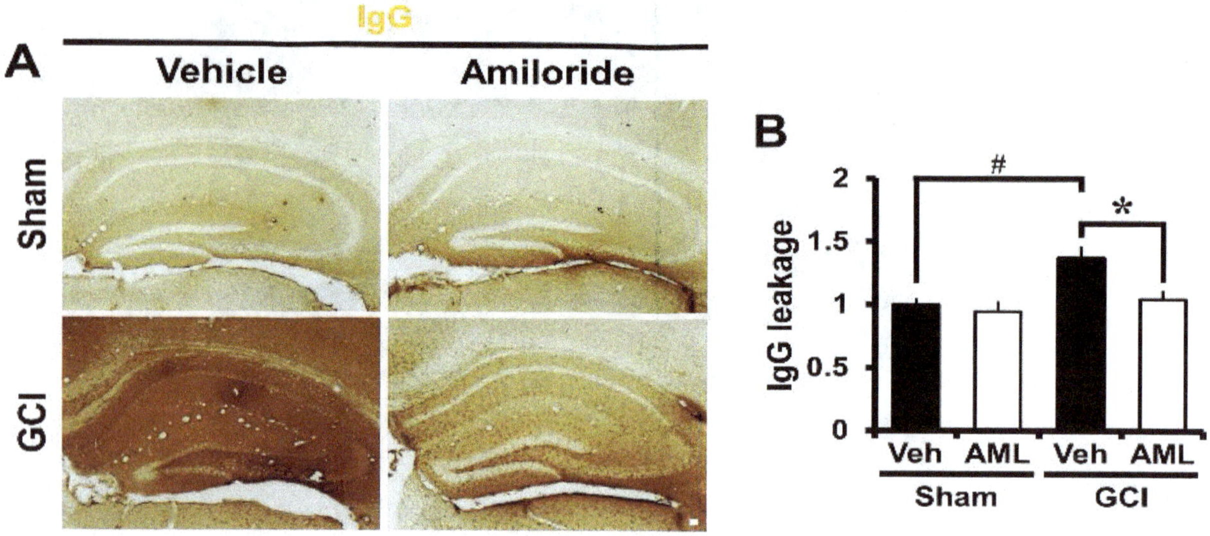

Figure 5. GCI-induced blood–brain barrier (BBB) disruption was decreased by amiloride administration. Brain sections were stained with antibodies against IgG to detect BBB disruption. (**A**) Indicates magnification (4×) of a microscopic image of IgG staining in the hippocampus in each group. These images indicate that BBB disruption occurred after GCI. The GCI-amiloride group had decreased leakage of serum IgG in the hippocampus compared with the GCI-vehicle group. Scale bar = 100 μm. (**B**) Bar graph shows the quantification of IgG serum extravasation in the hippocampus (sham-to-GCI ratio, sham-vehicle, $n = 6$; sham-amiloride, $n = 5$; GCI-vehicle, $n = 7$; GCI-amiloride, $n = 8$). Data are mean ± SEM. * Considerably different from the vehicle-treated group, $p < 0.05$; # sham versus vehicle-operated group; $p < 0.05$. (Kruskal–Wallis test (B) Chi square = 11.126, df = 3, $p = 0.011$).

2.7. Amiloride Improves Global Cerebral Ischemia-Induced Survival of Hippocampal Neurons at 3 Days Post-Insult

To investigate whether amiloride promotes neuronal survival after GCI-induced hippocampus, amiloride (10 mg/kg) was immediately injected to the intraperitoneal space after termination of the blood reperfusion process. Both vehicle- and amiloride-administrated cohorts were sacrificed at 3 days following ischemic insult. After the insult, a histological evaluation using NeuN staining to detect and quantify newly generated neurons was conducted in the hippocampal Sub, CA1, CA2, and CA3 regions. NeuN positive neurons were widespread in the hippocampal regions we examined ($p < 0.05$) and increased in number rapidly (Figure 6A). Figure 6B shows the counted NeuN (+) neurons in the hippocampal regions. Amiloride-administered groups displayed an increase of NeuN (+) neurons of 26% in the Sub (GCI-vehicle, 115.1 ± 4.0; GCI-amiloride, 156.4 ± 10.8), 17% in the CA1 (GCI-vehicle, 177.7 ± 3.5; GCI-amiloride, 213.4 ± 11.1), 17% in the CA2 (GCI-vehicle, 219.5 ± 5.9; GCI-amiloride, 265 ± 10.9), and 17% in the CA3 (GCI-vehicle, 251.2 ± 8.2; GCI-amiloride, 304.5 ± 13.2) regions compared with the vehicle-treated groups.

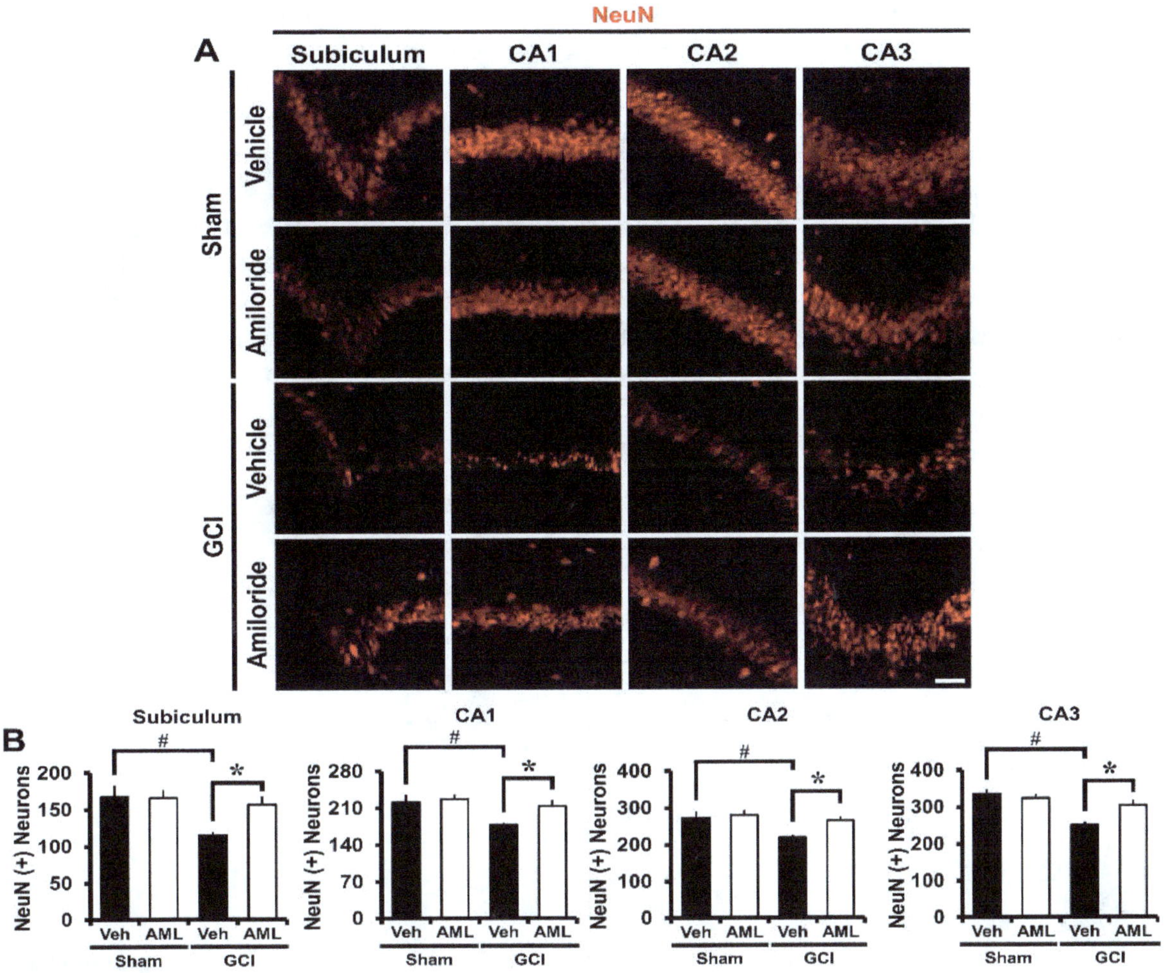

Figure 6. Amiloride treatment improves neuronal survival after GCI. The presence of live neurons after ischemic insult was confirmed in the Sub, CA1, CA2, and CA3 regions. (**A**) Fluorescent images show surviving neurons in the Sub, CA1, CA2, and CA3 regions. Intraperitoneal post-treatment with amiloride (10 mg/kg) increased the number of live neurons in the Sub, CA1, CA2, and CA3 regions at 3 days post-ischemia. Scale bar = 20 μm. (**B**) Bar graph displaying the quantification of surviving neurons in hippocampal subregions. The number of NeuN (+) neurons was increased in the amiloride-injected (10 mg/kg) group in the Sub, CA1, CA2, and CA3 regions compared with the vehicle-treated group (GCI-vehicle, $n = 8$; GCI-amiloride, $n = 6$). Data are mean ± SEM. * Considerably different from the vehicle-treated group, $p < 0.05$; # sham versus vehicle-operated group, $p < 0.05$. (Kruskal–Wallis test (B) Sub: Chi square = 14.214, df = 3, $p = 0.003$; CA1: Chi square = 13.422, df = 3, $p = 0.004$; CA2: Chi square = 14.249, df = 3, $p = 0.003$; CA3: Chi square = 16.158, df = 3, $p = 0.001$).

3. Discussion

Previous studies have demonstrated that amiloride showed neuroprotective effects in two different stroke models; middle cerebral artery occlusion (MCAO) in rat and transient forebrain ischemia in gerbil [27,37]. However, no studies have been performed with the global cerebral ischemia model with mice. The present study investigated whether amiloride administration has potential therapeutic effects for GCI-induced hippocampus neuronal damage and zinc accumulation via inhibition of NHE-1 in mice. Consequently, we found that amiloride significantly reduced zinc accumulation, neuronal degeneration, oxidative damage, microtubule damage, astrocyte and microglial activation, and BBB disruption.

Under ischemic conditions, blood flow to the brain is rapidly and dramatically reduced. This phenomenon leads to a lack of oxygen and other substrates to the nervous tissue.

Thus, the extracellular concentration of glucose is quickly reduced [38–40]. As a result, the physiological glycolysis process was disturbed, and glucose 6-phosphate altered ribulose 5-phosphate by the pentose phosphate pathway (PPP). While glucose is modified to ribulose 5-phosphate, hydrogen is released and triggers NHE-1 [41,42]. When the intracellular hydrogen ion concentration increases, NHE-1 is activated in the cell membrane. NHE-1 activation contributes to neuronal electron exchange via sodium and hydrogen ion exchange across the cell membrane [43]. Previous studies have shown that NHE-1 inhibitors reduced the activity of NCX [27,44–47]. Furthermore, additional studies demonstrated that zinc enters intracellularly through NCX [48,49]. Thus, we can speculate that NHE-1 inhibition may indirectly inhibit zinc influx into neurons. Also, ischemia-induced ROS formation degrades zinc-binding proteins in the intracellular space, thus significantly increasing free zinc levels within the intracellular space [18]. As this cycle becomes sustained, the accumulation of excessive amounts of zinc contributes to neuronal cell death [3,18,27,50] (Figure 7).

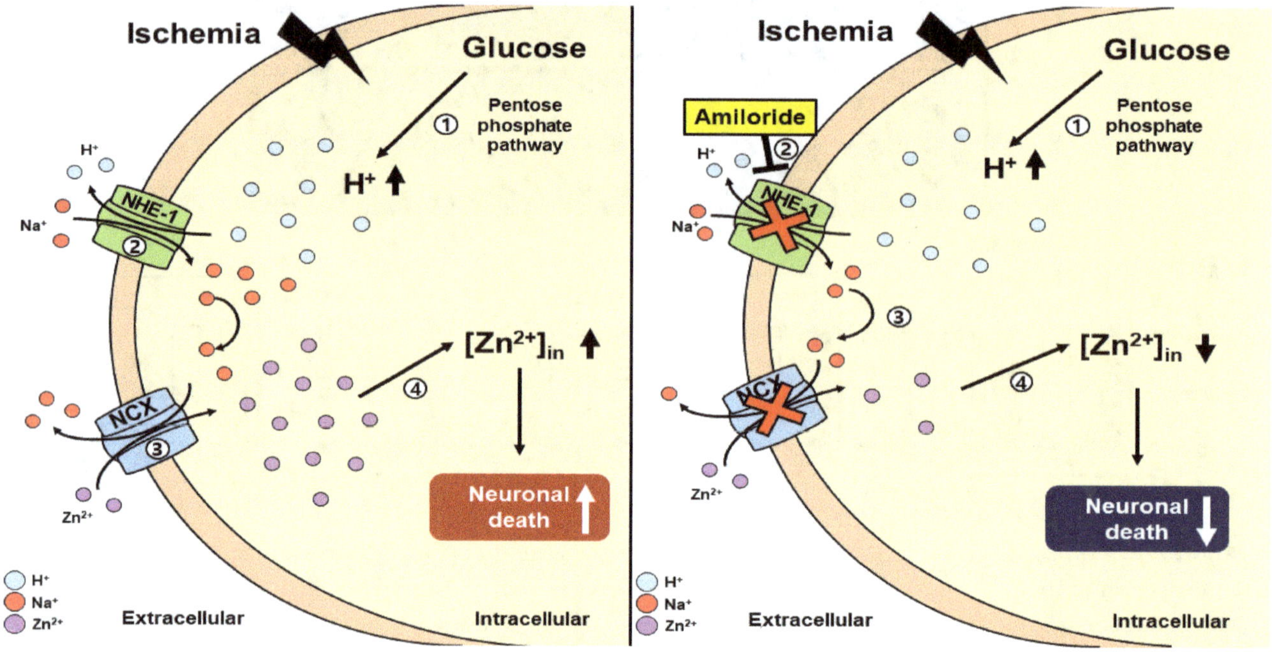

Figure 7. This schematic illustration shows amiloride action via inhibition and downregulation of the sodium–hydrogen exchanger-1 (NHE-1) channel. (**A**) [1] Global cerebral ischemia insult results in increasing levels of intracellular hydrogen. [2] Hydrogen ions are moved to the extracellular space via NHE-1. Sodium ions are moved to the intracellular space via NHE-1. [3] When sodium is overloaded in the intracellular space, it is released into the extracellular space through the sodium–calcium exchanger (NCX). Extracellular zinc enters the cell through NCX. [4] Intracellular zinc accumulation occurs, leading to neuronal death. (**B**) However, [1] after global cerebral ischemia, [2] amiloride administration inhibits intracellular sodium accumulation via the NHE-1 channel. [3] Sodium does not enter the intracellular space and becomes NCX inactivated. [4] Because of this agent's mechanism, zinc accumulation is reduced, resulting in reduced neuronal death after global cerebral ischemic insult.

Amiloride has previously been described as a diuretic and as a non-specific inhibitor for NHE-1. However, it has been used as an NHE-1 inhibitor in several studies [26,51]. Additionally, amiloride has been known to cross the blood–brain barrier and has neuroprotective effects against global cerebral ischemia. Several studies have demonstrated that amiloride has neuroprotective properties using a dose of 10 mg/kg [27,52–54]. Following this logic, we hypothesized that GCI-induced hippocampal damage can be protected by reducing intracellular zinc accumulation through inhibition of NHE-1 [27,55].

The histological evaluation, we performed further supports our hypothesis. The number of hippocampal degenerating neurons was estimated using FJB staining. The number of FJB fluorescence-signal-positive neurons in the hippocampal Sub, CA1, CA2, and CA3 regions was significantly reduced in the amiloride-administered group. Intraneuronal free zinc accumulation was displayed by TSQ staining. The number of the TSQ-positive neurons were significantly reduced in the amiloride-administered groups compared with the vehicle groups. These results demonstrated that the intraneuronal free zinc accumulation was reduced by inhibiting NHE-1 channels using amiloride. We confirmed that under ischemic conditions, zinc accumulation increases, and neuronal death occur. However, blocking NHE-1 by injection of amiloride reduces zinc accumulation and, subsequently, neuronal death was reduced. Additionally, we confirmed the presence of live neurons at 3 days following ischemic insult and stained for NeuN to identify neurons that survived the insult. The number of NeuN positive neurons in the hippocampal Sub, CA1, CA2 and CA3 regions were greater in the amiloride-administered group. So, we concluded that the administration of amiloride improved the survival of hippocampal neurons after 3 days post-insult.

Astrocytes and microglia play important roles in the brain. During neurological disorders such as ischemia, neuroinflammation, and neurodegenerative disease, astrocytes and microglia are over activated. Under ischemic conditions, activated astrocytes, together with reactive microglia, release several pro-inflammatory factors such as tumor necrosis factor-α (TNF-α), ROS, NO, and interleukin-1β (IL-1β), which exacerbate tissue damage [18,56–58]. Previous studies have demonstrated that NHE-1 expression occurs in astrocyte and microglial cells. In addition, NHE-1 activity caused by ischemia activates astrocyte and microglial cells, leading to neuronal death [18,59]. So, we thought that the administration of amiloride, an NHE-1 inhibitor, would reduce the activation of astrocytes and microglia, and thus reduce neuronal death. The present study verified astrocyte activation by GFAP and microglia activation by Iba-1 immunofluorescence staining in the hippocampal CA1 region. We found that amiloride administration reduced reactive astrocyte and microglial activation after GCI.

Ischemic damage leaded to microtubule damage and ROS production. In the present study, we found that amiloride administration reduced microtubule damage after GCI. ROS formation is caused via multiple intracellular signaling cascades, such as iron-associated free radical formation, depletion of antioxidant enzymes, and an increase in the breakdown of lipids and fatty acids after GCI [60]. Because of this, the zinc accumulation described above occurs and microtubules are damaged [18,61]. In addition, several previous studies have suggested that peroxynitrite (PN) toxicity is mediated by intracellular zinc release [62,63]. Peroxynitrite is produced by a combination of nitric oxide and superoxide. It has been reported that PN are endogenous reactive nitrogen species formed when superoxide radicals, or oxygen reacts with nitric oxide formed by inducible nitric oxide synthase (iNOS). Peroxynitrite can induce cytoplasmic free zinc release, mitochondria dysfunction, and lead to BBB disruption, and finally neuronal death, in several types of brain injuries [64–66]. To test whether ROS activation was reduced by amiloride, 4HNE staining was performed in the hippocampal Sub, CA1, CA2, and CA3 regions. The 4HNE fluorescence signal was significantly increased in the GCI-vehicle group. For the amiloride-administered group after GCI, the 4HNE fluorescence signal was significantly decreased in hippocampal regions compared with the GCI-vehicle group. Amiloride, which inhibits NHE-1 and decreases NCX activity, reduces ROS formation by regulating the intracellular ion balance.

Finally, we evaluated the BBB balance after GCI. Abnormal intracellular zinc accumulation and vesicular zinc release may mediate BBB disruption after brain insults such as ischemia, multiple sclerosis, and traumatic brain injury [67]. Thus, administration of amiloride may decrease zinc accumulation and reduces BBB disruption after GCI. After GCI insult, the BBB was destroyed, leading to extravasation of plasma components, such as erythrocytes, leukocytes, and several immunoglobulins. BBB disruption triggers neurodegenerative processes and produces neurotoxic substrates, which causes brain dysfunction that is deleterious to synapse function and disturbs neural transmission [68,69]. So, to evaluate the effects of amiloride on BBB disruption, we conducted IgG staining. As a result, we found that the IgG staining intensity was reduced in the amiloride-administered group compared with the vehicle group after GCI. This result indicates that the neuroprotective provided by amiloride administration might be mediated via protection against BBB disruption, which is one of the main mechanisms associated with GCI-induced neuronal death [70].

Taken together, we conclude that inhibition of NHE-1 by amiloride reduces neuronal death and zinc accumulation. We found that amiloride reduced various deleterious features associated with GCI, such as neurodegeneration, zinc accumulation, oxidative damage, microtubule damage, glial activation, and BBB disruption, which strongly indicates that amiloride administration has neuroprotective effects by decreasing ROS production and zinc accumulation in hippocampal neurons through the inhibition of NHE-1. Therefore, the present study suggests that amiloride can be a potential therapeutic tool to prevent ischemia-induced neuronal death.

4. Materials and Methods

4.1. Ethics Statement

The present study was performed in accordance with the protocols of the Guidelines for the Use and Care of Laboratory Animals, allowed by the National Institutes of Health. Animal studies were conducted in accordance with the guidelines of the Committee on Animal Use for Study and Education at Hallym University (protocol # Hallym-2018-32; Data of approval: July 19,2018). We sacrificed mice under isoflurane anesthesia to minimize any pain and suffering.

4.2. Experimental Animals

The present study used 2–3 month old adult male C57BL/6J mice (20–25 g, DBL Co., Chungcheongbuk-do, Eumseong-gun, Korea). The mice were housed three to four mice per cage under conditions of sustained temperature (20 ± 2 °C) and humidity (55% ± 5%). Animal room lights were managed automatically, turned on and off in a 12 h cycle (on at 6:00 a.m. and off at 6:00 p.m.).

4.3. Global Cerebral Ischemia Surgery

Male C57BL/6J mice (aged 2–3 months, weight 20–25 g) from DBL (Chungcheongbuk-do, Eumseong-gun, Korea) were used as controls. The mice were anesthetized with 2% isoflurane in a 75:25 mixture of oxygen and nitrous oxide. Core temperature was maintained at 36.7–37.5 °C with a homeothermic blanket control unit (Harvard Apparatus, Holliston, MA, USA). Bilateral common carotid arteries (BCCAs) were exposed through a midline neck incision. The BCCAs were loosely encircled with a 4/O silk suture before the occlusion. Aneurysmal clips were used to occlude BCCAs. Mice were subjected to common carotid artery occlusion for 30 min while anesthetized with 1% isoflurane [71–73]. The aneurysmal clips were removed, and the BCCAs were inspected for normal recovery of blood flow after the end of the 30 min ischemic period. Anesthetics were discontinued following the suture of the skin incision. When mice confirmed spontaneous respiration, they were returned to a recovery room retained at 37 °C. Sham-operated animals received the same neck skin incision under isoflurane anesthesia without BCCA occlusion.

4.4. Amiloride Administration

To confirm the effect of amiloride on GCI-induced neuronal death, the experimental groups were divided into four groups: sham (vehicle, amiloride) and global cerebral ischemia (vehicle, amiloride). The amiloride-treated groups were administrated amiloride (10 mg/kg, i.p.) dissolved in 0.9% normal saline. After GCI induction, we immediately injected the amiloride into the intraperitoneal space. The vehicle group was given 0.9% normal saline instead of amiloride. All experimental groups were sacrificed 24 h after GCI.

4.5. Brain Sample Preparation

Mice were sacrificed at 24 h or 3 days after GCI using urethane (1.5 g/kg, i.p.) to deeply anesthetize them. After anesthetizing, mice were perfused transcardially with 0.9% saline, followed by 4%

paraformaldehyde (PFA). Afterwards, harvested brains were post-fixed for approximately 1 h in 4% PFA. After fixation in PFA, brains were moved into a 30% sucrose solution overnight for cryoprotection. After the brain sank to the bottom of the sucrose solution, they were frozen in the freezing medium for 10 min and then cut with cryostats at 30 μm thicknesses. Brain slices were kept in storage solution until used for immunohistochemistry and immunofluorescence staining.

4.6. *Confirmation of Hippocampal Neuronal Death*

To confirm neuronal death after GCI, brain sections (30 μm) were put on gelatin-coated slides (Fisher Scientific, Pittsburgh, PA, USA). To detect degenerating neurons, brain slices were stained by the FJB staining method [74,75]. Firstly, a slide with a brain section was soaked in a 100% ethanol solution for 3 min, a 70% ethanol solution for 1 min, distilled water for 1 min, and then in 0.06% potassium permanganate for 15 min. Next, the slides were put into 0.001% FJB (Histo-Chem Inc., Jefferson, AR, USA) solution for 30 min and washed three times for 10 min in distilled water. After washing, slides were dried by a gentle air flow (Labtech, Co., Ltd., Namyangju, Korea), dehydrated in xylene for 2 min, and then mounted with DPX (Sigma-Aldrich Co., St. Louis, MO, USA). Slides were checked under a fluorescence microscope (Olympus, Japan) via blue (450–490 nm) excitation light. We chose about six to eight coronal brain sections that were collected from each mouse. A blinded observer counted the FJB-positive cells. The FJB-positive cells were counted and evaluated in the hippocampal Sub, CA1, CA2, and CA3 regions from the bilateral hemisphere. The total number of FJB-positive cells from the hippocampal region was used for statistical analysis. A blinded observer counted the FJB-positive cells. The FJB-positive cells were counted and evaluated in the hippocampal Sub, CA1, CA2, and CA3 regions from the bilateral hemisphere. The total number of FJB-positive cells from the hippocampal region was used for statistical analysis.

4.7. *Confirmation of Hippocampal Zinc Translocation*

Intracellular free zinc was verified using TSQ staining [76]. Mice were sacrificed 24 h after amiloride (10 mg/kg, i.p.) administration and the fresh frozen, but not fixed, brains were coronally sectioned at 10 μm thicknesses in a −15 °C cryostat, then mounted on gelatin-coated slides and dried. Five evenly spaced sections were chosen from the hippocampal region of each brain and soaked in a solution of 4.5 mmol/L TSQ (Enzo Life Science, Enzo Biochem, Inc, Farmingdale, New York, NY, USA, ENZ-52153) for 1 min, then washed for 1 min in 0.9% saline. Each sample was photographed with a microscope under 360 nm UV light and a 500 nm long-pass filter. We used the Image J (National Institute of Health, Bethesda, Rockville, MD, USA) program to measure zinc intensity and evaluated the mean gray value.

4.8. *Evaluation of Hippocampal Oxidative Stress*

To analyze oxidative damage induced by the lipid peroxidation product from the brain sections, 4HNE was detected by immunofluorescence staining. 4HNE antibodies (Alpha Diagnostic Intl. Inc., San Antonio, TX, USA) for immunohistochemical staining were used as in previous studies [77,78]. Brain sections were soaked in a monoclonal mouse anti-4HNE serum (diluted 1:500, Alpha Diagnostic Intl. Inc., San Antonio, TX, USA) with the PBS containing 0.3% TritonX-100 overnight in a 4 °C incubator. After overnight incubation, brain sections were washed three times for 10 min with 0.01 M PBS, and then the brain sections were also soaked in a solution of Alexa-Fluor-594-conjugated donkey anti-mouse IgG secondary antibody (diluted 1:250, Invitrogen, Grand Island, NY, USA) for 2 h at room temperature (RT). The brain sections were raised on gelatin-coated slides for analysis under a microscope. We used the Image J (NIH, Bethesda, Rockville, MD, USA) program to measure the oxidative injury and measured the mean gray value [79].

4.9. Evaluation of Hippocampal Microtubule Damage

To analyze microtubule damage from the brain sections, MAP2 was detected by immunofluorescence staining. MAP2 antibodies (Alpha Diagnostic Intl. Inc., San Antonio, TX, USA) for immunohistochemical staining were used as in a previous study [80]. Brain sections were soaked in a polyclonal rabbit anti-MAP2 serum (diluted 1:200, Alpha Diagnostic Intl. Inc., San Antonio, TX, USA) with PBS containing 0.3% TritonX-100 overnight in a 4 °C incubator. After overnight incubation, we washed the sections three times for 10 min with 0.01 M PBS, and then the brain sections were soaked in a solution of Alexa-Fluor-488-conjugated donkey anti-rabbit IgG secondary antibody (diluted 1:250, Invitrogen, Grand Island, NY, USA) for 2 h at RT. The brain sections were raised on gelatin-coated slides for analysis under a microscope. We used the Image J (NIH, Bethesda, Rockville, MD, USA) program to measure the microtubule damage and measured the mean gray value.

4.10. Evaluation of Hippocampal Astrocytes and Microglia

To analyze astrocyte and microglial activation, we performed Iba-1 and GFAP staining. Staining was used with a mixture of goat antibody to mouse Iba-1 (diluted 1:500, Abcam, Cambridge, UK) and rabbit antibody to mouse GFAP (diluted 1:1000, Abcam, Cambridge, UK). Following incubation in 0.01 M PBS containing 0.3% TritonX-100, we left it overnight in a 4 °C incubator. After overnight incubation, we washed the sections three times for 10 min with 0.01 M PBS. Then, the sections were soaked in a secondary antibody (Alexa-Fluor-488-conjugated donkey anti-rabbit IgG secondary antibody and Alexa-Fluor-594-conjugated donkey anti-goat IgG secondary antibody, both diluted 1:250, Invitrogen, Grand Island, NY, USA) for 2 h at RT. The brain sections were raised on gelatin-coated slides for analysis under a microscope. We used the Image J (NIH, Bethesda, Rockville, MD, USA) program to measure the astrocytes. In the case of microglia, five brain sections were scored with the same area (20× magnification) of the hippocampal CA1 region. The functional standards of microglia cells were their number, morphology, and intensity of microglia activation. Iba-1-immunoreactive cell score of 0: no cells are present; 1:1–9 cells; 2:10–20 cells; and 3:>20 cells with continuous processers per 100 μm^2. Morphology score of 0:no activated morphology (amoeboid morphology with enlarged soma and thickened processes); 1:1–45% of microglia activation; 2:45–90% of microglia activation; and 3: >90% of microglia with the activated morphology. The intensity of microglial activation was measured using the Image J (NIH, Bethesda, Rockville, MD, USA) program. After the measurements, an intensity score of 1:0–19% expression; 2:20–29% expression; and 3:>29% expression. Therefore, the total score summed up the three scores depending on the categories, ranging from 0 to 9 [18,81,82].

4.11. Evaluation of BBB Disruption

To analyze the putative breakdown of the BBB, we used immunohistochemistry to find serum IgG leakage [83]. To detect IgG-like immunoreactivity, the ABC immunoperoxidase protocol was used [84]. Mouse brains were fixed by transcardiac perfusion with 0.9% normal saline, followed by 4% paraformaldehyde. We used anti-mouse IgG (diluted 1:250, Burlingame, Vector, CA, USA) which can discover leakages of IgG when the BBB is damaged. After washing in 0.01 M PBS, brain sections were deeply soaked in the ABC complex mixture (Vector, Burlingame, CA, USA) for 2 h at RT. The immunoreactivity was visualized with 0.06% 3,3′-diaminobenzidine (DAB ager, Sigma–Aldrich Co., St. Louis, MO, USA) in 0.1 M PBS buffer. Leaked IgG extravasations were detected using a bright-field microscope.

4.12. Evaluation of Live Hippocampal Neurons

To assess the number of live neurons present in a sample, NeuN was detected by immunofluorescence staining. NeuN antibodies (diluted 1:500, EMD Millipore, Billerica, MA, USA) for immunohistochemical staining were used as in previous studies. Brain sections were soaked in a monoclonal rabbit anti-NeuN serum with PBS containing 0.3% TritonX-100 overnight in a 4 °C incubator. After overnight incubation, brain sections were washed three times for 10 min each with 0.01 M PBS, and then the brain sections were also soaked in a solution of Alexa-Fluor-594-conjugated donkey anti-rabbit IgG secondary antibody (diluted 1:250, Invitrogen, Grand Island, NY, USA) for 2 h at room temperature (RT). The brain sections were raised on gelatin-coated slides for analysis under a microscope. A blinded observer counted the NeuN-positive cells. NeuN-positive cells were counted and evaluated in the hippocampal Sub, CA1, CA2, and CA3 regions from each hemisphere. The total number of NeuN-positive cells from the hippocampal region was used for statistical analysis [18].

4.13. Statistical Analysis

We conducted nonparametric testing to confirm any statistical significance between the experimental groups. Data were analyzed using the Bonferroni post-hoc test, and the Kruskal–Wallis test was employed to compare among the four groups. For comparison across two groups, data were analyzed using the Mann–Whitey U test. Data are displayed as the mean ± SEM. Statistical significance is described as $p < 0.05$.

5. Conclusions

This present study supports the hypothesis that the administration of amiloride protects against hippocampal neuronal death and zinc accumulation after GCI. In addition, inhibition of NHE-1 by amiloride may have considerable therapeutic potential for the prevention of GCI.

Author Contributions: B.S.K. researched and collected the data and reviewed and edited the manuscript. B.Y.C. reviewed and edited the manuscript. A.R.K., S.H.L., D.K.H., J.H.J., D.H.K., and M.K.P. researched and collected the data. S.W.S. contributed to the discussion and wrote, reviewed, and edited the manuscript. All authors have read and agree to the published version of the manuscript.

References

1. Wan, L.; Cheng, Y.; Luo, Z.; Guo, H.; Zhao, W.; Gu, Q.; Yang, X.; Xu, J.; Bei, W.; Guo, J. Neuroprotection, learning and memory improvement of a standardized extract from Renshen Shouwu against neuronal injury and vascular dementia in rats with brain ischemia. *J. Ethnopharmacol.* **2015**, *165*, 118–126. [CrossRef] [PubMed]
2. Lee, R.H.C.; Lee, M.H.H.; Wu, C.Y.C.; Couto, E.S.A.; Possoit, H.E.; Hsieh, T.H.; Minagar, A.; Lin, H.W. Cerebral ischemia and neuroregeneration. *Neural Regen. Res.* **2018**, *13*, 373–385. [PubMed]
3. Hong, D.K.; Choi, B.Y.; Kho, A.R.; Lee, S.H.; Jeong, J.H.; Kang, B.S.; Kang, D.H.; Park, K.H.; Suh, S.W. Carvacrol attenuates hippocampal neuronal death after global cerebral ischemia via inhibition of transient receptor potential melastatin 7. *Cells* **2018**, *7*, 231. [CrossRef] [PubMed]
4. Ding, Q.; Liao, S.J.; Yu, J. Axon guidance factor netrin-1 and its receptors regulate angiogenesis after cerebral ischemia. *Neurosci. Bull.* **2014**, *30*, 683–691. [CrossRef] [PubMed]
5. Dirnagl, U.; Lindauer, U.; Them, A.; Schreiber, S.; Pfister, H.W.; Koedel, U.; Reszka, R.; Freyer, D.; Villringer, A. Global cerebral ischemia in the rat: Online monitoring of oxygen free radical production using chemiluminescence in vivo. *J. Cereb. Blood Flow Metab.* **1995**, *15*, 929–940. [CrossRef] [PubMed]
6. White, B.C.; Sullivan, J.M.; DeGracia, D.J.; O'Neil, B.J.; Neumar, R.W.; Grossman, L.I.; Rafols, J.A.; Krause, G.S. Brain ischemia and reperfusion: Molecular mechanisms of neuronal injury. *J. Neurol. Sci.* **2000**, *179*, 1–33. [CrossRef]
7. Rhee, S.G. Cell signaling. H_2O_2, a necessary evil for cell signaling. *Science* **2006**, *312*, 1882–1883. [CrossRef]
8. Klann, E. Cell-permeable scavengers of superoxide prevent long-term potentiation in hippocampal area CA1. *J. Neurophysiol.* **1998**, *80*, 452–457. [CrossRef]

9. Kalogeris, T.; Baines, C.P.; Krenz, M.; Korthuis, R.J. Cell biology of ischemia/reperfusion injury. *Int Rev. Cell Mol. Biol.* **2012**, *298*, 229–317.
10. Pan, J.; Konstas, A.A.; Bateman, B.; Ortolano, G.A.; Pile-Spellman, J. Reperfusion injury following cerebral ischemia: Pathophysiology, MR imaging, and potential therapies. *Neuroradiology* **2007**, *49*, 93–102. [CrossRef]
11. Rehncrona, S. Brain acidosis. *Ann. Emerg. Med.* **1985**, *14*, 770–776. [CrossRef]
12. Nedergaard, M.; Kraig, R.P.; Tanabe, J.; Pulsinelli, W.A. Dynamics of interstitial and intracellular pH in evolving brain infarct. *Am. J. Physiol.* **1991**, *260*, R581–R588. [CrossRef] [PubMed]
13. Siesjo, B.K.; Katsura, K.; Kristian, T. Acidosis-related damage. *Adv. Neurol.* **1996**, *71*, 209–233. [PubMed]
14. Cull, R.E. Role of axonal transport in maintaining central synaptic connections. *Exp. Brain Res.* **1975**, *24*, 97–101. [CrossRef] [PubMed]
15. Takeda, A.; Kodama, Y.; Ohnuma, M.; Okada, S. Zinc transport from the striatum and substantia nigra. *Brain Res. Bull.* **1998**, *47*, 103–106. [CrossRef]
16. Choi, D.W. Calcium-mediated neurotoxicity: Relationship to specific channel types and role in ischemic damage. *Trends Neurosci.* **1988**, *11*, 465–469. [CrossRef]
17. Chuah, M.I.; Tennent, R.; Jacobs, I. Response of olfactory Schwann cells to intranasal zinc sulfate irrigation. *J. Neurosci. Res.* **1995**, *42*, 470–478. [CrossRef]
18. Kho, A.R.; Choi, B.Y.; Lee, S.H.; Hong, D.K.; Lee, S.H.; Jeong, J.H.; Park, K.H.; Song, H.K.; Choi, H.C.; Suh, S.W. Effects of protocatechuic acid (PCA) on global cerebral ischemia-induced hippocampal neuronal death. *Int. J. Mol. Sci.* **2018**, *19*, 1420. [CrossRef]
19. Kim, J.H.; Jang, B.G.; Choi, B.Y.; Kwon, L.M.; Sohn, M.; Song, H.K.; Suh, S.W. Zinc chelation reduces hippocampal neurogenesis after pilocarpine-induced seizure. *PLoS ONE* **2012**, *7*, e48543. [CrossRef]
20. Inoue, K.; Branigan, D.; Xiong, Z.G. Zinc-induced neurotoxicity mediated by transient receptor potential melastatin 7 channels. *J. Biol. Chem.* **2010**, *285*, 7430–7439. [CrossRef]
21. Choi, B.Y.; Lee, B.E.; Kim, J.H.; Kim, H.J.; Sohn, M.; Song, H.K.; Chung, T.N.; Suh, S.W. Colchicine induced intraneuronal free zinc accumulation and dentate granule cell degeneration. *Metallomics* **2014**, *6*, 1513–1520. [CrossRef] [PubMed]
22. Yao, H.; Ma, E.; Gu, X.Q.; Haddad, G.G. Intracellular pH regulation of CA1 neurons in Na^+/H^+ isoform 1 mutant mice. *J. Clin. Invest.* **1999**, *104*, 637–645. [CrossRef] [PubMed]
23. Noel, J.; Pouyssegur, J. Hormonal regulation, pharmacology, and membrane sorting of vertebrate Na^+/H^+ exchanger isoforms. *Am. J. Physiol.* **1995**, *268*, C283–C296. [CrossRef] [PubMed]
24. Ohgaki, R.; Matsushita, M.; Kanazawa, H.; Ogihara, S.; Hoekstra, D.; van Ijzendoorn, S.C. The Na^+/H^+ exchanger NHE6 in the endosomal recycling system is involved in the development of apical bile canalicular surface domains in HepG2 cells. *Mol. Biol. Cell* **2010**, *21*, 1293–1304. [CrossRef] [PubMed]
25. Nakamura, N.; Tanaka, S.; Teko, Y.; Mitsui, K.; Kanazawa, H. Four Na^+/H^+ exchanger isoforms are distributed to Golgi and post-Golgi compartments and are involved in organelle pH regulation. *J. Biol. Chem.* **2005**, *280*, 1561–1572. [CrossRef] [PubMed]
26. Kleyman, T.R.; Cragoe, E.J., Jr. Amiloride and its analogs as tools in the study of ion transport. *J. Membr. Biol.* **1988**, *105*, 1–21. [CrossRef]
27. Hwang, I.K.; Yoo, K.Y.; An, S.J.; Li, H.; Lee, C.H.; Choi, J.H.; Lee, J.Y.; Lee, B.H.; Kim, Y.M.; Kwon, Y.G.; et al. Late expression of Na^+/H^+ exchanger 1 (NHE1) and neuroprotective effects of NHE inhibitor in the gerbil hippocampal CA1 region induced by transient ischemia. *Exp. Neurol.* **2008**, *212*, 314–323. [CrossRef]
28. Verma, V.; Bali, A.; Singh, N.; Jaggi, A.S. Implications of sodium hydrogen exchangers in various brain diseases. *J. Basic Clin. Physiol. Pharmacol.* **2015**, *26*, 417–426. [CrossRef] [PubMed]
29. Tai, K.K.; Truong, D.D. Amiloride but not memantine reduces neurodegeneration, seizures and myoclonic jerks in rats with cardiac arrest-induced global cerebral hypoxia and reperfusion. *PLoS ONE* **2013**, *8*, e60309. [CrossRef]
30. Ou-Yang, T.P.; Zhu, G.M.; Ding, Y.X.; Yang, F.; Sun, X.L.; Jiang, W. The effects of amiloride on seizure activity, cognitive deficits and seizure-induced neurogenesis in a novel rat model of febrile seizures. *Neurochem. Res.* **2016**, *41*, 933–942. [CrossRef]
31. Imai, T.; Katoh, H.; Suyama, K.; Kuroiwa, M.; Yanagisawa, S.; Watanabe, M. Amiloride promotes oligodendrocyte survival and remyelination after spinal cord injury in rats. *J. Clin. Med.* **2018**, *7*, 46. [CrossRef] [PubMed]

32. Foster, M.; Samman, S. Zinc and redox signaling: Perturbations associated with cardiovascular disease and diabetes mellitus. *Antioxid. Redox Signal.* **2010**, *13*, 1549–1573. [CrossRef] [PubMed]
33. Kho, A.R.; Choi, B.Y.; Lee, S.H.; Hong, D.K.; Jeong, J.H.; Kang, B.S.; Kang, D.H.; Park, K.H.; Park, J.B.; Suh, S.W. The effects of sodium dichloroacetate on mitochondrial dysfunction and neuronal death following hypoglycemia-induced injury. *Cells* **2019**, *8*, 405. [CrossRef] [PubMed]
34. Ali, S.M.; Dunn, E.; Oostveen, J.A.; Hall, E.D.; Carter, D.B. Induction of apolipoprotein E mRNA in the hippocampus of the gerbil after transient global ischemia. *Brain Res. Mol. Brain Res.* **1996**, *38*, 37–44. [CrossRef]
35. Hoane, M.R.; Kaplan, S.A.; Ellis, A.L. The effects of nicotinamide on apoptosis and blood-brain barrier breakdown following traumatic brain injury. *Brain Res.* **2006**, *1125*, 185–193. [CrossRef]
36. Tang, X.N.; Berman, A.E.; Swanson, R.A.; Yenari, M.A. Digitally quantifying cerebral hemorrhage using Photoshop and Image J. *J. Neurosci. Methods* **2010**, *190*, 240–243. [CrossRef]
37. Li, W.; Ward, R.; Dong, G.; Ergul, A.; O'Connor, P. Neurovascular protection in voltage-gated proton channel Hv1 knock-out rats after ischemic stroke: Interaction with Na^+/H^+ exchanger-1 antagonism. *Physiol. Rep.* **2019**, *7*, e14142. [CrossRef]
38. Sun, D.; Nguyen, N.; DeGrado, T.R.; Schwaiger, M.; Brosius, F.C., 3rd. Ischemia induces translocation of the insulin-responsive glucose transporter GLUT4 to the plasma membrane of cardiac myocytes. *Circulation* **1994**, *89*, 793–798. [CrossRef]
39. Tian, R.; Abel, E.D. Responses of GLUT4-deficient hearts to ischemia underscore the importance of glycolysis. *Circulation* **2001**, *103*, 2961–2966. [CrossRef]
40. Young, L.H.; Renfu, Y.; Russell, R.; Hu, X.; Caplan, M.; Ren, J.; Shulman, G.I.; Sinusas, A.J. Low-flow ischemia leads to translocation of canine heart GLUT-4 and GLUT-1 glucose transporters to the sarcolemma in vivo. *Circulation* **1997**, *95*, 415–422. [CrossRef]
41. Wang, Y.P.; Zhou, L.S.; Zhao, Y.Z.; Wang, S.W.; Chen, L.L.; Liu, L.X.; Ling, Z.Q.; Hu, F.J.; Sun, Y.P.; Zhang, J.Y.; et al. Regulation of G6PD acetylation by SIRT2 and KAT9 modulates NADPH homeostasis and cell survival during oxidative stress. *EMBO J.* **2014**, *33*, 1304–1320. [CrossRef] [PubMed]
42. Kruger, N.J.; von Schaewen, A. The oxidative pentose phosphate pathway: Structure and organisation. *Curr. Opin. Plant. Biol.* **2003**, *6*, 236–246. [CrossRef]
43. Orlowski, J.; Grinstein, S. Diversity of the mammalian sodium/proton exchanger SLC9 gene family. *Pflügers Arch.* **2004**, *447*, 549–565. [CrossRef] [PubMed]
44. Avkiran, M. Protection of the ischaemic myocardium by Na^+/H^+ exchange inhibitors: Potential mechanisms of action. *Basic Res. Cardiol.* **2001**, *96*, 306–311. [CrossRef] [PubMed]
45. Ferrazzano, P.; Shi, Y.; Manhas, N.; Wang, Y.; Hutchinson, B.; Chen, X.; Chanana, V.; Gerdts, J.; Meyerand, M.E.; Sun, D. Inhibiting the Na^+/H^+ exchanger reduces reperfusion injury: A small animal MRI study. *Front. Biosci. (Elite Ed.)* **2011**, *3*, 81–88. [CrossRef] [PubMed]
46. Yeves, A.M.; Ennis, I.L. Na^+/H^+ exchanger and cardiac hypertrophy. *Hipertens. Riesgo. Vasc.* **2020**, *37*, 22–32. [CrossRef]
47. Sensi, S.L.; Canzoniero, L.M.; Yu, S.P.; Ying, H.S.; Koh, J.Y.; Kerchner, G.A.; Choi, D.W. Measurement of intracellular free zinc in living cortical neurons: Routes of entry. *J. Neurosci.* **1997**, *17*, 9554–9564. [CrossRef]
48. Ohana, E.; Segal, D.; Palty, R.; Ton-That, D.; Moran, A.; Sensi, S.L.; Weiss, J.H.; Hershfinkel, M.; Sekler, I. A sodium zinc exchange mechanism is mediating extrusion of zinc in mammalian cells. *J. Biol. Chem.* **2004**, *279*, 4278–4284. [CrossRef]
49. Sekler, I.; Sensi, S.L.; Hershfinkel, M.; Silverman, W.F. Mechanism and regulation of cellular zinc transport. *Mol. Med.* **2007**, *13*, 337–343. [CrossRef]
50. Lee, B.K.; Jung, Y.S. The Na^+/H^+ exchanger-1 inhibitor cariporide prevents glutamate-induced necrotic neuronal death by inhibiting mitochondrial Ca^{2+} overload. *J. Neurosci Res.* **2012**, *90*, 860–869. [CrossRef]
51. Masereel, B.; Pochet, L.; Laeckmann, D. An overview of inhibitors of Na^+/H^+ exchanger. *Eur. J. Med. Chem.* **2003**, *38*, 547–554. [CrossRef]
52. Durham-Lee, J.C.; Mokkapati, V.U.; Johnson, K.M.; Nesic, O. Amiloride improves locomotor recovery after spinal cord injury. *J. Neurotrauma* **2011**, *28*, 1319–1326. [CrossRef] [PubMed]
53. Xiong, Z.G.; Zhu, X.M.; Chu, X.P.; Minami, M.; Hey, J.; Wei, W.L.; MacDonald, J.F.; Wemmie, J.A.; Price, M.P.; Welsh, M.J.; et al. Neuroprotection in ischemia: Blocking calcium-permeable acid-sensing ion channels. *Cell* **2004**, *118*, 687–698. [CrossRef] [PubMed]

54. Arias, R.L.; Sung, M.L.; Vasylyev, D.; Zhang, M.Y.; Albinson, K.; Kubek, K.; Kagan, N.; Beyer, C.; Lin, Q.; Dwyer, J.M.; et al. Amiloride is neuroprotective in an MPTP model of Parkinson's disease. *Neurobiol. Dis.* **2008**, *31*, 334–341. [CrossRef]
55. Lazarewicz, J.W.; Rybkowski, W.; Sadowski, M.; Ziembowicz, A.; Alaraj, M.; Wegiel, J.; Wisniewski, H.M. N-methyl-D-aspartate receptor-mediated, calcium-induced calcium release in rat dentate gyrus/CA4 in vivo. *J. Neurosci. Res.* **1998**, *51*, 76–84. [CrossRef]
56. Kreutzberg, G.W. Microglia: A sensor for pathological events in the CNS. *Trends Neurosci.* **1996**, *19*, 312–318. [CrossRef]
57. Jin, R.; Yang, G.; Li, G. Inflammatory mechanisms in ischemic stroke: Role of inflammatory cells. *J. Leukoc. Biol.* **2010**, *87*, 779–789. [CrossRef]
58. Yenari, M.A.; Kauppinen, T.M.; Swanson, R.A. Microglial activation in stroke: Therapeutic targets. *Neurotherapeutics* **2010**, *7*, 378–391. [CrossRef]
59. Shi, Y.; Chanana, V.; Watters, J.J.; Ferrazzano, P.; Sun, D. Role of sodium/hydrogen exchanger isoform 1 in microglial activation and proinflammatory responses in ischemic brains. *J. Neurochem.* **2011**, *119*, 124–135. [CrossRef]
60. Hua, J.S.; Li, L.P.; Zhu, X.M. Effects of moxibustion pretreating on SOD and MDA in the rat of global brain ischemia. *J. Tradit. Chin. Med.* **2008**, *28*, 289–292. [CrossRef]
61. Chen, H.; Yoshioka, H.; Kim, G.S.; Jung, J.E.; Okami, N.; Sakata, H.; Maier, C.M.; Narasimhan, P.; Goeders, C.E.; Chan, P.H. Oxidative stress in ischemic brain damage: Mechanisms of cell death and potential molecular targets for neuroprotection. *Antioxid. Redox Signal.* **2011**, *14*, 1505–1517. [CrossRef] [PubMed]
62. Choi, B.Y.; Jung, J.W.; Suh, S.W. The emerging role of zinc in the pathogenesis of multiple sclerosis. *Int. J. Mol. Sci.* **2017**, *18*, 2070. [CrossRef]
63. Li, S.; Vana, A.C.; Ribeiro, R.; Zhang, Y. Distinct role of nitric oxide and peroxynitrite in mediating oligodendrocyte toxicity in culture and in experimental autoimmune encephalomyelitis. *Neuroscience* **2011**, *184*, 107–119. [CrossRef] [PubMed]
64. Zhang, Y.; Wang, H.; Li, J.; Dong, L.; Xu, P.; Chen, W.; Neve, R.L.; Volpe, J.J.; Rosenberg, P.A. Intracellular zinc release and ERK phosphorylation are required upstream of 12-lipoxygenase activation in peroxynitrite toxicity to mature rat oligodendrocytes. *J. Biol. Chem.* **2006**, *281*, 9460–9470. [CrossRef] [PubMed]
65. Khan, M.; Dhammu, T.S.; Sakakima, H.; Shunmugavel, A.; Gilg, A.G.; Singh, A.K.; Singh, I. The inhibitory effect of S-nitrosoglutathione on blood-brain barrier disruption and peroxynitrite formation in a rat model of experimental stroke. *J. Neurochem.* **2012**, *123*, 86–97. [CrossRef]
66. Torreilles, F.; Salman-Tabcheh, S.; Guerin, M.; Torreilles, J. Neurodegenerative disorders: The role of peroxynitrite. *Brain Res. Brain Res. Rev.* **1999**, *30*, 153–163. [CrossRef]
67. Choi, B.Y.; Lee, S.H.; Choi, H.C.; Lee, S.K.; Yoon, H.S.; Park, J.B.; Chung, W.S.; Suh, S.W. Alcohol dependence treating agent, acamprosate, prevents traumatic brain injury-induced neuron death through vesicular zinc depletion. *Transl. Res.* **2019**, *207*, 1–18. [CrossRef]
68. Abbott, N.J.; Patabendige, A.A.; Dolman, D.E.; Yusof, S.R.; Begley, D.J. Structure and function of the blood-brain barrier. *Neurobiol. Dis.* **2010**, *37*, 13–25. [CrossRef]
69. Dalkara, T.; Gursoy-Ozdemir, Y.; Yemisci, M. Brain microvascular pericytes in health and disease. *Acta Neuropathol.* **2011**, *122*, 1–9. [CrossRef]
70. Woodruff, T.M.; Thundyil, J.; Tang, S.C.; Sobey, C.G.; Taylor, S.M.; Arumugam, T.V. Pathophysiology, treatment, and animal and cellular models of human ischemic stroke. *Mol. Neurodegener.* **2011**, *6*, 11. [CrossRef]
71. Won, S.J.; Yoo, B.H.; Brennan, A.M.; Shin, B.S.; Kauppinen, T.M.; Berman, A.E.; Swanson, R.A.; Suh, S.W. EAAC1 gene deletion alters zinc homeostasis and exacerbates neuronal injury after transient cerebral ischemia. *J. Neurosci.* **2010**, *30*, 15409–15418. [CrossRef]
72. Jang, B.G.; Won, S.J.; Kim, J.H.; Choi, B.Y.; Lee, M.W.; Sohn, M.; Song, H.K.; Suh, S.W. EAAC1 gene deletion alters zinc homeostasis and enhances cortical neuronal injury after transient cerebral ischemia in mice. *J. Trace Elem. Med. Biol.* **2012**, *26*, 85–88. [CrossRef] [PubMed]
73. Suh, S.W.; Shin, B.S.; Ma, H.; Van Hoecke, M.; Brennan, A.M.; Yenari, M.A.; Swanson, R.A. Glucose and NADPH oxidase drive neuronal superoxide formation in stroke. *Ann. Neurol.* **2008**, *64*, 654–663. [CrossRef]
74. Schmued, L.C.; Hopkins, K.J. Fluoro-Jade B: A high affinity fluorescent marker for the localization of neuronal degeneration. *Brain Res.* **2000**, *874*, 123–130. [CrossRef]

75. Suh, S.W.; Aoyama, K.; Chen, Y.; Garnier, P.; Matsumori, Y.; Gum, E.; Liu, J.; Swanson, R.A. Hypoglycemic neuronal death and cognitive impairment are prevented by poly(ADP-ribose) polymerase inhibitors administered after hypoglycemia. *J. Neurosci.* **2003**, *23*, 10681–10690. [CrossRef] [PubMed]
76. Frederickson, C.J.; Kasarskis, E.J.; Ringo, D.; Frederickson, R.E. A quinoline fluorescence method for visualizing and assaying the histochemically reactive zinc (bouton zinc) in the brain. *J. Neurosci. Methods* **1987**, *20*, 91–103. [CrossRef]
77. Suh, S.W.; Gum, E.T.; Hamby, A.M.; Chan, P.H.; Swanson, R.A. Hypoglycemic neuronal death is triggered by glucose reperfusion and activation of neuronal NADPH oxidase. *J. Clin. Invest.* **2007**, *117*, 910–918. [CrossRef] [PubMed]
78. Kim, J.H.; Jang, B.G.; Choi, B.Y.; Kim, H.S.; Sohn, M.; Chung, T.N.; Choi, H.C.; Song, H.K.; Suh, S.W. Post-treatment of an NADPH oxidase inhibitor prevents seizure-induced neuronal death. *Brain Res.* **2013**, *1499*, 163–172. [CrossRef] [PubMed]
79. Kho, A.R.; Choi, B.Y.; Kim, J.H.; Lee, S.H.; Hong, D.K.; Lee, S.H.; Jeong, J.H.; Sohn, M.; Suh, S.W. Prevention of hypoglycemia-induced hippocampal neuronal death by N-acetyl-L-cysteine (NAC). *Amino Acids* **2017**, *49*, 367–378. [CrossRef] [PubMed]
80. Lee, S.H.; Choi, B.Y.; Lee, S.H.; Kho, A.R.; Jeong, J.H.; Hong, D.K.; Suh, S.W. Administration of protocatechuic acid reduces traumatic brain injury-induced neuronal death. *Int. J. Mol. Sci.* **2017**, *18*, 2510. [CrossRef]
81. Kauppinen, T.M.; Swanson, R.A. Poly(ADP-ribose) polymerase-1 promotes microglial activation, proliferation, and matrix metalloproteinase-9-mediated neuron death. *J. Immunol.* **2005**, *174*, 2288–2296. [CrossRef] [PubMed]
82. Kauppinen, T.M.; Higashi, Y.; Suh, S.W.; Escartin, C.; Nagasawa, K.; Swanson, R.A. Zinc triggers microglial activation. *J. Neurosci.* **2008**, *28*, 5827–5835. [CrossRef] [PubMed]
83. Ruth, R.E.; Feinerman, G.S. Foreign and endogenous serum protein extravasation during harmaline tremors or kainic acid seizures in the rat: A comparison. *Acta Neuropathol.* **1988**, *76*, 380–387. [CrossRef] [PubMed]
84. Hsu, S.M.; Raine, L.; Fanger, H. Use of avidin-biotin-peroxidase complex (ABC) in immunoperoxidase techniques: A comparison between ABC and unlabeled antibody (PAP) procedures. *J. Histochem. Cytochem.* **1981**, *29*, 577–580. [CrossRef]

4

Nanomedicine for Ischemic Stroke

Xinyue Dong, Jin Gao, Yujie Su and Zhenjia Wang *

Department of Pharmaceutical Sciences, College of Pharmacy and Pharmaceutical Sciences, Washington State University, Spokane, WA 99202, USA; xinyue.dong@wsu.edu (X.D.); jin.gao3@wsu.edu (J.G.); yujie.su@wsu.edu (Y.S.)
* Correspondence: zhenjia.wang@wsu.edu

Abstract: Stroke is a severe brain disease leading to disability and death. Ischemic stroke dominates in stroke cases, and there are no effective therapies in clinic, partly due to the challenges in delivering therapeutics to ischemic sites in the brain. This review is focused on the current knowledge of pathogenesis in ischemic stroke, and its potential therapies and diagnosis. Furthermore, we present recent advances in developments of nanoparticle-based therapeutics for improved treatment of ischemic stroke using polymeric NPs, liposomes and cell-derived nanovesicles. We also address several critical questions in ischemic stroke, such as understanding how nanoparticles cross the blood brain barrier and developing in vivo imaging technologies to address this critical question. Finally, we discuss new opportunities in developing novel therapeutics by targeting activated brain endothelium and inflammatory neutrophils to improve the current therapies for ischemic stroke.

Keywords: ischemic stroke; blood brain barrier; nanoparticle-based drug delivery; brain targeting

1. Introduction

Stroke is an unexpected and acute brain disease. It is reported that one of nineteen deaths is related to stroke in the United States, and the mortality rate of stroke is as high as 30% [1]. Stroke is defined by a condition caused by a hemorrhage or occlusion of cerebral blood vessels. Lacking of blood flow in the brain causes dysfunctions of brain cells, oxidative stress, and neurological damage [2]. The symptoms of stroke include numbness, confusion, and aphasia, and those signs are related to injured areas in the brain [3]. Since 87% of strokes are related to ischemia in the brain and 13% are involved with the hemorrhage, this review will focus on discussing how nanotechnology improves therapies and diagnosis of ischemia stroke.

Cerebral ischemia initiates a cascade of pathological processes, eventually causing neuron death. Reperfusion is a clinical method to restore the blood flow in the brain by administration of tissue plasminogen activator (t-PA) or mechanical thrombectomy (MT) for treatment of ischemic stroke [4]. However, reperfusion often leads to tissue damage because oxygen influx of reperfusion generates reactive oxygen species (ROS), initiating inflammatory responses including cytokine production and leukocyte infiltration [5]. Many neuroprotectants have been developed to alleviate reperfusion-induced injury, but none of them were clinically approved. There are several reasons for this failure: (1) ineffective drug delivery into the brain because of blood brain barrier (BBB), (2) drugs with short circulation times, poor stability, and toxicity, (3) difficulty in choosing right drugs and doses due to the heterogenicity of stroke (e.g., disease locations and severity).

Recently, nanotechnology emerges as innovative tools in drug delivery and diagnosis to treat a wide range of diseases, such as cancer and inflammatory disorders [6–13]. In the case of ischemic stroke, nanoparticles could possibly deliver therapeutics across BBB, prolong the drug circulation, and increase the drug accumulation at diseased sites. In addition, nanoparticles can be utilized as innovative diagnostic systems to detect several biomarkers (such as ROS and neurotransmitters) in the brain for early-stage stroke diagnosis. In this review, we firstly describe the physiopathology of ischemic stroke and current limitations in therapy and diagnosis. Then, we discuss how nanotechnology offers opportunities in treating ischemic stroke, highlighting the recent progress on delivering neuroprotective agents, anti-inflammatory drugs, and small interfering RNA (siRNA) to alleviate ischemic injuries. We also review the applications of nanomaterials in stroke diagnosis. Finally, we describe new opportunities in translating nanoparticle-based therapies to clinic in the prevention and treatment of ischemic stroke.

2. Pathology of Stroke and Current Therapies

2.1. *Molecular Mechanisms for Pathology in Stroke*

Acute ischemic stroke and subsequent reperfusion cause a series of pathophysiological changes including neuronal damage, oxidative stress, local inflammation, and loss of blood brain barrier (BBB) integrity [14]. The cellular process and mechanism of ischemic stroke and the ischemic injury cascade is summarized in Figure 1. Herein, we mainly discuss neuronal damage, oxidative stress, and inflammation responses that contribute to the pathogenesis of ischemic stroke. These three events are intertwined, and each can result in brain damage.

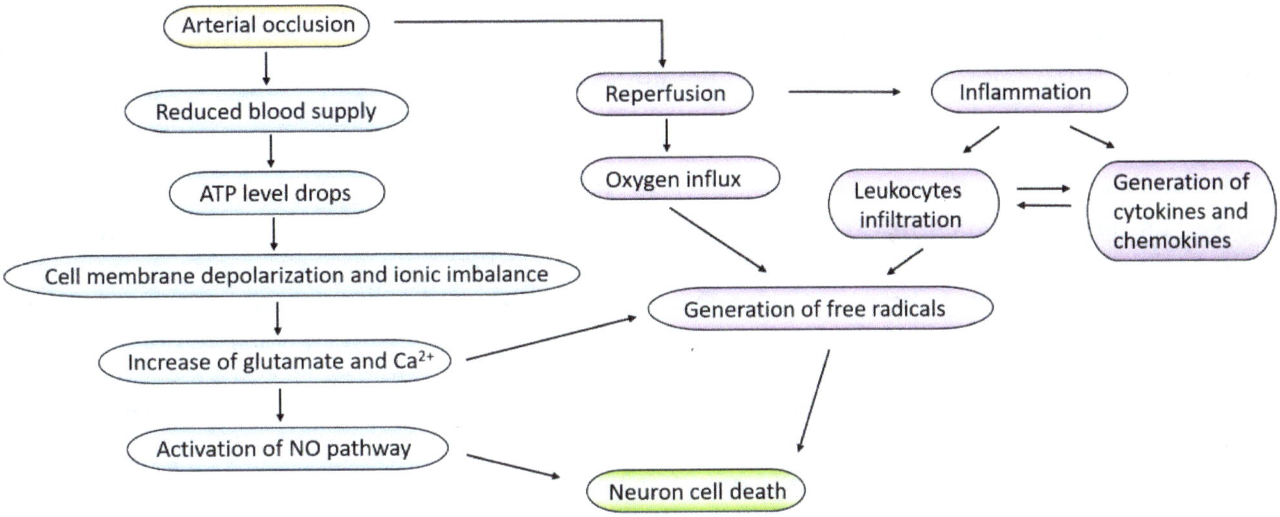

Figure 1. The cellular process and mechanism of ischemic stroke and the ischemic injury cascade.

2.1.1. Neuronal Damage

Neurons are the major components in brain and are particularly vulnerable to ischemia. Studies have shown that acute cerebral ischemia causes the vasculature infarction, thus leading to neuronal death in rodent models [15]. Due to reduced blood supply in the ischemic brain, adenosine triphosphate (ATP) level drops and lactate acidosis leads to the loss of ionic homeostasis in neurons [14]. Failure to maintain the ion gradients results in depolarization of cell membranes and therefore activating a variety of ion channels such as calcium and sodium channels. Those events also cause the excessive release of glutamate, which initiate more loss of neuronal cells [16]. Glutamate is a major excitatory neurotransmitter in nervous system regulating a variety of excitatory synapses, but high levels of extracellular glutamate can induce the cell death in the late stage. Dead neural cells release damage-associated molecular patterns (DAMPs), which activate the innate and adaptive immune system, initiating inflammatory pathways [17].

2.1.2. Oxidative Stress

Oxidative stress is involved with the production of reactive oxygen species (ROS), which activates apoptosis, necrosis, and autophagy pathways during ischemic stroke [18]. Oxidative stress also reduces the bioavailability of nitric oxide (NO) in endothelial cells. Nitric oxide is a potent chemical that inhibits platelet aggregation and leukocyte adhesion [19]. The loss of NO will exacerbate the coagulation, which aggravates the ischemic insult, leading to more blood flow reduction in the brain. In addition, cells under ischemia can increase the levels of calcium, sodium, and adenosine diphosphate (ADP) that produce oxygen species in mitochondria. Reperfusion is a commonly used method to treat ischemic stroke, but this also produces more ROS to cause the secondary damage in the brain. Furthermore, ROS damages lipids, proteins, and nucleic acid via lipid peroxidation, protein oxidation, and DNA fragmentation and leads to further cell death [20].

2.1.3. Inflammation Response

Inflammation response is an important event in ischemic stroke and the subsequent reperfusion. Ischemia and reperfusion activate immune system to respond to tissue injury including activation of endothelium and leukocytes. Specifically, the immune response is involved with the intravascular and parenchymal damage triggered by the interruption of blood supply. In other words, the immune system plays a central role in regulating the outcomes of stroke patients [21]. For the immune response, adhesion molecules on endothelial cells are upregulated during ischemia. For example, P-selectin was highly expressed when the mouse brain was damaged. P-selectin is a major adhesion molecule for the binding of platelets to endothelial cells, and this interaction causes proinflammatory signals [22]. ICAM-1 is another intercellular adhesion molecule and is upregulated during inflammation response. A study showed that knockdown of intercellular adhesion molecule-1 (ICAM-1) gene in mice reduced the infarction of the brain, suggesting that inflammation response plays a major role in pathogenesis of stroke [23].

Innate immune cells are major components during inflammation response because they sense endogenous danger signals through several receptors such as toll-like receptors (TLRs), retinoic acid-inducible gene (RIG)-1-like receptors, nucleotide oligomerization domain (NOD)-like receptors, C-type lectin receptors, and absent in melanoma (AIM2)-like receptors [24]. These receptors activate downstream signaling pathways, such as nuclear factor-κB (NF-κB), mitogen-activated protein kinase, and type 1 interferon pathways. These pathways upregulate proinflammatory cytokines, chemokines, and oxidative metabolites. The products including tumor necrosis factor alpha (TNF-α), interleukin-1β (IL-1β), IL-6, IL-18, and NO activate endothelial cells and astrocytes, and also act on leukocytes for their tissue infiltration in the brain, thus causing more tissue damage. Clinical studies found that in stroke patients, the increase of cytokines appeared in the cerebrospinal fluid and blood and this feature is correlated to patient survival [25]. In addition, the increased infiltration of leukocytes caused by the formation of fibrin and cytokines contributes to further tissue damage. Ischemia and reperfusion activate macrophages in the perivascular space. Activated macrophages release proinflammatory cytokines, which contribute to the expression of adhesion molecules in endothelium, promoting more leukocyte infiltration (especially neutrophils) to cause the BBB damage [26]. The large infiltration of neutrophils in a short period causes the release of proteases that can further destroy the BBB integrity and exacerbate oxidative stress, leading to severe brain damage.

2.2. *Blood Brain Barrier in Ischemic Stroke*

Blood brain barrier (BBB) plays an important role in ischemia/reperfusion (I/R). During ischemic stroke, there are two phases of BBB breaking. In the early phase of reperfusion (6 h), endothelial transcytosis dominates in increased permeability of BBB, and it may be associated with endothelial vesicle transport [27]. In the later phase, BBB is disrupted because of the loss of integrity of endothelial tight junctions (TJs). Studies showed that the structural changes of TJs occurred at 48–58 h after middle cerebral artery occlusion (MCAO) in mice [28], and these changes were associated with the degradation of TJs by matrix metalloproteinases (MMPs) [29]. MMPs also degraded extracellular matrix proteins of basal membrane of BBB, such as type IV collagen [30].

The immune response also causes the loss of BBB integrity, leading to cell death in stroke [31]. Microglia are macrophages existing in the brain, and they become activated in response to ischemic stroke, which cause the production of ROS, cytokines (e.g., TNF-α, IL-1β, and IL-6) and chemokines (e.g., macrophage inflammatory proteins-1alpha (MIP-1α)/CCL3, monocyte chemoattractant protein-1 (MCP-1)/CCL-2 and chemokine (C-X-C motif) ligand-1 (CXCL-1)). These inflammatory products act on endothelial cells to activate the NF-κB pathway for expression of adhesion molecules, such as vascular cell adhesion protein (VCAM), ICAM-1, and P-selectin. These molecules support leukocyte recruitment to invade brain parenchymal tissues [32], thus increasing the brain permeability [33].

Blood brain barrier maintains the brain homeostasis, but ischemic stroke disrupts this barrier, resulting in increased vascular permeability. As we discussed, the permeability is regulated by transcellular pathways in the early stage and the breaking TJs in the later stage [28]. Therapeutics delivery systems to ischemic stroke lesions can be designed based on its pathogenesis.

2.3. Current Treatment Options for Ischemic Stroke

Treating ischemic stroke is to restore blood flow to the brain as soon as possible, and reperfusion is a major tool to bring the blood back to the brain. The clinical methods include intravenous administration of tissue plasminogen activator (tPA) and mechanical thrombectomy (MT) [34]. Tissue plasminogen activator (tPA) is the gold standard treatment for ischemic stroke. The treatment window using tPA is in 4.5 h when patients show the stroke symptom, and the outcomes dramatically decrease beyond 4.5 h [35]. However, tPA treatment may potentially cause the intracerebral hemorrhage and lead to more mortality [36]. When patients appear with a large artery occlusion (the clot burden is high) or tPA treatment is beyond the best time window, the MT surgery is an alternative strategy to treat ischemic stroke. In MT surgery, a microcatheter is inserted to clotting blood vessels to remove the clots. The treatment procedure for stroke patients is summarized in Figure 2.

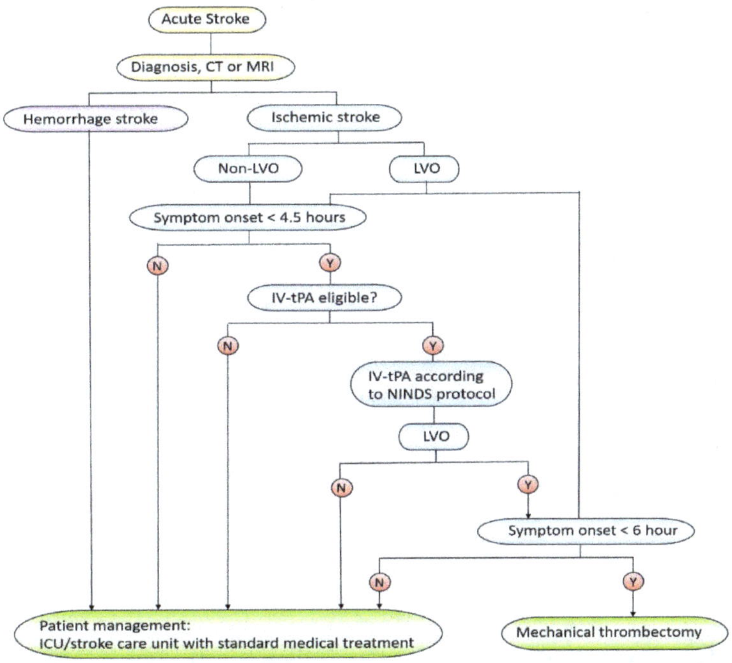

Figure 2. The procedure to treat stroke patients. CT: computed tomography; MRI: magnetic resonance imaging; LVO: large vessel occlusion; IV-tPA: intravenous injection of trans-plasminogen activator; ICU: intensive care unit; NIHSS: National Institutes of Health Stroke Scale; Y: yes; N: no.

Except for the reperfusion, supportive care is also very important. For example, 25% of patients may show neurological deficiency in 24–48 h, and care is needed to prevent further brain damage [37]. Although stroke and its pathogenesis have been investigated for many years, there are no pharmacological agents available in clinic to effectively treat ischemic stroke [38,39].

There are several drugs that have been tested to target inflammatory pathways in ischemic stroke. NXY-059 is a scavenger of free radicals and shows the neuroprotective effect in a pre-clinical stroke model [40]. However, NXY-059 was less effective in Stroke–Acute Ischemic NXY Treatment II (SAINT II) trial [41]. The failure may be due to the high water solubility of NXY-059 that has low permeability to BBB. Therefore, developing new drug delivery approaches are needed to solve the current issues on treating ischemic stroke.

3. Nanomedicine in Stroke Treatment

There are several challenges in treating ischemic stroke. Most therapeutics have short blood circulation and cannot easily cross the blood brain barrier to reach the ischemic tissues. In addition, controlling drug release and developing novel drug delivery vehicles are important factors to improve therapies of ischemic stroke. Nanotechnology is used to design nanoscale materials that can be applied in biomedical applications. Nanoparticles with the sizes of 50–200 nm are generated and can encapsulate drugs to increase drug water solubility and tissue targeting. Nanoparticles are smaller than a cell and larger than small molecules; thus, nanoparticles are excellent carriers to deliver therapeutics (drugs) and control their release for improved therapies in a wide range of diseases [42–44]. Nanoparticle-based drug delivery systems may solve the current challenges in ischemic stroke treatment. In this section, we present several nanoparticle-drug delivery systems used in treating ischemic stroke (Figure 3).

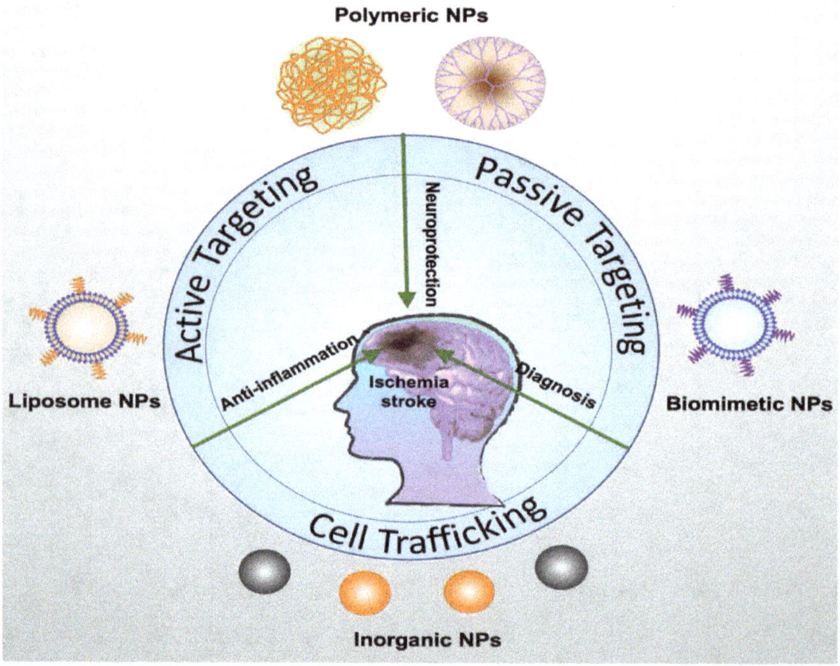

Figure 3. Nanoparticle-based delivery platforms for delivery of neuroprotectants, anti-inflammation reagents, and imaging probes for ischemic stroke therapy and diagnostics. Polymeric NPs include PLGA (poly(lactic-co-glycolic acid) NPs, chitosan NPs, and PAMAN dendrimer. Liposomes are made of a lipid bilayer and are loaded with therapeutics agents. Inorganic NPs include metallic NPs (such as platinum), ceria NPs, and Fe_2O_3 NPs. Biomimetic NPs are new drug delivery platforms generated from cell membrane vesicles. Each type of NPs has been discussed in the manuscript.

3.1. *Delivery of Neuroprotectants*

Early recanalization (thrombolysis) and neuroprotection are the two major steps for stroke patients [45]. Neuroprotection is an important strategy to protect the neurological damage from ischemic stroke. There are several approaches including reduced immune cell adhesion, blocking of proinflammatory cytokines, decreased lipid peroxidation, and decreased cell apoptosis. Many drugs, such as adenosine [46], have been developed and approved by the FDA to treat myocardial ischemia. However, they failed to be used in treating cerebral I/R injury [47] because they have the short plasma half-life time and lack of permeability to BBB. To address this issue, nanoparticle drug delivery systems have been developed to deliver drugs to cross BBB. The applications of nanoparticle-drug delivery systems have been summarized in Table 1.

Table 1. Studies of nanoparticle-based drug delivery in ischemic stroke.

Nanoparticles	Drugs/agents	Administration	Targeting	Stoke model	Results	Ref.
PEGylated liposomes	Asialo-erythropoietin	i.v.	Ischemic site	MCAO (1 h) * on rats	PEGylated liposomes increased the accumulation of AEPO at ischemia site and ameliorated cerebral I/R injury.	[48]
T7-conjugated liposomes	ZL006	i.v.	TfR over-expressed brain endothelium	MCAO (2 h) * on rats	T7 enhanced the transport of liposomes across the BBB and T7-PLPs/ZL006 reduced infarct volume and neurological deficit.	[49]
SHp and T7 conjugated-PEGylated liposomes	ZL006	i.v.	Ischemic endothelium and neurons	MCAO (2 h) * on rats	Dual targeting peptide enhanced the accumulation of NPs in brain and ameliorated ischemic injury.	[50]
Liposomes	Basic fibroblast growth factor (bFGF)	Intranasal injection	-	MCAO (2 h) * on rats	Liposomes improved bFGF accumulation in brain tissues and the system improved spontaneous locomotor activity of animals.	[51]
PEGylated liposomes	t-PA/fasudil	i.v.	-	MCAO (2 h) * on rats	Treatment of fasudil-lip before t-PA decreased the risk of t-PA-derived cerebral hemorrhage and extended the therapeutic time window of t-PA.	[52]

Table 1. *Cont.*

Nanoparticles	Drugs/agents	Administration	Targeting	Stoke model	Results	Ref.
DSPE-PEG2000 liposome	-	i.v.	Ischemic site	MCAO (20 min) * on mice	Liposomes accumulated in ischemic brain at both early stage (0.5) and late phase (48 h).	[53]
Cationic bovine serum albumin-conjugated PEG-PLA	Tanshinone IIA	i.v.	Brain microvessels	MCAO (2 h) * on rats	CBSA-PEG-TIIA-NPs reduced infarct volume and neurological deficits.	[54]
Cationic bovine serum albumin-conjugated PEG-PLA	Tanshinone IIA	i.v.	Brain microvessels	MCAO (2 h) * on rats	CBSA-PEG-TIIA-NPs suppressed neuronal apoptosis and inflammatory mediators (MMP-9 and COX-2) via MAPK signaling pathways.	[55]
SHp conjugated, red blood cell membrane shelled-polymer	NR2B9C	i.v.	Ischemic neurons	MCAO (2 h) * on rats	SHp-RBC-NP targeted to the ischemic site and ameliorate neuroscores and infarct volume.	[56]
Fas ligand conjugated-PEGylated-lipid NPs	3-n-Butylphthalide	i.v.	Microglia cells in ischaemic region	MCAO (45 min) on mice	By the help of Fas ligand, the NPs reached to ipsilateral region of ischemic brain and delivered the drug to improve brain injury.	[57]
AMD3100-conjugated PEG-T/M-PCL block copolymers (ASNPs)	Glyburide	i.v.	CXCR4 in the ischemic brain	MCAO on mice	ASNPs penetrated the ischemic brain and improve the neurological outcomes after ischemia.	[58]
TfRMAb-conjugated PEG-coated chitosan nanospheres	Z-DEVD-FMK, caspase-3 inhibitor	i.v.	TfR type 1 on the cerebral vasculature	MCAO (2 h) * on mice	Nano-system inhibited caspase activity and had subsequent neuroprotection effect.	[59]
T7-conjugated erythrocyte-coated Mn_3O_4 NPs	-	i.v.	Ischemic endothelium	MCAO (0.5 h) * on rats	The NPs scavenged free radical and restored the oxygen.	[60]

Table 1. *Cont.*

Nanoparticles	Drugs/agents	Administration	Targeting	Stoke model	Results	Ref.
Platelets coated-γ-Fe_2O_3 magnetic NPs	L-arginine	i.v.	Thrombus	Photochemical-induced thrombosis	L-arginine released at ischemic lesions disrupted the local platelets aggregation and recover blood flow.	[61]
PEGylated-ceria nanoparticles	-	i.v.	-	MCAO on rats	Ceria nanoparticles served as ROS scavenger and reduced ischemic brain damage.	[62]
Angiopep-2 and PEG modified Ceria nanoparticles	Edaravone	i.v.	LRP on BBB	MCAO on rats	E-A/P-CeO2 crossed BBB and delivered Edaravone to eliminate ROS, protected the BBB integrity and ameliorated ischemic injury.	[63]
Platinum nanoparticle (nPt)	-	i.v.	-	MCAO (1 h) * on mice	Platinum nanoparticle reduced ROS production and improved the neurological score.	[64]
Platinum nanoparticle (nPt)	-	i.v.	-	MCAO (1 h) * on mice	nPt protected the ischemic brain via reducing the MMP-9 activity and disruption of neurovascular unit.	[65]
c(RGDyK) peptide-conjugated exosomes	Curcumin	Stereotaxic injection	Ischemic site	MCAO (1 h)* on mice	They targeted the lesion region of the ischemic brain and entered microglia to suppress the inflammatory response and protect ischemic brain.	[66]
R3V6 peptides	Dexamethasone and heme oxygenase-1 siRNA	i.v.	-	MCAO (1 h) * on rats	Dexamethasone enhanced the delivery ability of R3V6 peptides for heme oxygenase-1 (HO-1) gene knockdown and reduced ischemic brain damage.	[67]

Nanoparticles	Drugs/agents	Administration	Targeting	Stoke model	Results	Ref.
Neutrophil membrane-derived nanovesicles	Resolvin D2	i.v.	Inflamed endothelium	MCAO (1 h) * on mice	Nanovesicles specifically targeted the ischemic endothelium and released Resolvin D2 to inhibit neutrophil infiltration and reduce inflammation in ischemic sites.	[68]
Functionalized carbon nanotubes (f-CNT)	Caspase-3 siRNA	Stereotaxic injection	Ischemic neurons	Endothelin Stroke Model	Gene silencing of Caspase-3 by f-CNT in neuronal tissue had neuroprotection effect and improved ischemic insult.	[69]
PAMAM dendrimer amide with basic L-arginine residues	HMGB1 siRNA	i.v.	HMGB1 mRNA in brain	MCAO (1 h) * on rats	HMGB1 siRNA delivered by e-PAM-R reduced neuronal death decreased infarct volume.	[70]

* The times represent the ischemic duration; (-) denotes that the information is not available in the studies.

3.1.1. Liposomes as Delivery Platforms

Liposomes are the first generation of nanocarriers for drug delivery used in academia and pharmaceutical industries [71]. Liposomes are made of biocompatible and biodegradable molecules that can protect drugs from enzymatic degradation and prevent drug clearance in blood.

Ishii and co-workers developed asialo-erythropoietin (AEPO)-modified PEGylated liposomes (AEPO-liposomes) to treat cerebral I/R injury [48]. Asialo-EPO (AEPO) is a neuroprotective agent that binds to EPO receptor (EPOR) on neuronal cells and activates MAPK and PI3K/Akt pathways for improved outcome of cerebral stroke. The results showed that AEPO-liposomes accumulated in the ischemic lesion for more than 24 h after injection, decreased infarct lesions, reduced the neuronal apoptosis, and ameliorated cerebral I/R injury in rats.

ZL006 is another neuroprotectant that can selectively block the ischemia-induced binding between nNOS (neuronal nitric oxide synthase) and PSD-95 (a scaffolding protein) to prevent ischemic damage [72]. However, this drug is limited to cross the BBB. To solve this problem, HAIYPRH (T7), a peptide for targeting transferrin receptor (TfR), was conjugated to PEGylated liposomes (T7-P-LPs) loaded with ZL006 (T7-P-LPs/ZL006), and the liposomes mediated the transport of ZL006 across BBB in the ischemic stroke model [49]. The results in ex vivo fluorescence imaging and particle biodistribution studies suggested that T7 enhanced the transport of liposomes across the BBB. T7-PLPs/ZL006 also significantly reduced infarct volume and prevented neurological deficit in the rat ischemic stroke model compared to free ZL006. The same group developed another dual targeting delivery system using T7 peptide and stroke homing peptide (SHp, CLEVSRKNC)-conjugated liposome (T7&SHp-P-LPs/ZL006) and demonstrated that this system can penetrate BBB to deliver ZL006 to the ischemia brain tissue. Administration of T7&SHp-P-LPs/ZL006 decreased the infarction sizes in the brain and ameliorated neurological damage [50].

Basic fibroblast growth factor (bFGF) has demonstrated the neuroprotective effect in acute stroke; however, bFGF encounters the same issue that it cannot cross the BBB. To overcome this problem, liposomes were developed to deliver bFGF (bFGF-NL) to the brain in a rat model of cerebral I/R. After treatment with bFGF-NL, in three consecutive days, mice showed improved neurological function, reduced infarct volume, and decreased nuclear fragmentation of neurons. The therapeutic effect is associated with PI3K/Akt activation by bFGF-NL [51].

To address the problem of narrow therapeutic time window of tPA (4.5 h), Fukuta et al. combined tPA and liposomal fasudil (fasudil-Lip) and examined whether they can increase the benefit of tPA to treat cerebral I/R. The results showed that the combined therapy increased neuroprotective effects compared to the administration of tPA or fasudil alone. In addition, the study indicated that administration of fasudil-Lip decreased the cerebral hemorrhage and extended the therapeutic time window of tPA compared to treatment with tPA [52].

To determine when drugs should be administered after reperfusion surgery, Al-Ahmady et al. selected a liposomal formulation made from HSPC:CHOL:DSPE-PEG2000 because PEGylated-liposomes have a long blood circulation. In the study, liposomes were intravenously administered at 0.5 or 48 h after reperfusion. Transmission electronic microscopy, histological, and immunostaining were performed, and the results indicated a higher accumulation of liposomes in cerebral ischemic mice than that in healthy mice. The possible mechanism was that the increased accumulation of liposomes in brain in the early phase (0.5 h) was due to transcellular transport. However, at 48 h after stroke, the liposome deposition was associated with both transcellular and paracellular pathways [53]. This is an interesting study, but it is needed to investigate the time course of liposome accumulation in ischemic stroke tissues to determine the therapeutic delivery time to improve the treatment of stroke.

3.1.2. Polymeric Nanoparticles as Delivery Platforms

Biodegradable polymeric NPs have also been developed as carriers for drug delivery to treat neurological diseases because they are not toxic and biocompatible, and they have the sustained-release feature [73]. Liu and co-workers developed tanshinone IIA PEGylated nanoparticles (CBSA-PEG-TIIA-NPs) conjugated with cationic bovine serum albumin (CBSA) to target negatively-charged lumens of brain microvessels [54]. The study demonstrated that NPs delivered tanshinone IIA into the rat brain in the cerebral I/R injury model, significantly suppressing the inflammation response. In addition, NPs reduced the infarcted volume and prevented the neuronal apoptosis. In another study, the same group investigated the mechanism of therapeutic effects using CBSA-PEG-TIIA-NPs. They found that NPs decreased neutrophil infiltration and prevented microglial activation. Furthermore, it is shown that prevention of neuronal apoptosis and suppression of inflammatory mediators (such as MMP-9 and COX-2) were regulated by mitogen-activated protein kinases (MAPK) signal pathways [55].

Nanoparticles were also bioengineered with ROS-responsive features that can control drug release in ischemic brain. In a study [56], Lv et al. designed nanoparticles to deliver NR2B9C (a neuroprotectant agent) to treat ischemic stroke. Nanoparticles (named SHp-RBC-NPs) composed of a red blood cell (RBC) membrane as a shell and a polymer nanoparticle with ROS-responsive boronic ester as a core. To target the ischemic brain, a peptide, SHp (CLEVSRKNC), was conjugated on the surface of nanoparticles. Triggered by high levels of ROS in ischemic region, the nanoparticles can control the release of NR2B9C in ischemic brain tissues. Ex vivo brain fluorescence imaging showed that SHp-RBC-NP can target the ischemic brain to significantly prevent neurological damage and reduce the brain infarction size.

3-n-Butylphthalide (dl-NBP) [74] has demonstrated the therapeutic value to treat ischemic stroke in clinic, but it is challenging to deliver it to the ischemic brain. To solve this problem, PEGylated-lipid nanoparticles (PLNs) conjugated with Fas ligand was developed to target the ischemic region of the brain and deliver 3-n-Butylphthalide (dl-NBP). The results are promising as the nanoparticle formulation alleviates the brain neurological injury [57].

Guo et al. designed AMD3100 (a targeting ligand)-conjugated and size-shrinkable nanoparticles (ASNPs) with the features of protease-responsiveness and brain-targeting. The nanoparticles specifically targeted the CXCR4 (C-X-C chemokine receptor type 4)-enriched ischemic brain tissue and penetrated the ischemic brain. Glyburide, a promising anti-stroke drug, was delivered by the nanoparticles, and this system enhanced the therapeutic outcomes in the ischemic stroke model [58].

Peptide inhibitors for caspases possess neuroprotection effects, but they also cannot cross the BBB. Based on this problem, Karatas et al. developed chitosan nanospheres loaded with N-benzyloxycarbonyl-Asp(OMe)-Glu(OMe)-Val-Asp(OMe)-fluoromethyl ketone (Z-DEVD-FMK), a caspase-3 inhibitor. Anti-mouse transferrin receptor monoclonal antibody (TfRMAb) was conjugated to polyethylene glycol-coated nanospheres because the antibody can selectively bind to TfR type 1 expressed on cerebral vasculature. Nanospheres suppressed the caspase-3 activity and improved neurological repair after ischemic stroke [59].

3.1.3. Biomimetic Nanoparticles as Delivery Platforms

Cell-derived biomimetic carriers have provided new options for drug delivery due to their advanced targeting abilities and better biosafety than artificial carriers. Shi et al. reported a T7 peptide (a brain targeting peptide)-linked erythrocyte membrane nanovesicles loaded with Mn_3O_4 nanoparticles (Mn_3O_4@nanoerythrocyte-T7, MNET), and this complex formulation may scavenge free radicals and change hypoxia environments in the ischemic brain. They found that MNET had a long circulation time and were capable of crossing BBB. In subsequent studies, MNET scavenged free radical and oxygen supply to rescue neurons during ischemic phase, and possibly MNET helped to remove oxygen generated by reperfusion [60].

Platelet membrane-derived nanovesicles were loaded with L-arginine, a nitric oxide (NO) donor, and γ-Fe_2O_3 magnetic nanoparticles (PAMNs) to achieve dual therapeutic and diagnostic purposes. The PAMNs were able to adhere to the damaged cerebral vessel induced by thrombosis and deliver L-arginine when the external magnetic field was applied. Furthermore, the release of L-arginine at ischemic lesions promoted vasodilation and the thrombosis was disrupted to restore the blood flow. This study showed that PAMNs may be a useful tool for both MRI imaging and targeted therapy for ischemic stroke [61].

3.1.4. Inorganic Nanoparticles as ROS Scavengers

Studies have showed that metallic NPs can function as scavengers of ROS. ROS includes superoxide anion, hydrogen peroxide, and hydroxyl radical, and they are generated during ischemic stroke. ROS is involved with oxidative tissue damage that is the mechanism responsible for brain injury in ischemic stroke.

It is reported that ceria nanoparticles can scavenge free radicals by reversibly reacting with oxygen to Ce^{4+} (oxidized) species from Ce^{3+} (reduced) species [62]. Kim et al. firstly reported that ceria nanoparticles reduced ROS production and prevented cell apoptosis, thus protecting the brain from ischemic damage. Although ceria nanoparticles are effective to scavenge ROS, the integrity of BBB is the barrier to prevent their brain deposition. Bao and coworkers developed ceria nanoparticles (E-A/P-CeO_2) modified with Angiopep-2 (ANG) and poly(ethylene glycol), which were able to cross BBB via receptor-mediated transcytosis (Figure 4A). In vitro transmigration assay (Figure 4B) showed that E-A/P-CeO_2 could cross the brain capillary endothelial cells (BCECs) compared to P-CeO_2 [63]. The BBB crossing capability of E-A/P-CeO_2 was also confirmed on healthy rats by determining the ratio of ceria nanoparticles in brain tissue and injected (Figure 4C). Finally, results showed that E-A/P-CeO_2 displayed ROS scavenging ability and decreased the infarct volume on rats (Figure 4D). The results showed that ceria nanoparticles might be promising in treating I/R injury.

Platinum nanoparticles (nPt) are novel ROS scavengers because the large surface area and the high electron density can potentiate their catalytic activity to quench ROS [75]. Takamiya et al. investigated whether nPt (2–3 nm) has the neuroprotection effect against I/R injury in the mouse model of transient middle cerebral artery occlusion (tMCAO) [64]. The results showed that treatment with nPt ameliorated the generation of superoxide via reduction of hydroethidine in the cerebral cortex and decreased the mouse infarct volume. The same group published another work to investigate whether nPt could ameliorate tissue plasminogen activator (tPA)-related ischemic injury since tPA treatment may upregulate the expression of MMP-9, which exacerbates cerebral infarction through low-density lipoprotein receptor-related protein [65]. They found that nPt decreased the MMP-9 activity and ameliorated the disrupted neurovascular unit (NVU) after tMCAO. Those results further strengthened that nPt could be combined with tPA reperfusion treatment to treat ischemic stroke patients.

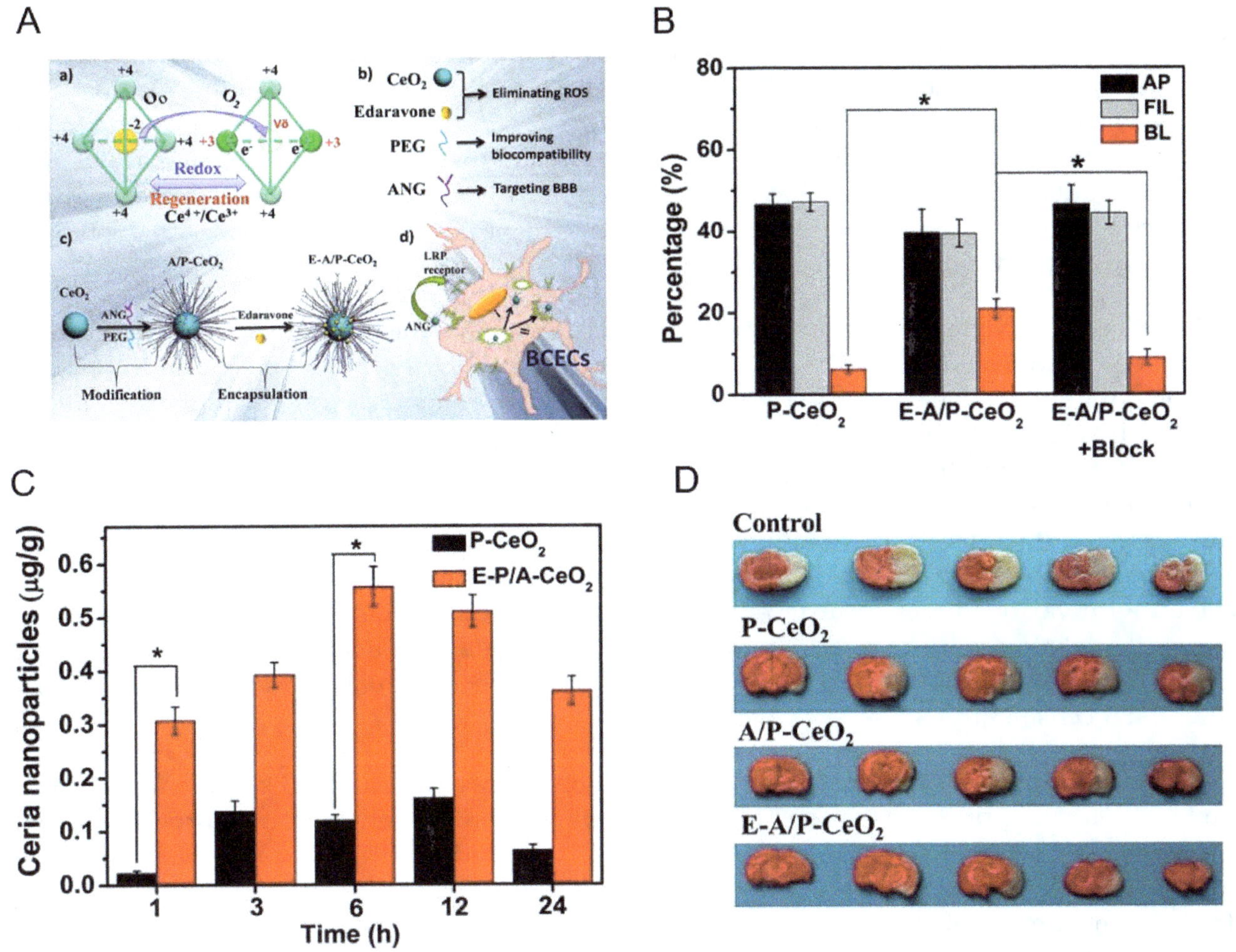

Figure 4. Edaravone-loaded ceria nanoparticles cross the blood brain barrier and protect the brain from ischemic stroke. (**A**) The nanoplatform is comprised of ceria nanoparticle core, PEG shell, and ANG as targeting peptide. (**a**) Transition between cerium(III) and cerium(IV) species in ceria NPs; (**b**) main components of the nanoparticle system; (**c**) synthetic procedure for E-A/P-CeO_2; (**d**) receptor-mediated (ANG-LRP) endocytosis of E-A/P-CeO_2. (**B**) Transmigrated amount of P-CeO_2 and E-A/P-CeO_2 in in vitro transmigration model. Free ANG was used as the blocking agent in group 3. (**C**) Concentrations (μg Ce/g brain tissue) of ceria nanoparticles in normal brain tissue. The injection dose was 0.5 mg/kg. (**D**) Representative TTC (triphenyl tetrazolium chloride)-stained brain sections after different treatments within 24 h of stroke. Data represent mean ± standard deviation (SD). * indicates $p < 0.05$. Reproduced with permission [63].

3.2. Delivery of Anti-inflammatory Reagents

Inflammation plays a central role in ischemic stroke, thus delivering anti-inflammatory drugs may be a novel strategy to treat ischemic stroke. Exosomes are endogenous vesicles made from cell membrane with cellular targeting features, therefore, they may be drug delivery tools [76–78]. In addition, exosomes have other properties, such as innate stability, biodegradability, low immunogenicity, and ability to cross BBB. Tian et al. used mesenchymal stromal cell (MSC)-derived exosomes conjugated with a c(RGDyK) peptide (called cRGD-Exo) to deliver curcumin to the ischemic brain [66]. Due to the high specific affinity of c(RGDyK) peptide to integrin $\alpha_v\beta_3$, highly expressed on cerebral vascular endothelial cells of ischemic tissues, cRGD-Exo was significantly accumulated in the stroke lesion. Administration of curcumin with exosomes (called cRGD-Exo-cur) suppressed the inflammatory response via the NF-κB pathway and protected the brain from ischemic injury.

Dexamethasone is an anti-inflammatory drug and can reduce proinflammatory cytokines, which prevent cellular damage in the ischemic brain [79]. Lee and co-workers incorporated dexamethasone to the hydrophobic component of a small peptide, R3V6 peptide (with a 3-arginine block and a 6-valine block), to form a stable micelle (named, R3V6-Dexa) used for gene delivery. R3V6-Dexa was loaded with a plasmid DNA, which expressed a heme oxygenase-1 (HO-1) as an antioxidant agent, and the complex of pSV-HO-1/R3V6-Dexa could target ischemic stroke tissues [67]. The authors stereotaxically injected the complex into rats and found that HO-1 expression was significantly increased. In addition, when mice were treated with the pSV-HO-1/R3V6-Dexa complex, the infarction size in the brain was significantly reduced compared to control groups.

Increased leukocyte infiltration is another factor to damage the brain in stroke. Within minutes after ischemia, adhesion molecules, such as P-selectin, are highly expressed on endothelial cells, and proinflammatory signals are rapidly generated [22]. Another strategy is to control the infiltration of neutrophils to alleviate the I/R injury in ischemic stroke. Targeting neutrophils may be a novel approach in treating ischemic stroke, but the methods in anti-neutrophil therapies and neutrophil depletion have failed in clinical studies. This failure may be associated with the complex signaling pathways and numerous receptors involved in neutrophil transmigration. For example, deactivating one receptor, such as anti-ICAM-1 therapy, may not be sufficient because neutrophil infiltration is involved with various types of surface proteins between neutrophils and endothelial cells [80,81]. Neutrophil depletion could be an effective approach, but systemic elimination of neutrophils can make the host vulnerable to bacterial and virus infections [82], and even impair other immune cells, such as natural killer cells [83].

Neutrophil infiltration is regulated by interactions between neutrophils and endothelial cells. Therefore, delivering drugs to the cerebral endothelium may effectively inhibit neutrophil infiltration without interfering neutrophils [77]. Dong et al. reported neutrophil cell membrane-derived nanovesicles (HVs), which can target inflamed endothelium at I/R injury sites and deliver therapeutics to treat the mouse I/R injury [68]. The nanovesicles were generated from differentiated HL-60 cells (neutrophil-like cells) using nitrogen cavitation. The nitrogen cavitation approach was used to disrupt cell membrane to eliminate nuclei and cytosols of cells. Figure 5A shows the scheme of experimental design. The TEM image showed the liposome-like structure of nanovesicles made from HL-60 cells and the size was 200 nm in diameter. In vivo imaging system (IVIS) and confocal microscopy (Figure 5B) showed that HVs (nanovesicles made from differentiated HL-60 cells) were specifically accumulated in the injured half of the brain rather than in the normal brain. To visualize how HVs interacted with brain vasculature, a cranial window was established and intravital microscopy was performed in live mice (Figure 5C). The real-time visualization images strongly indicated that HVs can specifically target ischemic vasculature. To examine the delivery of therapeutics with nanovesicles, Resolvin D2 (RvD2) was loaded into the membrane of nanovesicles because RvD2 is a new lipid mediator to resolve inflammatory responses [84]. After Resolvin D2-loaded nanovesicles (RvD2-HVs) were intravenously injected into mice, reduced neutrophil infiltration was observed using intravital microcopy in live mice, and brain homogenates also confirmed this observation (Figure 5D). Subsequently, the level cytokines, such as TNF-α (Figure 5E), were decreased after RvD2-HVs were administered. The data indicated that RvD2-HVs could alleviate inflammation responses in ischemic stroke. The diminished inflammatory responses reduced the infarction sizes and prevented neurological damage from ischemic stroke (Figure 5F).

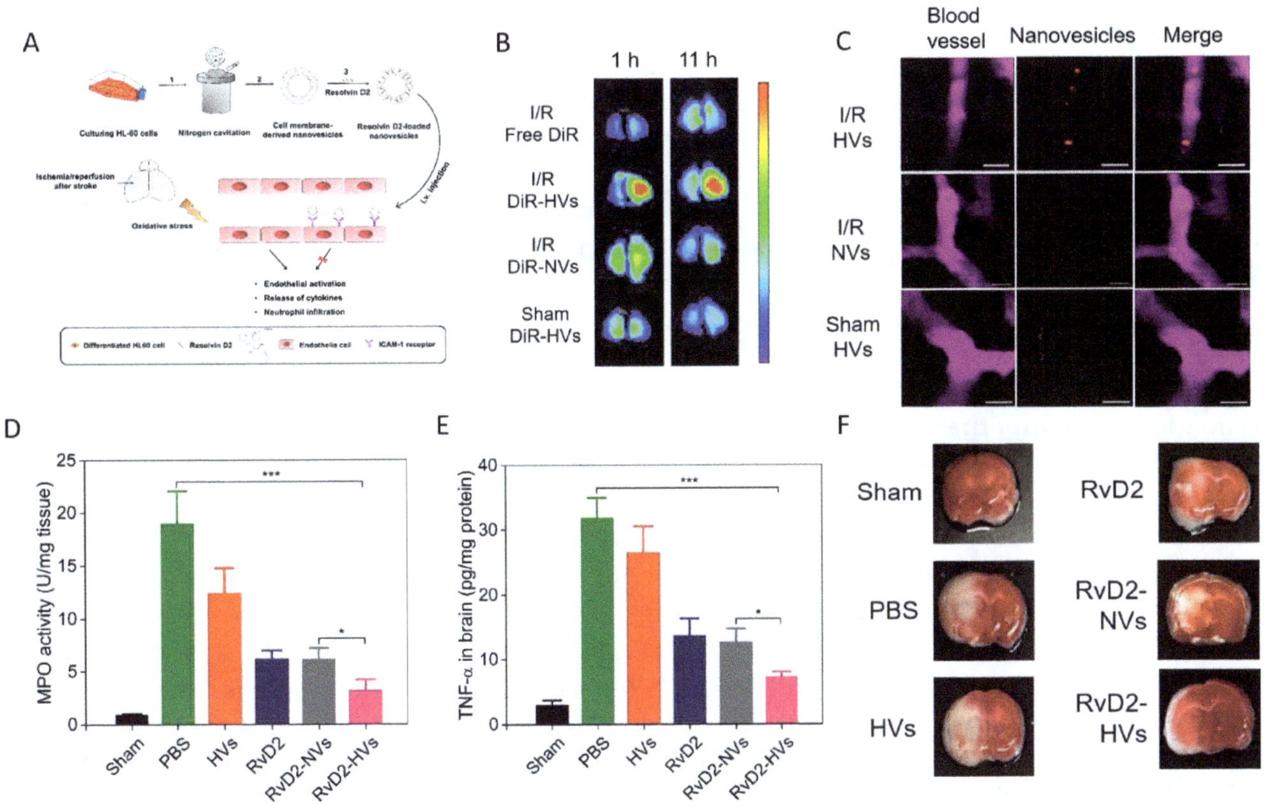

Figure 5. Neutrophil membrane-derived nanovesicles target ischemic endothelium and deliver therapeutics for ischemic stroke treatment. (**A**) A concept of nanovesicles binding to endothelium at ischemic/reperfusion injury sites and alleviating the I/R injury. Resolvin D2-loaded nanovesicles were prepared by: (1) nitrogen cavitation to break the cells; (2) purification; (3) Resolvin D2 loading. (**B**) Nanovesicles (HVs) specifically accumulated in I/R damaged half of brain. (**C**) Intravital microscopy images of HVs (red) specifically bind to I/R endothelium (top panel), instead of normal endothelium (bottom panel). Scale bar = 20 μm. (**D**) Myeloperoxidase (MPO) activity in the injured half of brain after different treatment, which indicates the neutrophil infiltration condition. (**E**) Level of TNF-α in the injured half of brain after different treatment. (**F**) TTC staining of brain sections in different groups. Data represent mean ± standard deviation (SD). * $p < 0.05$ and *** $p < 0.005$. Reproduced with permission [68].

3.3. Delivery of siRNA

Small interfering RNAs (siRNAs) can suppress the expression of a specific gene and are also used in ischemic stroke treatment [85]. Caspase-3 activation contributes to brain tissue loss and downstream biochemical events, which lead to programmed cell death in many brain injuries including ischemic stroke [86]. Khuloud et al. investigated whether using carbon nanotube-mediated in vivo RNA interference (RNAi) to silence Caspase-3 could offer a therapeutic opportunity against stroke. Peri-lesional stereotactic administration of functionalized carbon nanotubes (f-CNT) carrying Caspase-3 siRNA (siCas 3) decreased the neurodegeneration, improved behaviors, and reduced ischemic lesion in an endothelin-1 induced stroke model [69].

In another study, a gene delivery vector, PAMAM-Arg, consisting of a polyamidoamine (PAMAM) dendrimer amide grafted with basic L-arginine residues (e-PAM-R), was used to deliver the high mobility group box-1 (HGMB1) siRNA [70]. HMGB1 serves as a danger signal that evokes inflammatory responses in various types of cells. After the e-PAM-R/siRNA complex was administered in the rat MCAO model, HMGB1 levels and neuronal cell death were significantly decreased. In addition, the reduction of infarction sizes in the brain was also observed.

4. Stroke Diagnosis using Nanotechnology

Magnetic resonance imaging (MRI), computed tomography (CT), positron emission tomography (PET), and ultrasound are employed for the diagnosis of stroke. Brain CT and MRI imaging are important to detect the early stage of stroke in patients [87]. CT angiography can discover the arterial dissection in the brain vessels and changes of collateral blood flow. Diffusion-weighted imaging is a type of MRI methods used to detect the early stage of ischemic stroke because the imaging system can localize and measure the ischemic lesion to confirm the infarct sites [88]. I/R injury is associated with vascular inflammation, so fluorescence imaging can be used to investigate the changes of brain vessels using IV injection of fluorescent dyes such as dextran- or BSA-conjugates [89].

Shen's research groups developed a method to track administered stem cells and investigated cell-based therapies in ischemic stroke. Cationic polymersomes formed polymeric vesicles and they were loaded with superparamagnetic iron oxide nanoparticles (SPIONs) and quantum dots (QDs) as imaging agents. Cationic polymersome vesicles were incubated with neural stem cells (NSCs) to label the NSCs, thus NSCs could be tracked after they were injected to the striatum contralateral of the ischemic hemisphere. The migration and location of NSCs were monitored using MRI imaging in six weeks in a rat MCAO model and the optical imaging tracked the cells for four weeks [90]. Another example is that neural stem cells (NSCs) were labeled with an MRI reporter ferritin heavy chain (FTH) and enhanced green fluorescent protein (EGFP) to monitor the stem cells in the long-term for detecting ischemic stroke [91]. Those approaches are promising to understand how stem cells target the ischemic tissues and to develop the cell-based therapies to treat ischemic stroke.

Andreas et al. conducted a clinical phase II pilot trial using ultra small superparamagnetic iron oxide (USPIO)-enhanced MRI for macrophage imaging since USPIO particles have been introduced as a cell-specific MRI contrast agents taken up by macrophages. USPIO contrast agent was infused in ten patients 5 to 6 days after stroke onset, and MRI was performed within 24–36 h or 48–72 h after the infusion. Results showed that USPIO was much better than gadolinium (a clinically used imaging agent). The study indicates that USPIO-enhanced MRI may provide an in vivo tool to track cells in stroke and other CNS pathologies [92].

Theranostics nano-platform is a new way to combine diagnostics and therapeutics in ischemic stroke. In a study, HSP72 antibodies against HSP72, a specific molecular biomarker of the peri-infarct region, were conjugated to liposomes. Rhodamine/gadolinium labelled- and citicoline (CDP-Choline)-loaded liposomes specifically targeted the peri-infarct tissue in cerebral ischemia. MRI results demonstrated that the nanoparticles were accumulated in the injured brain and significantly reduced lesion volumes [93].

Clinically used gadolinium (Gd) chelates as contrast agents have several issues, such as short circulation time, rapid clearance, and low T1 signal. These issues limit the imaging time and resolution [94]. Upconversion nanoparticles doped with Gd ions can greatly enhance the T1 signals. In addition, upconversion nanoparticles can image the deep tissue and possess the photostability. Jing et al. reported synthetic UCNPs of core/shell structure ($NaYF_4$:Yb/Er@$NaGdF_4$) and coated with PEG (PEG-UCNPs). PEG-UCNPs showed the high diagnostic sensitivity to image acute ischemic stroke at a low dosage (5 mg Gd kg^{-1}) compared to the clinical dosage of 108 mg Gd kg^{-1} [95]. This new formulation may be promising in clinic.

5. New Opportunities and Perspectives

Stroke is an acute disease, therefore treating stroke requires the early diagnosis and immediate therapies. This review has highlighted the recent advances in design and engineering of new nanomaterials to target ischemic stroke tissues and new technologies used to image and monitor the disease progression in vivo.

Specifically delivering therapeutics to the injured brain is essential in treating ischemic stroke. While many nanoparticle-based formulations or cell-based platforms have been developed, the fundamental question of how they target ischemic stroke lesion has not been clearly addressed.

For example, BBB is the blood vessel barrier to prevent therapeutics across the blood vessels. Most studies showed the dramatic therapeutic effects of using nanoparticle-based formulations compared to free drugs. The enhanced outcomes claimed that nanoparticles transported therapeutics across BBB, but the direct in vivo experimental data were vague to support this conclusion. Developing advanced in vivo imaging systems [96,97] is needed to visualize the intact brain [68] and to address whether and how nanoparticles cross the BBB.

Brain vasculature during stroke shows the temporal opening, and this disruption of BBB may be a target to guide small molecules across the BBB. Further investigation is needed on the time course of BBB opening to design ideal drug delivery platforms. Although ischemic stroke increases brain vascular permeability, the endothelial gaps are unlikely to allow the efficient transport of nanoparticles because their size is usually larger than endothelial gaps. Therefore, developing new and novel concepts is needed to solve the drug delivery across BBB. Ischemic stroke and reperfusion cause acute inflammatory responses including neutrophil infiltration across blood vessels. Recent studies have shown that rational design of nanoparticles (gold nanoparticles, polymeric nanoparticles, or protein nanoparticles) enables neutrophils to transport nanoparticles across the blood vessel barrier in infection and cancer mouse models [6,98–101]. It is expected that this technology of hijacking neutrophils in vivo may transport nanotherapeutics across BBB for therapies of ischemic stroke.

Ischemic stroke is strongly correlated to inflammatory responses. Inflammatory responses include endothelial activation and neutrophil infiltration, which damages the brain tissues. Targeting activated endothelium using cell membrane-derived nanovesicles has demonstrated the value in delivering therapeutics to treat ischemic stroke [68]. To translate cell-derived nanovesicles, developing new technologies is needed to scale up their production. Recent studies show that nitrogen cavitation methods [77] and other approaches [102] could have the potential to scale up cell-derived nanovesicles for clinical applications. In addition, Dong [68] et al. reported an interesting study to deliver lipid mediators [84] (such as Resolvin D2) to treat ischemic stroke. This study is different from current therapies that mainly deliver anti-inflammatory agents. Anti-inflammatory therapies can cause side effects [103], but Resolvin D2 is a new drug to increase the host immune defense via increased neutrophil apoptosis and macrophage phagocytosis [104]. In the future, it is needed to investigate how to efficiently load lipid mediators in nanovesicles [105] for improved treatment of ischemic stroke. Another direction is the design of new nanoparticles in response to inflammatory environments (such as pH or enzymes) [8] to improve the treatment of ischemic stroke.

Targeting inflammatory neutrophils in situ to block brain neutrophil infiltration is a new opportunity to treat ischemic stroke. A recent study [7] shows that albumin protein-formed nanoparticles loaded with doxorubicin could induce neutrophil apoptosis, thus inhibiting neutrophil infiltration to prevent brain damage in a mouse ischemic stroke model. This is an exciting and new research area to develop novel therapies to solve the lacking pharmacological therapies for ischemic stroke in clinic.

In addition, developing new drugs that can target inflammatory pathways for management of the host injury during ischemic stroke is needed. The pathogenesis of ischemic stroke is complicated, and it is involved with multiple signaling pathways. The molecular mechanisms of ischemic stroke-induced brain injury are needed to be further determined. The timing of administering drugs or nanoparticle-based therapeutics is also very critical. Optimizing therapeutic windows in the future is needed.

Theranostics formulations are interesting and promising in treating ischemic stroke since they combine diagnosis and therapies. Nanoparticle-based platforms are novel constructs because they can contain imaging agents and drugs in single nanoparticle platforms. For instance, formulations with both neuroprotectants and Fe_2O_3 magnetic nanoparticles can achieve the therapy and imaging. In the future, developing more similar drug delivery systems is needed to treat ischemic stroke. However, considering that many inorganic materials do not naturally exist in the body (although iron oxide nanoparticles (IONPs) have been approved by the US food and drug administration (FDA) to treat anemia), fully evaluating the biodistribution and toxicity after systemic administration is required.

6. Conclusions

In summary, we have discussed various nanoparticle-based formulations and cell-based platforms used in treating ischemic stroke. It is essential to understand the pathogenesis of ischemic stroke and how nanoparticles interact with ischemic tissues. The fundamental question on how nanoparticles transport therapeutics across BBB is yet to be addressed, and advances in design and synthesis of nanoparticles and novel in vivo imaging systems (such as intravital microscopy) may address this question. The development of new drugs and novel nanoparticle-based therapeutics will improve the outcomes in treating ischemic stroke patients.

Author Contributions: X.D. was involved in literature review, writing the original draft and editing. J.G. was involved in figure creation and editing. Y.S. was involved in literature review and editing. Z.W. was involved in writing, editing, supervision and funding acquisition. All authors have read and agreed to the published version of the manuscript.

References

1. Virani, S.S.; Alonso, A.; Benjamin, E.J.; Bittencourt, M.S.; Callaway, C.W.; Carson, A.P.; Chamberlain, A.M.; Chang, A.R.; Cheng, S.; Delling, F.N.; et al. Heart Disease and Stroke Statistics-2020 Update: A Report From the American Heart Association. *Circulation* **2020**, *141*, e139–e596. [CrossRef] [PubMed]
2. Malik, R.; Dichgans, M. Challenges and opportunities in stroke genetics. *Cardiovasc. Res.* **2018**, *114*, 1226–1240. [CrossRef] [PubMed]
3. Fernandes, L.F.; Bruch, G.E.; Massensini, A.R.; Frézard, F. Recent Advances in the Therapeutic and Diagnostic Use of Liposomes and Carbon Nanomaterials in Ischemic Stroke. *Front. Neurosci.* **2018**, *12*, 453. [CrossRef] [PubMed]
4. Tsivgoulis, G.; Katsanos, A.H.; Alexandrov, A.V. Reperfusion therapies of acute ischemic stroke: Potentials and failures. *Front. Neurol.* **2014**, *5*, 215. [CrossRef]
5. Granger, D.N.; Kvietys, P.R. Reperfusion injury and reactive oxygen species: The evolution of a concept. *Redox. Biol.* **2015**, *6*, 524–551. [CrossRef]
6. Chu, D.; Dong, X.; Zhao, Q.; Gu, J.; Wang, Z. Photosensitization Priming of Tumor Microenvironments Improves Delivery of Nanotherapeutics via Neutrophil Infiltration. *Adv. Mater.* **2017**, *29*. [CrossRef]
7. Zhang, C.Y.; Dong, X.; Gao, J.; Lin, W.; Liu, Z.; Wang, Z. Nanoparticle-induced neutrophil apoptosis increases survival in sepsis and alleviates neurological damage in stroke. *Sci. Adv.* **2019**, *5*, eaax7964. [CrossRef] [PubMed]
8. Zhang, C.Y.; Gao, J.; Wang, Z. Bioresponsive Nanoparticles Targeted to Infectious Microenvironments for Sepsis Management. *Adv. Mater.* **2018**, *30*, e1803618. [CrossRef]
9. Wang, Z.; Tiruppathi, C.; Cho, J.; Minshall, R.D.; Malik, A.B. Delivery of nanoparticle: Complexed drugs across the vascular endothelial barrier via caveolae. *IUBMB Life* **2011**, *63*, 659–667. [CrossRef]
10. Wang, Z.; Tiruppathi, C.; Minshall, R.D.; Malik, A.B. Size and dynamics of caveolae studied using nanoparticles in living endothelial cells. *ACS Nano* **2009**, *3*, 4110–4116. [CrossRef]
11. Chauhan, V.P.; Jain, R.K. Strategies for advancing cancer nanomedicine. *Nat. Mater.* **2013**, *12*, 958–962. [CrossRef] [PubMed]
12. Zhao, Z.; Ukidve, A.; Kim, J.; Mitragotri, S. Targeting Strategies for Tissue-Specific Drug Delivery. *Cell* **2020**, *181*, 151–167. [CrossRef] [PubMed]
13. Cheng, C.J.; Tietjen, G.T.; Saucier-Sawyer, J.K.; Saltzman, W.M. A holistic approach to targeting disease with polymeric nanoparticles. *Nat. Rev. Drug Discov.* **2015**, *14*, 239–247. [CrossRef]
14. Xing, C.; Arai, K.; Lo, E.H.; Hommel, M. Pathophysiologic cascades in ischemic stroke. *Int. J. Stroke* **2012**, *7*, 378–385. [CrossRef] [PubMed]

15. Baron, J.C.; Yamauchi, H.; Fujioka, M.; Endres, M. Selective neuronal loss in ischemic stroke and cerebrovascular disease. *J. Cereb. Blood Flow Metab.* **2014**, *34*, 2–18. [CrossRef] [PubMed]
16. Nishizawa, Y. Glutamate release and neuronal damage in ischemia. *Life Sci.* **2001**, *69*, 369–381. [CrossRef]
17. Roh, J.S.; Sohn, D.H. Damage-Associated Molecular Patterns in Inflammatory Diseases. *Immune Netw.* **2018**, *18*, e27. [CrossRef]
18. Sun, M.S.; Jin, H.; Sun, X.; Huang, S.; Zhang, F.L.; Guo, Z.N.; Yang, Y. Free Radical Damage in Ischemia-Reperfusion Injury: An Obstacle in Acute Ischemic Stroke after Revascularization Therapy. *Oxid. Med. Cell Longev.* **2018**, *2018*, 3804979. [CrossRef]
19. Lubos, E.; Handy, D.E.; Loscalzo, J. Role of oxidative stress and nitric oxide in atherothrombosis. *Front. Biosci.* **2008**, *13*, 5323–5344. [CrossRef]
20. Nita, M.; Grzybowski, A. The Role of the Reactive Oxygen Species and Oxidative Stress in the Pathomechanism of the Age-Related Ocular Diseases and Other Pathologies of the Anterior and Posterior Eye Segments in Adults. *Oxid. Med. Cell Longev.* **2016**, *2016*, 3164734. [CrossRef]
21. Anrather, J.; Iadecola, C. Inflammation and Stroke: An Overview. *Neurotherapeutics* **2016**, *13*, 661–670. [CrossRef] [PubMed]
22. Iadecola, C.; Anrather, J. The immunology of stroke: From mechanisms to translation. *Nat. Med.* **2011**, *17*, 796–808. [CrossRef]
23. Connolly, E.S., Jr.; Winfree, C.J.; Springer, T.A.; Naka, Y.; Liao, H.; Yan, S.D.; Stern, D.M.; Solomon, R.A.; Gutierrez-Ramos, J.C.; Pinsky, D.J. Cerebral protection in homozygous null ICAM-1 mice after middle cerebral artery occlusion. Role of neutrophil adhesion in the pathogenesis of stroke. *J. Clin. Investig.* **1996**, *97*, 209–216. [CrossRef]
24. Kigerl, K.A.; de Rivero Vaccari, J.P.; Dietrich, W.D.; Popovich, P.G.; Keane, R.W. Pattern recognition receptors and central nervous system repair. *Exp. Neurol.* **2014**, *258*, 5–16. [CrossRef]
25. Chamorro, Á.; Meisel, A.; Planas, A.M.; Urra, X.; van de Beek, D.; Veltkamp, R. The immunology of acute stroke. *Nat. Rev. Neurol.* **2012**, *8*, 401–410. [CrossRef] [PubMed]
26. Jin, R.; Yang, G.; Li, G. Inflammatory mechanisms in ischemic stroke: Role of inflammatory cells. *J. Leukoc. Biol.* **2010**, *87*, 779–789. [CrossRef] [PubMed]
27. Haley, M.J.; Lawrence, C.B. The blood-brain barrier after stroke: Structural studies and the role of transcytotic vesicles. *J. Cereb. Blood Flow Metab.* **2017**, *37*, 456–470. [CrossRef] [PubMed]
28. Knowland, D.; Arac, A.; Sekiguchi, K.J.; Hsu, M.; Lutz, S.E.; Perrino, J.; Steinberg, G.K.; Barres, B.A.; Nimmerjahn, A.; Agalliu, D. Stepwise recruitment of transcellular and paracellular pathways underlies blood-brain barrier breakdown in stroke. *Neuron* **2014**, *82*, 603–617. [CrossRef] [PubMed]
29. Bauer, A.T.; Bürgers, H.F.; Rabie, T.; Marti, H.H. Matrix metalloproteinase-9 mediates hypoxia-induced vascular leakage in the brain via tight junction rearrangement. *J. Cereb. Blood Flow Metab.* **2010**, *30*, 837–848. [CrossRef]
30. Yang, Y.; Rosenberg, G.A. Blood-brain barrier breakdown in acute and chronic cerebrovascular disease. *Stroke* **2011**, *42*, 3323–3328. [CrossRef]
31. da Fonseca, A.C.; Matias, D.; Garcia, C.; Amaral, R.; Geraldo, L.H.; Freitas, C.; Lima, F.R. The impact of microglial activation on blood-brain barrier in brain diseases. *Front. Cell Neurosci.* **2014**, *8*, 362. [CrossRef] [PubMed]
32. Janardhan, V.; Qureshi, A.I. Mechanisms of ischemic brain injury. *Curr. Cardiol. Rep.* **2004**, *6*, 117–123. [CrossRef] [PubMed]
33. Mittal, M.; Siddiqui, M.R.; Tran, K.; Reddy, S.P.; Malik, A.B. Reactive oxygen species in inflammation and tissue injury. *Antioxid Redox Signal.* **2014**, *20*, 1126–1167. [CrossRef] [PubMed]
34. Bhaskar, S.; Stanwell, P.; Cordato, D.; Attia, J.; Levi, C. Reperfusion therapy in acute ischemic stroke: Dawn of a new era? *BMC Neurol.* **2018**, *18*, 8. [CrossRef] [PubMed]
35. Yoo, A.J.; Pulli, B.; Gonzalez, R.G. Imaging-based treatment selection for intravenous and intra-arterial stroke therapies: A comprehensive review. *Expert Rev. Cardiovasc. Ther.* **2011**, *9*, 857–876. [CrossRef]
36. Kurth, T.; Heuschmann, P.U.; Walker, A.M.; Berger, K. Mortality of stroke patients treated with thrombolysis: Analysis of nationwide inpatient sample. *Neurology* **2007**, *68*, 710. [CrossRef]

37. Powers, W.J.; Rabinstein, A.A.; Ackerson, T.; Adeoye, O.M.; Bambakidis, N.C.; Becker, K.; Biller, J.; Brown, M.; Demaerschalk, B.M.; Hoh, B.; et al. Guidelines for the Early Management of Patients With Acute Ischemic Stroke: 2019 Update to the 2018 Guidelines for the Early Management of Acute Ischemic Stroke: A Guideline for Healthcare Professionals From the American Heart Association/American Stroke Association. *Stroke* **2019**, *50*, e344–e418. [CrossRef]
38. Minnerup, J.; Sutherland, B.A.; Buchan, A.M.; Kleinschnitz, C. Neuroprotection for stroke: Current status and future perspectives. *Int J. Mol. Sci.* **2012**, *13*, 11753–11772. [CrossRef]
39. Ginsberg, M.D. Neuroprotection for ischemic stroke: Past, present and future. *Neuropharmacology* **2008**, *55*, 363–389. [CrossRef]
40. Diener, H.C.; Lees, K.R.; Lyden, P.; Grotta, J.; Davalos, A.; Davis, S.M.; Shuaib, A.; Ashwood, T.; Wasiewski, W.; Alderfer, V.; et al. NXY-059 for the treatment of acute stroke: Pooled analysis of the SAINT I and II Trials. *Stroke* **2008**, *39*, 1751–1758. [CrossRef]
41. Shuaib, A.; Lees, K.R.; Lyden, P.; Grotta, J.; Davalos, A.; Davis, S.M.; Diener, H.C.; Ashwood, T.; Wasiewski, W.W.; Emeribe, U. NXY-059 for the treatment of acute ischemic stroke. *N. Engl. J. Med.* **2007**, *357*, 562–571. [CrossRef]
42. Panagiotou, S.; Saha, S. Therapeutic benefits of nanoparticles in stroke. *Front. Neurosci.* **2015**, *9*, 182. [CrossRef]
43. Sarmah, D.; Saraf, J.; Kaur, H.; Pravalika, K.; Tekade, R.K.; Borah, A.; Kalia, K.; Dave, K.R.; Bhattacharya, P. Stroke Management: An Emerging Role of Nanotechnology. *Micromachines* **2017**, *8*, 262. [CrossRef]
44. Kyle, S.; Saha, S. Nanotechnology for the detection and therapy of stroke. *Adv. Healthc. Mater.* **2014**, *3*, 1703–1720. [CrossRef] [PubMed]
45. Shcharbina, N.; Shcharbin, D.; Bryszewska, M. Nanomaterials in stroke treatment: Perspectives. *Stroke* **2013**, *44*, 2351–2355. [CrossRef] [PubMed]
46. Williams-Karnesky, R.L.; Stenzel-Poore, M.P. Adenosine and stroke: Maximizing the therapeutic potential of adenosine as a prophylactic and acute neuroprotectant. *Curr. Neuropharmacol.* **2009**, *7*, 217–227. [CrossRef]
47. Chen, L.; Gao, X. The application of nanoparticles for neuroprotection in acute ischemic stroke. *Ther. Deliv.* **2017**, *8*, 915–928. [CrossRef] [PubMed]
48. Ishii, T.; Asai, T.; Oyama, D.; Fukuta, T.; Yasuda, N.; Shimizu, K.; Minamino, T.; Oku, N. Amelioration of cerebral ischemia-reperfusion injury based on liposomal drug delivery system with asialo-erythropoietin. *J. Control. Release* **2012**, *160*, 81–87. [CrossRef]
49. Wang, Z.; Zhao, Y.; Jiang, Y.; Lv, W.; Wu, L.; Wang, B.; Lv, L.; Xu, Q.; Xin, H. Enhanced anti-ischemic stroke of ZL006 by T7-conjugated PEGylated liposomes drug delivery system. *Sci. Rep.* **2015**, *5*, 12651. [CrossRef] [PubMed]
50. Zhao, Y.; Jiang, Y.; Lv, W.; Wang, Z.; Lv, L.; Wang, B.; Liu, X.; Liu, Y.; Hu, Q.; Sun, W.; et al. Dual targeted nanocarrier for brain ischemic stroke treatment. *J. Control. Release* **2016**, *233*, 64–71. [CrossRef] [PubMed]
51. Zhao, Y.Z.; Lin, M.; Lin, Q.; Yang, W.; Yu, X.C.; Tian, F.R.; Mao, K.L.; Yang, J.J.; Lu, C.T.; Wong, H.L. Intranasal delivery of bFGF with nanoliposomes enhances in vivo neuroprotection and neural injury recovery in a rodent stroke model. *J. Control. Release* **2016**, *224*, 165–175. [CrossRef] [PubMed]
52. Fukuta, T.; Asai, T.; Yanagida, Y.; Namba, M.; Koide, H.; Shimizu, K.; Oku, N. Combination therapy with liposomal neuroprotectants and tissue plasminogen activator for treatment of ischemic stroke. *FASEB J.* **2017**, *31*, 1879–1890. [CrossRef] [PubMed]
53. Al-Ahmady, Z.S.; Jasim, D.; Ahmad, S.S.; Wong, R.; Haley, M.; Coutts, G.; Schiessl, I.; Allan, S.M.; Kostarelos, K. Selective Liposomal Transport through Blood Brain Barrier Disruption in Ischemic Stroke Reveals Two Distinct Therapeutic Opportunities. *ACS Nano* **2019**, *13*, 12470–12486. [CrossRef] [PubMed]
54. Liu, X.; An, C.; Jin, P.; Liu, X.; Wang, L. Protective effects of cationic bovine serum albumin-conjugated PEGylated tanshinone IIA nanoparticles on cerebral ischemia. *Biomaterials* **2013**, *34*, 817–830. [CrossRef] [PubMed]
55. Liu, X.; Ye, M.; An, C.; Pan, L.; Ji, L. The effect of cationic albumin-conjugated PEGylated tanshinone IIA nanoparticles on neuronal signal pathways and neuroprotection in cerebral ischemia. *Biomaterials* **2013**, *34*, 6893–6905. [CrossRef]
56. Lv, W.; Xu, J.; Wang, X.; Li, X.; Xu, Q.; Xin, H. Bioengineered Boronic Ester Modified Dextran Polymer Nanoparticles as Reactive Oxygen Species Responsive Nanocarrier for Ischemic Stroke Treatment. *ACS Nano* **2018**, *12*, 5417–5426. [CrossRef]

57. Lu, Y.M.; Huang, J.Y.; Wang, H.; Lou, X.F.; Liao, M.H.; Hong, L.J.; Tao, R.R.; Ahmed, M.M.; Shan, C.L.; Wang, X.L.; et al. Targeted therapy of brain ischaemia using Fas ligand antibody conjugated PEG-lipid nanoparticles. *Biomaterials* **2014**, *35*, 530–537. [CrossRef] [PubMed]
58. Guo, X.; Deng, G.; Liu, J.; Zou, P.; Du, F.; Liu, F.; Chen, A.T.; Hu, R.; Li, M.; Zhang, S.; et al. Thrombin-Responsive, Brain-Targeting Nanoparticles for Improved Stroke Therapy. *ACS Nano* **2018**, *12*, 8723–8732. [CrossRef]
59. Karatas, H.; Aktas, Y.; Gursoy-Ozdemir, Y.; Bodur, E.; Yemisci, M.; Caban, S.; Vural, A.; Pinarbasli, O.; Capan, Y.; Fernandez-Megia, E.; et al. A nanomedicine transports a peptide caspase-3 inhibitor across the blood-brain barrier and provides neuroprotection. *J. Neurosci.* **2009**, *29*, 13761–13769. [CrossRef]
60. Shi, J.; Yu, W.; Xu, L.; Yin, N.; Liu, W.; Zhang, K.; Liu, J.; Zhang, Z. Bioinspired Nanosponge for Salvaging Ischemic Stroke via Free Radical Scavenging and Self-Adapted Oxygen Regulating. *Nano Lett.* **2020**, *20*, 780–789. [CrossRef]
61. Li, M.; Li, J.; Chen, J.; Liu, Y.; Cheng, X.; Yang, F.; Gu, N. Platelet Membrane Biomimetic Magnetic Nanocarriers for Targeted Delivery and in Situ Generation of Nitric Oxide in Early Ischemic Stroke. *ACS Nano* **2020**, *14*, 2024–2035. [CrossRef] [PubMed]
62. Kim, C.K.; Kim, T.; Choi, I.Y.; Soh, M.; Kim, D.; Kim, Y.J.; Jang, H.; Yang, H.S.; Kim, J.Y.; Park, H.K.; et al. Ceria nanoparticles that can protect against ischemic stroke. *Angew. Chem. Int. Ed. Engl.* **2012**, *51*, 11039–11043. [CrossRef] [PubMed]
63. Bao, Q.; Hu, P.; Xu, Y.; Cheng, T.; Wei, C.; Pan, L.; Shi, J. Simultaneous Blood-Brain Barrier Crossing and Protection for Stroke Treatment Based on Edaravone-Loaded Ceria Nanoparticles. *ACS Nano* **2018**, *12*, 6794–6805. [CrossRef] [PubMed]
64. Takamiya, M.; Miyamoto, Y.; Yamashita, T.; Deguchi, K.; Ohta, Y.; Ikeda, Y.; Matsuura, T.; Abe, K. Neurological and pathological improvements of cerebral infarction in mice with platinum nanoparticles. *J. Neurosci. Res.* **2011**, *89*, 1125–1133. [CrossRef] [PubMed]
65. Takamiya, M.; Miyamoto, Y.; Yamashita, T.; Deguchi, K.; Ohta, Y.; Abe, K. Strong neuroprotection with a novel platinum nanoparticle against ischemic stroke and tissue plasminogen activator-related brain damages in mice. *Neuroscience* **2012**, *221*, 47–55. [CrossRef] [PubMed]
66. Tian, T.; Zhang, H.X.; He, C.P.; Fan, S.; Zhu, Y.L.; Qi, C.; Huang, N.P.; Xiao, Z.D.; Lu, Z.H.; Tannous, B.A.; et al. Surface functionalized exosomes as targeted drug delivery vehicles for cerebral ischemia therapy. *Biomaterials* **2018**, *150*, 137–149. [CrossRef] [PubMed]
67. Lee, J.; Hyun, H.; Kim, J.; Ryu, J.H.; Kim, H.A.; Park, J.H.; Lee, M. Dexamethasone-loaded peptide micelles for delivery of the heme oxygenase-1 gene to ischemic brain. *J. Control. Release* **2012**, *158*, 131–138. [CrossRef]
68. Dong, X.; Gao, J.; Zhang, C.Y.; Hayworth, C.; Frank, M.; Wang, Z. Neutrophil Membrane-Derived Nanovesicles Alleviate Inflammation To Protect Mouse Brain Injury from Ischemic Stroke. *ACS Nano* **2019**, *13*, 1272–1283. [CrossRef]
69. Al-Jamal, K.T.; Gherardini, L.; Bardi, G.; Nunes, A.; Guo, C.; Bussy, C.; Herrero, M.A.; Bianco, A.; Prato, M.; Kostarelos, K.; et al. Functional motor recovery from brain ischemic insult by carbon nanotube-mediated siRNA silencing. *Proc. Natl. Acad. Sci. USA* **2011**, *108*, 10952–10957. [CrossRef]
70. Kim, I.D.; Lim, C.M.; Kim, J.B.; Nam, H.Y.; Nam, K.; Kim, S.W.; Park, J.S.; Lee, J.K. Neuroprotection by biodegradable PAMAM ester (e-PAM-R)-mediated HMGB1 siRNA delivery in primary cortical cultures and in the postischemic brain. *J. Control. Release* **2010**, *142*, 422–430. [CrossRef]
71. Sercombe, L.; Veerati, T.; Moheimani, F.; Wu, S.Y.; Sood, A.K.; Hua, S. Advances and Challenges of Liposome Assisted Drug Delivery. *Front. Pharmacol.* **2015**, *6*, 286. [CrossRef]
72. Zhou, L.; Li, F.; Xu, H.B.; Luo, C.X.; Wu, H.Y.; Zhu, M.M.; Lu, W.; Ji, X.; Zhou, Q.G.; Zhu, D.Y. Treatment of cerebral ischemia by disrupting ischemia-induced interaction of nNOS with PSD-95. *Nat. Med.* **2010**, *16*, 1439–1443. [CrossRef] [PubMed]
73. Masserini, M. Nanoparticles for brain drug delivery. *ISRN Biochem.* **2013**, *2013*, 238428. [CrossRef]
74. Zhang, Y.; Wang, L.; Li, J.; Wang, X.L. 2-(1-Hydroxypentyl)-benzoate increases cerebral blood flow and reduces infarct volume in rats model of transient focal cerebral ischemia. *J. Pharmacol. Exp. Ther.* **2006**, *317*, 973–979. [CrossRef] [PubMed]
75. Watanabe, A.; Kajita, M.; Kim, J.; Kanayama, A.; Takahashi, K.; Mashino, T.; Miyamoto, Y. In vitro free radical scavenging activity of platinum nanoparticles. *Nanotechnology* **2009**, *20*, 455105. [CrossRef] [PubMed]

76. Gao, J.; Chu, D.; Wang, Z. Cell membrane-formed nanovesicles for disease-targeted delivery. *J. Control. Release* **2016**, *224*, 208–216. [CrossRef]
77. Gao, J.; Wang, S.; Wang, Z. High yield, scalable and remotely drug-loaded neutrophil-derived extracellular vesicles (EVs) for anti-inflammation therapy. *Biomaterials* **2017**, *135*, 62–73. [CrossRef] [PubMed]
78. Fang, R.H.; Kroll, A.V.; Gao, W.; Zhang, L. Cell Membrane Coating Nanotechnology. *Adv. Mater.* **2018**, *30*, e1706759. [CrossRef]
79. Tuor, U.I.; Simone, C.S.; Barks, J.D.; Post, M. Dexamethasone prevents cerebral infarction without affecting cerebral blood flow in neonatal rats. *Stroke* **1993**, *24*, 452–457. [CrossRef]
80. Vinten-Johansen, J. Involvement of neutrophils in the pathogenesis of lethal myocardial reperfusion injury. *Cardiovasc. Res.* **2004**, *61*, 481–497. [CrossRef]
81. Chu, D.; Dong, X.; Shi, X.; Zhang, C.; Wang, Z. Neutrophil-Based Drug Delivery Systems. *Adv. Mater.* **2018**, *30*, e1706245. [CrossRef]
82. Fulurija, A.; Ashman, R.B.; Papadimitriou, J.M. Neutrophil depletion increases susceptibility to systemic and vaginal candidiasis in mice, and reveals differences between brain and kidney in mechanisms of host resistance. *Microbiology* **1996**, *142*, 3487–3496. [CrossRef]
83. Jaeger, B.N.; Donadieu, J.; Cognet, C.; Bernat, C.; Ordoñez-Rueda, D.; Barlogis, V.; Mahlaoui, N.; Fenis, A.; Narni-Mancinelli, E.; Beaupain, B.; et al. Neutrophil depletion impairs natural killer cell maturation, function, and homeostasis. *J. Exp. Med.* **2012**, *209*, 565–580. [CrossRef] [PubMed]
84. Serhan, C.N. Pro-resolving lipid mediators are leads for resolution physiology. *Nature* **2014**, *510*, 92–101. [CrossRef]
85. Pardridge, W.M. shRNA and siRNA delivery to the brain. *Adv. Drug Deliv. Rev.* **2007**, *59*, 141–152. [CrossRef] [PubMed]
86. Namura, S.; Zhu, J.; Fink, K.; Endres, M.; Srinivasan, A.; Tomaselli, K.J.; Yuan, J.; Moskowitz, M.A. Activation and cleavage of caspase-3 in apoptosis induced by experimental cerebral ischemia. *J. Neurosci.* **1998**, *18*, 3659–3668. [CrossRef]
87. Birenbaum, D.; Bancroft, L.W.; Felsberg, G.J. Imaging in acute stroke. *West. J. Emerg. Med.* **2011**, *12*, 67–76.
88. Okorie, C.K.; Ogbole, G.I.; Owolabi, M.O.; Ogun, O.; Adeyinka, A.; Ogunniyi, A. Role of Diffusion-weighted Imaging in Acute Stroke Management using Low-field Magnetic Resonance Imaging in Resource-limited Settings. *West. Afr. J. Radiol.* **2015**, *22*, 61–66. [CrossRef] [PubMed]
89. Misgeld, T.; Kerschensteiner, M. In vivo imaging of the diseased nervous system. *Nat. Rev. Neurosci.* **2006**, *7*, 449–463. [CrossRef]
90. Wen, X.; Wang, Y.; Zhang, F.; Zhang, X.; Lu, L.; Shuai, X.; Shen, J. In vivo monitoring of neural stem cells after transplantation in acute cerebral infarction with dual-modal MR imaging and optical imaging. *Biomaterials* **2014**, *35*, 4627–4635. [CrossRef]
91. Zhang, F.; Duan, X.; Lu, L.; Zhang, X.; Chen, M.; Mao, J.; Cao, M.; Shen, J. In Vivo Long-Term Tracking of Neural Stem Cells Transplanted into an Acute Ischemic Stroke model with Reporter Gene-Based Bimodal MR and Optical Imaging. *Cell Transpl.* **2017**, *26*, 1648–1662. [CrossRef] [PubMed]
92. Saleh, A.; Schroeter, M.; Jonkmanns, C.; Hartung, H.P.; Mödder, U.; Jander, S. In vivo MRI of brain inflammation in human ischaemic stroke. *Brain* **2004**, *127*, 1670–1677. [CrossRef] [PubMed]
93. Agulla, J.; Brea, D.; Campos, F.; Sobrino, T.; Argibay, B.; Al-Soufi, W.; Blanco, M.; Castillo, J.; Ramos-Cabrer, P. In vivo theranostics at the peri-infarct region in cerebral ischemia. *Theranostics* **2013**, *4*, 90–105. [CrossRef]
94. Estelrich, J.; Sánchez-Martín, M.J.; Busquets, M.A. Nanoparticles in magnetic resonance imaging: From simple to dual contrast agents. *Int. J. Nanomed.* **2015**, *10*, 1727–1741. [CrossRef]
95. Wang, J.; Zhang, H.; Ni, D.; Fan, W.; Qu, J.; Liu, Y.; Jin, Y.; Cui, Z.; Xu, T.; Wu, Y.; et al. High-Performance Upconversion Nanoprobes for Multimodal MR Imaging of Acute Ischemic Stroke. *Small* **2016**, *12*, 3591–3600. [CrossRef]
96. Wang, Z. Imaging Nanotherapeutics in Inflamed Vasculature by Intravital Microscopy. *Theranostics* **2016**, *6*, 2431–2438. [CrossRef]
97. Wang, Z.; Li, J.; Cho, J.; Malik, A.B. Prevention of vascular inflammation by nanoparticle targeting of adherent neutrophils. *Nat. Nanotechnol.* **2014**, *9*, 204–210. [CrossRef]
98. Chu, D.; Gao, J.; Wang, Z. Neutrophil-Mediated Delivery of Therapeutic Nanoparticles across Blood Vessel Barrier for Treatment of Inflammation and Infection. *ACS Nano* **2015**, *9*, 11800–11811. [CrossRef] [PubMed]

99. Chu, D.; Zhao, Q.; Yu, J.; Zhang, F.; Zhang, H.; Wang, Z. Nanoparticle Targeting of Neutrophils for Improved Cancer Immunotherapy. *Adv. Healthc. Mater.* **2016**, *5*, 1088–1093. [CrossRef]
100. Dong, X.; Chu, D.; Wang, Z. Leukocyte-mediated Delivery of Nanotherapeutics in Inflammatory and Tumor Sites. *Theranostics* **2017**, *7*, 751–763. [CrossRef]
101. Dong, X.; Chu, D.; Wang, Z. Neutrophil-mediated delivery of nanotherapeutics across blood vessel barrier. *Ther. Deliv.* **2018**, *9*, 29–35. [CrossRef] [PubMed]
102. Yurkin, S.T.; Wang, Z. Cell membrane-derived nanoparticles: Emerging clinical opportunities for targeted drug delivery. *Nanomedicine* **2017**, *12*, 2007–2019. [CrossRef] [PubMed]
103. Dinarello, C.A. Anti-inflammatory Agents: Present and Future. *Cell* **2010**, *140*, 935–950. [CrossRef] [PubMed]
104. Spite, M.; Norling, L.V.; Summers, L.; Yang, R.; Cooper, D.; Petasis, N.A.; Flower, R.J.; Perretti, M.; Serhan, C.N. Resolvin D2 is a potent regulator of leukocytes and controls microbial sepsis. *Nature* **2009**, *461*, 1287–1291. [CrossRef]
105. Gc, J.B.; Szlenk, C.T.; Gao, J.; Dong, X.; Wang, Z.; Natesan, S. Molecular Dynamics Simulations Provide Insight into the Loading Efficiency of Proresolving Lipid Mediators Resolvin D1 and D2 in Cell Membrane-Derived Nanovesicles. *Mol. Pharm.* **2020**, *17*, 2155–2164. [CrossRef] [PubMed]

5

Lipid Emulsion Improves Functional Recovery in an Animal Model of Stroke

Motomasa Tanioka [1,2], Wyun Kon Park [3], Joohyun Park [2,4], Jong Eun Lee [2,4] and Bae Hwan Lee [1,2,*]

1 Department of Physiology, Yonsei University College of Medicine, Seoul 03722, Korea; hpark@yuhs.ac
2 Brain Korea 21 PLUS Project for Medical Science, Yonsei University College of Medicine, Seoul 03722, Korea; jhpark922@yuhs.ac (J.P.); jelee@yuhs.ac (J.E.L.)
3 Department of Anesthesiology and Pain Medicine, Anesthesia and Pain Research Institute, Yonsei University College of Medicine, Seoul 03722, Korea; wkp7ark@yuhs.ac
4 Department of Anatomy, Yonsei University College of Medicine, Seoul 03722, Korea
* Correspondence: bhlee@yuhs.ac

Abstract: Stroke is a life-threatening condition that leads to the death of many people around the world. Reperfusion injury after ischemic stroke is a recurrent problem associated with various surgical procedures that involve the removal of blockages in the brain arteries. Lipid emulsion was recently shown to attenuate ischemic reperfusion injury in the heart and to protect the brain from excitotoxicity. However, investigations on the protective mechanisms of lipid emulsion against ischemia in the brain are still lacking. This study aimed to determine the neuroprotective effects of lipid emulsion in an in vivo rat model of ischemic reperfusion injury through middle cerebral artery occlusion (MCAO). Under sodium pentobarbital anesthesia, rats were subjected to MCAO surgery and were administered with lipid emulsion through intra-arterial injection during reperfusion. The experimental animals were assessed for neurological deficit wherein the brains were extracted at 24 h after reperfusion for triphenyltetrazolium chloride staining, immunoblotting and qPCR. Neuroprotection was found to be dosage-dependent and the rats treated with 20% lipid emulsion had significantly decreased infarction volumes and lower Bederson scores. Phosphorylation of Akt and glycogen synthase kinase 3-β (GSK3-β) were increased in the 20% lipid-emulsion treated group. The Wnt-associated signals showed a marked increase with a concomitant decrease in signals of inflammatory markers in the group treated with 20% lipid emulsion. The protective effects of lipid emulsion and survival-related expression of genes such as Akt, GSK-3β, Wnt1 and β-catenin were reversed by the intra-peritoneal administration of XAV939 through the inhibition of the Wnt/β-catenin signaling pathway. These results suggest that lipid emulsion has neuroprotective effects against ischemic reperfusion injury in the brain through the modulation of the Wnt signaling pathway and may provide potential insights for the development of therapeutic targets.

Keywords: neuroprotection; stroke; ischemia; middle cerebral artery occlusion; reperfusion injury; lipid emulsion; excitotoxicity

---

1. Introduction

Stroke is an acute life-threatening condition in which poor blood perfusion in the brain causes cell death. Life style modification and pharmacological interventions to manage risk factors have been used to lower the incidence of strokes worldwide [1]. Despite such efforts, stroke is still associated with high mortality and morbidity across the globe [2]. Ischemic reperfusion injury in the brain is detrimental and elicits major dysfunctions within the body, such as impairments in movement, cognition and other vital functions [3]. Ischemic reperfusion injury in the brain encompasses abnormal production of oxygen radicals that may exacerbate initial ischemic injuries [4]. Such injury can occur in the current clinical therapies for stroke, such as thrombectomy. These surgeries are effective to ameliorate ischemic damage in the brain by the elimination of blockages [5]. However, it is currently arduous to prevent further oxidative damage caused by reperfusion. Again, secondary damage caused by reperfusion is intractable and could render leaving the reversible areas, such as the penumbra, vulnerable to oxidative damage [6]. Meanwhile, increases in inflammatory markers have been shown to reflect ischemic injuries in clinical settings. Cytokines, such as interleukin-1β (IL-1β), interleukin-6 (IL-6), interleukin-8 (IL-8), tumor necrosis factor-α (TNF-α), ficolin-1 and others, have been reported to increase in relations with the incident of stroke [7–10]. Therefore, decreasing inflammatory activity may be a goal for effective therapies. In previous studies, the administration of recombinant interleukin-1 receptor antagonist in rat models of middle cerebral artery occlusion (MCAO) successfully provided protection against ischemic injury [11,12]. However, the protective effects of interleukin-1 receptor antagonist have not been able to translate to neuroprotection in clinical trials but remain as a potential therapy through continued research [7].

Previous studies have implicated the importance of the canonical Wnt signaling pathway in the case of ischemic reperfusion injury [13,14]. The activation of glycogen synthase kinase-3β (GSK-3β) and the downregulation of protein kinase B (Akt) have been reported as important factors that contribute to the death of neurons [15,16]. The modulation of these proteins has been reported to affect survival of neurons in excitotoxic conditions [16,17]. The activity of GSK-3β leads to the degradation of downstream survival markers such as β-catenin through ubiquitination. Furthermore, canonical Wnt signals, which are lipid-modified glycoproteins, have been reported to inactivate GSK-3β through phosphorylation and thereby promote cell survival [18]. A recent study reported that motor exercise stimulated the canonical Wnt/β-catenin pathway for recovering from focal cerebral ischemic reperfusion injury in juvenile rats. Motor activity regulated canonical Wnt/β-catenin pathway and promoted neurogenesis and myelin repair [19]. Another study reported that electroacupuncture in multiple acupoints of a paralyzed limb stimulated the proliferation of neural progenitor cells through the activation of the Wnt/β-catenin signaling pathway and suppression of GSK-3β [20].

Lipid emulsion (LE) was approved for clinical use as a component of parenteral nutrition in 1962 [21]. LE is composed of 20% soybean oil, 1.2% egg yolk phospholipids, 2.25% glycerin and water for injection (Intralipid™ 20%, Fresenius Kabi, Uppsala, Sweden). The major fatty acids that constitute soybean oil are linoleic acid (44–62%), oleic acid (19–30%), palmitic acid (7–14%), linolenic acid (4–11%) and stearic acid (1.4–5.5%). In 1998, Weinberg et al. [22] shed light on the cardioprotective properties of LE against local anesthetic toxicity. Clinical reports have utilized the administration of LE for resuscitation from cardiac toxicity induced by lidocaine [23], ropivacaine [24] or bupivacaine [25]. The mechanism of protection of cardiac cells from excitotoxic conditions by LE depends on the phosphorylation of Akt [26] and GSK-3β [27] that contributes to cell survival. LE also has been reported to provide cardioprotection against ischemic reperfusion injury in the isolated rat heart [28]. While research into the utilization of LE against various cardiotoxic conditions is being actively conducted, investigations delineating the protective properties of LE in the central nervous system are still lacking. Neurons and cardiomyocytes share key similarities such as excitability and conductibility, which lead to their vulnerability to excitotoxic conditions. Relevant reports have claimed that distinct cardioprotective properties of LE might provide therapeutic targets or diagnostic tools for neuroprotection [29,30]. Our recent study has reported the protective effects of LE against kainic acid-induced excitotoxicity when administered directly into the brain, thereby revealing the potential neuroprotective aspects of LE [31]. However, the neuroprotective effects of LE against ischemic reperfusion injury in the brain have not been clearly elucidated.

Therefore, the present study investigated the neuroprotective effects of LE against ischemic reperfusion injury and elucidates the mechanism involved in the protection process. We examined the neuroprotective roles of LE in an in vivo rat model of the middle cerebral artery occlusion (MCAO) and reperfusion. We assessed the neurological deficits using the modified Bederson score [32] and extracted the brain to measure the severity of infarctions in experimental groups. We assessed the changes in protein and mRNA expression of distinct genes related to cell survival, Wnt/β-catenin signaling pathway and inflammation. We verified that XAV939, a Wnt/β-catenin signaling pathway inhibitor, reversed the protective effects. Based on our results, we propose that LE provides neuroprotection against ischemic reperfusion injury in the brain by regulating the Wnt/β-catenin signaling pathway.

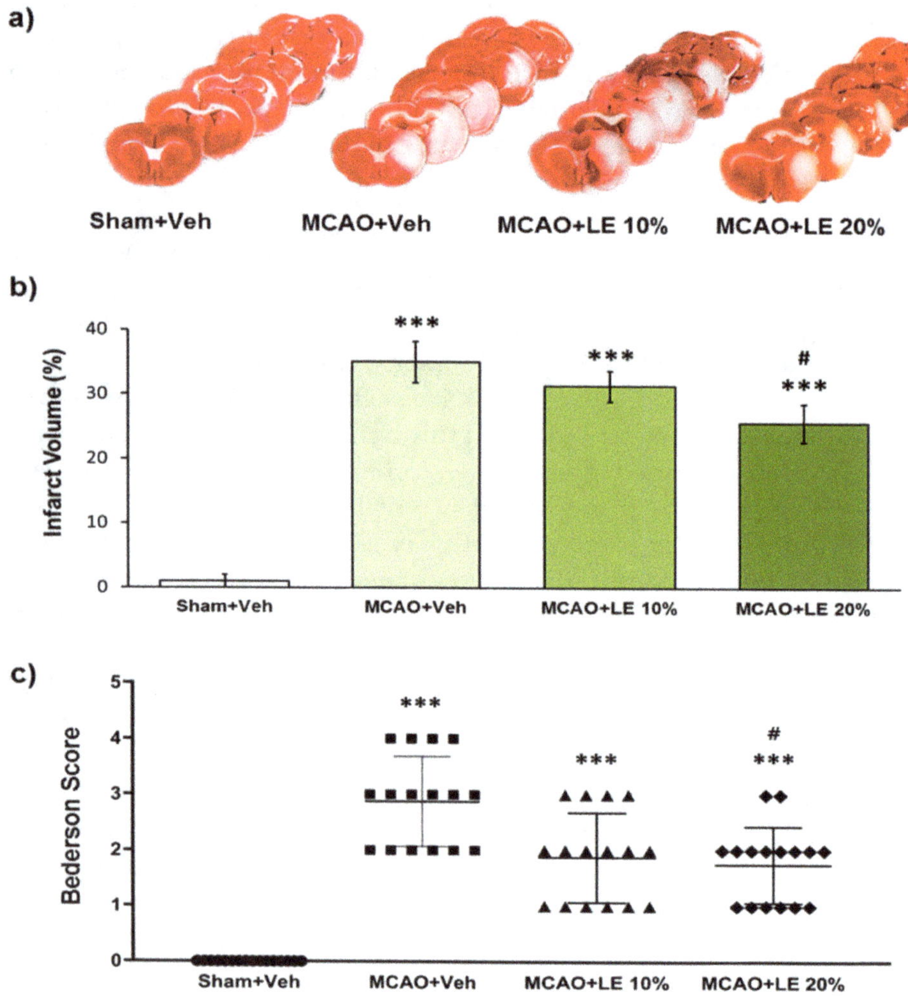

Figure 1. Neuroprotective effects of lipid emulsion (LE) or vehicle (Veh) after the middle cerebral artery occlusion (MCAO) and reperfusion injury. (**a**) Triphenyltetrazolium chloride (TTC)-stained brain slices for infarction measurement. Decrease in infarction volumes were observed in MCAO+LE 10% and MCAO+LE 20% groups. Sham group did not show ischemic reperfusion injury; (**b**) Measurement of infarction volume from TTC staining. The MCAO+Veh group increased significantly in infarction volume compared to Sham+Veh group. Both MCAO+LE 10% and MCAO+LE 20% decreased in infarction volume but only the MCAO+LE 20% group had significant difference compared to the MCAO+Veh group; (**c**) Bederson scores of the experimental groups. The MCAO+Veh group increased in Bederson score significantly compared to Sham+Veh group. Both MCAO+LE 10% and MCAO+LE 20% groups decreased in Bederson scores compared to MCAO+Veh group; however, only the MCAO+LE 20% group decreased significantly. Data are presented as mean ± standard error of the mean (SEM); $n = 16$ for each group; *** $p < 0.001$ vs. Sham+Veh, # $p < 0.05$ vs. MCAO+Veh. Statistical analysis for the measurement of infarction volume was performed using one-way analysis of variance (ANOVA) followed by Tukey's multiple comparison test. Statistical analysis for Bederson scores was performed using Kruskal-Wallis non-parametric test followed by Dunn's post hoc test.

2. Results

2.1. Dosage-Dependent Reduction in Infarction and Behavior by LE

The severity of infarction was measured by triphenyltetrazolium chloride (TTC) staining and neurological deficit assessment. The severity of infarction was visible through the unstained areas of the brain in Figure 1a. The Sham+Vehicle (Veh) group did not experience notable infarction. The MCAO+Veh group suffered an injury of approximately 35% of the left hemisphere. The MCAO+LE 10% group exhibited decrease in infarction volume to about 31%, which was not significant compared to MCAO+Veh group ($p > 0.05$, one-way ANOVA). There was a significant decrease in infarction to about 26% in the MCAO+LE 20% group compared to the MCAO+Veh group ($p < 0.05$, one-way ANOVA followed by Tukey's multiple comparison test) (Figure 1b). In behavioral test, all experimental groups suffered a certain degree of behavioral deficit except for the Sham+Veh group. The MCAO+Veh group had an average Bederson score of 3. The MCAO+LE 10% group scored lower in the behavior test and did not differ significantly compared to the MCAO+Veh group ($p > 0.05$, Kruskal-Wallis non-parametric test). The administration of LE 20% significantly decreased the average Bederson score to approximately 2 ($p < 0.05$, Kruskal-Wallis non-parametric test followed by Dunn's post hoc test). The majority of the MCAO+LE 20% group achieved a Bederson score of 2 or under, while the majority MCAO+Veh group recorded between 2 and 4. (Figure 1c).

2.2. Wnt/β-Catenin-Dependent Reduction in Infarction and Behavior by LE

Experimental groups were administered with intra-peritoneal (i.p.) injection of XAV939 to inhibit the Wnt/β-catenin signaling pathway induced by LE. The control group was administered with DMSO instead of XAV939. The severity of infarction was visible through the unstained areas of the brain as depicted in Figure 2a. The DMSO+Sham+Veh group did not experience notable infarction. Approximately 33% of the left hemisphere of the DMSO+MCAO+Veh group suffered an injury, while a significant decrease in infarction to about 24% was observed in the DMSO+MCAO+LE 20% group ($p < 0.05$, one-way ANOVA followed by Tukey's multiple comparison test). The XAV939+MCAO+LE 20% failed to protect the brain with approximately 29% infarction volume, which was not significantly different from the DMSO+MCAO+Veh group ($p > 0.05$, one-way ANOVA followed by Tukey's multiple comparison test) (Figure 2b). All experimental groups suffered a certain degree of infarction except for the DMSO+Sham+Veh group. The DMSO+Sham+Veh group did not experience notable neurological deficits. The DMSO+MCAO+Veh group recorded an average Bederson score of 3. The administration of LE 20% decreased the Bederson score to approximately 2 ($p < 0.05$, Kruskal-Wallis non-parametric test followed by Dunn's post hoc test). The XAV939+MCAO+Veh group achieved an average Bederson score of 3, which was similar to the DMSO+MCAO+Veh group ($p > 0.05$, Kruskal-Wallis non-parametric test) (Figure 2c). The i.p. injection of DMSO did not induce significant differences in the experimental group.

2.3. LE Dosage-Dependent Alleviation of Ischemic Reperfusion Injury through the Wnt/β-Catenin Signaling Pathway and Reduction of Inflammatory Protein Markers

The administration of LE affected the protein expression of survival and inflammation-related signals (Figure 3a). The expression of total Akt did not differ among the experimental groups (Figure 3b). The MCAO+Veh group showed significant decrease in phosphorylation of Akt levels (pAkt) compared to the Sham+Veh group ($p < 0.05$, one-way ANOVA followed by Tukey's multiple comparison test). The MCAO+LE 10% group also exhibited an increase in pAkt levels. However, such an increase was not statistically significant compared to the MCAO+Veh group ($p > 0.05$, one-way ANOVA). The significantly elevated level of pAkt in MCAO+LE 20% group compared to the MCAO+Veh group indicated the increased survival of neurons after ischemic reperfusion injury ($p < 0.05$, one-way ANOVA followed by Tukey's multiple comparison test) (Figure 3c). The ratio of pAkt and Akt was markedly decreased in the MCAO+Veh group compared to the Sham+Veh group ($p < 0.05$, one-way

ANOVA followed by Tukey's multiple comparison test). pAkt/Akt increased in expression in a dosage dependent manner in MCAO+LE 10% and MCAO+LE 20% groups; but only the MCAO+LE 20% group was significantly different from the MCAO+Veh group ($p < 0.05$, one-way ANOVA followed by Tukey's multiple comparison test) (Figure 3d).

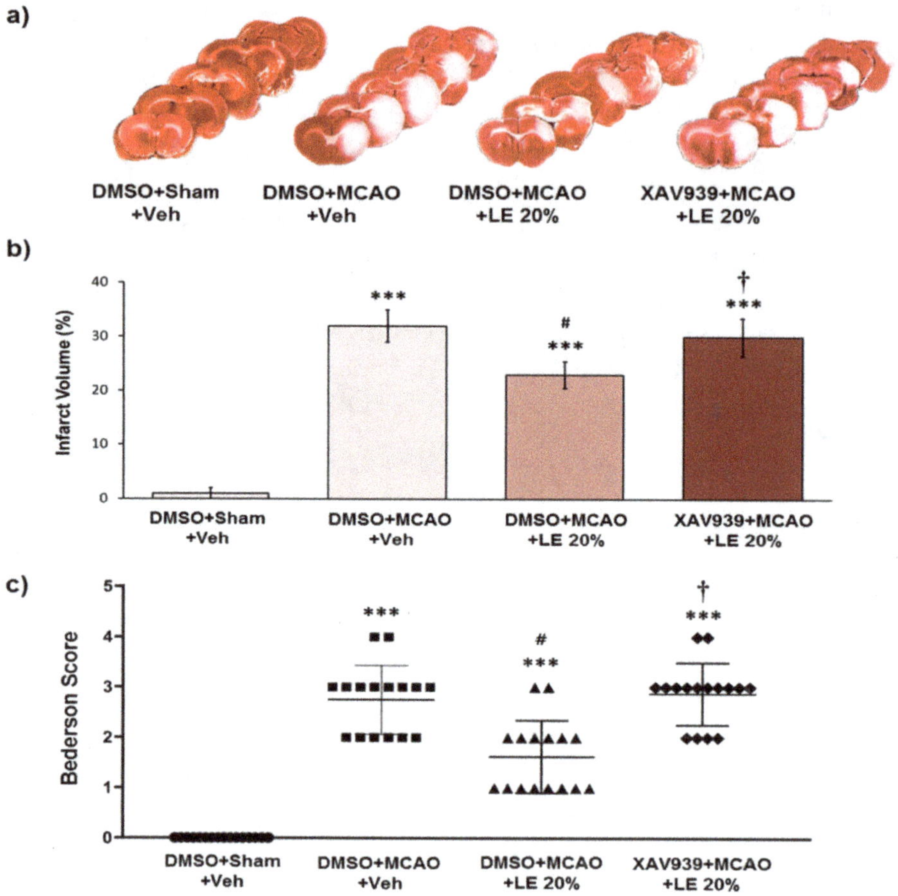

Figure 2. Neuroprotective effects of LE or vehicle on the MCAO and reperfusion injury after the administration of DMSO or XAV939. (**a**) TTC-stained brain slices for infarction measurement. Decrease in infarction volume was observed in the DMSO+MCAO+LE 20% group but not in the XAV939+MCAO+LE 20% group. Sham group (DMSO+Sham+Veh) did not experience ischemic reperfusion injury; (**b**) Measurement of infarction volume by TTC staining. The DMSO+MCAO+Veh group exhibited significant increase in infarction volume compared to the DMSO+Sham+Veh group. DMSO+MCAO+LE 20% group decreased significantly with respect to infarction volume when compared to the DMSO+MCAO+Veh. The XAV939+MCAO+LE 20% group had significantly increased infraction volume compared to the DMSO+MCAO+LE 20% group; (**c**) Bederson scores of experimental groups. The DMSO+MCAO+Veh group significantly increased in Bederson scores compared to the DMSO+Sham+Veh group. The DMSO+MCAO+LE 20% group showed significant decrease in Bederson scores compared to the DMSO+MCAO+Veh groups. The XAV939+MCAO+LE 20% group significantly increased in Bederscon scores compared to the DMSO+MCAO+LE 20% group. Data are presented as mean ± standard error of the mean (SEM); $n = 16$ for each group; *** $p < 0.001$ vs. DMSO+Sham+Veh, $^{\#}$ $p < 0.05$ vs. DMSO+MCAO+Veh, $^{+}$ $p < 0.05$ vs. DMSO+MCAO+LE 20%. Statistical analysis for the measurement of infarction volume was performed using one-way ANOVA followed by Tukey's multiple comparison test. Statistical analysis for Bederson scores was performed using Kruskal-Wallis non-parametric test followed by Dunn's post hoc test.

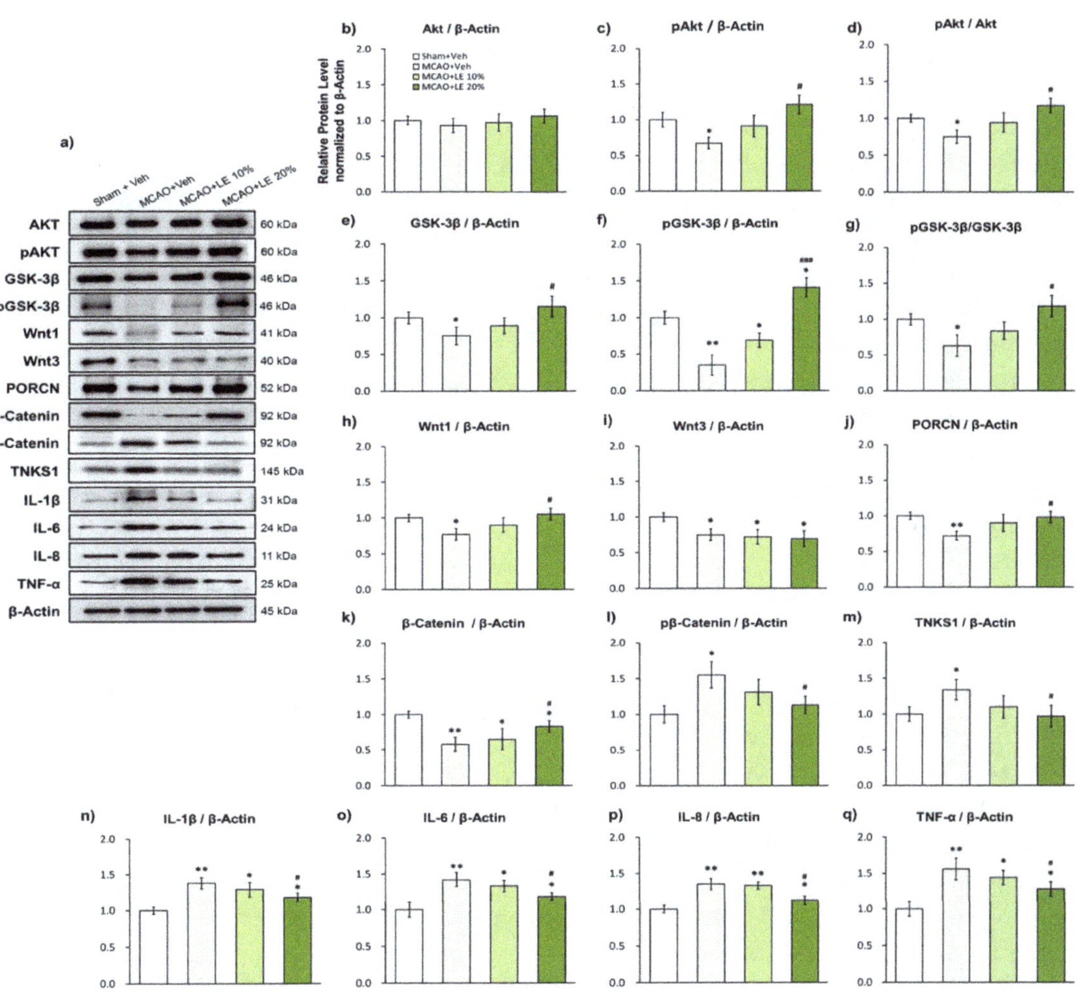

Figure 3. Effects of LE or vehicle on protein expressions after MCAO and reperfusion injury. (**a**) Representative Western blots indicating the expression of specific proteins in the penumbra region of the left hemisphere; (**b**–**d**) Expression and phosphorylation of Akt in the experimental groups. pAkt levels in MCAO+Veh group decreased significantly compared to the Sham+Veh group. pAkt was significantly increased in the MCAO+LE 20% group compared to the MCAO+Veh group; (**e**–**g**) Expression and phosphorylation levels of GSK-3β (pGSK-3β) in the experimental groups. pGSK-3β and GSK-3β levels in the MCAO+Veh group was significantly lower than the Sham+Veh group. The MCAO+LE 20% had significantly increased pGSK-3β and GSK-3β levels compared to the MCAO+Veh group; (**h**–**m**) Wnt signal-related protein expressions of experimental groups. Decreased levels of Wnt1, Wnt3, PORCN and β-catenin were observed in the MCAO+Veh group compared to the Sham+Veh group. The MCAO+LE 20% group had significantly increased protein levels of Wnt1, PORCN and β-catenin compared to MCAO+Veh group. Increased levels of pβ-catenin and tankyrase 1 were observed in the MCAO+Veh group compared to the Sham+Veh group. The MCAO+LE 20% group had significantly decreased levels of pβ-catenin and tankyrase 1 compared to the MCAO+Veh group; (**n**–**q**) Inflammatory protein expressions of experimental groups. Significantly increased expressions of inflammatory markers were observed in MCAO-injured groups compared to the Sham+Veh group. The MCAO+LE 20% group had significantly decreased inflammatory protein expression levels compared to the MCAO+Veh group. Data are presented as mean ± standard error of the mean (SEM); $n = 8$ for each group; * $p < 0.05$, ** $p < 0.01$ vs. Sham+Veh, $^{\#}$ $p < 0.05$, $^{\#\#\#}$ $p < 0.001$ vs. MCAO+Veh, one-way ANOVA followed by Tukey's multiple comparison test.

Significant decrease in total GSK-3β expression was observed in the MCAO+Veh group compared to the Sham+Veh group ($p < 0.05$, one-way ANOVA followed by Tukey's multiple comparison test). The MCAO+LE 10% group showed substantial increase in GSK-3β levels but this increment was not statistically significant compared to the MCAO+Veh group ($p > 0.05$, one-way ANOVA). The total GSK-3β expression of the MCAO+LE 20% was also significantly increased compared to the MCAO+Veh group ($p < 0.05$, one-way ANOVA followed by Tukey's multiple comparison test) (Figure 3e). The phosphorylation of GSK-3β (pGSK-3β) was significantly decreased in the MCAO+Veh group compared to the Sham+Veh group ($p < 0.01$, one-way ANOVA), which might be indicating a diminished Wnt activity. The phosphorylation of GSK-3β was significantly increased in the MCAO+LE 10% ($p < 0.05$, one-way ANOVA followed by Tukey's multiple comparison test) and MCAO+LE 20% ($p < 0.001$, one-way ANOVA followed by Tukey's multiple comparison test) group when compared to the MCAO+Veh group. There was also a significant increase in pGSK-3β in the MCAO+LE 20% group compared to the Sham+Veh group ($p < 0.05$, one-way ANOVA followed by Tukey's multiple comparison test), thereby indicating an increased activity of the Wnt/β-catenin signaling pathway (Figure 3f). The pGSK-3β/GSK-3β activity exhibited marked decrease in the MCAO+Veh group compared to the Sham+Veh group ($p < 0.05$, one-way ANOVA followed by Tukey's multiple comparison test). The pGSK-3β/GSK-3β expression for MCAO+LE 10% did not differ significantly compared to the MCAO+Veh group ($p > 0.05$, one-way ANOVA). pGSK-3β/GSK-3β activity significantly increased in the MCAO+LE 20% group compared to the MCAO+Veh group ($p < 0.05$, one-way ANOVA followed by Tukey's multiple comparison test) (Figure 3g).

Wnt1, a canonical Wnt signal and upstream marker of GSK-3β, was significantly decreased in the MCAO+Veh group compared to the Sham+Veh group ($p < 0.05$, one-way ANOVA followed by Tukey's multiple comparison test) and significantly increased in the MCAO+LE 20% group compared to the MCAO+Veh group ($p < 0.05$, one-way ANOVA followed by Tukey's multiple comparison test) (Figure 3h). All experimental groups ($p < 0.05$, one-way ANOVA followed by Tukey's multiple comparison test), excluding the Sham+Veh group, displayed robust decrease in the neurogenesis marker, Wnt3. Although Wnt3 is one of canonical Wnt signals, it does not seem to affect the Wnt/β-catenin signaling pathway induced by LE (Figure 3i). Porcupine (PORCN), a key regulator of Wnt proteins [33], decreased significantly in the MCAO+Veh group compared to the Sham+Veh group ($p < 0.05$, one-way ANOVA followed by Tukey's multiple comparison test). PORCN expression increased in the MCAO+LE 20% group compared to the MCAO+Veh group, implying elevated activity in the modulation of Wnt proteins (Figure 3j). The downstream survival marker of GSK-3β, β-catenin, was decreased in all MCAO injury groups compared to the Sham+Veh group due to infarction. However, β-catenin was significantly preserved in the MCAO+LE 20% group compared to the MCAO+Veh group ($p < 0.05$, one-way ANOVA followed by Tukey's multiple comparison test) (Figure 3k). Phosphorylation of β-catenin (pβ-catenin) was increased significantly in the MCAO+Veh group compared to the Sham+Veh group ($p < 0.05$, one-way ANOVA followed by Tukey's multiple comparison test), indicating an elevated level of β-catenin degradation. The MCAO+LE 20% group had a significantly lower expression level of pβ-catenin compared to the MCAO+Veh group ($p < 0.05$, one-way ANOVA followed by Tukey's multiple comparison test), which supported the survival of cells (Figure 3l). The expression level of tankyrase 1 was significantly increased in the MCAO+Veh group compared to the Sham+Veh group ($p < 0.05$, one-way ANOVA followed by Tukey's multiple comparison test), indicating the accumulation of tankyrase 1 through increased axis inhibition protein (AXIN) stabilization for β-catenin degradation. The MCAO+LE 20% group had a significantly lower expression level of tankyrase 1 compared to the MCAO+Veh group ($p < 0.05$, one-way ANOVA followed by Tukey's multiple comparison test) (Figure 3m).

Inflammatory protein markers of ischemic reperfusion damage, IL-1β, IL-6, IL-8 and TNF-α [34,35], increased significantly for all MCAO-injured groups when compared to the Sham+Veh group. However, attenuated levels of inflammatory markers were observed in the MCAO+LE 20% group compared to the MCAO+Veh group ($p < 0.05$, one-way ANOVA followed by Tukey's multiple comparison test), indicating the reduction of ischemic reperfusion injury (Figure 3n–q).

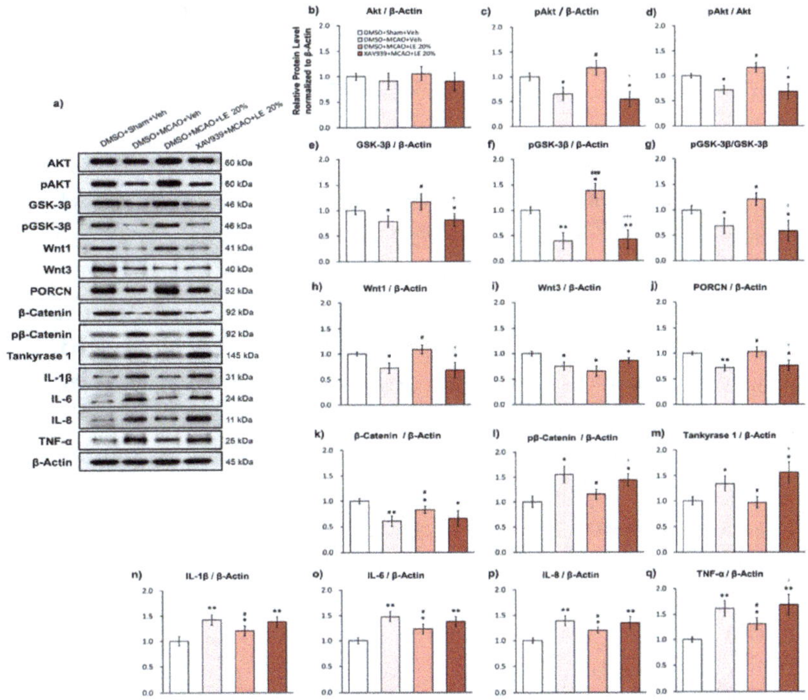

Figure 4. Effects of LE or vehicle on protein expression on the MCAO and reperfusion injury after the administration of DMSO or XAV939. (**a**) Representative Western blots of proteins in the penumbra region of the left hemisphere; (**b–d**) Levels of Akt and pAkt in the experimental groups. The DMSO+MCAO+Veh group and XAV939+MCAO+LE 20% group decreased significantly in pAkt level compared to DMSO+Sham+Veh group. pAkt was significantly increased in the DMSO+MCAO+LE 20% group compared to the DMSO+MCAO+Veh group and XAV939+MCAO+LE 20% group; (**e–g**) Levels of GSK-3β and pGSK-3β in the experimental groups. GSK-3β and pGSK-3β levels of DMSO+MCAO+Veh group and XAV939+MCAO+LE 20% group were significantly lower than the DMSO+Sham+Veh group. The DMSO+MCAO+LE 20% had significantly increased pGSK-3β and GSK-3β levels compared to the DMSO+MCAO+Veh and XAV939+MCAO+LE 20% groups; (**h–m**) Wnt signal-related protein expressions of experimental groups. Significantly decreased levels of Wnt1, Wnt3, PORCN and β-catenin were observed in the DMSO+MCAO+Veh group compared to the DMSO+Sham+Veh group. The DMSO+MCAO+LE 20% group had significantly increased protein levels of Wnt1 and PORCN compared to the DMSO+MCAO+Veh group. The XAV939+MCAO+LE 20% group had decreased expression levels of Wnt1 and PORCN compared to the DMSO+MCAO+LE 20% group. The β–catenin expression level in the DMSO+MCAO+LE 20% and XAV939+MCAO+LE 20% groups did not differ significantly. There was a significant increase in pβ–catenin and tankyrase 1 in the DMSO+MCAO+Veh compared to the DMSO+Sham+Veh group. Pβ–catenin and tankyrase1 was significantly decreased in the DMSO+MCAO+LE 20% compared to the DMSO+MCAO+Veh group. The XAV939+MCAO+LE 20% group had significantly increased pβ–catenin and tankyrase 1 expression levels compared to the DMSO+MCAO+LE 20% group; (**n–q**) Inflammatory protein expressions in the experimental groups. Significantly increased expressions of inflammatory markers were observed in the MCAO-injured groups compared to the DMSO+Sham+Veh group. The DMSO+MCAO+LE 20% group had significantly decreased inflammatory protein expression levels compared to the DMSO+MCAO+Veh group. Significant decrease in inflammatory protein expressions were observed in the XAV939+MCAO+LE 20% group compared to the DMSO+Sham+Veh group. TNF-α expression level was increased significantly in the XAV939+MCAO+LE 20% group compared to the DMSO+MCAO+LE 20% group. Data are presented as mean ± standard error of the mean (SEM); $n = 8$ for each group; * $p < 0.05$, ** $p < 0.01$ vs. DMSO+Sham+Veh, # $p < 0.05$, ### $p < 0.001$ vs. DMSO+MCAO+Veh, † $p < 0.05$, ††† $p < 0.001$ vs. DMSO+MCAO+LE 20%, one-way ANOVA followed by Tukey's multiple comparison test.

2.4. Wnt/β-Catenin-Dependent Alleviation of Ischemic Reperfusion Injury and Reversal of Protection-Related Proteins

The administration of XAV939 inhibited the activity of the Wnt/β-catenin signaling pathway, which was reflected in the protein expression (Figure 4a) of distinct genes. The expression of total Akt did not differ among the experimental groups (Figure 4b). The DMSO+MCAO+Veh group and XAV939+MCAO+LE 20% group significantly showed substantial decrease in pAkt levels compared to the DMSO+Sham+Veh group ($p < 0.05$, one-way ANOVA followed by Tukey's multiple comparison test). There was significant elevation in the level of pAkt in DMSO+MCAO+LE 20% group compared to the DMSO+MCAO+Veh group ($p < 0.05$, one-way ANOVA followed by Tukey's multiple comparison test) and XAV939+MCAO+LE 20% group ($p < 0.01$, one-way ANOVA followed by Tukey's multiple comparison test) (Figure 4c). The pAkt/Akt expression was decreased significantly in the DMSO+MCAO+Veh and XAV939+MCAO+LE 20% groups compared to the DMSO+Sham+Veh group ($p < 0.05$, one-way ANOVA followed by Tukey's multiple comparison test). The expression of pAkt/Akt in the DMSO+MCAO+LE 20% group was significantly increased compared to DMSO+MCAO+Veh and XAV939+MCAO+LE 20% groups ($p < 0.05$, one-way ANOVA followed by Tukey's multiple comparison test) (Figure 4d).

Significant decrease in total GSK-3β expression was observed in the DMSO+MCAO+Veh and XAV939+MCAO+LE 20% groups when compared to the DMSO+Sham+Veh group ($p < 0.05$, one-way ANOVA followed by Tukey's multiple comparison test). Total GSK-3β expression of the DMSO+MCAO+LE 20% group was also significantly increased compared to the DMSO+MCAO+Veh and XAV939+MCAO+LE 20% groups ($p < 0.05$, one-way ANOVA followed by Tukey's multiple comparison test) (Figure 4e). The level of pGSK-3β was significantly decreased in the DMSO+MCAO+Veh and XAV939+MCAO+LE 20% groups compared to the DMSO+Sham+Veh group ($p < 0.01$, one-way ANOVA followed by Tukey's multiple comparison test), which might be indicative of a compromised Wnt activity. The phosphorylation of GSK-3β was significantly increased in the DMSO+MCAO+LE 20% group compared to the DMSO+Sham+Veh group ($p < 0.05$, one-way ANOVA followed by Tukey's multiple comparison test). There was also a significant increase in the pGSK-3β levels in the DMSO+MCAO+LE 20% group compared to the DMSO+MCAO+Veh and XAV939+MCAO+LE 20% groups ($p < 0.001$, one-way ANOVA followed by Tukey's multiple comparison test) (Figure 4f). The pGSK-3β/GSK-3β activity was significantly decreased in the DMSO+MCAO+Veh and XAV939+MCAO+LE 20% groups when compared to the DMSO+Sham+Veh group ($p < 0.05$, one-way ANOVA followed by Tukey's multiple comparison test) and significantly increased in the DMSO+MCAO+LE 20% group compared to the DMSO+MCAO+Veh and XAV939+MCAO+LE 20% groups ($p < 0.05$, one-way ANOVA followed by Tukey's multiple comparison test). The administration of XAV939 effectively decreased the phosphorylation GSK-3β induced by LE (Figure 4g).

Wnt1 was significantly decreased in the DMSO+MCAO+Veh and XAV939+MCAO+LE 20% groups compared to the DMSO+Sham+Veh group ($p < 0.05$, one-way ANOVA followed by Tukey's multiple comparison test) and significantly increased in the DMSO+MCAO+LE 20% group compared to the DMSO+MCAO+Veh and XAV939+MCAO+LE 20% groups ($p < 0.05$, one-way ANOVA followed by Tukey's multiple comparison test) (Figure 4h). All experimental groups, excluding the DMSO+Sham+Veh group, showed steep decrease ($p < 0.05$, one-way ANOVA followed by Tukey's multiple comparison test) in Wnt3 (Figure 4i). PORCN decreased significantly in the DMSO+MCAO+Veh group ($p < 0.01$, one-way ANOVA followed by Tukey's multiple comparison test) and XAV939+MCAO+LE 20% group ($p < 0.05$, one-way ANOVA followed by Tukey's multiple comparison test) compared to the DMSO+Sham+Veh group. PORCN expression increased in expression in the DMSO+MCAO+LE 20% group compared to the DMSO+MCAO+Veh and XAV939+MCAO+LE 20% groups ($p < 0.05$, one-way ANOVA followed by Tukey's multiple comparison test) (Figure 4j). β-catenin was decreased in all MCAO injury groups compared to the DMSO+Sham+Veh group due to infarction. Significantly attenuated level of β-catenin was also observed in the XAV939+MCAO+LE 20% group, while DMSO+MCAO+LE 20% group were preserved significantly compared to DMSO+MCAO+Veh group ($p < 0.05$, one-way ANOVA followed by Tukey's multiple comparison test). Average β-catenin expression decreased in the XAV939+MCAO+LE 20% group compared to the DMSO+MCAO+LE 20% group but not to a significant level ($p > 0.05$ one-way ANOVA) (Figure 4k). pβ-Catenin was increased in the DMSO+MCAO+Veh group compared to the DMSO+Sham+Veh group ($p < 0.05$, one-way ANOVA followed by Tukey's multiple comparison test), indicating lowered cellular survival. The level of pβ-catenin was significantly decreased in the DMSO+MCAO+LE 20% group compared to the DMSO+MCAO+Veh group ($p < 0.05$, one-way ANOVA followed by Tukey's multiple comparison test). The pβ-catenin expression level was significantly increased in the XAV939+MCAO+LE 20% group compared to the DMSO+MCAO+LE 20% group ($p < 0.05$, one-way ANOVA followed by Tukey's multiple comparison test) (Figure 4l). The accumulation of tankyrase 1 was significant in the DMSO+MCAO+Veh compared to DMSO+Sham+Veh ($p < 0.05$, one-way ANOVA followed by Tukey's multiple comparison test). The tankyrase 1 expression of DMSO+MCAO+LE 20% group significantly decreased compared to the DMSO+MCAO+Veh group ($p < 0.05$, one-way ANOVA followed by Tukey's multiple comparison test). The XAV939+MCAO+LE 20% group had significantly higher levels of tankyrase 1 expression levels compared to the DMSO+MCAO+LE 20% group ($p < 0.05$, one-way ANOVA followed by Tukey's multiple comparison test). The administration of XAV939 successfully inhibited tankyrase 1 activity which increased degradation of β-catenin (Figure 4m).

Inflammatory protein markers of ischemic reperfusion damage, IL-1β, IL-6, IL-8 and TNF-α, also significantly increased for all MCAO-injured groups compared to the DMSO+Sham+Veh group. Attenuated levels of inflammatory markers were observed in the DMSO+MCAO+LE 20% group compared to the DMSO+MCAO+Veh group ($p < 0.05$, one-way ANOVA followed by Tukey's multiple comparison test). The expression levels of the XAV939+MCAO+LE 20% group were not significantly different from the DMSO+MCAO+Veh group ($p > 0.05$, one-way ANOVA) The TNF-α expression level of the XAV939+MCAO+LE 20% group increased significantly compared to the DMSO+MCAO+LE 20% group ($p < 0.05$, one-way ANOVA followed by Tukey's multiple comparison test) (Figure 4n–q).

2.5. LE Dosage-Dependent mRNA Expression Against Ischemic Reperfusion Injury

According to the results of qPCR, Wnt1 can be implicated as one of the main regulators for neuroprotection. in the MCAO+Veh group, Wnt1 expression level was approximately 0.4 folds compared to the Sham+Veh group ($p < 0.05$, one-way ANOVA followed by Tukey's multiple comparison test). The mRNA expression of Wnt1 signals of MCAO+LE 20% was upregulated by approximately 2.4 folds compared to the Sham+Veh group ($p < 0.01$, one-way ANOVA followed by Tukey's multiple comparison test) and 4 folds compared to the MCAO+Veh group ($p < 0.001$, one-way ANOVA followed by Tukey's multiple comparison test) (Figure 5a). Wnt3 expression was attenuated in all MCAO-injured groups compared to the Sham+Veh group. The MCAO+LE 10% ($p < 0.05$, one-way ANOVA followed by Tukey's multiple comparison test) and MCAO+LE 20% groups' ($p < 0.001$, one-way ANOVA followed by Tukey's multiple comparison test) Wnt3 expression levels were significantly decreased compared to the MCAO+Veh group (Figure 5b). Mki67, a cell proliferation marker, increased in all MCAO-injured groups compared to the Sham+Veh group. The Mki67 expression level increased significantly in the MCAO+LE 20% group compared to the MCAO+Veh group ($p < 0.05$, one-way ANOVA followed by Tukey's multiple comparison test), which may have been affected by the elevated expression level of Wnt1 (Figure 5c). The Wnt regulator, Porcn, decreased significantly in the MCAO+Veh group compared to the Sham+Veh group ($p < 0.05$, one-way ANOVA followed by Tukey's multiple comparison test). Significant increase of Porcn was observed in the MCAO+LE 20% group compared to the MCAO+Veh group ($p < 0.05$, one-way ANOVA followed by Tukey's multiple comparison test), which may be induced by the increase in Wnt1 activity (Figure 5d). Inflammatory markers, IL-1β, IL-6, IL-8 and TNF-α, significantly increased in MCAO-injured groups compared to the Sham+Veh group. Significantly lower inflammatory mRNA markers were observed in the MCAO+LE 20%

group compared to the MCAO+Veh group ($p < 0.05$, one-way ANOVA followed by Tukey's multiple comparison test) (Figure 5e–h).

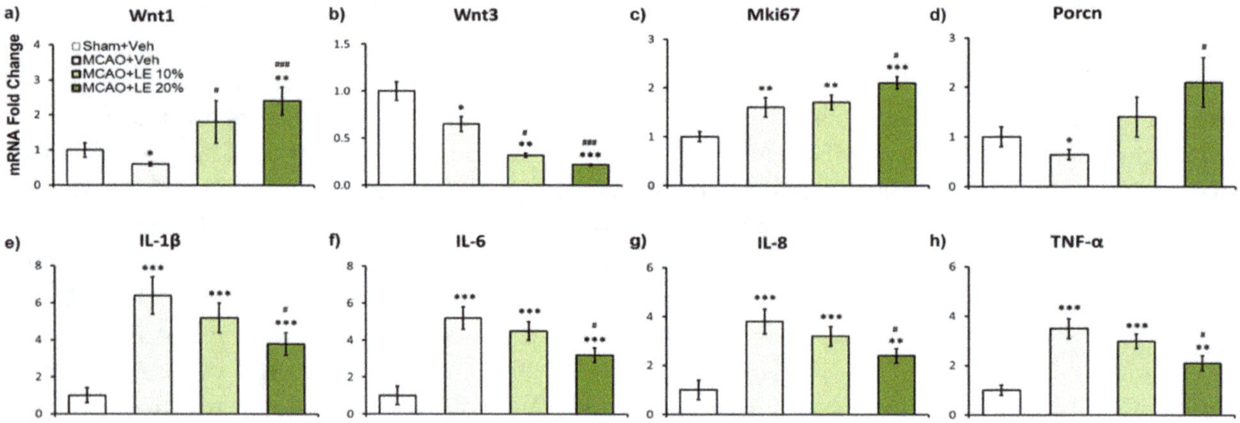

Figure 5. Effects of LE or vehicle on mRNA expression after the MCAO and reperfusion injury. (**a**,**b**) Wnt expressions in experimental groups. The Wnt1 mRNA expression of the MCAO+Veh group was significantly decreased compared to the Sham+Veh group. Significantly increased expression of Wnt1 was expressed in the MCAO+LE 10% and MCAO+LE 20% groups compared to the MCAO+Veh group. Wnt3 expressions were significantly lower in MCAO injury groups compared to the Sham+Veh group. Significantly decreased Wnt3 expressions were observed in the MCAO+LE 10% and MCAO+LE 20% groups compared to the MCAO+Veh group; (**c**) Mki67 expression was increased in all MCAO-injury groups compared to the Sham+Veh group. Significant increase in Mki67 expression was observed in the MCAO+LE 20% group compared to the MCAO+Veh group; (**d**) Porcn expression was significantly decreased in the MCAO+Veh group compared to the Sham+Veh group. Significant increase of Porcn was observed in the MCAO+LE 20% group compared to the MCAO+Veh group; (**e**–**h**) mRNA expression of inflammatory markers. MCAO-injury groups expressed significantly increased levels of inflammatory markers compared to the Sham+Veh group. Significantly decreased inflammatory expression levels were observed in the MCAO+LE 20% group compared to the MCAO+Veh group. Data are presented as mean ± standard error of the mean (SEM); $n = 8$ for each group; * $p < 0.05$, ** $p < 0.01$, *** $p < 0.001$ vs. Sham+Veh, # $p < 0.05$, ### $p < 0.001$ vs. MCAO+Veh, one-way ANOVA followed by Tukey's multiple comparison test. Wnt subfamily mRNA expressions are shown in Supplementary Materials S1.

2.6. *Wnt-Dependent mRNA Expression of LE Against Ischemic Reperfusion Injury*

XAV939 injection inhibited Wnt activity in mRNA levels to reverse neuroprotection. in the DMSO+MCAO+Veh group ($p < 0.05$, one-way ANOVA followed by Tukey's multiple comparison test) and XAV939+MCAO+LE 20% group, Wnt1 mRNA expression levels were approximately 0.5 folds and 0.6 folds compared to the DMSO+Sham+Veh group, respectively. Expression of Wnt1 signals in the DMSO+MCAO+LE 20% was upregulated by approximately 2.2 folds compared to the DMSO+Sham+Veh group ($p < 0.01$, one-way ANOVA followed by Tukey's multiple comparison test) and 4.2 folds compared to the DMSO+MCAO+Veh group ($p < 0.001$, one-way ANOVA followed by Tukey's multiple comparison test). There was a significant decrease in Wnt1 expression in the XAV939+MCAO+LE 20% group compared to the DMSO+MCAO+LE 20% group ($p < 0.01$, one-way ANOVA followed by Tukey's multiple comparison test) (Figure 6a). Wnt3 expression was attenuated in all MCAO-injured groups compared to the DMSO+Sham+Veh group. The DMSO+MCAO+LE 20% group's Wnt3 expression was significantly decreased compared to the DMSO+MCAO+Veh group ($p < 0.001$, one-way ANOVA followed by Tukey's multiple comparison test). The XAV939+MCAO+LE 20% group was also showed significant decreased in Wnt3 expression level compared to the DMSO+Sham+Veh group ($p < 0.01$, one-way ANOVA followed by Tukey's multiple comparison test) but displayed marked increase when compared to the DMSO+MCAO+LE

20% group ($p < 0.001$, one-way ANOVA followed by Tukey's multiple comparison test) (Figure 6b). Mki67 levels increased in all MCAO-injured groups compared to the DMSO+Sham+Veh group. in the DMSO+MCAO+LE 20% group, Mki67 expression level increased significantly compared to the DMSO+MCAO+Veh group ($p < 0.05$, one-way ANOVA followed by Tukey's multiple comparison test); while in the XAV939+MCAO+LE 20% group, it was significantly downregulated compared to the DMSO+MCAO+LE 20% group ($p < 0.05$, one-way ANOVA followed by Tukey's multiple comparison test) (Figure 6c). Porcn decreased significantly in the DMSO+MCAO+Veh group ($p < 0.05$, one-way ANOVA followed by Tukey's multiple comparison test) and XAV939+MCAO+LE 20% group compared to the DMSO+Sham+Veh group. Significant increase of Porcn was observed in the DMSO+MCAO+LE 20% group when compared to the DMSO+MCAO+Veh group ($p < 0.05$, one-way ANOVA followed by Tukey's multiple comparison test). The XAV939+MCAO+LE 20% group decreased in Porcn compared to the DMSO+Sham+Veh group but did not differ significantly. The XAV939+MCAO+LE 20% group expression levels of Porcn were significantly decreased compared to the DMSO+MCAO+LE 20% group ($p < 0.05$, one-way ANOVA followed by Tukey's multiple comparison test) (Figure 6d). Inflammatory markers, IL-1β, IL-6, IL-8 and TNF-α, significantly increased in MCAO-injured groups compared to the DMSO+Sham+Veh group. Significantly lower inflammatory mRNA markers were observed in the DMSO+MCAO+LE 20% group compared to the DMSO+MCAO+Veh group ($p < 0.05$, one-way ANOVA). XAV939 injection significantly reversed attenuated levels of inflammation by LE 20% (Figure 6e–h).

3. Discussion

Our results suggest that LE provides neuroprotection against ischemic reperfusion injury in a dosage-dependent manner. Intra-arterial injection of 20% LE during reperfusion after MCAO was able to reduce infarction significantly. The decreases in infarction volumes have been reflected in the improved performance in the neurological deficit assessment. Rats injected with LE 20% possessed better control over their paralyzed limb. Increased levels of Wnt1 signaling in both protein and mRNA levels in 20% LE-treated rats were observed, which in turn enhanced the resistance to reperfusion injury following ischemia. Especially, a notable increase in Wnt1 mRNA expression was observed, which may have led to increased Wnt1 protein expression. The elevated levels of Wnt1 are consistent with previous studies that have indirectly stimulated Wnt/β-catenin signaling pathway for cell survival after ischemic injury [20,36]. The expression levels of Wnt3 decreased in all MCAO groups which may be due to a decline in cell populations as a result of ischemic reperfusion injury [37]. Although Wnt3 is also known as a canonical Wnt signal, not all canonical Wnt signals seem to be involved in the protection process. As in our previous study [31], Wnt3 did not seem to be involved in protection process in response to the administration of LE. In addition, the phosphorylation of GSK-3β increased due to 20% LE injection, which inactivated the β-catenin destruction complex. β-catenin was preserved to promote cell survival, which resulted in enhanced resistance to the ischemic reperfusion damage. Elevation of PORCN expression may have been due to the increase in demand for Wnt1 to resist damage; however, a clear link between PORCN and LE cannot be formulated at this stage. A previous study on the ischemic reperfusion injury in the heart has reported that palmitic acid of LE affects the lipid-modification of Wnt ligands for protection [38]. Clear distinctions between cardiac cells and neurons exist but Wnt modifications seem to occur regardless of their metabolic factors. Inflammatory markers, IL-1β, IL-6, IL-8 and TNF-α, are known to increase after ischemic reperfusion injury [34,35]. Inflammation by oxidative stress was significantly decreased in the 20% LE-treated group, indicating an anti-inflammatory action of LE in the central nervous system. The preservation of β-catenin through the activation of the Wnt signaling pathway induces the transcription of T cell factor/lymphoid enhancer factor, which results in decreased inflammatory activity [39]. Therefore, the expressions of inflammatory cytokines, including IL-1β, IL-6 and TNF-α, might be reduced. The decrease in the expression of IL-8 is assumed to be reduced by an overall decline in inflammatory activity.

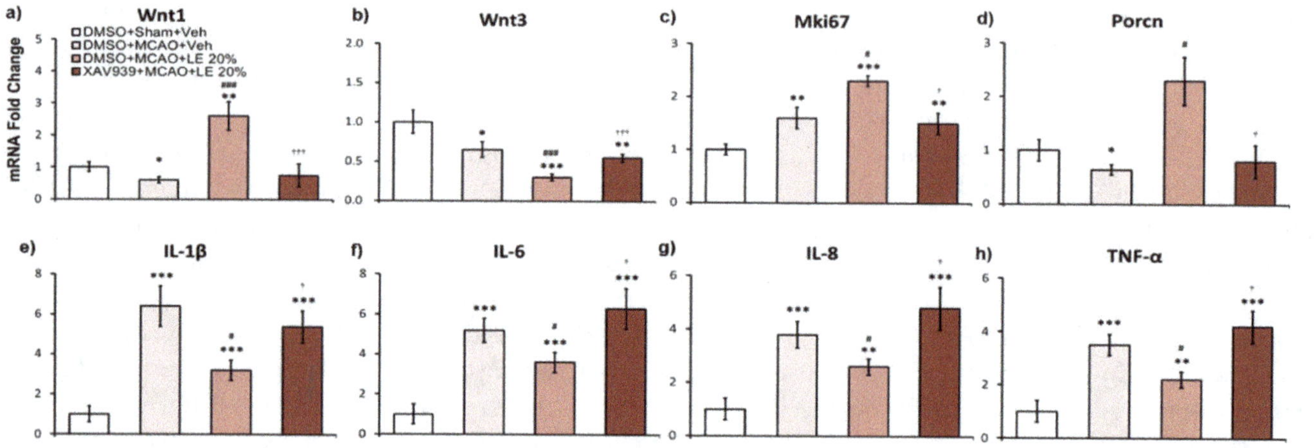

Figure 6. Effects of LE or vehicle on mRNA expression on the MCAO and reperfusion injury after the administration of DMSO or XAV939. (**a**,**b**) Wnt expressions in experimental groups. The Wnt1 mRNA expression of the DMSO+MCAO+Veh group was significantly decreased compared to the DMSO+Sham+Veh group. Significantly increased expression of Wnt1 was expressed Wnt1 decreased significantly in the XAV939+MCAO+LE 20% group compared to the DMSO+MCAO+LE 20% group. There was no significant difference in Wnt1 expression in the XAV939+MCAO+LE 20% group compared to the DMSO+MCAO+Veh group. Wnt3 expressions were significantly lower in MCAO-injury groups compared to the DMSO+Sham+Veh group. Significantly decreased Wnt3 expressions were observed in the DMSO+MCAO+LE 20% group compared to the DMSO+MCAO+Veh and XAV939+MCAO+LE 20% groups; (**c**) Mki67 expression was increased in all MCAO-injury groups compared to the DMSO+Sham+Veh group. Significant increase in Mki67 expression was observed in the DMSO+MCAO+LE 20% group compared to the DMSO+MCAO+Veh. The XAV939+MCAO+LE 20% group had a significant decrease in Mki67 expression compared to the DMSO+MCAO+LE 20% group; (**d**) Porcn expression was significantly decreased in the DMSO+MCAO+Veh group compared to the DMSO+Sham+Veh group. Significant increase of Porcn was observed in the DMSO+MCAO+LE 20% group compared to the DMSO+MCAO+Veh. The XAV939+MCAO+LE 20% group had a significant decrease in Porcn expression compared to the DMSO+MCAO+LE 20% group. There was no significant difference in Porcn expression in the XAV939+MCAO+LE 20% group compared to the DMSO+MCAO+Veh group; (**e**–**h**) The mRNA expression of inflammatory markers. MCAO injury groups expressed significantly increased levels of inflammatory markers compared to the DMSO+Sham+Veh group. Significantly decreased inflammatory expression levels were observed in the DMSO+MCAO+LE 20% group compared to DMSO+MCAO+Veh group. Significantly increased levels of inflammatory markers were observed in the XAV939+MCAO+LE 20% group compared to the DMSO+MCAO+LE 20% group and DMSO+Sham+Veh group but there was no significant difference compared to the DMSO+MCAO+Veh group. Data are presented as mean ± standard error of mean (SEM); $n = 8$ for each group; * $p < 0.05$, ** $p < 0.01$, *** $p < 0.001$ vs. DMSO+Sham+Veh, $^{\#}$ $p < 0.05$, $^{\#\#\#}$ $p < 0.001$ vs. DMSO+MCAO+Veh, † $p < 0.05$, ††† $p < 0.001$ vs. DMSO+MCAO+LE 20%, one-way ANOVA followed by Tukey's multiple comparison test. Wnt subfamily mRNA expressions are shown in Supplementary Materials S1.

The Wnt/β-catenin signaling pathway has been considered a potential therapeutic target in preventing cell death for an extensive amount of time [18,40,41]. The down-regulation of Wnt ligands and increased antagonistic activity have been observed in neurodegenerative and excitotoxic disorders [42–44]. In order to verify the protective mechanism of LE, which increased Wnt1, we were required to interrupt the protective process. XAV939, a Wnt/β-catenin signaling pathway inhibitor, has been commonly utilized to inhibit Wnt activity in many studies [45,46]. in the present study, the i.p. injection of XAV939 successfully inhibited Wnt activity and reversed the protective effects induced by LE. The XAV939+MCAO+LE 20% group exhibited infarction volumes nearly as arge as our control, the DMSO+MCAO+Veh group. Akin to earlier studies, our results show that the Wnt/β-catenin signaling pathway might be a potential therapeutic target for neuroprotection. The administration of XAV939 inhibited the mRNA expression level of Wnt1, indicating that Wnt1 may be dependent on the activity of GSK-3β. XAV939 is known to inhibit tankyrase 1, which prevents the degradation of axis inhibition protein 2 (AXIN2), allowing the accumulation of the GSK-3β destruction complex [47]. Therefore, pGSK-3β was attenuated in the XAV939+MCAO+LE 20% group, which reversed the protective effect of LE by the degradation of the downstream survival marker, β-catenin (Figure 4k). We can infer that LE has effects on the upstream signals of GSK-3β and not on the downstream signals of GSK-3β (Figure 7). If LE affected the GSK-3β downstream marker, β-catenin, XAV939 might not have affected the protection effect. In addition, if LE affected GSK-3β directly, a less effective or partial reversal of protection may have occurred. We observed that the infarction damage was not significantly different between the DMSO+MCAO+Veh group and XAV939+MCAO+LE 20% group, implying an effective reversal from the effects of 20% LE injection.

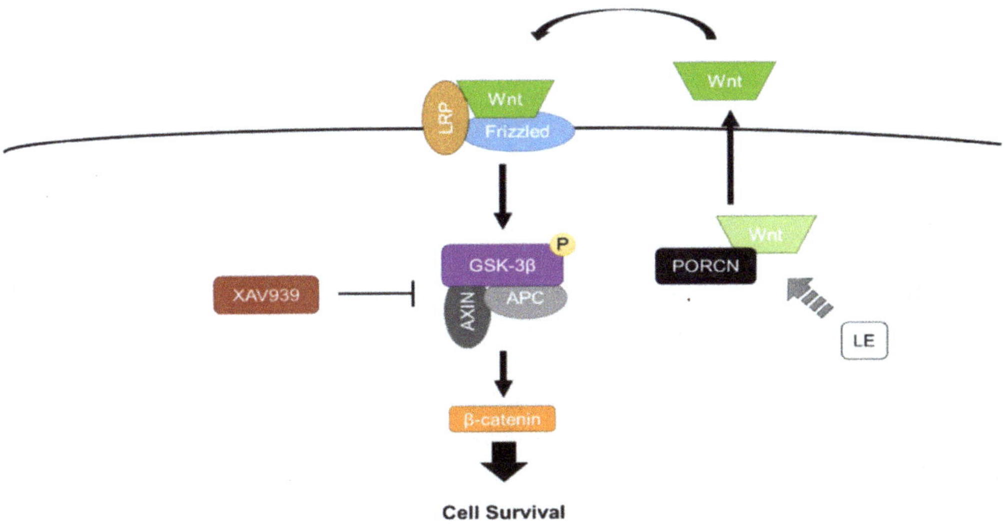

Figure 7. Schematic diagram of the protective mechanism of LE in ischemic reperfusion injury. LE increases the lipid modification of Wnt proteins by PORCN. Lipid-modified/active Wnt proteins are released to the extra-cellular space for the binding to Frizzled/LRP receptors. The activated receptors induce the phosphorylation of GSK-3β, which prevents the destruction complex from the degradation of β-catenin by proteasomes. Preserved levels of β-catenin lead to cell survival. The injection of XAV939 prevents the phosphorylation of GSK-3β, which allows β-catenin degradation for cell death. Abbreviations: PORCN—porcupine, Wnt—wingless integration, LRP—low-density lipoprotein receptor-related protein, GSK-3β—glycogen synthase kinase 3β, APC—adenomatous polyposis coli, AXIN—axis inhibition protein.

The protective roles of fatty acids have received much attention in studies regarding stroke. Different compositions of lipid emulsions, such as omega-3, have been reported to provide neuroprotection against ischemic stroke injuries [48]. Emulsions of n-3 fatty acids have been shown to effectively reduce infarction volume and inflammation in the ischemic brain in neonatal mice [49]. in the present study, we observed significant neuroprotective effects of LE against ischemic reperfusion injury but limitations exist. Although we were able to investigate protective properties of LE regarding the Wnt/β-catenin signaling pathway, we are yet to discover specific targets of LE. Further studies should consider other signals that are involved in the Wnt/β-catenin signaling pathway, such as frizzled-1, low-density lipoprotein receptor-related protein 5/6 or PORCN, that can be subjected for inhibition. Elucidation of specific signals may lead to more effective therapeutic targets in the brain. Through our study, we suggested that the neuroprotective mechanism of LE is dependent on the Wnt/β-catenin signaling pathway through the inhibition of GSK-3β phosphorylation. We assumed that lipid modification occurs through PORCN through the constituents of LE that interact with the protein.

As a result, the expression levels of Wnt1 increased, which also affects its downstream signals. The scope for future studies is considerable: LE may be utilized with other lipophilic anti-inflammatory drugs to further extend its neuroprotective properties. Furthermore, the investigation of different routes of delivery may also be considered with regard to invasiveness and safety.

In conclusion, the intra-arterial administration of 20% LE alleviated ischemic reperfusion injury induced by MCAO and reperfusion. Infarction volumes and Bederson scores were attenuated in a dosage-dependent manner. Protein and mRNA expression levels of the Wnt/β-catenin signaling pathway were elevated and inflammatory markers decreased significantly in the 20% LE-treated group. Especially, GSK-3β was phosphorylated significantly, which in turn preserved β-catenin to promote cell survival. The protective actions were reversed by the administration of XAV939 indicating that the protection mechanism of LE has been induced through the Wnt/β-catenin signaling pathway. These findings regarding the anti-inflammatory and neuroprotective properties of LE may provide a foundation for further research regarding excitotoxic neural injuries and functional recovery.

4. Materials and Methods

4.1. Animals

Adult Sprague-Dawley rats weighing 260-300 g (Koatec, Pyeongtaek, South Korea) were used for experiments in this study. Animals were housed in groups of three per cage under 12-h light/dark cycles, with free access to food and water. Animals were subjected to 7 days of acclimatization upon arrival at the Association for Assessment and Accreditation of Laboratory Animal Care (AAALAC)-accredited Yonsei University College of Medicine Animal Care Facilities. All experimental procedures were approved by the Institutional Animal Care and Use Committee of Yonsei University Health System (permit no.: 2019-0263, approval date: 22 January 2020) and performed according to the National Institutes of Health Guide for Care.

4.2. Middle Cerebral Artery Occlusion and Reperfusion

Rats were anesthetized by i.p. injection of 50 mg/kg sodium pentobarbital (Hanlim Pharmaceutical, Seoul, South Korea) and were placed on a heated mat to maintain body temperature of 37.0 ± 1.0 °C. The surgical and injection process is illustrated in Figure 8. The Koizumi method [50] of MCAO was used for inducing ischemic reperfusion injury. Cervical skin incision was made to expose the common carotid artery (CCA), external carotid artery (ECA) and internal carotid artery (ICA). The CCA was permanently ligated below the bifurcation to the ECA and ICA. The ECA was temporarily ligated while a small incision was made in the CCA to insert a silicone coated nylon filament (403723PK10Re, Doccol Corporation, Sharon, MA, USA) into the ICA until a mild resistance stopped the insertion. The length of the insertion was approximately 18-20 mm (Figure 8a). The rat was occluded for 90 min. and the filament was removed. The experimental group undergoing sham surgery did not have the filament inserted. Polyethylene tubing with an inner diameter of 0.28 mm and outer diameter of 0.61 mm (427401, Becton, Dickson and Company, Sparks, MD, USA) was inserted for injection of LE or vehicle (Figure 8b). Injections were made at 0.5 mL/min over 2 min. The polyethylene tubing was removed after the injection and the CCA above the incision was permanently ligated. The temporary ligation of the ECA was removed. A total of 374 rats were used for this study. The MCAO surgery was conducted on 310 rats and sham surgery was conducted on 64 rats. 84 rats that deceased during MCAO, reperfusion or intra-arterial injection were excluded from the experiment. None of Sham-operated rats deceased. 34 rats that underwent MCAO and reperfusion but did not show infarction due to surgical errors were also excluded from the study.

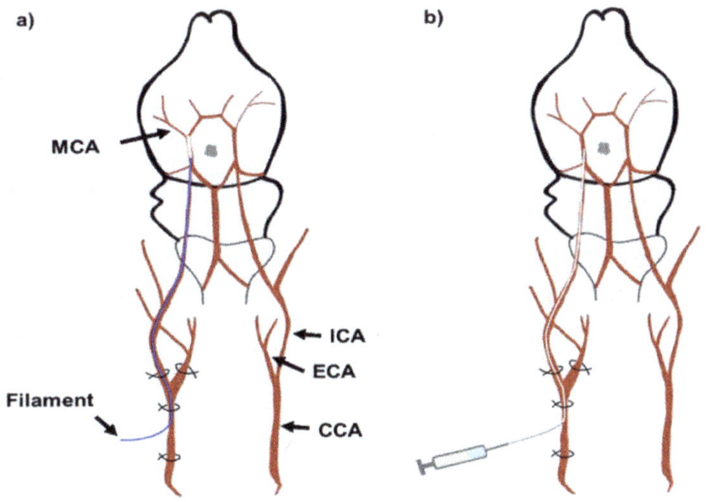

Figure 8. Illustration of middle cerebral artery occlusion and injection. (**a**) Insertion of nylon filament for MCAO. The CCA was ligated permanently while the ECA and ICA were temporarily ligated to stop blood flow. A small incision was made in the CCA for the filament insertion. The silicone-coated filament was inserted until it reached the MCA. The artery was occluded for 90 min. Then the filament was removed for reperfusion; (**b**) Insertion of polyethylene tubing for injection of LE or vehicle. The polyethylene tubing was inserted near to the MCA. After injection, the tubing was removed and the CCA near the bifurcation was permanently ligated. The temporary ligations on the ICA and ECA were removed. Abbreviations: CCA—common carotid artery, ECA—external carotid artery, ICA—internal carotid artery, MCA—middle cerebral artery.

4.3. Drug Treatment

LE (Intralipid™ 20%, Fresenius Kabi, Uppsala, Sweden) was dissolved in sterile 0.9% NaCl to a final concentration of 10% for the injection of the LE 10% group. Vehicle, 10% LE and 20% LE were intra-arterially administered during reperfusion after 90 min. of MCAO. Intra-peritoneal injection XAV939 (S1180, Selleck Chemicals, Houston, TX, USA) 40mg/kg or DMSO were injected for 2 days prior to the MCAO surgery and on the day of the surgery before MCAO.

4.4. Neurological Deficit Assessment

A neurological examination of experimental animals was performed in accordance with the modified Bederson method [51] 24 h after MCAO or sham surgery by a blinded researcher. The scoring criteria are as follows: score 0: no deficit; score 1: lost forelimb flexion; score 2: as for 1, plus decreased resistance to lateral push; score 3: unidirectional circling; score 4: longitudinal spinning or seizure activity; score 5: no movement.

4.5. Infarction Volume Assessment

The infarction volume was assessed by TTC staining of consecutive 2.0 mm coronal sections from bregma +4 mm to −6.0 mm. The sections were immersed into 2% TTC (T8877, Sigma Aldrich, St. Louis, MO, USA) solution for 30 min at 37.0 °C. The sections were transferred into 4% paraformaldehyde solution for 24 h. The sections were then photographed and analyzed using the ImageJ software (ImageJ, National Institute of Health, Bethesda, MD, USA). The infarction volume was calculated using the following formula [50]: (contralateral volume − non-infarct ipsilateral volume)/contralateral volume × 100%. The contralateral volume refers to the opposite brain hemisphere of the infarcted side.

4.6. Western Blotting

Frozen samples were homogenized for protein extraction in lysis buffer (ProPrep; Intron Biotechnology, Pyeongtaek, South Korea) with phosphatase inhibitors (Phosstop; Roche, Mannheim,

Germany). Supernatants were collected from homogenized samples that were centrifuged at 15,000 rpm for 15 min at 4 °C. Total protein concentrations were measured using a spectrophotometer (Nano Drop ND-1000, NanoDrop Technologies Inc., Wilmington, DE, USA) and equal amount of protein (30 mg per well) were resolved on 10% sodium dodecyl sulfate-polyacrylamide gel electrophoresis (SDS-PAGE) and transferred to a polyvinylidene difluoride membrane (Merck Millipore, Darmstadt, Germany) for 2 h. Phospho-proteins were detected by immunoblotting prior to their corresponding total protein levels, which were detected after the membrane had been stripped. Transferred proteins on membranes were fixed using 0.05% glutaraldehyde in Tris-buffered saline containing 0.05% Tween-20 (TBST) for 15 min at room temperature. The membrane was stained with Ponceau S (P7170, Sigma-Aldrich, St. Louis, MO, USA) for visualization of the transferred proteins and cut into strips according to the size of the target protein to minimize interactions between antibodies. Membranes were blocked with 5% bovine serum albumin (BSA) dissolved in TBST for 1 h at room temperature. The membranes were incubated overnight with primary antibodies diluted in 5% BSA in TBST at 4 °C. Rabbit was the host of all primary antibodies used for immunoblotting. The following antibodies were used—anti-Wnt1 (ab15251, 1:1000, Abcam, Cambridge, UK), anti-Wnt3 (ab32249, Abcam), anti-PORCN (ab105543, Abcam), anti-β-catenin (#9562, 1:3000, Cell Signaling Technology, Beverly, MA, USA), anti-Akt (#4691, 1:3000, Cell Signaling Technology), anti-Phospho-Akt (#9271, 1:1000, Cell Signaling Technology), anti-GSK3-β (#9315, 1:3000, Cell Signaling Technology), anti-Phospho-GSK3-β (#9336, 1:1000, Cell Signaling Technology), anti-pβ-catenin (#9561, 1:1000, Cell Signaling Technology), anti-tankyrase 1 (MBS8531631, 1:1000, MyBioSource, San Diego, CA, USA), anti-IL-1β (AB1832P, 1:1000, Sigma Aldrich), anti-IL-6 (ARC0062, 1:500, Invitrogen, Carlsbad, CA, USA), anti-IL-8 (MBS9385550, 1:500, MyBioSource), anti-TNF-α (AAR33, 1:1000, Bio-Rad, Hercules, CA, USA) and anti-β-actin (#4967, 1:10,000, Cell Signaling Technology). After overnight incubation of primary antibodies, the membranes were incubated with anti-rabbit horseradish peroxidase-conjugated secondary antibody (#7074, 1:10,000, Cell Signaling Technology). Visualization of immunoreactive proteins was performed with the application of chemiluminescent detection reagent (ECL™ Prime, GE Healthcare, Little Chalfont, UK) and images were taken by ImageQuant™ LAS 4000 (GE Healthcare). Protein immunoreactivity was measured using Multi-gauge software (Fuji Film Inc., Tokyo, Japan).

Table 1. Primer pairs for qPCR.

Gene Name	Forward Primer (5′-3′)	Reverse Primer (5′-3′)
Wnt1	GCAACCAAAGTCGCCAGAA	TATGTTCACGATGCCCCACCA
Wnt2b	GCTACCCAGACATCATGCG	ACACTCTCGGATCCATTCCC
Wnt3	AATTTGGTGGTCCCTGGC	GATAGAGCCGCAGAGCAGAG
Wnt4	GTTTCCAGTGGTCAGGATGC	AGGACTGTGAGAAGGCTACGC
Wnt5a	AAGGGAACGAATCCACGCC	ATACTGTCCTGCGACCTGCTTC
Wnt7a	CCAAGGTCTTCGTGGATGC	TGTAAGTTCATGAGGGTTCGG
Wnt7b	CGTGTTTCTCTGCTTTGGC	CACCACGGATGACAATGC
Wnt9a	GTACAGCAGCAAGTTTGTCAAGG	CACGAGGTTGTTGTGGAAGTCC
Wnt10a	CGGAACAAAGTCCCCTACG	AGGCGAAAGCACTCTCTCG
Wnt16	GCACTCTGTAACCAGGTCATGC	TGCAAGGTGGTGTCACAGG
Mki67	TTCAGTTCCGCCAATCCAAC	CCGTGCTGGTTCCTTTCCA
Porcn	CCTACCTCTTCCCCTACTTCA	CTTTGCGTTTCTTGTTGCGA
IL-1β	AATGCCTCGTGCTGTCTG	TCCATTGAGGTGGAGAGC
IL-6	ATGAAGTTTCTCTCCGCAAG	CAACAACATCAGTCCCAAG
IL-8	AGCCTTCCTGATTTCTGC	AGCACTCCTTGGCAAAAC
TNFα	CAGCCGATTTGCCATTTC	TCTTGATGGCAGAGAGGAG
β-Actin	GTCCACCCGCGAGTACAAC	TATCGTCATCCATGGCGAACTGG

4.7. qPCR

RNA was extracted by using the Hybrid-R kit (305-010; GeneAll Biotechnology, Seoul, Korea). The concentration of RNA was measured using a spectrophotometer (Nano Drop ND-1000, NanoDrop

Technologies Inc.). cDNA was prepared from 1 μg of total RNA using the PrimeScript 1st strand cDNA synthesis kit (Takara Bio, Shiga, Japan). PCR amplification was executed using the SYBR-Green reagent (Takara Bio) in the ABI 7500 real-time PCR system (Applied Biosystems, Foster City, CA, USA). PCR amplification was performed in 20 μL reaction volumes. Sequences for oligonucleotide primers were selected using the Gene Database of National Center for Biotechnology Information (NCBI) and Primer Express™ Software v3.0.1 (Thermo Fisher Scientific, Waltham, MA, USA). Primer pairs are listed in Table 1.

4.8. Statistical Analysis

Statistical evaluations were performed using one-way ANOVA or unpaired *t*-test, as indicated in figure legends. Post hoc analyses were performed using the Tukey's multiple comparisons test or as otherwise specified in the figure legends. All statistical analyses were performed using GraphPad Prism software (GraphPad Software Inc., San Diego, CA, USA). A *p*-value less than 0.05 was considered statistically significant for all analyses.

Author Contributions: Conceptualization, M.T., W.K.P., J.P., J.E.L. and B.H.L.; Data curation, M.T. and J.P.; Formal analysis, M.T. and J.P.; Funding acquisition, B.H.L.; Investigation, M.T. and J.P.; Methodology, M.T., J.P. and J.E.L.; Project administration, M.T. and B.H.L.; Resources, M.T., W.K.P., J.P. and J.E.L.; Supervision, W.K.P., J.E.L. and B.H.L.; Validation, M.T., W.K.P., J.P., J.E.L. and B.H.L.; Visualization, M.T.; Writing—original draft, M.T.; Writing—review & editing, M.T., W.K.P. and B.H.L. All authors have read and agreed to the published version of the manuscript.

Abbreviations

AAALAC	Association and Accreditation of Laboratory Animal Care
ANOVA	analysis of variance
APC	adenomatous polyposis coli
AXIN	axis inhibition protein
CCA	common carotid artery
DMSO	dimethyl sulfoxide
ECA	external carotid artery
GSK3-β	glycogen synthase kinase-3β
ICA	internal carotid artery
IL	interleukin
LE	lipid emulsion
LRP	low-density lipoprotein receptor-related protein
MCA	middle cerebral artery
MCAO	middle cerebral artery occlusion
mRNA	messenger ribonucleic acid
PORCN	porcupine
qPCR	quantitative polymerase chain reaction
SEM	standard error of mean
TNF-α	tumor necrosis factor-α
Veh	vehicle
Wnt	wingless integration
XAV939	2-[4-(trifluoromethyl)phenyl]-7,8-dihydro-5H-thiino [4,3-d]pyrimidin-4-ol

References

1. Romero, J.R.; Morris, J.; Pikula, A. Stroke prevention: Modifying risk factors. *Ther. Adv. Cardiovasc. Dis.* **2008**, *2*, 287–303. [CrossRef] [PubMed]
2. Feigin, V.L.; Forouzanfar, M.H.; Krishnamurthi, R.; Mensah, G.A.; Connor, M.; Bennett, D.A.; Moran, A.E.; Sacco, R.L.; Anderson, L.; Truelsen, T.; et al. Global and regional burden of stroke during 1990–2010: Findings from the global burden of disease study 2010. *Lancet* **2014**, *383*, 245–254. [CrossRef]

3. Gottesman, R.F.; Hillis, A.E. Predictors and assessment of cognitive dysfunction resulting from ischaemic stroke. *Lancet Neurol.* **2010**, *9*, 895–905. [CrossRef]
4. Sun, M.-S.; Jin, H.; Sun, X.; Huang, S.; Zhang, F.-L.; Guo, Z.-N.; Yang, Y. Free radical damage in ischemia-reperfusion injury: An obstacle in acute ischemic stroke after revascularization therapy. *Oxid. Med. Cell Longev.* **2018**, *2018*, 3804979. [CrossRef] [PubMed]
5. Wardlaw, J.M.; Murray, V.; Berge, E.; del Zoppo, G.J. Thrombolysis for acute ischaemic stroke. *Cochrane Database Syst. Rev.* **2014**, *2014*, Cd000213. [CrossRef] [PubMed]
6. Pan, J.; Konstas, A.A.; Bateman, B.; Ortolano, G.A.; Pile-Spellman, J. Reperfusion injury following cerebral ischemia: Pathophysiology, MR imaging and potential therapies. *Neuroradiology* **2007**, *49*, 93–102. [CrossRef]
7. Sobowale, O.A.; Parry-Jones, A.R.; Smith, C.J.; Tyrrell, P.J.; Rothwell, N.J.; Allan, S.M. Interleukin-1 in stroke: From bench to bedside. *Stroke* **2016**, *47*, 2160–2167. [CrossRef]
8. Aref, H.M.A.; Fahmy, N.A.; Khalil, S.H.; Ahmed, M.F.; ElSadek, A.; Abdulghani, M.O. Role of interleukin-6 in ischemic stroke outcome. *Egypt J. Neurol. Psychiatr. Neurosurg.* **2020**, *56*, 12. [CrossRef]
9. Domac, F.M.; Misirli, H. The role of neutrophils and interleukin-8 in acute ischemic stroke. *Neurosciences (Riyadh)* **2008**, *13*, 136–141.
10. Zangari, R.; Zanier, E.R.; Torgano, G.; Bersano, A.; Beretta, S.; Beghi, E.; Casolla, B.; Checcarelli, N.; Lanfranconi, S.; Maino, A.; et al. Early ficolin-1 is a sensitive prognostic marker for functional outcome in ischemic stroke. *J. Neuroinflammation* **2016**, *13*, 16. [CrossRef]
11. Relton, J.K.; Rothwell, N.J. Interleukin-1 receptor antagonist inhibits ischaemic and excitotoxic neuronal damage in the rat. *Brain Res. Bull.* **1992**, *29*, 243–246. [CrossRef]
12. Yamasaki, Y.; Matsuura, N.; Shozuhara, H.; Onodera, H.; Itoyama, Y.; Kogure, K. Interleukin-1 as a pathogenetic mediator of ischemic brain damage in rats. *Stroke* **1995**, *26*, 676–680. [CrossRef] [PubMed]
13. Shruster, A.; Ben-Zur, T.; Melamed, E.; Offen, D. Wnt signaling enhances neurogenesis and improves neurological function after focal ischemic injury. *PLoS ONE* **2012**, *7*, e40843. [CrossRef] [PubMed]
14. Jean LeBlanc, N.; Menet, R.; Picard, K.; Parent, G.; Tremblay, M.-È.; ElAli, A. Canonical Wnt pathway maintains blood-brain barrier integrity upon ischemic stroke and its activation ameliorates tissue plasminogen activator therapy. *Mol. Neurobiol.* **2019**, *56*, 6521–6538. [CrossRef]
15. Endo, H.; Nito, C.; Kamada, H.; Yu, F.; Chan, P.H. Akt/GSK3beta survival signaling is involved in acute brain injury after subarachnoid hemorrhage in rats. *Stroke* **2006**, *37*, 2140–2146. [CrossRef]
16. Kim, U.J.; Lee, B.H.; Lee, K.H. Neuroprotective effects of a protein tyrosine phosphatase inhibitor against hippocampal excitotoxic injury. *Brain Res.* **2019**, *1719*, 133–139. [CrossRef]
17. Lee, K.H.; Won, R.; Kim, U.J.; Kim, G.M.; Chung, M.A.; Sohn, J.H.; Lee, B.H. Neuroprotective effects of FK506 against excitotoxicity in organotypic hippocampal slice culture. *Neurosci. Lett.* **2010**, *474*, 126–130. [CrossRef]
18. Wang, W.; Li, M.; Wang, Y.; Wang, Z.; Zhang, W.; Guan, F.; Chen, Q.; Wang, J. GSK-3β as a target for protection against transient cerebral ischemia. *Int. J. Med. Sci.* **2017**, *14*, 333–339. [CrossRef]
19. Cheng, J.; Shen, W.; Jin, L.; Pan, J.; Zhou, Y.; Pan, G.; Xie, Q.; Hu, Q.; Wu, S.; Zhang, H.; et al. Treadmill exercise promotes neurogenesis and myelin repair via upregulating Wnt/β-catenin signaling pathways in the juvenile brain following focal cerebral ischemia/reperfusion. *Int. J. Mol. Med.* **2020**, *45*, 1447–1463. [CrossRef]
20. Chen, B.; Tao, J.; Lin, Y.; Lin, R.; Liu, W.; Chen, L. Electro-acupuncture exerts beneficial effects against cerebral ischemia and promotes the proliferation of neural progenitor cells in the cortical peri-infarct area through the Wnt/β-catenin signaling pathway. *Int. J. Mol. Med.* **2015**, *36*, 1215–1222. [CrossRef]
21. Isaksson, B.; Hambraeus, L.; Vinnars, E.; Samuelson, G.; Larsson, J.; Asp, N.-G. In memory of Arvid Wretlind 1919–2002. *J. Food Nutr. Res.* **2002**, *46*, 117–118.
22. Weinberg, G.L.; VadeBoncouer, T.; Ramaraju, G.A.; Garcia-Amaro, M.F.; Cwik, M.J. Pretreatment or resuscitation with a lipid infusion shifts the dose-response to bupivacaine-induced asystole in rats. *Anesthesiology* **1998**, *88*, 1071–1075. [CrossRef] [PubMed]
23. Tierney, K.J.; Murano, T.; Natal, B. Lidocaine-induced cardiac arrest in the emergency department: Effectiveness of lipid therapy. *Int. J. Emerg. Med.* **2016**, *50*, 47–50. [CrossRef] [PubMed]
24. Litz, R.J.; Popp, M.; Stehr, S.N.; Koch, T. Successful resuscitation of a patient with ropivacaine-induced asystole after axillary plexus block using lipid infusion. *Anaesthesia* **2006**, *61*, 800–801. [CrossRef] [PubMed]

25. Rosenblatt, M.A.; Abel, M.; Fischer, G.W.; Itzkovich, C.J.; Eisenkraft, J.B. Successful use of a 20% lipid emulsion to resuscitate a patient after a presumed bupivacaine-related cardiac arrest. *Anesthesiology* **2006**, *105*, 217–218. [CrossRef]
26. Zaugg, M.; Lou, P.H.; Lucchinetti, E.; Gandhi, M.; Clanachan, A.S. Postconditioning with Intralipid emulsion protects against reperfusion injury in post-infarct remodeled rat hearts by activation of ROS-Akt/Erk signaling. *Transl. Res.* **2017**, *186*, 36–51. [CrossRef]
27. Rahman, S.; Li, J.; Bopassa, J.C.; Umar, S.; Iorga, A.; Partownavid, P.; Eghbali, M. Phosphorylation of GSK-3β mediates intralipid-induced cardioprotection against ischemia/reperfusion injury. *Anesthesiology* **2011**, *115*, 242–253. [CrossRef]
28. Li, J.; Ruffenach, G.; Kararigas, G.; Cunningham, C.M.; Motayagheni, N.; Barakai, N.; Umar, S.; Regitz-Zagrosek, V.; Eghbali, M. Intralipid protects the heart in late pregnancy against ischemia/reperfusion injury via Caveolin2/STAT3/GSK-3β pathway. *J. Mol. Cell Cardiol.* **2017**, *102*, 108–116. [CrossRef]
29. Anna, R.; Rolf, R.; Mark, C. Update of the organoprotective properties of xenon and argon: From bench to beside. *Intensive Care Med. Exp.* **2020**, *8*, 11. [CrossRef]
30. Auzmendi, J.; Puchulu, M.B.; Rodríguez, J.C.G.; Balaszczuk, A.M.; Lazarowski, A.; Merelli, A. EPO and EPO-receptor system as potential actionable mechanism for the protection of brain and heart in refractory epilepsy and SUDEP. *Curr. Pharm. Des.* **2020**, *26*, 1356–1364. [CrossRef]
31. Tanioka, M.; Park, W.K.; Shim, I.; Kim, K.; Choi, S.; Kim, U.J.; Lee, K.H.; Hong, S.K.; Lee, B.H. Neuroprotection from excitotoxic injury by local administration of lipid emulsion into the brain of rats. *Int. J. Mol. Sci.* **2020**, *21*, 2706. [CrossRef] [PubMed]
32. Fan, Y.; Luo, Q.; Wei, J.; Lin, R.; Lin, L.; Li, Y.; Chen, Z.; Lin, W.; Chen, Q. Mechanism of salvianolic acid B neuroprotection against ischemia/reperfusion induced cerebral injury. *Brain Res.* **2018**, *1679*, 125–133. [CrossRef] [PubMed]
33. Torres, V.I.; Godoy, J.A.; Inestrosa, N.C. Modulating Wnt signaling at the root: Porcupine and Wnt acylation. *Pharmacol. Therapeut.* **2019**, *198*, 34–45. [CrossRef] [PubMed]
34. Huang, L.; Ma, Q.; Li, Y.; Li, B.; Zhang, L. Inhibition of microRNA-210 suppresses pro-inflammatory response and reduces acute brain injury of ischemic stroke in mice. *Exp. Neurol.* **2018**, *300*, 41–50. [CrossRef]
35. Tarkowski, E.; Rosengren, L.; Blomstrand, C.; Wikkelsö, C.; Jensen, C.; Ekholm, S.; Tarkowski, A. Intrathecal release of pro- and anti-inflammatory cytokines during stroke. *Clin. Exp. Immunol.* **1997**, *110*, 492–499. [CrossRef]
36. Chong, Z.Z.; Shang, Y.C.; Hou, J.; Maiese, K. Wnt1 neuroprotection translates into improved neurological function during oxidant stress and cerebral ischemia through AKT1 and mitochondrial apoptotic pathways. *Oxid. Med. Cell Longev.* **2010**, *3*, 153–165. [CrossRef]
37. Morris, D.C.; Zhang, Z.G.; Wang, Y.; Zhang, R.L.; Gregg, S.; Liu, X.S.; Chopp, M. Wnt expression in the adult rat subventricular zone after stroke. *Neurosci. Lett.* **2007**, *418*, 170–174. [CrossRef]
38. Lou, P.-H.; Lucchinetti, E.; Zhang, L.; Affolter, A.; Schaub, M.C.; Gandhi, M.; Hersberger, M.; Warren, B.E.; Lemieux, H.; Sobhi, H.F.; et al. The mechanism of Intralipid®-mediated cardioprotection complex IV inhibition by the active metabolite, palmitoylcarnitine, generates reactive oxygen species and activates reperfusion injury salvage kinases. *PLoS ONE* **2014**, *9*, e87205. [CrossRef]
39. Suryawanshi, A.; Tadagavadi, R.K.; Swafford, D.; Manicassamy, S. Modulation of inflammatory responses by Wnt/β-Catenin signaling in dendritic cells: A novel immunotherapy target for autoimmunity and cancer. *Front. Immunol.* **2016**, *7*, 460. [CrossRef]
40. Yu, Z.; Cheng, C.; Liu, Y.; Liu, N.; Lo, E.H.; Wang, X. Neuroglobin promotes neurogenesis through Wnt signaling pathway. *Cell Death Dis.* **2018**, *9*, 945. [CrossRef]
41. Jia, L.; Piña-Crespo, J.; Li, Y. Restoring Wnt/β-catenin signaling is a promising therapeutic strategy for Alzheimer's disease. *Mol. Brain* **2019**, *12*, 104. [CrossRef] [PubMed]
42. Scott, E.L.; Brann, D.W. Estrogen regulation of Dkk1 and Wnt/β-Catenin signaling in neurodegenerative disease. *Brain Res.* **2013**, *1514*, 63–74. [CrossRef] [PubMed]
43. Rosi, M.C.; Luccarini, I.; Grossi, C.; Fiorentini, A.; Spillantini, M.G.; Prisco, A.; Scali, C.; Gianfriddo, M.; Caricasole, A.; Terstappen, G.C.; et al. Increased Dickkopf-1 expression in transgenic mouse models of neurodegenerative disease. *J. Neurochem.* **2010**, *112*, 1539–1551. [CrossRef] [PubMed]
44. Purro, S.A.; Galli, S.; Salinas, P.C. Dysfunction of Wnt signaling and synaptic disassembly in neurodegenerative diseases. *J. Mol. Cell Biol.* **2014**, *6*, 75–80. [CrossRef]

45. Ragab, N.; Viehweger, F.; Bauer, J.; Geyer, N.; Yang, M.; Seils, A.; Belharazem, D.; Brembeck, F.H.; Schildhaus, H.-U.; Marx, A.; et al. Canonical WNT/β-catenin signaling plays a subordinate role in rhabdomyosarcomas. *Front. Pediatr.* **2018**, *6*, 378. [CrossRef] [PubMed]
46. Wei, Z.Z.; Zhang, J.Y.; Taylor, T.M.; Gu, X.; Zhao, Y.; Wei, L. Neuroprotective and regenerative roles of intranasal Wnt-3a administration after focal ischemic stroke in mice. *J. Cereb. Blood Flow Metab.* **2018**, *38*, 404–421. [CrossRef] [PubMed]
47. Bao, R.; Christova, T.; Song, S.; Angers, S.; Yan, X.; Attisano, L. Inhibition of tankyrases induces Axin stabilization and blocks Wnt signalling in breast cancer cells. *PLoS ONE* **2012**, *7*, e48670. [CrossRef] [PubMed]
48. Berressem, D.; Koch, K.; Franke, N.; Klein, J.; Eckert, G.P. Intravenous treatment with a long-chain omega-3 lipid emulsion provides neuroprotection in a murine model of ischemic stroke—A pilot study. *PLoS ONE* **2016**, *11*, e0167329. [CrossRef]
49. Williams, J.J.; Mayurasakorn, K.; Vannucci, S.J.; Mastropietro, C.; Bazan, N.G.; Ten, V.S.; Deckelbaum, R.J. N-3 fatty acid rich triglyceride emulsions are neuroprotective after cerebral hypoxic-ischemic injury in neonatal mice. *PLoS ONE* **2013**, *8*, e56233. [CrossRef]
50. Morris, G.P.; Wright, A.L.; Tan, R.P.; Gladbach, A.; Ittner, L.M.; Vissel, B. A comparative study of variables influencing ischemic injury in the Longa and Koizumi methods of intraluminal filament middle cerebral artery occlusion in mice. *PLoS ONE* **2016**, *11*, e0148503. [CrossRef]
51. Lyu, C.; Zhang, Y.; Gu, M.; Huang, Y.; Liu, G.; Wang, C.; Li, M.; Chen, S.; Pan, S.; Gu, Y. IRAK-M deficiency exacerbates ischemic neurovascular injuries in experimental stroke mice. *Front. Cell Neurosci.* **2018**, *12*, 504. [CrossRef] [PubMed]

6

Adiponectin: The Potential Regulator and Therapeutic Target of Obesity and Alzheimer's Disease

Jong Youl Kim [1,†], Sumit Barua [1,†], Ye Jun Jeong [1] and Jong Eun Lee [1,2,*]

1 Department of Anatomy, Yonsei University College of Medicine, Seoul 120-752, Korea; jongyoul74@gmail.com (J.Y.K.); drsbarua@gmail.com (S.B.); jyj4453@naver.com (Y.J.J.)

2 BK21 Plus Project for Medical Sciences, and Brain Research Institute, Yonsei University College of Medicine, Seoul 120-752, Korea

* Correspondence: jelee@yuhs.ac

† co-first authors.

Abstract: Animal and human mechanistic studies have consistently shown an association between obesity and Alzheimer's disease (AD). AD, a degenerative brain disease, is the most common cause of dementia and is characterized by the presence of extracellular amyloid beta (Aβ) plaques and intracellular neurofibrillary tangles disposition. Some studies have recently demonstrated that Aβ and tau cannot fully explain the pathophysiological development of AD and that metabolic disease factors, such as insulin, adiponectin, and antioxidants, are important for the sporadic onset of nongenetic AD. Obesity prevention and treatment can be an efficacious and safe approach to AD prevention. Adiponectin is a benign adipokine that sensitizes the insulin receptor signaling pathway and suppresses inflammation. It has been shown to be inversely correlated with adipose tissue dysfunction and may enhance the risk of AD because a range of neuroprotection adiponectin mechanisms is related to AD pathology alleviation. In this study, we summarize the recent progress that addresses the beneficial effects and potential mechanisms of adiponectin in AD. Furthermore, we review recent studies on the diverse medications of adiponectin that could possibly be related to AD treatment, with a focus on their association with adiponectin. A better understanding of the neuroprotection roles of adiponectin will help clarify the precise underlying mechanism of AD development and progression.

Keywords: Alzheimer's disease; metabolic disease; adiponectin; insulin; antioxidants

---

1. Introduction

The global prevalence of obesity has increased at an alarming rate over the years. In 2016, it was estimated that nearly 39% of adults aged ≥18 years were overweight worldwide, and 13% were obese [WHO, 2016]. Obesity is generally defined as a body mass index of >30 kg/m^2 and is mainly caused by physical inactivity and westernized dietary habits. Obesity is a major concern because it is a risk factor for a plethora of metabolic diseases that increase mortality rates. Since obesity causes insulin resistance, it is one of the major risk factors for type 2 diabetes (T2DM). After years of obesity-associated hyperinsulinemia, the insulin secretory function in the pancreas could falter and eventually lead to hyperglycemia. A previous study has suggested that obesity and diabetes are linked to Alzheimer's disease (AD) [1]. The pooled effect size for AD in relation to obesity and diabetes was calculated at 1.59 and 1.54 in longitudinal epidemiological studies of body mass, metabolic syndrome (dyslipidemia, hypertension, abdominal obesity, and insulin resistance), diabetes, and glucose and insulin levels [2]. A clinical study has also shown that an increased number of metabolic and vascular risk factors in midlife is critical for amyloid deposition and could lead to the risk of developing AD during old age [3].

Recently, the World Alzheimer Report estimated that the total number of people with AD and dementia is set to triple to 132–152 million cases worldwide by 2050 (World Alzheimer Report 2015). About 60%–70% of dementia cases are caused by AD, a chronic neurodegenerative disease. These dementia cases are often associated with extracellular amyloid beta (Aβ) plaques and intraneuronal deposits of neurofibrillary tangles (NFTs) in the brain. Hyperphosphorylation of tau protein leads to the formation of NFTs, whereas the accumulation of Aβ forms hard, insoluble plaques (Aβ peptide) [4]. For over two decades, these two proteins have been the main target for AD therapeutics; currently, available treatments for AD are symptomatic and do not decelerate or prevent the progression of the disease. However, these therapies demonstrate modest but particularly consistent benefits for cognition, global status, and functional ability. The abovementioned studies have suggested that another approach should be considered for the development of AD treatment based on the relationship between AD, obesity, and T2DM. According to the Mayo Clinic AD Patient Registry, 80% of AD patients had either diabetes or showed impairment in glucose tolerance [5]. Many studies are being conducted to decipher the underlying mechanisms responsible for the association between obesity, T2DM, and AD. In some studies that used a rodent model, a high-fat diet was shown to cause AD pathology due to the accumulation of Aβ peptides and phosphorylated tau proteins, as well as cognitive impairment [6,7].

Adiponectin secreted from the adipose tissue sensitizes the insulin receptor signaling pathway and prevents inflammation. Adiponectin is a protein that modulates a number of metabolic diseases (Figure 1), including diabetes, dyslipidemia, atherosclerosis, and comorbid metabolic dysfunction that occur in cardiovascular diseases such as hypertension. Many studies have indicated that alteration levels of adiponectin in the plasma and cerebrospinal fluid (CSF) correspond to a distinctive condition of mild cognitive impairment (MCI) and AD [8–13]. The reason for the discrepancies among these studies is unclear, but adiponectin may be considered to be a metabolic biomarker for AD.

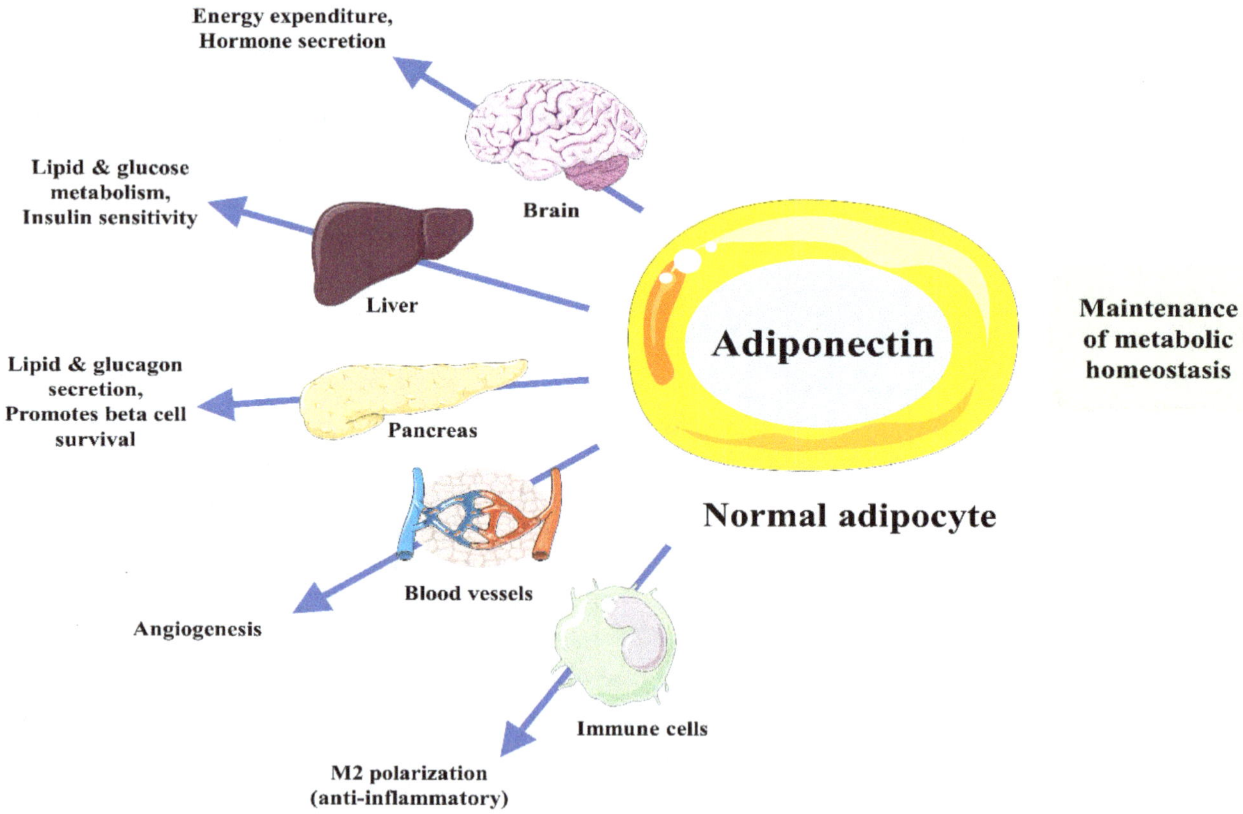

Figure 1. Major mechanisms of adiponectin's actions in the maintenance of metabolic homeostasis.

In this review, we will discuss the potential mechanisms that bridge the relationship between adiponectin and AD. Understanding these mechanisms could narrow down the process of AD's therapeutic window and also help to design novel therapeutic applications against AD and related neurodegenerative diseases.

2. Relationship between Metabolic Disorder and Alzheimer's Disease

The most common age-related neurodegenerative disease is AD, which accounts for the most predominant form (about 60–70%) of dementia, as mentioned by WHO. It is characterized by a gradual loss of learning and memory, particularly episodic memory, and may lead to death within 10 years of onset [14,15]. Limited information is known about the etiology and associated nongenetic risk factors of AD. However, some modifiable events, such as dietary habits, lifestyle, and environmental exposure (toxic chemicals), and the nonmodifiable event of aging are common global factors for AD pathology [16,17]. The prevalence of AD is higher in developed countries than in developing countries, and >40% of AD cases are known to occur in individuals aged ≥80 years.

AD was named after Alois Alzheimer, the first person to describe that extensive neuronal tangles and amyloid plaques, considered to be important hallmarks of the disease, can be found in the AD brain. However, recent studies have shown that AD patients have an insidious loss of neurons and increased reactive gliosis in different parts of the brain, comprising the cerebral cortex and the limbic system, including the amygdala and hippocampus [18]. Cellular changes in the basal ganglia, cerebellum, brain stem, and spinal cord are relatively spared in AD. According to pathological findings of affected AD brain regions, two different types of aggregates are commonly found in the intracellular and extracellular compartments—the intracellular aggregates are known as NFTs and the extracellular aggregates are known as senile plaques that consist of insoluble paired helical filaments of hyperphosphorylated tau protein [19,20]. The major component of the senile plaque is known as Aβ aggregation, which occurs before other pathological events such as NFT formation and neuronal death [21]. Thus, Aβ aggregation is considered the central player of neuronal death, which has also been observed in in-vitro neuronal cells subjected to synthetic Aβ peptide (Aβ1-42/43) treatment [22]. Over the years, the amyloid hypothesis, a process where extracellular Aβ accumulation is followed by the loss of synapses and subsequent neuronal loss, has become the popular concept of AD pathogenesis and has been used by many AD research groups [23].

It has been suggested that metabolic impairment and modification of the AD-related protein levels can contribute to a higher prevalence of AD. Dyslipidemia, hypertension, abdominal obesity, and insulin resistance are the popular hallmarks of metabolic abnormalities, which are collectively known as metabolic syndrome (MetS) [24]. Individuals with higher life expectancy (above 80 years) have a higher prevalence of MetS, which is a potential cause of neurodegenerative diseases, especially cognitive impairment and dementia. Other studies have also found that MetS is not solely responsible for AD progression in elderly people, regardless of their backgrounds. Higher MetS could bridge inappropriate regulation of the central nervous system (CNS) function (especially part of the limbic system, such as the prefrontal cortex, hippocampus, and amygdala) and metabolic regulatory responses that result in functional cognitive impairments [25]. Metabolic products that are produced in peripheral organs, such as estrogen, insulin, cortisol, and leptin, can cross the blood–brain barrier (BBB) and influence cognitive function. However, neuropeptides such as orexin (mice), allastostatin (drosophila), and neuropeptide Y (grass carp) modulate metabolic processes in different animals [26]. In a recent review, Yi et al. suggested that neuropeptide Y receptors in humans can be a promising target for metabolic disorders [27]. Furthermore, food intake and weight gain can be increased by lesions in oxytocin-containing hypothalamic nuclei [28].

Some studies on metabolic diseases have reported that metabolic diseases, such as T2DM and obesity, are associated with AD. Metabolic alteration of substances such as T2DM-related insulin receptors [29] and obesity-related adiponectin [30,31] could alter the process of aging and age-related dementia, such as in AD. In a recent study, Nasoohi et al. suggested the relationship of "type 3 diabetes" to AD pathology, in which the metabolic syndrome consisting of oxidative stress and neuroinflammation leads to brain insulin resistance [32]. This concept suggests that the thioredoxin-interacting protein (TXNIP) is a key regulator of oxidative stress and inflammasome activation, which is associated with impaired insulin function in the brain. Brain insulin resistance is found to be related to the progressive atrophy of the brain regions of early AD progression, which are cingulate cortices, medial temporal lobe, prefrontal gyri, and other regions [33]. Along with the discussion above, brain insulin resistance due to metabolic disorders such as diabetes mellitus, metabolic syndrome, and nonalcoholic fatty liver disease are considered to be a prominent component of AD pathology; the maintenance of brain insulin supply should also be a target of AD therapy for individuals with metabolic disorder [34]. Thus, metabolism and neurological disorders are closely related to each other.

3. Adiponectin as a Modulator of Metabolic Disorder

Adiponectin is secreted with the bioactive molecule leptin from normal adipose tissues (together, they are called adipokines) [35]. It regulates glucose and fatty acid metabolism by increasing insulin sensitivity of peripheral organs [36–38]. However, small amounts of adiponectin, an adipose-tissue-specific protein, can also be synthesized by other cell types. Paradoxically, the adiponectin level decreases with the increase of central adiposity, which causes obesity [39–41]. Obesity causes damage to several organ systems because it regulates MetS, which can be characterized physiologically as excess weight and pathologically as high triglyceride levels and insulin resistance [42]. Moreover, obesity is related to an increase in cognitive decline and AD [43]. Recently, our laboratory has shown that touchscreen-based behavioral testing of high-fat diet mice led to an impairment in cognitive function compared with cognitive function in normal diet mice [44]. MetS, including obesity, cardiovascular disease, type 2 diabetes, and neurodegenerative disorders, is associated with the regulation of adiponectin expression [8,45,46]. Like other hormonal proteins, adiponectin also functions through specific receptors known as adiponectin receptors. Adiponectin receptors have been classified into adiponectin receptor (AdipoR) 1, AdipoR2, and T-cadherin. Through the recruitment of adaptor protein APPL1 by AdipoRs activation, adiponectin signaling regulates a series of signaling pathways [47]. AMP-activated protein kinase (AMPK), peroxisome proliferator-activated receptor-α (PPARα), IkB kinase (IKK)/NF-κB/PTEN, IRS1/2–Akt, and Ras-ERK1/2 signaling are examples of downstream adiponectin signaling [48–52]. Adiponectin receptors are found to be expressed throughout the whole brain. Thundyil et al. suggested that in the cortical neurons, AdipoR1 expression is more prominent than AdipoR2 expression [53]. On the other hand, T-cadherin acts as the coreceptor of a unidentified receptor, through which the adiponectin can transmit the metabolic signals [54].

4. Adiponectin's Potential Role in Alzheimer's Disease

4.1. Adiponectin and Brain

Adiponectin gives a beneficial effect on synaptic regulation and memory in AD (Figure 2). It also promotes synaptic plasticity in AD by improving the hippocampal's long-term potentiation [55]. Adiponectin and its homolog, osmotin, enhance neurite outgrowth and synaptic complexity and improve learning and memory defects in mouse AD models [56–59]. Furthermore, chronic adiponectin deficiency in aged mice leads to AD-like cognitive impairments and pathologies [60]. In a recent clinical study, individuals with higher-than-normal adiponectin levels performed better in cognitive tests, indicating the protective effect of adiponectin against cognitive failure. Furthermore, the study showed that adiponectin could be used to identify the risk of cognitive dysfunction [61]. The upregulation of serum adiponectin expression has been found to be associated with MCI and AD [8]. The adiponectin receptors AdipoR1 and AdipoR2 have approximately 95% homology between human and mice. They are ubiquitously expressed and structurally related in humans and mice, with variable affinity to different isoforms and predominance in some tissues [62]. The expression of AdipoR1 and AdipoR2 is mainly localized to neurons in the hypothalamus, brainstem, and cortex [22], as well as the nucleus basalis of Meynert and the hippocampus, the two main targeted structures in AD [63]. In the hypothalamus and the brainstem, adiponectin is thought to regulate food intake and energy expenditure via AdipoR1-mediated AMPK signaling [23]. However, low levels of adiponectin in CSF may be compensated by the presence of two high-affinity receptors, AdipoR1 and AdipoR2, in the brain [64,65]. Suppression of AdipoR1 can result in metabolic diseases such as obesity and diabetes, which also potentiate spatial learning deficit, memory impairment, and AD pathologies [30]. Hence, studies have evaluated adiponectin and its receptors as therapeutic alternatives for AD.

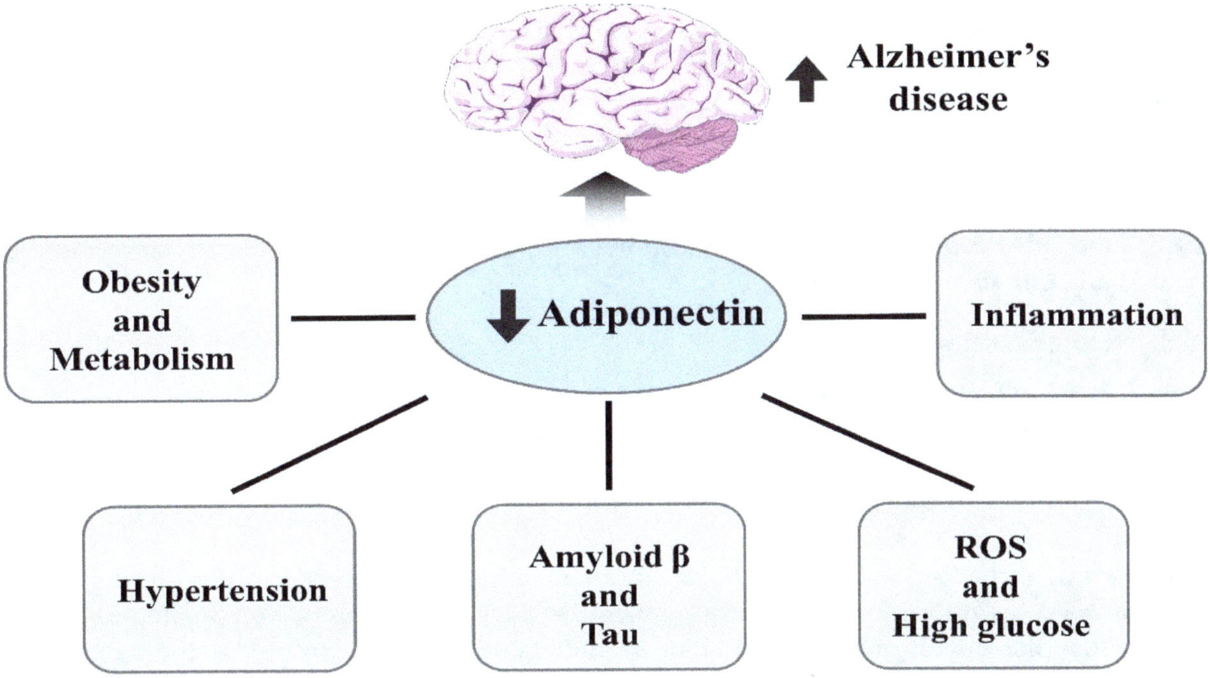

Figure 2. Downregulation of adiponectin involved in the mechanism of Alzheimer's disease exacerbates AD pathology and impairment.

In AD, Aβ has to cross BBB to be transported in the brain, where it is regulated by specific receptors and transporters [66]. Therefore, it is necessary to protect BBB disruption. Adiponectin protects BBB disruption by inhibiting apoptosis of endothelial cells, protecting tight junction integrity via the AdipoR1-mediated NF-κB pathway, and maintaining the balance of Aβ transporters in endothelial cells [67].

4.2. *Adiponectin Improves Insulin Signaling*

Recently, many studies have provided evidence that insulin signaling dysfunction plays a key role in cognitive decline, such as in MCI and AD [68–70]. It is well known that T2DM is independently associated with cognitive dysfunction and loss of hippocampus volume [71]. Further, insulin signaling prevents Aβ oligomer toxicity [72]. Adiponectin has been found to be beneficial for T2DM because of its ability to enhance insulin sensitivity, and it has been used in T2DM treatment [73]. A few studies have reported the relationship between increased diabetes prevalence and decreased levels of adiponectin [74]. In T2DM patients with low adiponectin, the hippocampus volume is significantly decreased [75]. Lower levels of adiponectin in T2DM have also been associated with lower gray matter volume and reduced cerebral glucose metabolism in the temporal brain regions [76]. In addition, adiponectin-deficient mice have been used as models of insulin resistance and the associated memory pathology [60]. In a rat cognitive-deficient model induced by streptozocin, which is commonly used to induce diabetes, adiponectin attenuated tau hyperphosphorylation and alleviated cognitive function by activating the PI3K/Akt/GSK-3β signaling pathway [77].

4.3. *Adiponectin Regulates Glucose/Fatty Acid Metabolism*

Deterioration of cerebral glucose metabolism is an important feature in age-related AD and is key to the progression of AD pathogenesis [78–81]. Adiponectin modulates glucose metabolism in hippocampal neurons by increasing glucose uptake, glycolysis, and adenosine triphosphate production rates [82]. Glucose and lactate are considered major energy sources in the brain. However, the amounts of glucose consumption and oxygen utilization in the brain are not the same [83]. In addition, lactate cannot generate energy because of the fast removal of lactate from cells and activated tissues [84]. A study conducted by Dhopeshwarka et al. suggested that there are gaps between glucose consumption and oxygen utilization by the brain and that fatty acids can enter the brain and mitochondria and can be oxidized to produce energy [85]. About 20% (maximum) of the total energy in the brain can be produced from mitochondrial oxidation of fatty acids [86]. Moreover, fatty acids are regarded as key players in the homeostasis of glucose [87]. Fatty acid metabolism has been found to be related to MCI and to adiponectin and its receptors in mice fed a high-fat diet [44,88,89]. Therefore, changes in adiponectin levels can alter the brain metabolism and progression of AD. Adiponectin also activates the AMPK and PPARα pathways through AdipoR1 and AdipoR2, respectively, which reduce hepatic lipogenesis and enhance β-oxidation [90].

4.4. *Adiponectin Alleviates Inflammation*

One of the key factors for cognitive decline (MCI) and AD is chronic neuroinflammation [91–93]. Amongst renowned anti-inflammatory molecules, adiponectin is considered to be an active contributor to chronic inflammation in obesity and T2DM [91,92,94,95]. Chronic inflammation, which induces AD and metabolic-distress-related pathologies such as neuronal insulin resistance, endoplasmic reticulum stress, synaptotoxicity, and neurodegeneration, is caused by the secretion of proinflammatory cytokines by microglial cell activation [92,96]. In an adiponectin-knockout mouse model, activation of proinflammatory cytokines such as interleukin (IL)-1β, IL-6, and tumor necrotic factor-α has been shown to cause the development of AD-like pathology [60]. Furthermore, adiponectin prevents neuroinflammation by decreasing microglia and regulating the brain macrophage proinflammatory phenotype [97,98]. Therefore, changes in adiponectin levels may be closely related to neuroinflammation in AD.

4.5. *Adiponectin Has Protective Effect on Oxidative Stress/Hypoxia*

Studies have shown that oxidative stress and hypoxia conditions render an important role in the pathogenesis of age-related neurodegenerative diseases such as AD [78,99,100]. Adiponectin alleviates oxidative stress and oxidative-stress-mediated cytotoxicity [101,102] and has a protective effect in high glucose concentrations in blood [26]. Many of these effects have been reported to occur because of upregulated AMPK signaling [101,103]. Since AMPK is considered the general energy sensor in the brain, inhibition of adiponectin may influence the AMPK pathway, which in turn could affect brain metabolism [104,105]. Similarly, in a hypoxic environment in obese individuals, hypertrophic adipocytes upregulate the expression of hypoxia-inducible factor-1α (HIF-1α) [106]. Upregulation of HIF-1α has been found to inhibit the production of adiponectin. This phenomenon has been confirmed by the expression of high levels of adiponectin mRNA in adipocyte-specific HIF-1α-deficient mice fed a high-fat diet for 7 weeks compared with control mice [107]. With the above study, adiponectin can be considered a modulator of neurocognitive disorders, which might suggest adiponectin as a potential therapeutic target for AD.

4.6. *Adiponectin and Neuroprotection/Neurogenesis*

Adiponectin has a neuroprotective effect in various conditions. It shows a protective effect in brain injury caused by ischemic stroke and intracerebral hemorrhage [108,109]. Neuroprotective effects of adiponectin have also been demonstrated in a kainite-induced excitotoxicity model [103].

Furthermore, adiponectin plays a role in many deleterious conditions such as Aβ deposition/tau phosphorylation, neuroinflammation, and oxidative stress by protecting neurons and glial cells. Hippocampal neurogenesis is crucial for maintaining cognitive function; however, it is impaired in AD patients [110,111]. In this respect, it seems necessary to pay attention to the neuroproliferative effect of adiponectin in the adult brain. Intracerebroventricular injection of adiponectin has shown neurogenic and proliferative effects in an adiponectin-deficient mice model [55]. An in-vitro and in-vivo study has also indicated that adiponectin stimulates neurogenesis through AdipoR1 [112].

5. Adiponectin-Associated Therapeutic Strategy against AD Induced by Metabolic Diseases

A number of in-vitro, animal, and clinical studies have been conducted to find molecular targets that prevent protein aggregation, oxidative stress, and inflammation for AD treatment. However, a therapeutic target is still unclear. Adiponectin can be considered a protein of interest in the search for new neuroprotective targets for AD. Previous studies have attempted to use adiponectin levels as an AD marker [8–10,13,113] (Table). In addition, numerous therapeutic agents that are being considered new paradigms in AD therapy have been found to be related to adiponectin signaling. These therapeutic agents do not only include adiponectin and AdipoR homologs but also conventional AD drugs, anti-insulin resistance drugs, and cardiovascular drugs.

5.1. *Adiponectin as an AD Marker*

In some recent studies, the relationship between plasma and CSF adiponectin levels in MCI or AD has been reported. However, there are discrepancies in their results. Some studies have shown decreased adiponectin levels in AD or MCI [113–115], while others have shown increased levels or insignificant changes [9,11–13,116,117]. The reason for the discrepancies among these studies might be because of the ambiguous criteria for classifying AD and MCI patients or failure to exclude other factors that may have affected adiponectin levels. As mentioned earlier, conventional AD medications (acetylcholinesterase inhibitors) can increase serum adiponectin levels. Furthermore, there is also a possibility that increased adiponectin levels may have served as a compensatory mechanism for the progress of AD. Thus, to establish the relationship between adiponectin levels and AD, more controlled studies should be conducted.

5.2. *Adiponectin and Adiponectin Receptor Homolog*

Osmotin, a protein found in tobacco that structurally and functionally mimics adiponectin, positively modulates the AdipoR1/AMPK/SIRT1 pathway and reduces the AD-related protein Aβ expression (Figure 3) [59]. SIRT1 and AMPK are known for their metabolic activities and cellular energy homeostasis; they positively regulate each [118,119]. Osmotin treatment has been found to inhibit the expression of AD markers, such as amyloid precursor protein, p-tau, and Aβ, in inflammation-induced mouse brains [82,120]. In addition, adiponectin also enhances neurite outgrowth and synaptic complexity via AdipoR1/NgR1 signaling [57].

Adiporon, an agonist of adiponectin receptors that bind AdipoRs, has been known to play a vital role in many neurological diseases. Its ability as an anti-depressive agent and metabolic regulator has been demonstrated in a mouse model of depression, where it also regulated dopaminergic neurons [121]. It has also been shown to modulate fear and intrinsic excitability in the hippocampus [122]. These beneficial neurological effects are possible because of the BBB-penetrating property of this molecule. More recently, Liu et al. have reported that adiporon improves cognitive dysfunction, inhibits Aβ deposition, and restores impaired hippocampal neuron proliferation activation in AD mice by activating the AdipoR1/AMPK pathway [123]. Ultimately, osmotin and adiporon can be effective and realistic therapeutic alternatives for adiponectin-based AD treatment in patients.

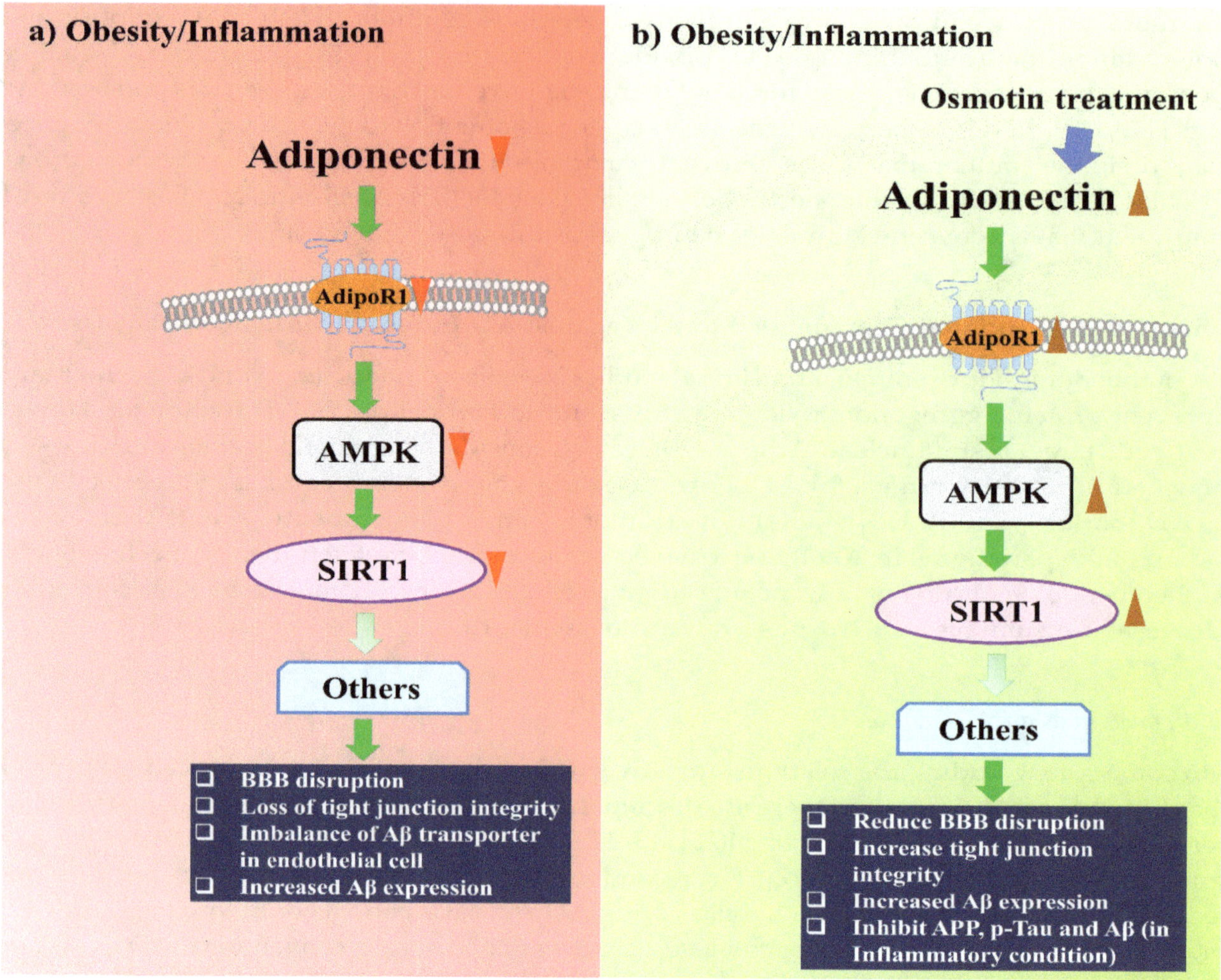

Figure 3. Osmotin treatment positively modulates AD through the AdipoR1/AMPK/SIRT1 pathway. (**a**) Obesity reduces adiponectin and AdipoR1 expressions, which negatively modulate the AMPK/SIRT1 pathway and increase the AD biomarkers. (**b**) Osmotin treatment increases adiponectin and AdipoR1 expressions and reduces AD biomarkers through the AMPK/SIRT1 pathway.

5.3. *Adiponectin and Conventional AD Drug*

The US Food and Drug Administration (FDA) has approved only two types of medications for the treatment of cognitive dysfunction of AD—acetylcholinesterase inhibitors (AChEI; donepezil and galantamine) and memantine [124]. One study has shown that donepezil increases serum adiponectin levels in AD patients, while another study has shown that galantamine increases serum adiponectin levels in a type 2 diabetes rat model [125]. A recent study has also reported a significant weight loss after AChEI treatment and that AChEI treatment exerts an insulin-sensitizing effect via the activation of IR/PI3K/Akt/GLUT2,4 and Wnt/GSK3β/β-catenin signaling [126]. Although more studies are needed, the beneficial effect of AChEI on AD is thought to be possibly mediated by adiponectin.

Memantine is another FDA-approved medication for AD. Although it cannot be factually claimed that its therapeutic mechanism is directly associated with adiponectin, there are some interesting points that suggest a connection between them. Memantine is an *N*-methyl-D-aspartate (NMDA) receptor antagonist that modulates glutamatergic dysfunction and inhibits excitotoxicity mediated by NMDA [127]. Its therapeutic ability in AD is attributed to this mechanism. Similarly, adiponectin has been shown to have a neuroprotective effect by inhibiting NMDA-mediated excitotoxicity [128]. In addition, adiponectin and memantine play a protective role in glutamate-induced excitotoxicity (shown in both animal/in-vitro models) [129,130]. Furthermore, memantine also has the ability to attenuate insulin resistance and improve brain function in high-fat diet-induced models. Given these similarities, there is a possibility that the comprehensive role of adiponectin in AD could be a hint in conducting research on memantine.

5.4. Adiponectin and Type 2 Diabetes Medications

Several studies have suggested that AD and T2DM are related to each other; thus, T2DM drugs and their potential to be used as AD treatment are drawing attention [131,132]. There are several types of type 2 diabetes drugs, such as biguanide derivatives (metformin), PPARγ agonists (thiazolidinedione [TZD] derivatives), glucagon-like peptide-1 receptor (GLP-1R) agonists, dipeptidyl peptidases 4 (DPP-4) inhibitors, sodium-glucose transport protein 2 inhibitors, and second-generation sulfonylureas [133]. In addition to these drugs' ability to improve cognitive function, some of these drugs are capable of increasing adiponectin levels.

Metformin, the drug used as first-line pharmacologic therapy in T2DM, has been shown to attenuate AD-like pathology in both in-vitro and in-vivo studies [134–136]. An improvement in cognitive function has been observed in many studies on mild cognitive function and dementia patients [60,137,138]. Many studies have shown that metformin increases serum adiponectin levels in various conditions [139–141]. Furthermore, like adiponectin, metformin plays a neuroprotective role by activating AMPK signaling [142,143].

TZD derivatives, including rosiglitazone and pioglitazone, act as PPARγ agonists and are used for T2DM treatment because of their insulin sensitization activity [144,145]. They have also been researched as alternative AD treatments [146,147]. Increased adiponectin by TZD might play a key role in the insulin sensitization activity induced by TZD [132,148]. Thus, TZD's beneficial effect on AD might be related to the increased adiponectin levels.

An insulin-releasing hormone in hyperglycemic conditions, GLP-1, has been found to have a neuroprotective effect [149–151]. GLP-1 receptors are responsible for controlling food intake and body weight and are widely distributed in the brain and special neurons (pyramidal neurons of the hippocampus and neocortex), which means that it plays an important role in neural function and synaptic transmission [149,151–154]. In an AD mice model, Val(8)GLP-1, liraglutide, and exidin-4 (GLP-1 analogs, well known for the upregulation of adiponectin) treatments rescued synaptic plasticity by preventing synaptic degradation, which is also correlated with the increased learning ability of new spatial tasks [155–158]. Several studies have also shown the beneficiary effect of GLP-1 analogs for AD [159–161].

Inhibitors of DPP-4 also increase GLP-1 signaling activation by inhibiting the degradation of GLP-1 [162]. Therefore, they potentially act on AD, like other GLP-1 analogs [163]. They also lead to increased adiponectin and are thought to be alternative medications for AD [164–167]. Accordingly, the GLP-1 functional facilitator, GLP-1 analogs, and DPP-4 inhibitors might be good candidates for AD treatment because of their ability to increase adiponectin.

5.5. Drugs for Cardiovascular Disease and Adiponectin

A recent study has suggested that medications aimed at cardiovascular diseases may also decrease the risk of dementia caused by AD [168]. Several neuroprotective pleiotropic agents have been shown to increase plasma adiponectin levels [169]. In studies with animal models, angiotensin II receptor blockers have shown beneficial effects on cognitive function related to AD [170–172]. Improvements in AD progress and cognitive function have also been observed in human clinical trials [173–175]. Moreover, angiotensin II receptor blockers can reduce neuroinflammation directly or by regulating the infiltration of inflammatory cytokines because of their ability to restore the blood-brain barrier [176–178]. Altogether, angiotensin II receptor blockers may be beneficial in AD therapy because it upregulates adiponectin [179–181].

Angiotensin-converting enzyme inhibitors (ACEIs) regulate the renin–angiotensin system and angiotensin II receptor blockers. Upregulation of blood adiponectin has been observed after treatment with ACEIs [182,183]. Some clinical and meta-analysis studies have also shown that ACEIs reduce the progression and risk of AD [184–187]. This result has also been observed in several animal model studies [188–190]. However, in one meta-analysis study, ACEIs had no effect on cognitive decline [191], and some studies have shown a negative effect of ACEIs in in-vivo AD models [192–194]. Thus, ACEI treatment is controversial for its effect on AD.

Another cardiovascular medication, fibrate, a PPARα agonist, has been shown to increase adiponectin levels [195,196]. Since ligand-activated PPARα decreases tau phosphorylation, Aβ pathology, and neuroinflammation, fibrate might be a good candidate for AD treatment [197].

Statins (such as simvastatin, paravastatin, and atorvastatin) have been reported to increase blood adiponectin levels [198–200]. Statins are well known for their anti-inflammatory properties in diabetic patients [201,202]. According to the above studies, statins might also be useful in the treatment of AD by increasing blood adiponectin levels and reducing neuroinflammation.

6. Conclusions

The conventional approach to developing therapeutics for AD has been focused on the Aβ hypothesis, which insists that Aβ causes AD pathologies. However, this approach has yet to provide a successful treatment or prevention method for AD. Based on the metabolic alterations that occur in the pathological markers of AD, this review suggests that the adipocyte metabolite adiponectin can be considered a therapeutic option for the treatment of AD.

Author Contributions: J.E.L. provided concept, design, and overall supervision of this study. J.Y.K. and S.B. contributed to the writing and drawing. Y.J.J. participated in the discussion and revision. All authors have read and agreed to the published version of the manuscript.

References

1. Pugazhenthi, S.; Qin, L.; Reddy, P.H. Common neurodegenerative pathways in obesity, diabetes, and Alzheimer's disease. *Biochim. Biophys. Acta Mol. Basis Dis.* **2017**, *1863*, 1037–1045. [CrossRef] [PubMed]
2. Profenno, L.A.; Porsteinsson, A.P.; Faraone, S.V. Meta-analysis of Alzheimer's disease risk with obesity, diabetes, and related disorders. *Biol. Psychiatry.* **2010**, *67*, 505–512. [CrossRef] [PubMed]
3. Gottesman, R.F.; Schneider, A.L.; Zhou, Y.; Coresh, J.; Green, E.; Gupta, N.; Knopman, D.S.; Mintz, A.; Rahmim, A.; Sharrett, A.R.; et al. Association between midlife vascular risk factors and estimated brain amyloid deposition. *JAMA* **2017**, *317*, 1443–1450. [CrossRef] [PubMed]
4. Mucke, L. Neuroscience: Alzheimer's disease. *Nature* **2009**, *461*, 895–897. [CrossRef] [PubMed]
5. Janson, J.; Laedtke, T.; Parisi, J.E.; O'Brien, P.; Petersen, R.C.; Butler, P.C. Increased risk of type 2 diabetes in Alzheimer disease. *Diabetes* **2004**, *53*, 474–481. [CrossRef]
6. Niu, L.; Han, D.W.; Xu, R.L.; Han, B.; Zhou, X.; Wu, H.W.; Li, S.H.; Qu, C.X.; Liu, M. A high-sugar high-fat diet induced metabolic syndrome shows some symptoms of Alzheimer's disease in rats. *J. Nutr. Health Aging.* **2016**, *20*, 509–513. [CrossRef]
7. Ledreux, A.; Wang, X.; Schultzberg, M.; Granholm, A.C.; Freeman, L.R. Detrimental effects of a high fat/high cholesterol diet on memory and hippocampal markers in aged rats. *Behav. Brain Res.* **2016**, *312*, 294–304. [CrossRef]
8. Une, K.; Takei, Y.A.; Tomita, N.; Asamura, T.; Ohrui, T.; Furukawa, K.; Arai, H. Adiponectin in plasma and cerebrospinal fluid in MCI and Alzheimer's disease. *Eur. J. Neurol.* **2011**, *18*, 1006–1009. [CrossRef]
9. Van Himbergen, T.M.; Beiser, A.S.; Ai, M.; Seshadri, S.; Otokozawa, S.; Au, R.; Thongtang, N.; Wolf, P.A.; Schaefer, E.J. Biomarkers for insulin resistance and inflammation and the risk for all-cause dementia and alzheimer disease: Results from the framingham heart study. *Arch. Neurol.* **2012**, *69*, 594–600. [CrossRef]

10. Waragai, M.; Adame, A.; Trinh, I.; Sekiyama, K.; Takamatsu, Y.; Une, K.; Masliah, E.; Hashimoto, M. Possible involvement of adiponectin, the anti-diabetes molecule, in the pathogenesis of Alzheimer's disease. *J. Alzheimers Dis.* **2016**, *52*, 1453–1459. [CrossRef]
11. Khemka, V.K.; Bagchi, D.; Bandyopadhyay, K.; Bir, A.; Chattopadhyay, M.; Biswas, A.; Basu, D.; Chakrabarti, S. Altered serum levels of adipokines and insulin in probable Alzheimer's disease. *J. Alzheimer Dis. JAD* **2014**, *41*, 525–533. [CrossRef] [PubMed]
12. Ma, J.; Zhang, W.; Wang, H.F.; Wang, Z.X.; Jiang, T.; Tan, M.S.; Yu, J.T.; Tan, L. peripheral blood adipokines and insulin levels in patients with Alzheimer's disease: A replication study and meta-analysis. *Curr. Alzheimer Res.* **2016**, *13*, 223–233. [CrossRef] [PubMed]
13. Wennberg, A.M.; Gustafson, D.; Hagen, C.E.; Roberts, R.O.; Knopman, D.; Jack, C.; Petersen, R.C.; Mielke, M.M. Serum adiponectin levels, neuroimaging, and cognition in the mayo clinic study of aging. *J. Alzheimers Dis.* **2016**, *53*, 573–581. [CrossRef] [PubMed]
14. Albert, M.S.; DeKosky, S.T.; Dickson, D.; Dubois, B.; Feldman, H.H.; Fox, N.C.; Gamst, A.; Holtzman, D.M.; Jagust, W.J.; Petersen, R.C.; et al. The diagnosis of mild cognitive impairment due to Alzheimer's disease: Recommendations from the national institute on aging-Alzheimer's association workgroups on diagnostic guidelines for Alzheimer's disease. *Alzheimers Dement.* **2011**, *7*, 270–279. [CrossRef]
15. Sacks, D.; Baxter, B.; Campbell, B.C.V.; Carpenter, J.S.; Cognard, C.; Dippel, D.; Hirchs, J. Multisociety consensus quality improvement revised consensus statement for endovascular therapy of acute ischemic stroke. *Int. J. Stroke* **2018**, *13*, 612–632. [CrossRef] [PubMed]
16. Alzheimer's, Assotiation. Alzheimer's disease facts and figures. *Alzheimers Dement.* **2016**, *12*, 459–509. [CrossRef]
17. Van Cauwenberghe, C.; van Broeckhoven, C.; Sleegers, K. The genetic landscape of Alzheimer disease: Clinical implications and perspectives. *Genet. Med.* **2016**, *18*, 421–430. [CrossRef]
18. Lee, E.B. Obesity, leptin, and Alzheimer's disease. *Ann. N. Y. Acad. Sci.* **2011**, *1243*, 15–29. [CrossRef]
19. Lee, V.M.; Goedert, M.; Trojanowski, J.Q. Neurodegenerative tauopathies. *Annu. Rev. Neurosci.* **2001**, *24*, 1121–1159. [CrossRef]
20. Mattson, M.P. Pathways towards and away from Alzheimer's disease. *Nature* **2004**, *430*, 631–639. [CrossRef]
21. Morishima, M.; Ihara, Y. Posttranslational modifications of tau in paired helical filaments. *Dementia* **1994**, *5*, 282–288. [CrossRef] [PubMed]
22. Han, X.J.; Hu, Y.Y.; Yang, Z.J.; Jiang, L.P.; Shi, S.L.; Li, Y.R.; Guo, M.Y.; Wu, H.L.; Wan, Y.Y. Amyloid beta-42 induces neuronal apoptosis by targeting mitochondria. *Mol. Med. Rep.* **2017**, *16*, 4521–4528. [CrossRef] [PubMed]
23. Selkoe, D.J.; Hardy, J. The amyloid hypothesis of Alzheimer's disease at 25 years. *EMBO Mol. Med.* **2016**, *8*, 595–608. [CrossRef] [PubMed]
24. Bussler, S.; Penke, M.; Flemming, G.; Elhassan, Y.S.; Kratzsch, J.; Sergeyev, E.; Lipek, T.; Vogel, M.; Spielau, U.; Korner, A.; et al. Novel insights in the metabolic syndrome in childhood and adolescence. *Horm. Res. Paediatr.* **2017**, *88*, 181–193. [CrossRef]
25. Pugazhenthi, S. Metabolic syndrome and the cellular phase of Alzheimer's disease. *Prog. Mol. Biol. Transl. Sci.* **2017**, *146*, 243–258. [CrossRef]
26. Blais, A.; Drouin, G.; Chaumontet, C.; Voisin, T.; Couvelard, A.; Even, P.C.; Couvineau, A. Impact of Orexin-A treatment on food intake, energy metabolism and body weight in mice. *PLoS ONE* **2017**, *12*, e0169908. [CrossRef]
27. Yi, M.; Li, H.; Wu, Z.; Yan, J.; Liu, Q.; Ou, C.; Chen, M. A promising therapeutic target for metabolic diseases: Neuropeptide Y receptors in humans. *Cell Physiol. Biochem.* **2018**, *45*, 88–107. [CrossRef]
28. Lawson, E.A. The effects of oxytocin on eating behaviour and metabolism in humans. *Nat. Rev. Endocrinol.* **2017**, *13*, 700–709. [CrossRef]
29. Frolich, L.; Blum-Degen, D.; Bernstein, H.G.; Engelsberger, S.; Humrich, J.; Laufer, S.; Muschner, D.; Thalheimer, A.; Turk, A.; Hoyer, S.; et al. Brain insulin and insulin receptors in aging and sporadic Alzheimer's disease. *J. Neural. Transm.* **1998**, *105*, 423–438. [CrossRef]
30. Kim, M.W.; Abid, N.B.; Jo, M.H.; Jo, M.G.; Yoon, G.H.; Kim, M.O. Suppression of adiponectin receptor 1 promotes memory dysfunction and Alzheimer's disease-like pathologies. *Sci. Rep.* **2017**, *7*, 12435. [CrossRef]
31. Song, J.; Lee, J.E. Adiponectin as a new paradigm for approaching Alzheimer's disease. *Anat. Cell Biol.* **2013**, *46*, 229–234. [CrossRef]

32. Nasoohi, S.; Parveen, K.; Ishrat, T. Metabolic syndrome, brain insulin resistance, and Alzheimer's disease: Thioredoxin interacting protein (TXNIP) and inflammasome as core amplifiers. *J. Alzheimers Dis.* **2018**, *66*, 857–885. [CrossRef] [PubMed]
33. Willette, A.A.; Xu, G.; Johnson, S.C.; Birdsill, A.C.; Jonaitis, E.M.; Sager, M.A.; Hermann, B.P.; la Rue, A.; Asthana, S.; Bendlin, B.B.; et al. Insulin resistance, brain atrophy, and cognitive performance in late middle-aged adults. *Diabetes Care* **2013**, *36*, 443–449. [CrossRef] [PubMed]
34. De la Monte, S.M. Insulin resistance and neurodegeneration: Progress towards the development of new therapeutics for Alzheimer's disease. *Drugs* **2017**, *77*, 47–65. [CrossRef] [PubMed]
35. Cao, H. Adipocytokines in obesity and metabolic disease. *J. Endocrinol.* **2014**, *220*, T47–T59. [CrossRef]
36. Hotta, K.; Funahashi, T.; Bodkin, N.L.; Ortmeyer, H.K.; Arita, Y.; Hansen, B.C.; Matsuzawa, Y. Circulating concentrations of the adipocyte protein adiponectin are decreased in parallel with reduced insulin sensitivity during the progression to type 2 diabetes in rhesus monkeys. *Diabetes* **2001**, *50*, 1126–1133. [CrossRef]
37. Yamauchi, T.; Kamon, J.; Waki, H.; Terauchi, Y.; Kubota, N.; Hara, K.; Mori, Y.; Ide, T.; Murakami, K.; Tsuboyama-Kasaoka, N.; et al. The fat-derived hormone adiponectin reverses insulin resistance associated with both lipoatrophy and obesity. *Nat. Med.* **2001**, *7*, 941–946. [CrossRef]
38. Yamauchi, T.; Nio, Y.; Maki, T.; Kobayashi, M.; Takazawa, T.; Iwabu, M.; Okada-Iwabu, M.; Kawamoto, S.; Kubota, N.; Kubota, T.; et al. Targeted disruption of AdipoR1 and AdipoR2 causes abrogation of adiponectin binding and metabolic actions. *Nat. Med.* **2007**, *13*, 332–339. [CrossRef]
39. Scherer, P.E.; Williams, S.; Fogliano, M.; Baldini, G.; Lodish, H.F. A novel serum protein similar to C1q, produced exclusively in adipocytes. *J. Biol. Chem.* **1995**, *270*, 26746–26749. [CrossRef]
40. Arita, Y.; Kihara, S.; Ouchi, N.; Takahashi, M.; Maeda, K.; Miyagawa, J.; Hotta, K.; Shimomura, I.; Nakamura, T.; Miyaoka, K.; et al. Paradoxical decrease of an adipose-specific protein, adiponectin, in obesity. *Biochem. Biophys. Res. Commun.* **1999**, *257*, 79–83. [CrossRef]
41. Turer, A.T.; Scherer, P.E. Adiponectin: Mechanistic insights and clinical implications. *Diabetologia* **2012**, *55*, 2319–2326. [CrossRef] [PubMed]
42. Pataky, Z.; Bobbioni-Harsch, E.; Golay, A. Obesity: A complex growing challenge. *Exp. Clin. Endocrinol. Diabetes* **2010**, *118*, 427–433. [CrossRef] [PubMed]
43. Emmerzaal, T.L.; Kiliaan, A.J.; Gustafson, D.R. 2003–2013: A decade of body mass index, Alzheimer's disease, and dementia. *J. Alzheimers Dis.* **2015**, *43*, 739–755. [CrossRef] [PubMed]
44. Lee, S.; Kim, J.Y.; Kim, E.; Seo, K.; Kang, Y.J.; Kim, J.Y.; Kim, C.H.; Song, H.T.; Saksida, L.M.; Lee, J.E.; et al. Assessment of cognitive impairment in a mouse model of high-fat diet-induced metabolic stress with touchscreen-based automated battery system. *Exp. Neurobiol.* **2018**, *27*, 277–286. [CrossRef]
45. Okada-Iwabu, M.; Yamauchi, T.; Iwabu, M.; Honma, T.; Hamagami, K.; Matsuda, K.; Yamaguchi, M.; Tanabe, H.; Kimura-Someya, T.; Shirouzu, M.; et al. A small-molecule AdipoR agonist for type 2 diabetes and short life in obesity. *Nature* **2013**, *503*, 493–499. [CrossRef]
46. Sekiyama, K.; Waragai, M.; Akatsu, H.; Sugama, S.; Takenouchi, T.; Takamatsu, Y.; Fujita, M.; Sekigawa, A.; Rockenstein, E.; Inoue, S.; et al. Disease-modifying effect of adiponectin in model of alpha-synucleinopathies. *Ann. Clin. Transl. Neurol.* **2014**, *1*, 479–489. [CrossRef]
47. Mao, X.; Kikani, C.K.; Riojas, R.A.; Langlais, P.; Wang, L.; Ramos, F.J.; Fang, Q.; Christ-Roberts, C.Y.; Hong, J.Y.; Kim, R.Y.; et al. APPL1 binds to adiponectin receptors and mediates adiponectin signalling and function. *Nat. Cell Biol.* **2006**, *8*, 516–523. [CrossRef]
48. XiaoTian, L.; QiNan, W.; XiaGuang, G.; WuQuan, D.; Bing, C.; ZiWen, L. Exenatide Activates the APPL1-AMPK-PPARalpha axis to prevent diabetic cardiomyocyte apoptosis. *J. Diabetes Res.* **2016**, *2016*, 4219735. [CrossRef]
49. Cheng, K.K.; Lam, K.S.; Wang, Y.; Huang, Y.; Carling, D.; Wu, D.; Wong, C.; Xu, A. Adiponectin-induced endothelial nitric oxide synthase activation and nitric oxide production are mediated by APPL1 in endothelial cells. *Diabetes* **2007**, *56*, 1387–1394. [CrossRef]
50. Chandrasekar, B.; Boylston, W.H.; Venkatachalam, K.; Webster, N.J.; Prabhu, S.D.; Valente, A.J. Adiponectin blocks interleukin-18-mediated endothelial cell death via APPL1-dependent AMP-activated protein kinase (AMPK) activation and IKK/NF-kappaB/PTEN suppression. *J. Biol. Chem.* **2008**, *283*, 24889–24898. [CrossRef]
51. Coope, A.; Milanski, M.; Araujo, E.P.; Tambascia, M.; Saad, M.J.; Geloneze, B.; Velloso, L.A. AdipoR1 mediates the anorexigenic and insulin/leptin-like actions of adiponectin in the hypothalamus. *FEBS Lett.* **2008**, *582*, 1471–1476. [CrossRef] [PubMed]

52. Lee, M.H.; Klein, R.L.; El-Shewy, H.M.; Luttrell, D.K.; Luttrell, L.M. The adiponectin receptors AdipoR1 and AdipoR2 activate ERK1/2 through a Src/Ras-dependent pathway and stimulate cell growth. *Biochemistry* **2008**, *47*, 11682–11692. [CrossRef] [PubMed]
53. Thundyil, J.; Tang, S.C.; Okun, E.; Shah, K.; Karamyan, V.T.; Li, Y.I.; Woodruff, T.M.; Taylor, S.M.; Jo, D.G.; Mattson, M.P.; et al. Evidence that adiponectin receptor 1 activation exacerbates ischemic neuronal death. *Exp. Transl. Stroke. Med.* **2010**, *2*, 15. [CrossRef]
54. Parker-Duffen, J.L.; Nakamura, K.; Silver, M. T-cadherin is essential for adiponectin-mediated revascularization. *J. Biol. Chem.* **2013**, *288*, 24886–24897. [CrossRef] [PubMed]
55. Wang, M.; Jo, J.; Song, J. Adiponectin improves long-term potentiation in the 5XFAD mouse brain. *Sci. Rep.* **2019**, *9*, 8918. [CrossRef]
56. Zhang, D.; Wang, X.; Lu, X.Y. Adiponectin exerts neurotrophic effects on dendritic arborization, spinogenesis, and neurogenesis of the dentate gyrus of male mice. *Endocrinology* **2016**, *157*, 2853–2869. [CrossRef]
57. Yoon, G.; Shah, S.A.; Ali, T.; Kim, M.O. The adiponectin homolog osmotin enhances neurite outgrowth and synaptic complexity via AdipoR1/NgR1 Signaling in Alzheimer's Disease. *Mol. Neurobiol.* **2018**, *55*, 6673–6686. [CrossRef]
58. Ali, T.; Yoon, G.H.; Shah, S.A.; Lee, H.Y.; Kim, M.O. Osmotin attenuates amyloid beta-induced memory impairment, tau phosphorylation and neurodegeneration in the mouse hippocampus. *Sci. Rep.* **2015**, *5*, 11708. [CrossRef]
59. Shah, S.A.; Yoon, G.H.; Chung, S.S.; Abid, M.N.; Kim, T.H.; Lee, H.Y.; Kim, M.O. Novel osmotin inhibits SREBP2 via the AdipoR1/AMPK/SIRT1 pathway to improve Alzheimer's disease neuropathological deficits. *Mol. Psychiatry* **2017**, *22*, 407–416. [CrossRef]
60. Ng, R.C.; Cheng, O.Y.; Jian, M.; Kwan, J.S.; Ho, P.W.; Cheng, K.K.; Yeung, P.K.; Zhou, L.L.; Hoo, R.L.; Chung, S.K.; et al. Chronic adiponectin deficiency leads to Alzheimer's disease-like cognitive impairments and pathologies through AMPK inactivation and cerebral insulin resistance in aged mice. *Mol. Neurodegener.* **2016**, *11*, 71. [CrossRef]
61. Cezaretto, A.; Suemoto, C.K.; Bensenor, I.; Lotufo, P.A.; de Almeida-Pititto, B.; Ferreira, S.R.G.; Group, E.R. Association of adiponectin with cognitive function precedes overt diabetes in the Brazilian Longitudinal Study of Adult Health: ELSA. *Diabetol. Metab. Syndr.* **2018**, *10*, 54. [CrossRef] [PubMed]
62. Yamauchi, T.; Iwabu, M.; Okada-Iwabu, M.; Kadowaki, T. Adiponectin receptors: A review of their structure, function and how they work. *Best Pract. Res. Clin. Endocrinol. Metab.* **2014**, *28*, 15–23. [CrossRef] [PubMed]
63. Thundyil, J.; Pavlovski, D.; Sobey, C.G.; Arumugam, T.V. Adiponectin receptor signalling in the brain. *Br. J. Pharmacol.* **2012**, *165*, 313–327. [CrossRef]
64. Ebinuma, H.; Miida, T.; Yamauchi, T.; Hada, Y.; Hara, K.; Kubota, N.; Kadowaki, T. Improved ELISA for selective measurement of adiponectin multimers and identification of adiponectin in human cerebrospinal fluid. *Clin. Chem.* **2007**, *53*, 1541–1544. [CrossRef]
65. Yamauchi, T.; Kamon, J.; Ito, Y.; Tsuchida, A.; Yokomizo, T.; Kita, S.; Sugiyama, T.; Miyagishi, M.; Hara, K.; Tsunoda, M.; et al. Cloning of adiponectin receptors that mediate antidiabetic metabolic effects. *Nature* **2003**, *423*, 762–769. [CrossRef]
66. Deane, R.; Bell, R.D.; Sagare, A.; Zlokvic, B.V. Clearance of amyloid-β peptide across the blood-brain barrier: Implication for therapies in Alzheimer's disease. *CNS Neurol. Disord. Drug Targets* **2009**, *8*, 16–30. [CrossRef]
67. Varhelyi, Z.P.; Kalman, J.; Olah, Z.; Ivitz, E.V.; Fodor, E.K.; Santha, M.; Datki, Z.L.; Pakaski, M. Adiponectin receptors are less sensitive to stress in a transgenic mouse model of Alzheimer's Disease. *Front. Neurosci.* **2017**, *11*, 199. [CrossRef] [PubMed]
68. Steen, E.; Terry, B.M.; Rivera, E.J.; Cannon, J.L.; Neely, T.R.; Tavares, R.; Xu, X.J.; Wands, J.R.; de la Monte, S.M. Impaired insulin and insulin-like growth factor expression and signaling mechanisms in Alzheimer's disease-Is this type 3 diabetes? *J. Alzheimers Dis.* **2005**, *7*, 63–80. [CrossRef]
69. Arnold, S.E.; Arvanitakis, Z.; Macauley-Rambach, S.L.; Koenig, A.M.; Wang, H.Y.; Ahima, R.S.; Craft, S.; Gandy, S.; Buettner, C.; Stoeckel, L.E.; et al. Brain insulin resistance in type 2 diabetes and Alzheimer disease: Concepts and conundrums. *Nat. Rev. Neurol.* **2018**, *14*, 168–181. [CrossRef] [PubMed]
70. De Felice, F.G. Alzheimer's disease and insulin resistance: Translating basic science into clinical applications. *J. Clin. Investig.* **2013**, *123*, 531–539. [CrossRef]

71. Jack, C.R., Jr.; Petersen, R.C.; Xu, Y.; O'Brien, P.C.; Smith, G.E.; Ivnik, R.J.; Tangalos, E.G.; Kokmen, E. Rate of medial temporal lobe atrophy in typical aging and Alzheimer's disease. *Neurology* **1998**, *51*, 993–999. [CrossRef] [PubMed]
72. De Felice, F.G.; Vieira, M.N.; Bomfim, T.R.; Decker, H.; Velasco, P.T.; Lambert, M.P.; Viola, K.L.; Zhao, W.Q.; Ferreira, S.T.; Klein, W.L. Protection of synapses against Alzheimer's-linked toxins: Insulin signaling prevents the pathogenic binding of Abeta oligomers. *Proc. Natl. Acad. Sci. USA* **2009**, *106*, 1971–1976. [CrossRef] [PubMed]
73. Lopez-Jaramillo, P.; Gomez-Arbelaez, D.; Lopez-Lopez, J.; Lopez-Lopez, C.; Martinez-Ortega, J.; Gomez-Rodriguez, A.; Triana-Cubillos, S. The role of leptin/adiponectin ratio in metabolic syndrome and diabetes. *Horm. Mol. Biol. Clin. Investig.* **2014**, *18*, 37–45. [CrossRef] [PubMed]
74. Berg, A.H.; Combs, T.P.; Du, X.; Brownlee, M.; Scherer, P.E. The adipocyte-secreted protein Acrp30 enhances hepatic insulin action. *Nat. Med.* **2001**, *7*, 947–953. [CrossRef]
75. Masaki, T.; Anan, F.; Shimomura, T.; Fujiki, M.; Saikawa, T.; Yoshimatsu, H. Association between hippocampal volume and serum adiponectin in patients with type 2 diabetes mellitus. *Metabolism* **2012**, *61*, 1197–1200. [CrossRef]
76. Garcia-Casares, N.; Garcia-Arnes, J.A.; Rioja, J.; Ariza, M.J.; Gutierrez, A.; Alfaro, F.; Nabrozidis, A.; Gonzalez-Alegre, P.; Gonzalez-Santos, P. Alzheimer's like brain changes correlate with low adiponectin plasma levels in type 2 diabetic patients. *J. Diabetes Complicat.* **2016**, *30*, 281–286. [CrossRef]
77. Xu, Z.P.; Gan, G.S.; Liu, Y.M.; Xiao, J.S.; Liu, H.X.; Mei, B.; Zhang, J.J. adiponectin attenuates streptozotocin-induced tau hyperphosphorylation and cognitive deficits by rescuing PI3K/Akt/GSK-3beta pathway. *Neurochem. Res.* **2018**, *43*, 316–323. [CrossRef]
78. Butterfield, D.A.; Halliwell, B. Oxidative stress, dysfunctional glucose metabolism and Alzheimer disease. *Nat. Rev. Neurosci.* **2019**, *20*, 148–160. [CrossRef]
79. Cunnane, S.; Nugent, S.; Roy, M.; Courchesne-Loyer, A.; Croteau, E.; Tremblay, S.; Castellano, A.; Pifferi, F.; Bocti, C.; Paquet, N.; et al. Brain fuel metabolism, aging, and Alzheimer's disease. *Nutrition* **2011**, *27*, 3–20. [CrossRef]
80. Jack, C.R., Jr.; Knopman, D.S.; Jagust, W.J.; Shaw, L.M.; Aisen, P.S.; Weiner, M.W.; Petersen, R.C.; Trojanowski, J.Q. Hypothetical model of dynamic biomarkers of the Alzheimer's pathological cascade. *Lancet Neurol.* **2010**, *9*, 119–128. [CrossRef]
81. Small, G.W.; Mazziotta, J.C.; Collins, M.T.; Baxter, L.R.; Phelps, M.E.; Mandelkern, M.A.; Kaplan, A.; La Rue, A.; Adamson, C.F.; Chang, L.; et al. Apolipoprotein E type 4 allele and cerebral glucose metabolism in relatives at risk for familial Alzheimer disease. *JAMA* **1995**, *273*, 942–947. [CrossRef]
82. Cisternas, P.; Martinez, M.; Ahima, R.S.; William Wong, G.; Inestrosa, N.C. Modulation of Glucose Metabolism in Hippocampal Neurons by Adiponectin and Resistin. *Mol. Neurobiol.* **2019**, *56*, 3024–3037. [CrossRef]
83. Dienel, G.A.; Cruz, N.F. Nutrition during brain activation: Does cell-to-cell lactate shuttling contribute significantly to sweet and sour food for thought? *Neurochem. Int.* **2004**, *45*, 321–351. [CrossRef]
84. Dienel, G.A.; Hertz, L. Glucose and lactate metabolism during brain activation. *J. Neurosci. Res.* **2001**, *66*, 824–838. [CrossRef] [PubMed]
85. Dhopeshwarkar, G.A.; Mead, J.F. Fatty acid uptake by the brain. 3. Incorporation of (1-14C)oleic acid into the adult rat brain. *Biochim. Biophys. Acta* **1970**, *210*, 250–256. [CrossRef]
86. Panov, A.; Orynbayeva, Z.; Vavilin, V.; Lyakhovich, V. Fatty acids in energy metabolism of the central nervous system. *Biomed. Res. Int.* **2014**, *2014*, 472459. [CrossRef] [PubMed]
87. Schonfeld, P.; Reiser, G. Why does brain metabolism not favor burning of fatty acids to provide energy? Reflections on disadvantages of the use of free fatty acids as fuel for brain. *J. Cereb. Blood Flow. Metab.* **2013**, *33*, 1493–1499. [CrossRef]
88. Se Oliveira, C.; de Mattos, A.B.; Biz, C.; Oyama, L.M.; Ribeiro, E.B.; do Nascimento, C.M. High-fat diet and glucocorticoid treatment cause hyperglycemia associated with adiponectin receptor alterations. *Lipids Health Dis.* **2011**, *10*, 11. [CrossRef]
89. Yanai, H.; Yoshida, H. Beneficial effects of adiponectin on glucose and lipid metabolism and atherosclerotic progression: Mechanisms and perspectives. *Int. J. Mol. Sci.* **2019**, *20*, 1190. [CrossRef]
90. Yamauchi, T.; Kadowaki, T. Adiponectin receptor as a key player in healthy longevity and obesity-related diseases. *Cell Metab.* **2013**, *17*, 185–196. [CrossRef]

91. Elfeky, M.; Kaede, R.; Okamatsu-Ogura, Y.; Kimura, K. Adiponectin inhibits LPS-induced HMGB1 release through an AMP kinase and heme oxygenase-1-dependent pathway in RAW 264 macrophage cells. *Mediators Inflamm.* **2016**, *2016*, 5701959. [CrossRef] [PubMed]
92. Rizzo, F.R.; Musella, A.; de Vito, F.; Fresegna, D.; Bullitta, S.; Vanni, V.; Guadalupi, L.; Stampanoni Bassi, M.; Buttari, F.; Mandolesi, G.; et al. Tumor necrosis factor and interleukin-1beta modulate synaptic plasticity during neuroinflammation. *Neural. Plast.* **2018**, *2018*, 8430123. [CrossRef] [PubMed]
93. Ferreira, S.T.; Clarke, J.R.; Bomfim, T.R.; De Felice, F.G. Inflammation, defective insulin signaling, and neuronal dysfunction in Alzheimer's disease. *Alzheimers Dement.* **2014**, *10*, S76–S83. [CrossRef] [PubMed]
94. Fruhbeck, G.; Catalan, V.; Rodriguez, A.; Ramirez, B.; Becerril, S.; Salvador, J.; Portincasa, P.; Colina, I.; Gomez-Ambrosi, J. Involvement of the leptin-adiponectin axis in inflammation and oxidative stress in the metabolic syndrome. *Sci. Rep.* **2017**, *7*, 6619. [CrossRef] [PubMed]
95. Yokota, T.; Oritani, K.; Takahashi, I.; Ishikawa, J.; Matsuyama, A.; Ouchi, N.; Kihara, S.; Funahashi, T.; Tenner, A.J.; Tomiyama, Y.; et al. Adiponectin, a new member of the family of soluble defense collagens, negatively regulates the growth of myelomonocytic progenitors and the functions of macrophages. *Blood* **2000**, *96*, 1723–1732. [CrossRef]
96. Lourenco, M.V.; Clarke, J.R.; Frozza, R.L.; Bomfim, T.R.; Forny-Germano, L.; Batista, A.F.; Sathler, L.B.; Brito-Moreira, J.; Amaral, O.B.; Silva, C.A.; et al. TNF-alpha mediates PKR-dependent memory impairment and brain IRS-1 inhibition induced by Alzheimer's beta-amyloid oligomers in mice and monkeys. *Cell Metab.* **2013**, *18*, 831–843. [CrossRef] [PubMed]
97. Nicolas, S.; Cazareth, J.; Zarif, H.; Guyon, A.; Heurteaux, C.; Chabry, J.; Petit-Paitel, A. Globular adiponectin limits microglia pro-inflammatory phenotype through an AdipoR1/NF-kappaB signaling pathway. *Front. Cell Neurosci.* **2017**, *11*, 352. [CrossRef]
98. Chabry, J.; Nicolas, S.; Cazareth, J.; Murris, E.; Guyon, A.; Glaichenhaus, N.; Heurteaux, C.; Petit-Paitel, A. Enriched environment decreases microglia and brain macrophages inflammatory phenotypes through adiponectin-dependent mechanisms: Relevance to depressive-like behavior. *Brain Behav. Immun.* **2015**, *50*, 275–287. [CrossRef]
99. Tonnies, E.; Trushina, E. Oxidative stress, synaptic dysfunction, and Alzheimer's disease. *J. Alzheimers Dis.* **2017**, *57*, 1105–1121. [CrossRef]
100. Snyder, B.; Shell, B.; Cunningham, J.T.; Cunningham, R.L. Chronic intermittent hypoxia induces oxidative stress and inflammation in brain regions associated with early-stage neurodegeneration. *Physiol. Rep.* **2017**, *5*. [CrossRef] [PubMed]
101. Chan, K.H.; Lam, K.S.; Cheng, O.Y.; Kwan, J.S.; Ho, P.W.; Cheng, K.K.; Chung, S.K.; Ho, J.W.; Guo, V.Y.; Xu, A. Adiponectin is protective against oxidative stress induced cytotoxicity in amyloid-β neurotoxicity. *PLoS ONE* **2012**, *7*, e52354. [CrossRef] [PubMed]
102. Park, M.; Youn, B.; Zheng, X.L.; Wu, D.; Xu, A.; Sweeney, G. Globular adiponectin, acting via AdipoR1/APPL1, protects H9c2 cells from hypoxia/reoxygenation-induced apoptosis. *PLoS ONE* **2011**, *6*, e19143. [CrossRef] [PubMed]
103. Qiu, G.; Wan, R.; Hu, J.; Mattson, M.P.; Spangler, E.; Liu, S.; Yau, S.Y.; Lee, T.M.; Gleichmann, M.; Ingram, D.K.; et al. Adiponectin protects rat hippocampal neurons against excitotoxicity. *Age* **2011**, *33*, 155–165. [CrossRef] [PubMed]
104. Ramamurthy, S.; Ronnett, G.V. Developing a head for energy sensing: AMP-activated protein kinase as a multifunctional metabolic sensor in the brain. *J. Physiol.* **2006**, *574*, 85–93. [CrossRef]
105. Kubota, N.; Yano, W.; Kubota, T.; Yamauchi, T.; Itoh, S.; Kumagai, H.; Kozono, H.; Takamoto, I.; Okamoto, S.; Shiuchi, T.; et al. Adiponectin stimulates AMP-activated protein kinase in the hypothalamus and increases food intake. *Cell Metab.* **2007**, *6*, 55–68. [CrossRef]
106. Girgis, C.M.; Cheng, K.; Scott, C.H.; Gunton, J.E. Novel links between HIFs, type 2 diabetes, and metabolic syndrome. *Trends Endocrinol. Metab.* **2012**, *23*, 372–380. [CrossRef]
107. Jiang, C.; Kim, J.H.; Li, F.; Qu, A.; Gavrilova, O.; Shah, Y.M.; Gonzalez, F.J. Hypoxia-inducible factor 1α regulates a SOCS3-STAT3-adiponectin signal transduction pathway in adipocytes. *J. Biol. Chem.* **2013**, *288*, 3844–3857. [CrossRef]
108. Bai, H.; Zhao, L.; Liu, H.; Guo, H.; Guo, W.; Zheng, L.; Liu, X.; Wu, X.; Luo, J.; Li, X.; et al. Adiponectin confers neuroprotection against cerebral ischemia-reperfusion injury through activating the cAMP/PKA-CREB-BDNF signaling. *Brain Res. Bull.* **2018**, *143*, 145–154. [CrossRef]

109. Wang, S.; Li, D.; Huang, C.; Wan, Y.; Wang, J.; Zan, X.; Yang, B. Overexpression of adiponectin alleviates intracerebral hemorrhage-induced brain injury in rats via suppression of oxidative stress. *Neurosci. Lett.* **2018**, *681*, 110–116. [CrossRef]
110. Choi, S.H.; Bylykbashi, E.; Chatila, Z.K.; Lee, S.W.; Pulli, B.; Clemenson, G.D.; Kim, E.; Rompala, A.; Oram, M.K.; Asselin, C.; et al. Combined adult neurogenesis and BDNF mimic exercise effects on cognition in an Alzheimer's mouse model. *Science* **2018**, *361*, eaan8821. [CrossRef]
111. Moreno-Jiménez, E.P.; Flor-García, M.; Terreros-Roncal, J.; Rábano, A.; Cafini, F.; Pallas-Bazarra, N.; Ávila, J.; Llorens-Martín, M. Adult hippocampal neurogenesis is abundant in neurologically healthy subjects and drops sharply in patients with Alzheimer's disease. *Nat. Med.* **2019**, *25*, 554–560. [CrossRef] [PubMed]
112. Song, J.; Kang, S.M.; Kim, E.; Kim, C.H.; Song, H.T.; Lee, J.E. Adiponectin receptor-mediated signaling ameliorates cerebral cell damage and regulates the neurogenesis of neural stem cells at high glucose concentrations: An in vivo and in vitro study. *Cell Death Dis.* **2015**, *6*, e1844. [CrossRef] [PubMed]
113. Teixeira, A.L.; Diniz, B.S.; Campos, A.C.; Miranda, A.S.; Rocha, N.P.; Talib, L.L.; Gattaz, W.F.; Forlenza, O.V. Decreased levels of circulating adiponectin in mild cognitive impairment and Alzheimer's disease. *Neuromol. Med.* **2013**, *15*, 115–121. [CrossRef] [PubMed]
114. Kamogawa, K.; Kohara, K.; Tabara, Y.; Uetani, E.; Nagai, T.; Yamamoto, M.; Igase, M.; Miki, T. Abdominal fat, adipose-derived hormones and mild cognitive impairment: The J-SHIPP study. *Dement. Geriatr. Cogn. Disord.* **2010**, *30*, 432–439. [CrossRef]
115. Gorska-Ciebiada, M.; Saryusz-Wolska, M.; Borkowska, A.; Ciebiada, M.; Loba, J. Adiponectin, leptin and IL-1 β in elderly diabetic patients with mild cognitive impairment. *Metab. Brain Dis.* **2016**, *31*, 257–266. [CrossRef]
116. Kitagawa, K.; Miwa, K.; Okazaki, S.; Sakaguchi, M.; Mochizuki, H. Serum high-molecular-weight adiponectin level and incident dementia in patients with vascular risk factors. *Euro. J. Neurol.* **2016**, *23*, 641–647. [CrossRef]
117. Bigalke, B.; Schreitmüller, B.; Sopova, K.; Paul, A.; Stransky, E.; Gawaz, M.; Stellos, K.; Laske, C. Adipocytokines and CD34 progenitor cells in Alzheimer's disease. *PLoS ONE* **2011**, *6*, e20286. [CrossRef]
118. Hardie, D.G. AMP-activated protein kinase: An energy sensor that regulates all aspects of cell function. *Genes Dev.* **2011**, *25*, 1895–1908. [CrossRef]
119. Ruderman, N.B.; Xu, X.J.; Nelson, L.; Cacicedo, J.M.; Saha, A.K.; Lan, F.; Ido, Y. AMPK and SIRT1: A long-standing partnership? *Am. J. Physiol Endocrinol. Metab.* **2010**, *298*, E751–E760. [CrossRef]
120. Badshah, H.; Ali, T.; Kim, M.O. Osmotin attenuates LPS-induced neuroinflammation and memory impairments via the TLR4/NFkappaB signaling pathway. *Sci. Rep.* **2016**, *6*, 24493. [CrossRef]
121. Nicolas, S.; Debayle, D.; Bechade, C.; Maroteaux, L.; Gay, A.S.; Bayer, P.; Heurteaux, C.; Guyon, A.; Chabry, J. Adiporon, an adiponectin receptor agonist acts as an antidepressant and metabolic regulator in a mouse model of depression. *Transl. Psychiatry* **2018**, *8*, 159. [CrossRef] [PubMed]
122. Zhang, D.; Wang, X.; Wang, B.; Garza, J.C.; Fang, X.; Wang, J.; Scherer, P.E.; Brenner, R.; Zhang, W.; Lu, X.Y. Adiponectin regulates contextual fear extinction and intrinsic excitability of dentate gyrus granule neurons through AdipoR2 receptors. *Mol. Psychiatry* **2017**, *22*, 1044–1055. [CrossRef] [PubMed]
123. Liu, B.; Liu, J.; Wang, J.G.; Liu, C.L.; Yan, H.J. AdipoRon improves cognitive dysfunction of Alzheimer's disease and rescues impaired neural stem cell proliferation through AdipoR1/AMPK pathway. *Exp. Neurol.* **2020**, *327*, 113249. [CrossRef]
124. FDA approves memantine drug for treating AD. *Am. J. Alzheimers Dis. Other Demen.* **2003**, *18*, 329–330.
125. Pákáski, M.; Fehér, A.; Juhász, A.; Drótos, G.; Fazekas, O.C.; Kovács, J.; Janka, Z.; Kálmán, J. Serum adipokine levels modified by donepezil treatment in Alzheimer's disease. *J. Alzheimers Dis.* **2014**, *38*, 371–377. [CrossRef]
126. Ali, M.A.; El-Abhar, H.S.; Kamel, M.A.; Attia, A.S. Antidiabetic Effect of Galantamine: Novel Effect for a Known centrally acting drug. *PLoS ONE* **2015**, *10*, e0134648. [CrossRef]
127. Song, X.; Jensen, M.O.; Jogini, V.; Stein, R.A.; Lee, C.H.; McHaourab, H.S.; Shaw, D.E.; Gouaux, E. Mechanism of NMDA receptor channel block by MK-801 and memantine. *Nature* **2018**, *556*, 515–519. [CrossRef]
128. Liu, B.; Liu, J.; Wang, J.; Sun, F.; Jiang, S.; Hu, F.; Wang, D.; Liu, D.; Liu, C.; Yan, H. Adiponectin protects against cerebral ischemic injury through AdipoR1/AMPK pathways. *Front. Pharmacol.* **2019**, *10*, 597. [CrossRef]
129. Yue, L.; Zhao, L.; Liu, H.; Li, X.; Wang, B.; Guo, H.; Gao, L.; Feng, D.; Qu, Y. Adiponectin Protects against Glutamate-Induced Excitotoxicity via Activating SIRT1-Dependent PGC-1alpha Expression in HT22 Hippocampal Neurons. *Oxid. Med. Cell Longev.* **2016**, *2016*, 2957354. [CrossRef]

130. Shah, S.A.; Lee, H.Y.; Bressan, R.A.; Yun, D.J.; Kim, M.O. Novel osmotin attenuates glutamate-induced synaptic dysfunction and neurodegeneration via the JNK/PI3K/Akt pathway in postnatal rat brain. *Cell Death Dis.* **2014**, *5*, e1026. [CrossRef]
131. Tumminia, A.; Vinciguerra, F.; Parisi, M.; Frittitta, L. Type 2 Diabetes mellitus and Alzheimer's disease: Role of insulin signalling and therapeutic implications. *Int. J. Mol. Sci.* **2018**, *19*, 3306. [CrossRef] [PubMed]
132. Li, J.; Xue, Y.M.; Zhu, B.; Pan, Y.H.; Zhang, Y.; Wang, C.; Li, Y. rosiglitazone elicits an adiponectin-mediated insulin-sensitizing action at the adipose tissue-liver axis in otsuka long-evans tokushima fatty rats. *J. Diabetes Res.* **2018**, *2018*, 4627842. [CrossRef] [PubMed]
133. American Diabetes, A. 9. Pharmacologic approaches to glycemic treatment: Standards of medical care in diabetes-2019. *Diabetes Care* **2019**, *42*, S90–S102. [CrossRef] [PubMed]
134. Kickstein, E.; Krauss, S.; Thornhill, P.; Rutschow, D.; Zeller, R.; Sharkey, J.; Williamson, R.; Fuchs, M.; Kohler, A.; Glossmann, H.; et al. Biguanide metformin acts on tau phosphorylation via mTOR/protein phosphatase 2A (PP2A) signaling. *Proc. Natl. Acad. Sci. USA* **2010**, *107*, 21830–21835. [CrossRef]
135. Gupta, A.; Bisht, B.; Dey, C.S. Peripheral insulin-sensitizer drug metformin ameliorates neuronal insulin resistance and Alzheimer's-like changes. *Neuropharmacology* **2011**, *60*, 910–920. [CrossRef]
136. Li, J.; Deng, J.; Sheng, W.; Zuo, Z. Metformin attenuates Alzheimer's disease-like neuropathology in obese, leptin-resistant mice. *Pharmacol. Biochem. Behav.* **2012**, *101*, 564–574. [CrossRef]
137. Luchsinger, J.A.; Perez, T.; Chang, H.; Mehta, P.; Steffener, J.; Pradabhan, G.; Ichise, M.; Manly, J.; Devanand, D.P.; Bagiella, E. Metformin in amnestic mild cognitive impairment: Results of a pilot randomized placebo controlled clinical trial. *J. Alzheimer Disease JAD* **2016**, *51*, 501–514. [CrossRef]
138. Hsu, C.C.; Wahlqvist, M.L.; Lee, M.S.; Tsai, H.N. Incidence of dementia is increased in type 2 diabetes and reduced by the use of sulfonylureas and metformin. *J. Alzheimer Disease JAD* **2011**, *24*, 485–493. [CrossRef]
139. Abbas, N.A.T.; El Salem, A. Metformin, sitagliptin, and liraglutide modulate serum retinol-binding protein-4 level and adipocytokine production in type 2 diabetes mellitus rat model. *Can. J. Physiol. Pharmacol.* **2018**, *96*, 1226–1231. [CrossRef]
140. Su, J.R.; Lu, Z.H.; Su, Y.; Zhao, N.; Dong, C.L.; Sun, L.; Zhao, S.F.; Li, Y. relationship of serum adiponectin levels and metformin therapy in patients with type 2 diabetes. *Horm. Metab. Res.* **2016**, *48*, 92–98. [CrossRef]
141. Chiang, M.C.; Cheng, Y.C.; Chen, S.J.; Yen, C.H.; Huang, R.N. Metformin activation of AMPK-dependent pathways is neuroprotective in human neural stem cells against Amyloid-beta-induced mitochondrial dysfunction. *Exp. Cell Res.* **2016**, *347*, 322–331. [CrossRef] [PubMed]
142. Kong, W.; Niu, X.; Zeng, T.; Lu, M.; Chen, L. Impact of treatment with metformin on adipocytokines in patients with polycystic ovary syndrome: A meta-analysis. *PLoS ONE* **2015**, *10*, e0140565. [CrossRef]
143. Chung, M.M.; Chen, Y.L.; Pei, D.; Cheng, Y.C.; Sun, B.; Nicol, C.J.; Yen, C.H.; Chen, H.M.; Liang, Y.J.; Chiang, M.C. The neuroprotective role of metformin in advanced glycation end product treated human neural stem cells is AMPK-dependent. *Biochim. Biophys. Acta* **2015**, *1852*, 720–731. [CrossRef] [PubMed]
144. Saltiel, A.R.; Olefsky, J.M. Thiazolidinediones in the treatment of insulin resistance and type II diabetes. *Diabetes* **1996**, *45*, 1661–1669. [CrossRef]
145. Malinowski, J.M.; Bolesta, S. Rosiglitazone in the treatment of type 2 diabetes mellitus: A critical review. *Clin. Ther.* **2000**, *22*, 1151–1168. [CrossRef]
146. Jojo, G.M.; Kuppusamy, G. Scope of new formulation approaches in the repurposing of pioglitazone for the management of Alzheimer's disease. *J. Clin. Pharm. Ther.* **2019**, *44*, 337–348. [CrossRef] [PubMed]
147. Silva-Abreu, M.; Gonzalez-Pizarro, R.; Espinoza, L.C.; Rodriguez-Lagunas, M.J.; Espina, M.; Garcia, M.L.; Calpena, A.C. Thiazolidinedione as an alternative to facilitate oral administration in geriatric patients with Alzheimer's disease. *Eur. J. Pharm. Sci.* **2019**, *129*, 173–180. [CrossRef]
148. Tsuchida, A.; Yamauchi, T.; Takekawa, S.; Hada, Y.; Ito, Y.; Maki, T.; Kadowaki, T. Peroxisome proliferator-activated receptor (PPAR)alpha activation increases adiponectin receptors and reduces obesity-related inflammation in adipose tissue: Comparison of activation of PPARα, PPARγ, and their combination. *Diabetes* **2005**, *54*, 3358–3370. [CrossRef]
149. Holscher, C. Potential role of glucagon-like peptide-1 (GLP-1) in neuroprotection. *CNS Drugs* **2012**, *26*, 871–882. [CrossRef]
150. Kakimura, J.; Kitamura, Y.; Takata, K.; Umeki, M.; Suzuki, S.; Shibagaki, K.; Taniguchi, T.; Nomura, Y.; Gebicke-Haerter, P.J.; Smith, M.A.; et al. Microglial activation and amyloid-beta clearance induced by exogenous heat-shock proteins. *FASEB J.* **2002**, *16*, 601–603. [CrossRef]

151. Perry, T.; Holloway, H.W.; Weerasuriya, A.; Mouton, P.R.; Duffy, K.; Mattison, J.A.; Greig, N.H. Evidence of GLP-1-mediated neuroprotection in an animal model of pyridoxine-induced peripheral sensory neuropathy. *Exp. Neurol.* **2007**, *203*, 293–301. [CrossRef]
152. Baggio, L.L.; Drucker, D.J. Glucagon-like peptide-1 receptors in the brain: Controlling food intake and body weight. *J. Clin. Investig.* **2014**, *124*, 4223–4226. [CrossRef]
153. During, M.J.; Cao, L.; Zuzga, D.S.; Francis, J.S.; Fitzsimons, H.L.; Jiao, X.; Bland, R.J.; Klugmann, M.; Banks, W.A.; Drucker, D.J.; et al. Glucagon-like peptide-1 receptor is involved in learning and neuroprotection. *Nat. Med.* **2003**, *9*, 1173–1179. [CrossRef]
154. Hamilton, A.; Holscher, C. Receptors for the incretin glucagon-like peptide-1 are expressed on neurons in the central nervous system. *Neuroreport* **2009**, *20*, 1161–1166. [CrossRef]
155. Wang, A.; Li, T.; An, P.; Yan, W.; Zheng, H.; Wang, B.; Mu, Y. Exendin-4 upregulates adiponectin level in adipocytes via Sirt1/Foxo-1 signaling pathway. *PLoS ONE* **2017**, *12*, e0169469. [CrossRef] [PubMed]
156. Ryan, D.; Acosta, A. GLP-1 receptor agonists: Nonglycemic clinical effects in weight loss and beyond. *Obesity* **2015**, *23*, 1119–1129. [CrossRef]
157. Gault, V.A.; Holscher, C. GLP-1 agonists facilitate hippocampal LTP and reverse the impairment of LTP induced by beta-amyloid. *Eur. J. Pharmacol.* **2008**, *587*, 112–117. [CrossRef]
158. Han, W.N.; Holscher, C.; Yuan, L.; Yang, W.; Wang, X.H.; Wu, M.N.; Qi, J.S. Liraglutide protects against amyloid-beta protein-induced impairment of spatial learning and memory in rats. *Neurobiol. Aging.* **2013**, *34*, 576–588. [CrossRef]
159. Batista, A.F.; Forny-Germano, L.; Clarke, J.R.; Lyra, E.S.N.M.; Brito-Moreira, J.; Boehnke, S.E.; Winterborn, A.; Coe, B.C.; Lablans, A.; Vital, J.F.; et al. The diabetes drug liraglutide reverses cognitive impairment in mice and attenuates insulin receptor and synaptic pathology in a non-human primate model of Alzheimer's disease. *J. Pathol.* **2018**, *245*, 85–100. [CrossRef]
160. Wicinski, M.; Socha, M.; Malinowski, B.; Wodkiewicz, E.; Walczak, M.; Gorski, K.; Slupski, M.; Pawlak-Osinska, K. Liraglutide and its neuroprotective properties-focus on possible biochemical mechanisms in Alzheimer's disease and cerebral ischemic events. *Int. J. Mol. Sci.* **2019**, *20*, 1050. [CrossRef]
161. Zhang, Y.; Xie, J.Z.; Xu, X.Y.; Hu, J.; Xu, T.; Jin, S.; Yang, S.J.; Wang, J.Z. Liraglutide ameliorates hyperhomocysteinemia-induced alzheimer-like pathology and memory deficits in rats via multi-molecular targeting. *Neurosci. Bull.* **2019**, *35*, 724–734. [CrossRef] [PubMed]
162. Cahn, A.; Cernea, S.; Raz, I. An update on DPP-4 inhibitors in the management of type 2 diabetes. *Expert Opin. Emerg. Drugs* **2016**, *21*, 409–419. [CrossRef] [PubMed]
163. Chen, S.; Zhou, M.; Sun, J.; Guo, A.; Fernando, R.L.; Chen, Y.; Peng, P.; Zhao, G.; Deng, Y. DPP-4 inhibitor improves learning and memory deficits and AD-like neurodegeneration by modulating the GLP-1 signaling. *Neuropharmacology* **2019**, *157*, 107668. [CrossRef] [PubMed]
164. Sahebkar, A.; Ponzo, V.; Bo, S. Effect of dipeptidyl peptidase-4 inhibitors on plasma adiponectin: A systematic review and meta-analysis of randomized controlled trials. *Curr. Med. Chem.* **2016**, *23*, 1356–1369. [CrossRef]
165. Kosaraju, J.; Holsinger, R.M.D.; Guo, L.; Tam, K.Y. Linagliptin, a dipeptidyl peptidase-4 inhibitor, mitigates cognitive deficits and pathology in the 3xTg-AD mouse model of Alzheimer's disease. *Mol. Neurobiol.* **2017**, *54*, 6074–6084. [CrossRef]
166. Isik, A.T.; Soysal, P.; Yay, A.; Usarel, C. The effects of sitagliptin, a DPP-4 inhibitor, on cognitive functions in elderly diabetic patients with or without Alzheimer's disease. *Diabetes Res. Clin. Pract.* **2017**, *123*, 192–198. [CrossRef]
167. Angelopoulou, E.; Piperi, C. DPP-4 inhibitors: A promising therapeutic approach against Alzheimer's disease. *Ann. Transl. Med.* **2018**, *6*, 255. [CrossRef]
168. Claassen, J.A. New cardiovascular targets to prevent late onset Alzheimer disease. *Eur. J. Pharmacol.* **2015**, *763*, 131–134. [CrossRef]
169. Montecucco, F.; Mach, F. Update on therapeutic strategies to increase adiponectin function and secretion in metabolic syndrome. *Diabetes Obes. Metab.* **2009**, *11*, 445–454. [CrossRef]
170. Mogi, M.; Li, J.M.; Tsukuda, K.; Iwanami, J.; Min, L.J.; Sakata, A.; Fujita, T.; Iwai, M.; Horiuchi, M. Telmisartan prevented cognitive decline partly due to PPAR-gamma activation. *Biochem. Biophys. Res. Commun.* **2008**, *375*, 446–449. [CrossRef]

171. Takeda, S.; Sato, N.; Takeuchi, D.; Kurinami, H.; Shinohara, M.; Niisato, K.; Kano, M.; Ogihara, T.; Rakugi, H.; Morishita, R. Angiotensin receptor blocker prevented beta-amyloid-induced cognitive impairment associated with recovery of neurovascular coupling. *Hypertension* **2009**, *54*, 1345–1352. [CrossRef]
172. Ongali, B.; Nicolakakis, N.; Tong, X.K.; Aboulkassim, T.; Papadopoulos, P.; Rosa-Neto, P.; Lecrux, C.; Imboden, H.; Hamel, E. Angiotensin II type 1 receptor blocker losartan prevents and rescues cerebrovascular, neuropathological and cognitive deficits in an Alzheimer's disease model. *Neurobiol. Dis.* **2014**, *68*, 126–136. [CrossRef]
173. Saavedra, J.M. Evidence to consider angiotensin II receptor blockers for the treatment of early Alzheimer's disease. *Cell Mol. Neurobiol.* **2016**, *36*, 259–279. [CrossRef] [PubMed]
174. Li, W.; Zhang, J.W.; Lu, F.; Ma, M.M.; Wang, J.Q.; Suo, A.Q.; Bai, Y.Y.; Liu, H.Q. Effects of telmisartan on the level of Aβ1-42, interleukin-1β, tumor necrosis factor α and cognition in hypertensive patients with Alzheimer's disease. *Zhonghua Yi Xue Za Zhi* **2012**, *92*, 2743–2746.
175. Hsu, C.Y.; Huang, C.C.; Chan, W.L.; Huang, P.H.; Chiang, C.H.; Chen, T.J.; Chung, C.M.; Lin, S.J.; Chen, J.W.; Leu, H.B. Angiotensin-receptor blockers and risk of Alzheimer's disease in hypertension population-A nationwide cohort study. *Circ. J.* **2013**, *77*, 405–410. [CrossRef]
176. Benicky, J.; Sánchez-Lemus, E.; Pavel, J.; Saavedra, J.M. Anti-inflammatory effects of angiotensin receptor blockers in the brain and the periphery. *Cell Mol. Neurobiol.* **2009**, *29*, 781–792. [CrossRef] [PubMed]
177. Panahpour, H.; Nekooeian, A.A.; Dehghani, G.A. Candesartan attenuates ischemic brain edema and protects the blood-brain barrier integrity from ischemia/reperfusion injury in rats. *Iran. Biomed. J.* **2014**, *18*, 232–238. [CrossRef]
178. So, G.; Nakagawa, S.; Morofuji, Y.; Hiu, T.; Hayashi, K.; Tanaka, K.; Suyama, K.; Deli, M.A.; Nagata, I.; Matsuo, T.; et al. Candesartan improves ischemia-induced impairment of the blood-brain barrier in vitro. *Cell Mol. Neurobiol.* **2015**, *35*, 563–572. [CrossRef]
179. Clasen, R.; Schupp, M.; Foryst-Ludwig, A.; Sprang, C.; Clemenz, M.; Krikov, M.; Thone-Reineke, C.; Unger, T.; Kintscher, U. PPARgamma-activating angiotensin type-1 receptor blockers induce adiponectin. *Hypertension* **2005**, *46*, 137–143. [CrossRef]
180. Zorad, S.; Dou, J.T.; Benicky, J.; Hutanu, D.; Tybitanclova, K.; Zhou, J.; Saavedra, J.M. Long-term angiotensin II AT1 receptor inhibition produces adipose tissue hypotrophy accompanied by increased expression of adiponectin and PPARgamma. *Eur. J. Pharmacol.* **2006**, *552*, 112–122. [CrossRef] [PubMed]
181. Makita, S.; Abiko, A.; Naganuma, Y.; Moriai, Y.; Nakamura, M. Potential effects of angiotensin II receptor blockers on glucose tolerance and adiponectin levels in hypertensive patients. *Cardiovasc. Drugs Ther.* **2007**, *21*, 317–318. [CrossRef] [PubMed]
182. Kohlstedt, K.; Gershome, C.; Trouvain, C.; Hofmann, W.K.; Fichtlscherer, S.; Fleming, I. Angiotensin-converting enzyme (ACE) inhibitors modulate cellular retinol-binding protein 1 and adiponectin expression in adipocytes via the ACE-dependent signaling cascade. *Mol. Pharmacol.* **2009**, *75*, 685–692. [CrossRef] [PubMed]
183. Fontana, V.; de Faria, A.P.C.; Oliveira-Paula, G.H.; Silva, P.S.; Biagi, C.; Tanus-Santos, J.E.; Moreno, H. Effects of angiotensin-converting enzyme inhibition on leptin and adiponectin levels in essential hypertension. *Basic. Clin. Pharmacol. Toxicol.* **2014**, *114*, 472–475. [CrossRef] [PubMed]
184. Hajjar, I.M.; Keown, M.; Lewis, P.; Almor, A. Angiotensin converting enzyme inhibitors and cognitive and functional decline in patients with Alzheimer's disease: An observational study. *Am. J. Alzheimer Dis. Other Dement.* **2008**, *23*, 77–83. [CrossRef]
185. Soto, M.E.; van Kan, G.A.; Nourhashemi, F.; Gillette-Guyonnet, S.; Cesari, M.; Cantet, C.; Rolland, Y.; Vellas, B. Angiotensin-converting enzyme inhibitors and Alzheimer's disease progression in older adults: Results from the Réseau sur la Maladie d'Alzheimer Français cohort. *J. Am. Geriatr. Soc.* **2013**, *61*, 1482–1488. [CrossRef]
186. De Oliveira, F.F.; Chen, E.S.; Smith, M.C.; Bertolucci, P.H.F. Pharmacogenetics of angiotensin-converting enzyme inhibitors in patients with Alzheimer's disease dementia. *Curr. Alzheimer Res.* **2018**, *15*, 386–398. [CrossRef]
187. Zhuang, S.; Wang, X.; Wang, H.F.; Li, J.; Wang, H.Y.; Zhang, H.Z.; Xing, C.M. Angiotensin converting enzyme serum activities: Relationship with Alzheimer's disease. *Brain Res.* **2016**, *1650*, 196–202. [CrossRef]
188. AbdAlla, S.; El Hakim, A.; Abdelbaset, A.; Elfaramawy, Y.; Quitterer, U. Inhibition of ACE Retards Tau hyperphosphorylation and signs of neuronal degeneration in aged rats subjected to chronic mild stress. *Biomed. Res. Int.* **2015**, *2015*, 917156. [CrossRef]

189. AbdAlla, S.; Langer, A.; Fu, X.; Quitterer, U. ACE inhibition with captopril retards the development of signs of neurodegeneration in an animal model of Alzheimer's disease. *Int. J. Mol. Sci.* **2013**, *14*, 16917–16942. [CrossRef]

190. Dong, Y.F.; Kataoka, K.; Tokutomi, Y.; Nako, H.; Nakamura, T.; Toyama, K.; Sueta, D.; Koibuchi, N.; Yamamoto, E.; Ogawa, H.; et al. Perindopril, a centrally active angiotensin-converting enzyme inhibitor, prevents cognitive impairment in mouse models of Alzheimer's disease. *FASEB J.* **2011**, *25*, 2911–2920. [CrossRef]

191. Zhuang, S.; Wang, H.F.; Wang, X.; Li, J.; Xing, C.M. The association of renin-angiotensin system blockade use with the risks of cognitive impairment of aging and Alzheimer's disease: A meta-analysis. *J. Clin. Neurosci.* **2016**, *33*, 32–38. [CrossRef]

192. Bernstein, K.E.; Koronyo, Y.; Salumbides, B.C.; Sheyn, J.; Pelissier, L.; Lopes, D.H.J.; Shah, K.H.; Bernstein, E.A.; Fuchs, D.T.; Yu, J.J.Y.; et al. Angiotensin-converting enzyme overexpression in myelomonocytes prevents Alzheimer's-like cognitive decline. *J. Clin. Investig.* **2014**, *124*, 1000–1012. [CrossRef] [PubMed]

193. Liu, S.; Liu, J.; Miura, Y.; Tanabe, C.; Maeda, T.; Terayama, Y.; Turner, A.J.; Zou, K.; Komano, H. Conversion of Aβ43 to Aβ40 by the successive action of angiotensin-converting enzyme 2 and angiotensin-converting enzyme. *J. Neurosci. Res.* **2014**, *92*, 1178–1186. [CrossRef] [PubMed]

194. Zou, K.; Yamaguchi, H.; Akatsu, H.; Sakamoto, T.; Ko, M.; Mizoguchi, K.; Gong, J.-S.; Yu, W.; Yamamoto, T.; Kosaka, K.; et al. Angiotensin-converting enzyme converts amyloid beta-protein 1-42 (Abeta(1-42)) to Abeta(1-40), and its inhibition enhances brain Abeta deposition. *J. Neurosci.* **2007**, *27*, 8628–8635. [CrossRef] [PubMed]

195. Okopien, B.; Buldak, L.; Boldys, A. Fibrates in the management of atherogenic dyslipidemia. *Expert Rev. Cardiovasc. Ther.* **2017**, *15*, 913–921. [CrossRef] [PubMed]

196. Sahebkar, A.; Watts, G.F. Fibrate therapy and circulating adiponectin concentrations: A systematic review and meta-analysis of randomized placebo-controlled trials. *Atherosclerosis* **2013**, *230*, 110–120. [CrossRef]

197. D'Orio, B.; Fracassi, A.; Ceru, M.P.; Moreno, S. Targeting PPARalpha in Alzheimer's Disease. *Curr. Alzheimer Res.* **2018**, *15*, 345–354. [CrossRef]

198. Kai, T.; Arima, S.; Taniyama, Y.; Nakabou, M.; Kanamasa, K. Comparison of the effect of lipophilic and hydrophilic statins on serum adiponectin levels in patients with mild hypertension and dyslipidemia: Kinki Adiponectin Interventional (KAI) Study. *Clin. Exp. Hypertens* **2008**, *30*, 530–540. [CrossRef]

199. Qu, H.Y.; Xiao, Y.W.; Jiang, G.H.; Wang, Z.Y.; Zhang, Y.; Zhang, M. Effect of atorvastatin versus rosuvastatin on levels of serum lipids, inflammatory markers and adiponectin in patients with hypercholesterolemia. *Pharm. Res.* **2009**, *26*, 958–964. [CrossRef]

200. Tsutamoto, T.; Yamaji, M.; Kawahara, C.; Nishiyama, K.; Fujii, M.; Yamamoto, T.; Horie, M. Effect of simvastatin vs. rosuvastatin on adiponectin and haemoglobin A1c levels in patients with non-ischaemic chronic heart failure. *Eur. J. Heart Fail.* **2009**, *11*, 1195–1201. [CrossRef]

201. Guimaraes, E.S.; Cerda, A.; Dorea, E.L.; Bernik, M.M.S.; Gusukuma, M.C.; Pinto, G.A.; Fajardo, C.M.; Hirata, M.H.; Hirata, R.D.C. Effects of short-term add-on ezetimibe to statin treatment on expression of adipokines and inflammatory markers in diabetic and dyslipidemic patients. *Cardiovasc. Ther.* **2017**, *35*. [CrossRef] [PubMed]

202. Hu, Y.; Tong, G.; Xu, W.; Pan, J.; Ryan, K.; Yang, R.; Shuldiner, A.R.; Gong, D.W.; Zhu, D. Anti-inflammatory effects of simvastatin on adipokines in type 2 diabetic patients with carotid atherosclerosis. *Diab. Vasc. Dis. Res.* **2009**, *6*, 262–268. [CrossRef] [PubMed]

7

Transient Receptor Potential Melastatin 2 (TRPM2) Inhibition by Antioxidant, *N*-Acetyl-L-Cysteine, Reduces Global Cerebral Ischemia-Induced Neuronal Death

Dae Ki Hong [1], A Ra Kho [1], Song Hee Lee [1], Jeong Hyun Jeong [1], Beom Seok Kang [1], Dong Hyeon Kang [2], Min Kyu Park [1], Kyoung-Ha Park [3], Man-Sup Lim [4], Bo Young Choi [1,*] and Sang Won Suh [1,*]

1 Department of Physiology, College of Medicine, Hallym University, Chuncheon 24252, Korea; zxnm01220@gmail.com (D.K.H.); rnlduadkfk136@hallym.ac.kr (A.R.K.); sshlee@hallym.ac.kr (S.H.L.); jd1422@hanmail.net (J.H.J.); ttiger1993@gmail.com (B.S.K.); bagmingyu50@gmail.com (M.K.P.)

2 Department of Medical Science, College of Medicine, Hallym University, Chuncheon 24252, Korea; ehdgus6312@gmail.com

3 Division of Cardiovascular Diseases, Hallym University Medical Center, Anyang 14068, Korea; pkhmd@naver.com

4 Department of Medical Education, College of Medicine, Hallym University, Chuncheon 24252, Korea; ellemes@hallym.ac.kr

* Correspondence: bychoi@hallym.ac.kr (B.Y.C.); swsuh@hallym.ac.kr (S.W.S.)

Abstract: A variety of pathogenic mechanisms, such as cytoplasmic calcium/zinc influx, reactive oxygen species production, and ionic imbalance, have been suggested to play a role in cerebral ischemia induced neurodegeneration. During the ischemic state that occurs after stroke or heart attack, it is observed that vesicular zinc can be released into the synaptic cleft, and then translocated into the cytoplasm via various cation channels. Transient receptor potential melastatin 2 (TRPM2) is highly distributed in the central nervous system and has high sensitivity to oxidative damage. Several previous studies have shown that TRPM2 channel activation contributes to neuroinflammation and neurodegeneration cascades. Therefore, we examined whether anti-oxidant treatment, such as with *N*-acetyl-L-cysteine (NAC), provides neuroprotection via regulation of TRPM2, following global cerebral ischemia (GCI). Experimental animals were then immediately injected with NAC (150 mg/kg/day) for 3 and 7 days, before sacrifice. We demonstrated that NAC administration reduced activation of GCI-induced neuronal death cascades, such as lipid peroxidation, microglia and astroglia activation, free zinc accumulation, and TRPM2 over-activation. Therefore, modulation of the TRPM2 channel can be a potential therapeutic target to prevent ischemia-induced neuronal death.

Keywords: global cerebral ischemia; *N*-acetyl-L-cysteine; transient receptor potential melastatin 2; zinc; neurodegeneration

---

1. Introduction

Recent decades have seen a dramatic increase in the attention and focus on the study of brain disease. In particular, cerebral ischemia is a global problem and is the leading cause of brain disease and morbidity [1,2]. There are many reasons why cerebral ischemia is so widespread, in part due to the diverse number of individual pathologies that converge on the emergence of the ischemic state; the largest risk factor for development of cerebral ischemia is occlusion of blood vessels to the brain.

Upon the occlusion of these blood vessels, cerebral blood flow is considerably reduced to regions of the brain and essential supplies of oxygen, nutrients, glucose, and many other cellular substrates are reduced [3]. Cerebral ischemia is divided into two sub-categories. The first, focal cerebral ischemia, involves transiently or permanently reduced blood flow and nutrient supply to particular brain areas that are directly fed by the occluded vasculature. Damage to the brain after focal ischemia is thus focused on the affected areas and injury occurs locally [4]. Global cerebral ischemia (GCI) is similar to focal cerebral ischemia, although the mechanisms of induction and patterns of damage to specific brain regions are different. This brain injury occurs due to several reasons, but is best described by a sudden and near-complete stop in cerebral blood-flow, such as is seen under cardiac arrest-induced cessation of blood circulation [5].

Once the ischemic insult has occurred, abnormal physiological changes to brain function have already began to occur. Under the ischemic condition, disruption of brain homeostasis is disturbed and cell death mechanisms are initiated. This cerebral injury leads to an alteration in ionic balance within the intra-extracellular space [6], reactive oxygen species (ROS) production [7], microglia [8] and astrocyte [9] activation, zinc accumulation [10], and neuronal cell degeneration [11–13] in the brain. Blockage of blood flow to the brain by ischemic insult causes tissue infarction, dysfunction of ionic balance, and intracellular calcium overload [14]. In a previous study, excessive release of calcium ions from synaptic vesicles after brain ischemia was shown to have deleterious effects on neurons and glia [15]. Overloaded intracellular calcium ions trigger glutamate release, proteolysis, mitochondrial dysfunction, and other deleterious cascades [16]. As discussed above, calcium overload contributes to ischemic injury-induced cell death mechanisms. According to a recent report, the cation zinc has an essential role in brain ischemia, in addition to the calcium ion [17].

Zinc is the most widely distributed metal ion in the central nervous system, and is especially abundant in the hippocampus. Zinc has many important roles in enzymes and transcription factors, and its concentration in neurons and glia is controlled by binding proteins, known as metallothionein, as well as several transporters and channels [17–19]. In addition, zinc regulates neural synaptic transmission, innate and adaptive immunity, signal transduction, and cell proliferation, particularly for DNA synthesis [20,21]. In the pre-synaptic vesicles, chelatable zinc is abundant. It is released into the synaptic cleft, moved into pre-synaptic neurons via several transporters, and subsequently undergoes reuptake from the synaptic cleft under normal physiological conditions [22,23]. Under abnormal physiological conditions, such as neurological disorders, zinc homeostasis is disturbed and dysregulated. In the case of neurological disorders, vesicular zinc is excessively released and largely accumulates within post-synaptic neurons. In addition to releasing zinc from synaptic vesicles, zinc that is loosely bound by proteins can be divided into the categories of chelatable free zinc and proteins [12,24,25]. Pathological zinc accumulation can influence cellular dysfunction in several ways. In a previous study, it was demonstrated that zinc-treated cultured neurons produce ROS from their mitochondria [18] and trigger microglial activation [26]. In addition, previous studies by our group have observed that excessive zinc accumulation within brain hippocampal regions can lead to neurodegeneration after cerebral insult, such as ischemia [10,27], head trauma [25], hypoglycemia [28], and cultured neurons [29].

N-acetyl-L-cysteine (NAC), which contains an acetylated cysteine residue, acts as a powerful antioxidant by supplementation of cysteine and promotion of glutathione biosynthesis [30,31]. Injury-induced oxidative damage plays a primary role in central nervous system dysfunction and contributes to neurodegenerative cascades [32,33]. To protect against brain injury-induced oxidative damage, our group has previously used NAC to treat hypoglycemia and traumatic brain injury. NAC stabilized glutathione concentrations, reduced degenerating neurons, and decreased oxidative damage within hippocampal regions [24,34]. Hippocampal neurodegeneration can be prevented or reduced when oxidative damage and other deleterious cascades are prevented by regulating physiologic concentrations of glutathione via providing ample cysteine, which is supplied from NAC [35]. Moreover, NAC has binding sites for trace metals that include copper, magnesium, and zinc. These studies demonstrate that NAC can neutralize toxically accumulated trace metals occurring in neuropathies [24,36].

Transient receptor potential melastatin 2 (TRPM2) is one of the non-selective cationic channels, and the activity of this channel is triggered by ROS production promoted by deleterious cell death mechanisms in several neurological disorders. Recently, the TRPM2 channel has been reported to be included in both physiological and pathological conditions [37,38]. Several previous studies have shown that the TRPM2 channel is expressed in the central nervous system (CNS), which is largely expressed within the hippocampus, stratum, and cortex [39]. These studies found that several divalent cations, for example, calcium and magnesium, moved into the intracellular space via TRPM2, and that its activity was regulated by external stimuli such as ROS, hydrogen peroxide, and tumor necrosis factor-α (TNF-α) [40–42]. In addition, TRPM2 is distributed in both neurons and glia, and is involved in pathophysiological conditions of nitric oxide (NO) and ROS production signaling [38,43]. Following several neurological injuries, excessive calcium influx via TRPM2 can trigger release of diverse cytokines and thus contributes to the inflammatory response [44]. Several brain diseases, such as stroke or head trauma, lead to excitotoxicity, which is caused by the inappropriate activation of voltage-dependent calcium channels and excitatory amino acid release from the dendritic and presynaptic space into the extracellular cleft. Previous studies verified that in a rodent disease model of ischemia, TRPM2 mRNA levels were significantly increased. Interestingly, a recent study demonstrated that TRPM2 deficiency in mice decreased cytosolic zinc concentrations and reduced zinc influx from the extracellular space [45]. These findings suggest that, during several brain diseases, TRPM2 is activated and this contributes to cell death mechanisms [44,46].

In the present study, we tested the hypothesis that if ischemia-induced oxidative damage leads to TRPM2 activation, inhibition of this channel may have therapeutic effects through blockade of zinc influx-induced cell damage, which is supported by evidence that NAC administration decreased brain damage in several other neurological diseases [24,34]. Following this logic, we hypothesized that if the TRPM2 level was increased by global cerebral ischemia-induced cell death cascades, regulation of TRPM2 as a potential target for preventing ischemia-induced injury could ameliorate a diverse number of cerebral pathologies associated with ischemia. In addition, we speculated that the zinc ion is closely related to TRPM2 and is excessively moved into the intracellular space via this channel. To test our hypothesis, we used a GCI brain disease model in adult rats and conducted several types of histological evaluations and behavioral assessments.

2. Results

2.1. *Global Cerebral Ischemia-Induced Neuronal Death and Zinc Accumulation Is Attenuated by Post-Administration of NAC*

Timeline showing the experimental design for 3 days and 7 days (Figure 1A). Whole GCI conducted experimental animals were monitored for arterial blood pressure and electroencephalography continuously during the before-isoelectric, isoelectric, and after-blood reperfusion condition (Figure 1B–D).

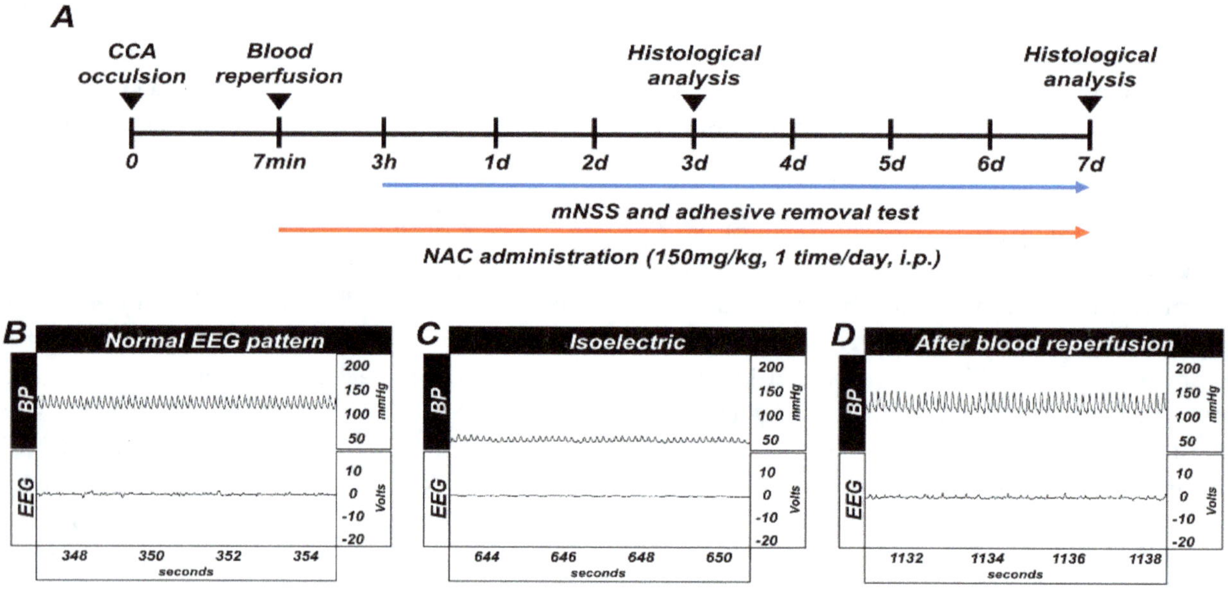

Figure 1. (**A**) Timeline representing the experimental design for 3 and 7 days following global cerebral ischemia (GCI). Experimental animals were given vehicle and *N*-acetyl-L-cysteine (NAC) (dosage: 150 mg/kg) once per day for 3 and 7 days. During the 7 days of the experiment, animals were subjected to behavioral outcome assessment by adhesive removal test and modified neurological severity score measurement. Global cerebral ischemia (GCI) induces electroencephalograph (EEG) and blood pressure changes, and timeline of experiment. (**B**) Normal blood pressure, resting EEG pattern. (**C**) Blood pressure decreased up to 40 (diastolic)–50 (systolic) mmHg, and EEG displayed isoelectric pattern. (**D**) Blood pressure and EEG pattern completely normalized after blood reperfusion.

To determine whether GCI-induced neuronal death and zinc accumulation was attenuated by NAC post-administration, we used FJB (Fluoro-Jade B) and TSQ (*N*-(6-methoxy-8-quinolyl)-para-toluenesulfonamide staining at 3 days after GCI. The degenerating neurons were strongly present in the GCI–vehicle groups. When compared with vehicle-treated groups, NAC-treated groups showed significantly reduced numbers of degenerating neurons (Figure 2A). Quantified numbers of degenerating neurons are displayed using bar graphs (vehicle: subiculum, 168.48 ± 19.63; CA1, 140.03 ± 16.81; CA2, 132.75 ± 14.96; NAC: subiculum, 52.17 ± 20.09; CA1, 54.97 ± 19.74; CA2, 54.98 ± 19.24; Figure 2B). Consequently, GCI-induced zinc accumulation in post-synaptic neurons was observed in vehicle-treated groups. However, NAC administration after GCI reduced zinc accumulation in hippocampal areas (Figure 2C). Representative bar graph shows number of quantified TSQ-positive cells in both GCI–vehicle and GCI–NAC groups (vehicle: subiculum, 84.6 ± 4.29; CA1, 76.28 ± 5.32; CA2, 76.53 ± 3.18; NAC: subiculum, 37.66 ± 2.18; CA1, 32.63 ± 10.52; CA2, 27.77 ± 4.77; Figure 2D).

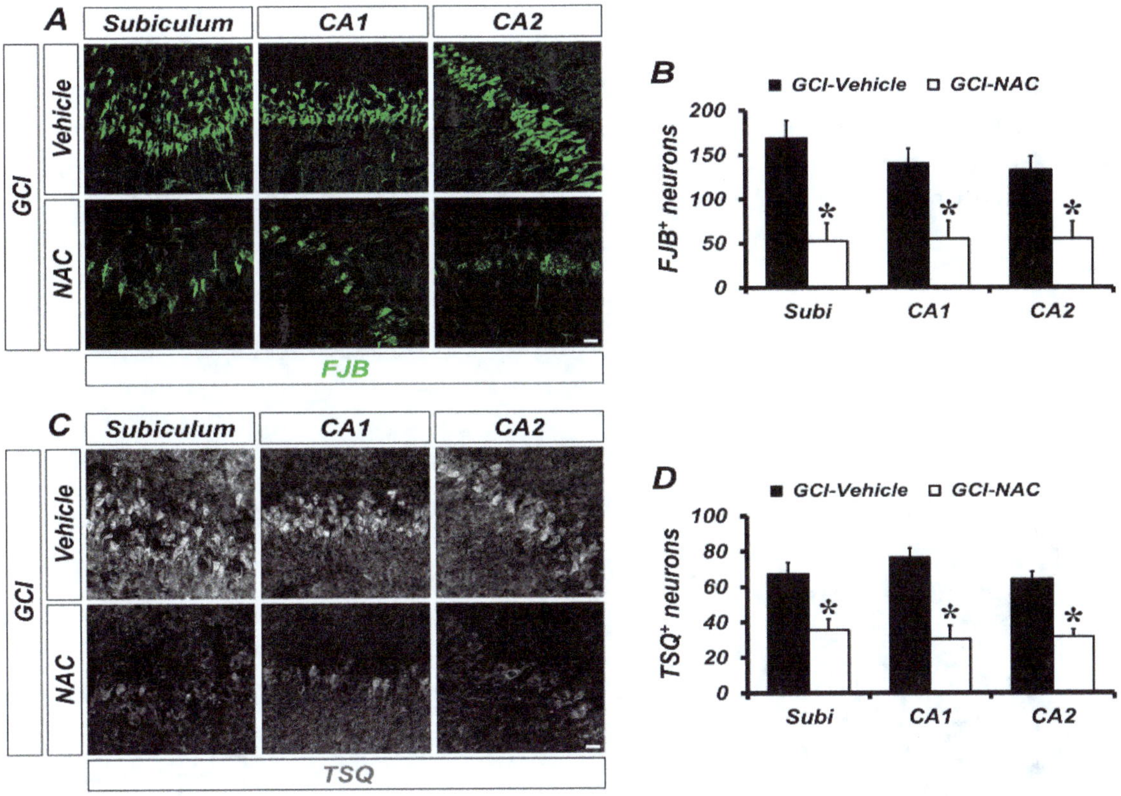

Figure 2. Number of GCI-induced degenerating neurons and zinc accumulation was attenuated by NAC treatment. (**A**) Brain sections were stained with fluorescence dye for detection of degenerating neurons, Fluoro-Jade B (FJB, green signal) in the hippocampal subiculum, cornus ammonis (CA) 1 and CA2 regions. Brain tissues that suffered GCI condition have numerous degenerating neurons in hippocampal regions and administration of NAC reduces the number of FJB-positive neurons in the same regions. Scale bar = 20 µm. (**B**) Quantification of FJB-positive neurons counted in each hippocampal region. Data are mean ± standard error of mean (SEM), $n = 6$ each group, * $p < 0.05$ versus vehicle-treated group (Mann–Whitney U test, Subiculum: z = 2.562, $p = 0.010$; CA1: z = 2.402, $p = 0.016$; CA2: z = 2.082, $p = 0.037$). (**C**) Fluorescence microscopic images of free zinc stained by *N*-(6-methoxy-8-quinolyl)-para-toluenesulfonamide (TSQ) staining. Bright blue fluorescence signal means ischemic condition-induced excessive zinc release and translocation into hippocampal neurons. The NAC-administered group had a remarkably reduced number of TSQ-positive neurons. Scale bar = 20 µm. (**D**) Quantification of TSQ fluorescence signal-positive neurons counted from the hippocampus. Data are mean ± SEM, $n = 4$–5 each group, * $p < 0.05$ versus vehicle-treated group (Mann–Whitney U test, Subiculum: z = 2.205, $p = 0.027$; CA1: z = 2.449, $p = 0.014$; CA2: z = 2.449, $p = 0.014$).

2.2. NAC Post-Treatment Regulates Global Cerebral Ischemia-Induced Loss of Neuronal Glutathione and Lipid Peroxidation

One strategy to solve the problem of ischemic injury is to focus on reducing oxidative damage. We speculated that post-administration of NAC can supply cysteine to produce the powerful anti-oxidant glutathione and influence neuronal oxidative damage. Representative images show glutathione (GS-NEM) levels (Figure 3A). Sham groups show a wide distribution of glutathione within neurons, but the GCI–vehicle group shows a loss of glutathione after injury, particularly oxidative damage. NAC treatment after GCI elevates glutathione concentration in damaged neurons. Based on the above results, we confirmed whether NAC administration directly protects against ROS-induced neuronal oxidative damage by enhancing glutathione levels. ROS triggers lipid peroxidation, and 4-hydroxy-2-nonenal (4-HNE) is a histological marker for lipid peroxidation. GCI led to an increase in ROS, and 4-HNE-positive fluorescence signal was largely increased in the hippocampal subiculum, CA1, and CA2 regions (Figure 3B). Increased lipid peroxidation by GCI-induced ROS production was significantly attenuated following post-treatment of NAC (mean gray value, GCI–vehicle: subiculum, 25.93 ± 2.08; CA1, 28.89 ± 1.69; CA2, 26.36 ± 2.41; GCI–NAC: subiculum, 17.20 ± 0.97; CA1, 16.34 ± 0.99; CA2, 16.90 ± 0.31; Figure 3C). Sham groups had no differences in 4-HNE signal (sham–vehicle: subiculum, 11.12 ± 0.37; CA1, 9.76 ± 0.64; CA2, 11.12 ± 0.97; sham NAC: subiculum, 10.10 ± 0.92; CA1, 8.65 ± 0.43; CA2, 10.89 ± 1.21; Figure 3C).

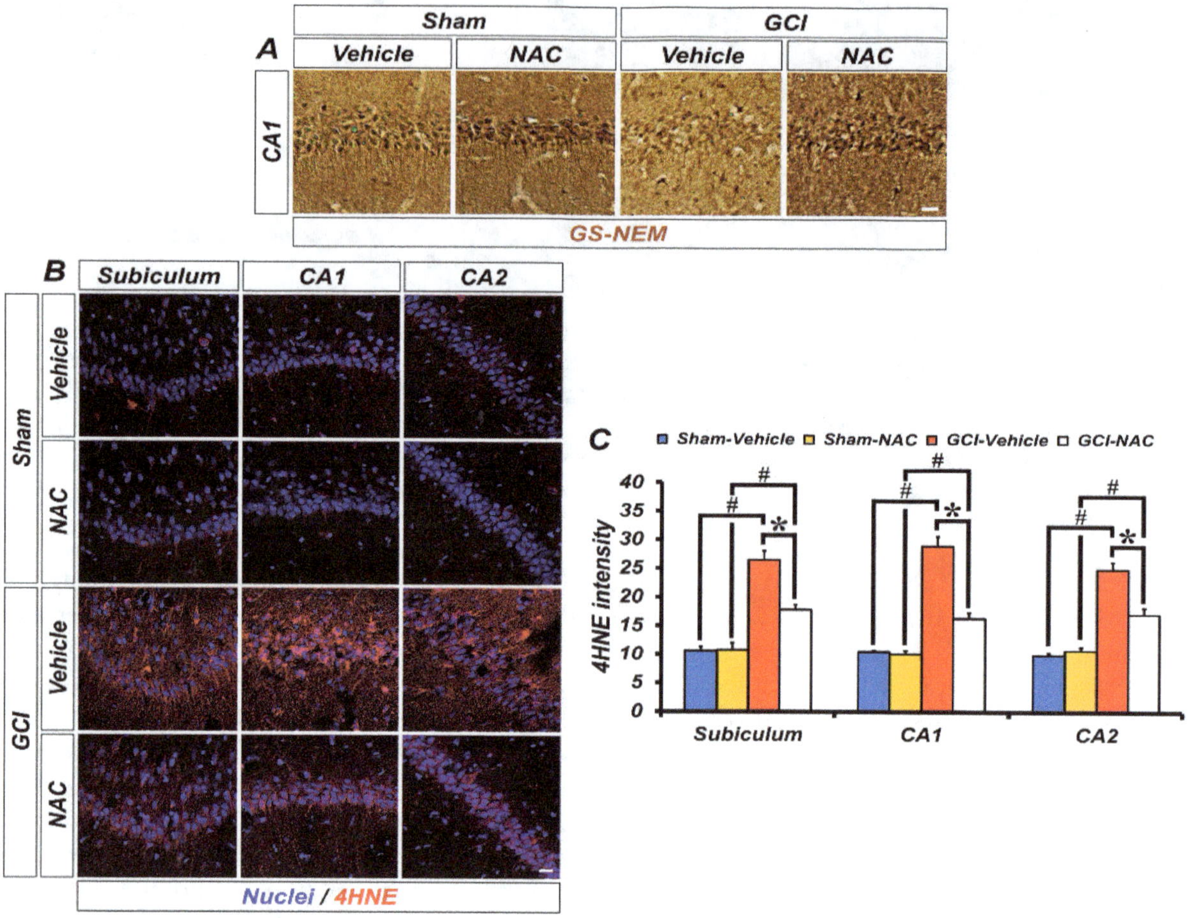

Figure 3. GCI-induced decreasing concentration of glutathione and increasing oxidative damage was restored by anti-oxidant, NAC. (**A**) Representative histological images show concentration of glutathione marker GS-NEM in the hippocampal CA1. Neuronal glutathione level was remarkably reduced after GCI and was restored to normal levels. Scale bar = 20 μm. (**B**) 4-hydroxy-2-nonenal (4-HNE) immunofluorescence staining was used as a marker for lipid peroxidation. Sham–vehicle and NAC groups show minimized 4-HNE-positive signal (red color) in hippocampal regions. It was remarkably increased in the GCI–vehicle group and NAC administration after GCI attenuates oxidative damage-induced lipid peroxidation. Scale bar = 20 μm. (**C**) Bar graph means intensity of 4-HNE signal in the hippocampal regions. Data are mean ± SEM, $n = 4$–7 each group, * $p < 0.05$ versus vehicle-treated group; # $p < 0.05$ versus sham-operated group (Kruskal–Wallis test followed by Bonferroni post-hoc test, Subiculum: chi square = 18.688, df = 3, $p < 0.001$; CA1: chi square = 18.783, df = 3, $p < 0.001$; CA2: chi square = 18.229, df = 3, $p < 0.001$).

2.3. NAC Attenuates TRPM2 Activation in Hippocampal Neurons and Glial Cells

GCI activates TRPM2 channels in the brain, which is localized to glial cells in addition to hippocampal neurons. To demonstrate whether TRPM2 is located within neurons or glial cells in our experimental setting, we conducted immuno-fluorescence staining. Figure 4A shows distribution of TRPM2 channels in the hippocampal pyramidal layer CA1 region, where it was co-localized with neuronal nuclei (NeuN). There was no difference in TRPM2-positive fluorescence signals in sham groups (mean gray value, sham–vehicle: 11.08 ± 0.58; sham NAC: 11.09 ± 0.62; Figure 4B). However, the ischemic condition contributes to activation of TRPM2 in the brain and this is highly localized to the hippocampal pyramidal CA1 layer, which is also known to be especially vulnerable to ischemic injury. The TRPM2-positive signal was dramatically increased in the GCI–vehicle group and significantly decreased in the NAC post-treatment group (GCI–vehicle: 29.55 ± 1.15; GCI–NAC: 18.25 ± 1.76, Figure 4B).

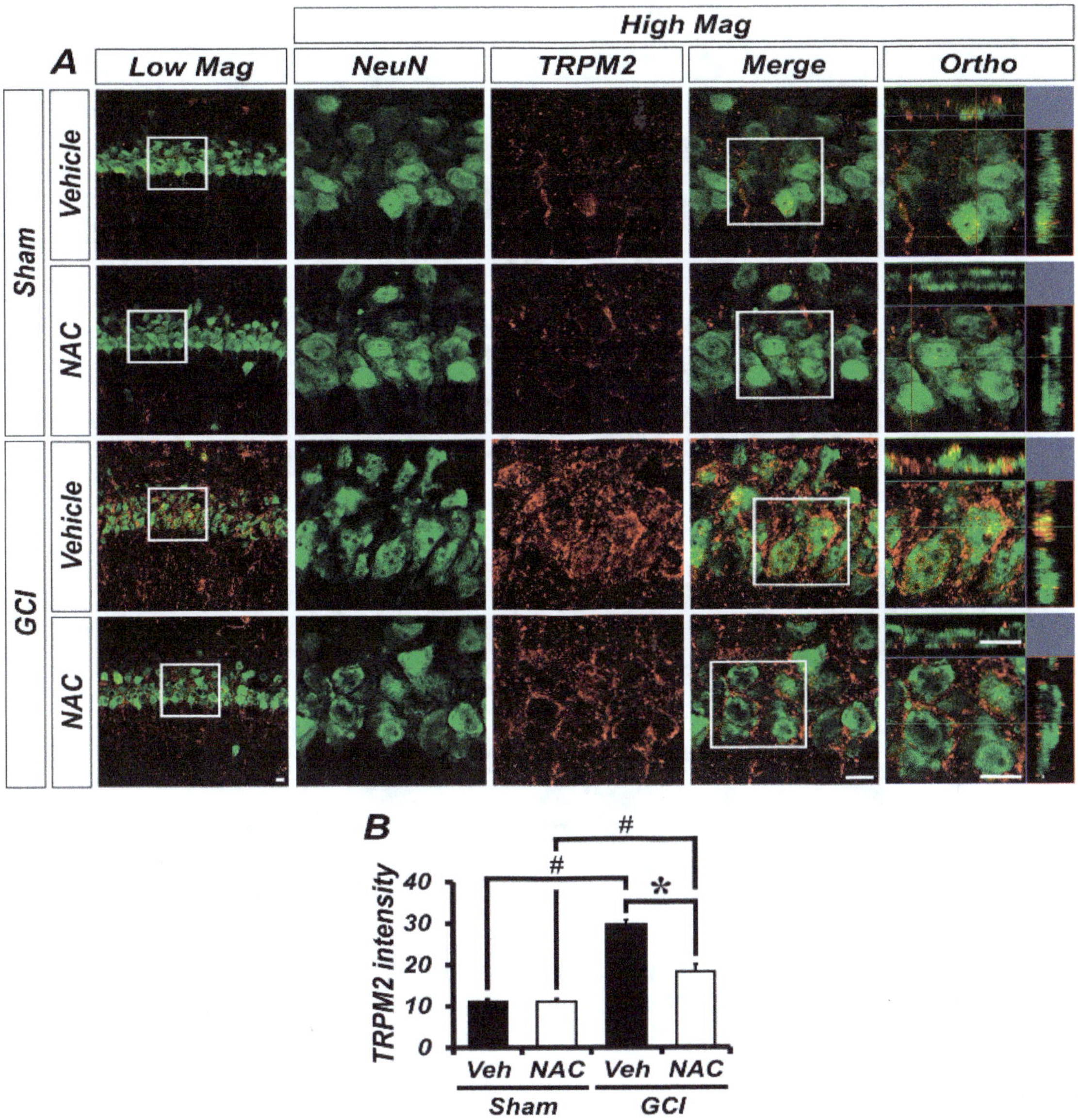

Figure 4. GCI-induced transient receptor potential melastatin 2 (TRPM2) activation was attenuated by NAC treatment. (**A**) Representative histological images of TRPM2-positive signal in the hippocampal CA1. The neuronal TRPM2 level was remarkably increased in the GCI–vehicle group and NAC administration after GCI reduced TRPM2 activation. Scale bar = 20 µm. (**B**) Bar graph shows intensity of TRPM2-positive signal (red color) within the hippocampal pyramidal layer. Data are mean ± SEM, $n = 5$ each group, * $p < 0.05$ versus vehicle-treated group; # $p < 0.05$ versus sham-operated group (Kruskal–Wallis test followed by Bonferroni post-hoc test: chi square = 16.097, df = 3, $p = 0.001$).

To explore the localization of TRPM2 in non-neuronal cells, we conducted glial cell immunostaining. Sham groups showed that Iba-1-positive microglia were distributed throughout the hippocampus in an inactivated state. However, GCI triggers microglial activation, which was significantly decreased by NAC post-treatment (Figure 5A). The bar graph shows quantified microglia intensity (mean gray value, sham–vehicle, 7.59 ± 0.70; sham NAC, 7.82 ± 0.54; GCI–vehicle, 48.35 ± 4.60; GCI–NAC, 23.59 ± 1.01; Figure 5B). Figure 5C shows co-localized TRPM2 with microglia in GCI–vehicle groups. Similarly, astrocytes were distributed throughout the hippocampus, and there were no differences in sham groups. GCI triggers astrocyte activation, which was significantly reduced by NAC post-treatment (Figure 5D). The bar graph shows quantified astrocyte activation (mean gray value, sham–vehicle, 12.52 ± 1.29; sham NAC, 11.88 ± 1.96; GCI–vehicle, 61.46 ± 5.21; GCI–NAC, 36.75 ± 4.58; Figure 5E). Figure 5F shows co-localized TRPM2 with astrocyte in GCI–vehicle groups.

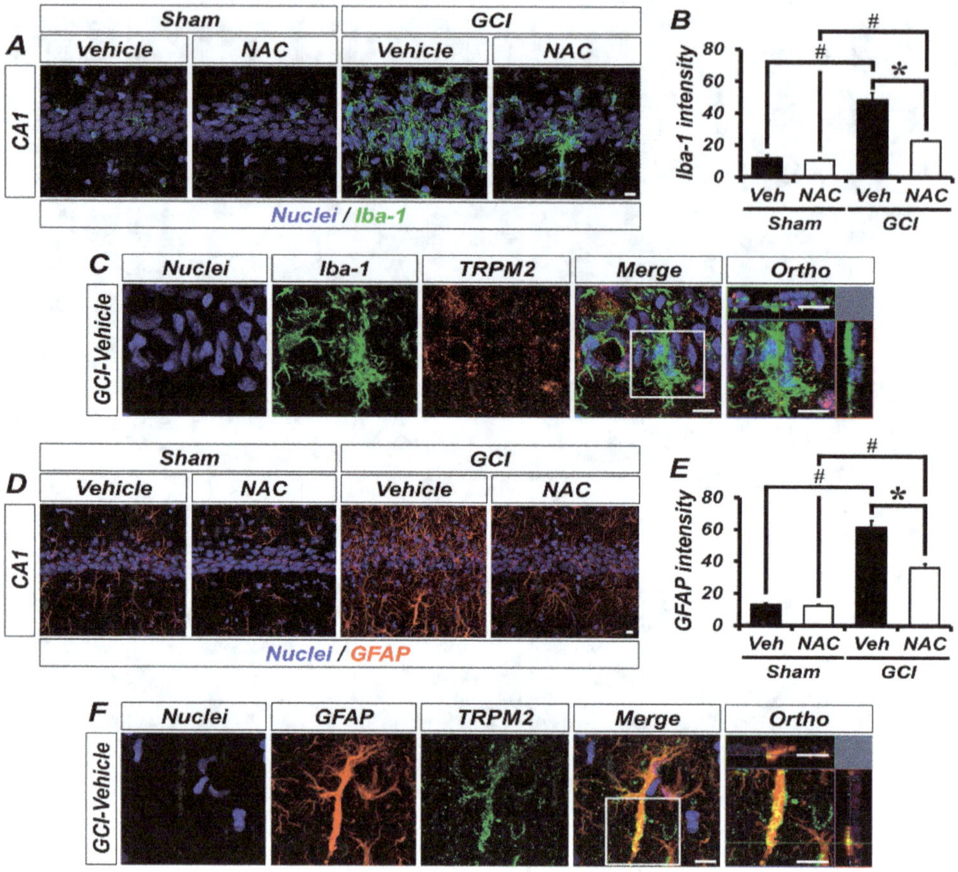

Figure 5. GCI-induced glial cell activation was attenuated by NAC treatment. (**A**) Microglial activation was estimated by Iba-1 immuno-staining. Sham groups (vehicle and NAC) had no difference in Iba-1-positive signal (green color). GCI triggers excessive microglial activation in the hippocampal pyramidal layer, and this was attenuated by NAC administration for 3 days after onset of GCI. Scale bar = 10 μm. (**B**) Bar graph representing intensity of Iba-1-positive signals from hippocampal pyramidal layer administered with vehicle and NAC for 3 days after sham and GCI surgery. Data are mean ± SEM, $n = 5$–7 each group, * $p < 0.05$ versus vehicle-treated group; # $p < 0.05$ versus sham-operated group (Kruskal–Wallis test followed by Bonferroni post-hoc test: chi square = 20.248, df = 3, $p < 0.001$). (**C**) Distribution of TRPM2 in microglial cells (merged image). (**D**) Astrocyte activation was evaluated by GFAP immuno-staining. Sham groups had no difference in GFAP-positive signal (red color). Astrocyte activation was stimulated by GCI, and reduced by NAC administration. Scale bar = 10 μm. (**E**) Bar graph displaying intensity of GFAP-positive signals from the hippocampal pyramidal layer in vehicle and NAC-treated groups after sham and GCI surgery. Data are mean ± SEM, $n = 5$–6 each group, * $p < 0.05$ versus vehicle-treated group; # $p < 0.05$ versus sham-operated group (Kruskal–Wallis test followed by Bonferroni post-hoc test: chi square = 18.747, df = 3, $p < 0.001$). (**F**) Distribution of TRPM2 in astrocyte following GCI (merged image).

2.4. NAC Restores Global Cerebral Ischemia-Induced Sensorimotor Deficit, Neurologic Decline, and Neurodegeneration

To investigate the effects of NAC post-administration on GCI-induced sensorimotor deficit and loss of neurological function, experimental animals were analyzed using the adhesive removal test and modified neurological severity score (mNSS) methods. First, to evaluate sensorimotor deficit after ischemic damage we used the adhesive removal test method. The GCI–vehicle-treated groups spent longer periods of time recognizing adhesive tapes on palms than the GCI–NAC-treated groups after ischemic insult. Sham–vehicle and NAC groups had no difference in removal time during the test days. These results showed that GCI-induced sensorimotor deficit was restored by NAC treatment (Figure 6A). Next, we also assessed whether NAC administration restored GCI-induced neurological decline. Because the sham groups had no impairment, the mNSS count was zero. Following GCI, neurological impairment lead to high scores in the vehicle group and NAC administration attenuated this neurologic decline (Figure 6B). In addition, we determined whether post-administration of NAC provides neuroprotective effects on GCI-induced neurodegeneration following 7 days of consecutive treatment (Figure 6C). Sham groups show numerous neuronal nuclei (NeuN)-positive cells in hippocampal subiculum, CA1, and CA2 regions. There were no significant differences in the number of NeuN-positive cells between the sham–vehicle and NAC group (sham–vehicle: subiculum, 170.5 ± 5.5; CA1, 180.5 ± 5.5; CA2, 210 ± 11, sham-NAC: subiculum, 177 ± 7; CA1, 179 ± 10; CA2, 205 ± 7; Figure 6D). In contrast, the number of NeuN-positive cells was dramatically decreased in the GCI–vehicle group. However, NAC administration significantly restored the number of NeuN-positive cells in the hippocampal regions (GCI–vehicle: subiculum, 79.95 ± 7.69; CA1, 62.74 ± 11.15; CA2, 66.82 ± 4.91, GCI–NAC: subiculum, 110.47 ± 6.42; CA1, 108.12 ± 9.87; CA2, 110.31 ± 7.81; Figure 6D).

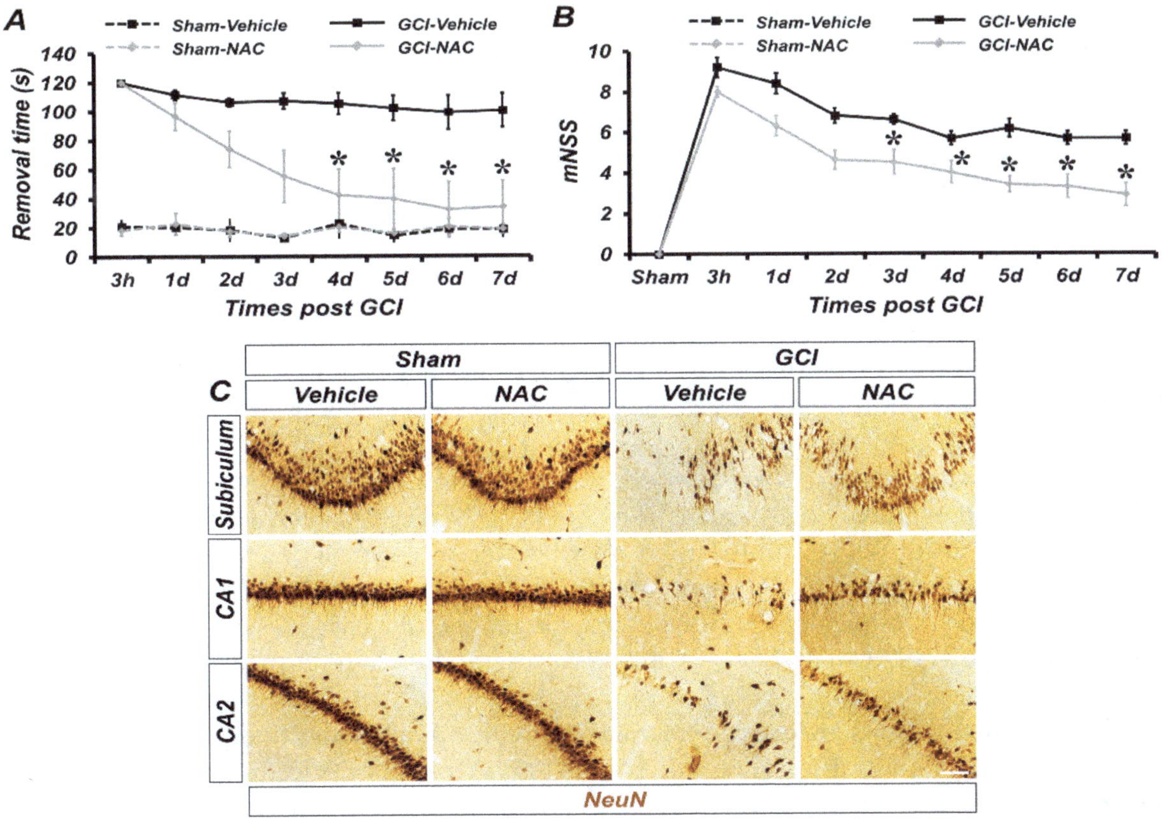

Figure 6. *Cont.*

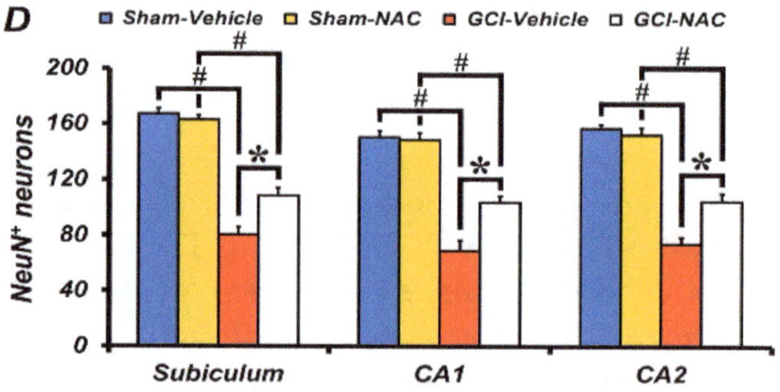

Figure 6. Post administration of NAC reduces GCI-induced behavioral outcome deficits and delays neuronal loss. (**A**) The adhesive removal test to assess sensorimotor deficit was conducted at both 3 h and 7 days after sham and GCI surgery. Sham groups showed no difference in time to remove the adhesive tape during the test. GCI–vehicle group took significantly longer to remove the tape. Post treatment of NAC after GCI reduces removal time (time dependently). Data are mean ± SEM, $n = 5$–8 each group, * $p < 0.05$ versus vehicle-treated group; # $p < 0.05$ versus sham-operated group (repeated measure test followed by ANOVA, time: $F = 6.365$, $p < 0.001$; group: $F = 33.354$, $p < 0.001$; time * group: $F = 3.061$, $p < 0.001$). (**B**) The mNSS was conducted at 3 h and 7 consecutive days after sham and GCI surgery. Sham groups indicate a 0 score which means all tasks were performed completely without defect. Under the ischemic condition, the vehicle group showed a failure of mNSS sessions. Post administration, NAC improved mNSS procedures and reduced failure of tasks. Data are mean ± SEM, $n = 6$–8 each group, * $p < 0.05$ versus the vehicle-treated group (repeated measure test followed by ANOVA, time: $F = 35.621$, $p < 0.001$; group: $F = 17.576$, $p = 0.001$; time * group: $F = 2.322$, $p = 0.032$). (**C**) Immunohistochemistry images show NeuN-positive neurons in the hippocampal subiculum, CA1, and CA2 regions. Scale bar = 50 μm. (**D**) Bar graph shows analysis of NeuN-positive cells in each hippocampal region. Post treatment of NAC restores GCI-induced delayed neuronal loss in the following 7 days. Data are mean ± SEM, $n = 5$–6 each group, * $p < 0.05$ versus vehicle-treated group; # $p < 0.05$ versus sham-operated group (Kruskal–Wallis test followed by Bonferroni post-hoc test, Subiculum: chi square = 17.792, df = 3, $p < 0.001$; CA1: chi square = 17.958, df = 3, $p < 0.001$; CA2: chi square = 17.735, df = 3, $p < 0.001$).

3. Discussion

In the present study, we verified whether NAC administration attenuates GCI-induced neuronal death via inhibition of TRPM2 channels. Our findings indicate that NAC reduces accumulation of intracellular free zinc and TRPM2 over-activation by maintaining a sufficient supply of glutathione production. Cysteine is the rate-limiting substrate required for the biosynthesis of glutathione and the cysteine residue present in NAC can serve as an immediate source of cellular cysteine to maintain high levels of intracellular glutathione, which in turn protects against oxidative damage arising from free radicals. In addition, daily administration of NAC for 3 days after GCI also clearly attenuated several GCI-induced cell death cascades involving neurodegeneration, intracellular free zinc accumulation, oxidative damage-induced lipid peroxidation, loss of glutathione, TRPM2 over-activation, and glial activation. Furthermore, post-treatment of NAC for 7 days prevented GCI-induced delayed hippocampal neuron death, sensorimotor impairment, and neurological deficits. Taken together, these results suggest that reduction of intracellular free zinc and restoration of neuronal GSH concentration by NAC administration attenuates GCI-induced neurodegenerative cascades and promotes behavioral impairments. Therefore, NAC may be an outstanding therapeutic agent for preventing GCI-induced neuronal death.

In general, ionic gradients are actively maintained within finely tuned ranges via several selective and non-selective ion channels throughout the central nervous system, and this process is fundamental to preserving healthy brain function. However, during many neurological injuries that include ischemic stroke [12] and traumatic brain injury [25] damage leads to an ionic imbalance, which in turn allows for the initiation of multiple neurodegenerative cascades. Our previous studies have focused on these mechanisms that follow ionic imbalance in several neurological diseases, such as global ischemia [13,47], hypoglycemia [48], and traumatic brain injury [49]. In particular, we have focused on the abnormal phenomenon of excessive release of vesicular zinc ions following brain injuries and its subsequent cellular pathology. Chelatable zinc that is liberated in this manner moves into post-synaptic neurons through non-selective cation channels, TRPM2 [50], and once chelatable zinc has accumulated within post-synaptic neurons it acts as a neurotoxin [51]. TRPM2 is one of the non-selective cation channels that regulates physiological and pathological processes in the central nervous system via modulation of numerous signaling pathways [38]. In addition, brain disease-induced ROS production triggers TRPM2 activation, leading to calcium influx from the extracellular space, and finally triggers cell death cascades that include PARP-1/PARG and caspase-dependent cell-death pathways [50,52,53]. In this present study, we focused on attenuating the effects of excessively released free zinc ions from synaptic vesicles after GCI that translocate into post-synaptic neurons via the TRPM2 channel. Hence, we hypothesized and verified that by reducing ROS production through supplementation of cysteine by NAC administration to maximize glutathione production, one can reduce hippocampal neurodegeneration through inhibition of zinc accumulation and TRPM2 activation.

N-acetyl-L-cysteine (NAC) is a derivative of cysteine and acts as a scavenger for elimination of free radicals [54]. In the present study, we focused on NAC as a cysteine donor to improve glutathione synthesis, and also as a chelator of heavy metal ions. Excessively released and accumulated free zinc ions after ischemic stroke have a deleterious effect on the nervous system. Previous studies determined that NAC can bind heavy metals (nickel, copper, zinc) because NAC has a thiol group (-SH), which allows it to bind cationic metal ions [55]. In addition, NAC can restore neuronal glutathione concentrations and protect against brain injuries. Kho et al. recently demonstrated that hypoglycemic brain disease-induced hippocampal neurodegeneration, lipid peroxidation, and zinc accumulation were restored to pre-insult levels by NAC administration [24]. Furthermore, Choi et al. recently verified that genetic deletion of the cysteine-related transporter, excitatory amino acid carrier 1 (EAAC1), exacerbates traumatic brain injury (TBI)-induced neurological damage, compared with wild type controls. These cell death cascades were attenuated by NAC treatment in both wild type and EAAC1 gene deletion animals [34]. In light of the abovementioned results, we hypothesized that NAC treatment after GCI may chelate zinc ions, and reduce accumulation of zinc-induced neurotoxicity and downregulation of the TRPM2 channel by reducing ROS production.

The post-global ischemic neuro-inflammatory response contributes to formation of the glial scar and exacerbates neuronal damage. Both microglia and astrocytes play an essential role in maintaining ionic gradients within the extracellular space and in supporting neurotransmission in neighboring neurons. In general, inactivated (resting) microglia and astrocytes regulate the maintenance of central nervous system homeostasis [56]. However, neurodegenerative diseases, such as head trauma, multiple sclerosis, epilepsy and stroke, trigger gliosis which is a non-specific alteration of glial cells and this can lead to glial scar formation if unchecked [57]. Lakhan et al. demonstrated that stroke-induced excitotoxicity and oxidative damage triggers activation of microglia and astrocytes, and these cells secrete several cytokines, chemokines, and matrix metalloproteases [58]. In addition, Kauppinen et al. verified that the zinc-overloaded condition alters the morphology of resting microglia to an activated form in cultured microglia, which was attenuated by treatment with the extracellular zinc chelator, CaEDTA, during the ischemic condition [59]. Barreto et al. reported that astrocyte viability was important for the restoration of neurons following ischemic damage. Furthermore, they asserted that although reactive astrocytes trigger the production of pro-inflammatory cytokines, they also perform functions for maintaining neuronal survival [9].

In the present study, our findings indicate that TRPM2 activation in neurons and glial cells were found after GCI, but were significantly correlated with astrocytes. Astrocytes have a dual nature when activated that can both alleviate or exacerbate the effects of brain damage depending on a sensitive mix of cellular factors. Accordingly, Barreto et al. assert that any solution that adequately addresses the problem of stroke-induced neurodegenerative must involve astrocytes [9]. No details about the interaction of TRPM2 and astrocytes has been reported, but we assumed that there must be some ischemia-related cascades between TRPM2 channels and astrocytes, and began to test this hypothesis. In the case of our research, TRPM2 activation in microglia was only mildly observed compared with astrocytes. However, microglia have a strong influence on CNS diseases, and it is also necessary to consider them for understanding injury-induced neuroinflammation and neurodegeneration in several neurological conditions. Malko et al. reported that calcium influx via TRPM2 after external stimuli triggers microglial activation and generates pro-inflammatory mediators from activated microglial cells, which further exacerbate damage. Furthermore, the TRPM2 activation process was closely related with NADPH oxidase-mediated ROS production, and PARP-1 (poly ADP-ribose polymerase-1) and ADPR (ADP-ribose) activation [60]. As mentioned in the introduction, oxidative damage following ischemic stroke is an essential factor for understanding brain damage, and is closely related with regulation of cation channel activity.

Based on our study and other previous studies, we speculated that a possible neuronal death cascade could be triggered by zinc influx via TRPM2 (Figure 7). In Figure 7A, schematic drawings describe the process of GCI-induced zinc accumulation, ROS production, and TRPM2 activation. Predicted steps of zinc-related neuronal death are as follows. (1) GCI induces vesicular zinc release from the pre-synaptic terminal to the synaptic cleft [10,13], where it translocated into post-synaptic neurons via the non-selective cation channel, TRPM2 [50,61]. In the post-synaptic neurons, translocated zinc contributes several deleterious cascades such as apoptosis [62,63], necrosis [63], as well as ROS-producing signaling. (2) Following ischemia zinc aggravates ROS production via neuronal NADPH oxidase activation [64]. Synaptically released zinc after GCI stimulates protein kinase C (PKC), and PKC contributes NADPH oxidase activation [65]. (3) A major activator of TRPM2 is ADP-ribose (ADPR), which is released upon oxidative stress including ROS [66,67]. (4) ROS-induced TRPM2 activation triggers increased secondary zinc influx [61]. (5) Secondary translocation of zinc promotes increased ROS production [59,68]. (6) Zinc and ROS induce neuronal death. In Figure 7B, the predicted mechanism of NAC on TRPM2 is shown, as follows. (7) GCI induces zinc translocation from the synaptic terminal into neurons through TRPM. Zinc increases ROS production via NADPH oxidase activation. (8) NAC-supplied cysteine enters into post-synaptic neurons through EAAC1. EAAC1 acts as a cysteine carrier in the brain. (9) Cysteine is converted to glutathione, which has an anti-oxidative effect. ROS production is attenuated by glutathione. (10) Reduction of ROS production decreases TRPM2 activation. (11) Reduced TRPM2 induces diminished secondary zinc influx. Zinc influx reduction contributes neuroprotection. (12) NAC administration induced reduced ROS production and diminished zinc influx, which finally attenuates neuronal death. Thus, as discussed above, steps (1)–(6) shown in the Figure 7A have been demonstrated by our and other group's previous studies. However, steps (7)–(12) in the Figure 7B have been verified in this study; it is shown in Figures 2–6 that NAC treatment reduced GCI-induced zinc accumulation, oxidative stress, TRPM2 activation and neuronal death.

Taken together, the present study demonstrates the efficacy of NAC in preventing GCI-induced neuronal death, sensorimotor deficits, and neurological pathology via several signaling cascades. NAC inhibits GCI-induced zinc accumulation and influx via TRPM2 into postsynaptic neurons. Therefore, we speculate that inhibition of zinc influx and TRPM2 activation by NAC may have a potential for the treatment of ischemic stroke.

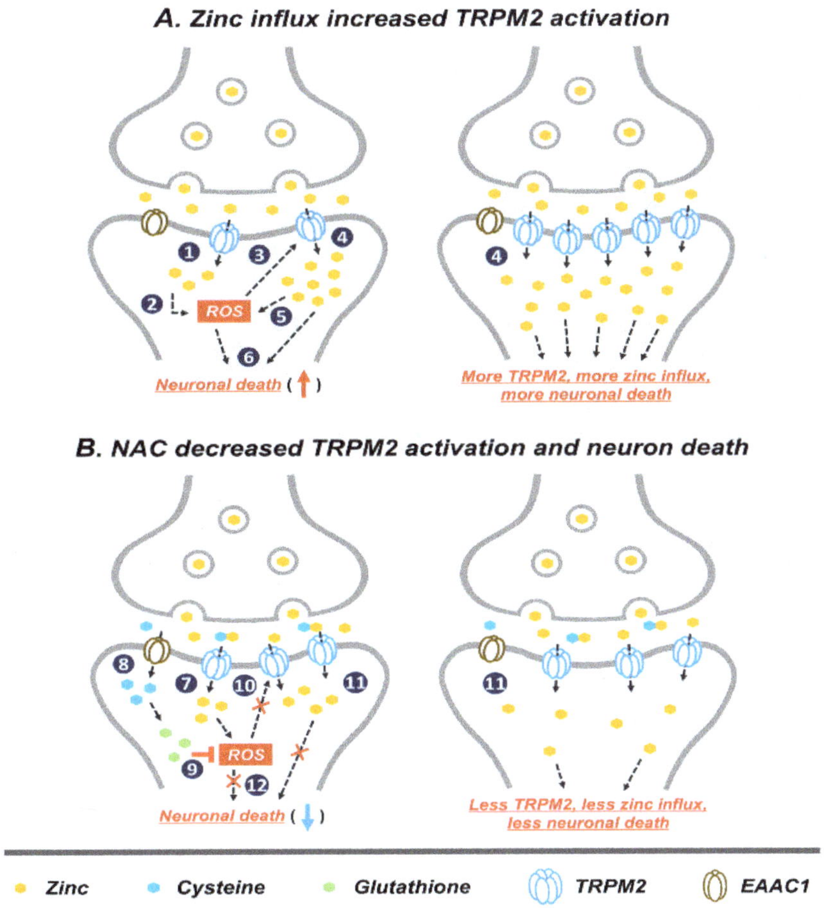

Figure 7. Predicted reactions of NAC post treatment on GCI-induced neuronal death. Representative schematic illustration indicates NAC action via reduction of reactive oxygen species (ROS) production and subsequent decrease in TRPM2 activation. (**A**) (1) Released zinc after GCI moves into the post-synaptic neurons through TRPM2. (2) Translocated zinc contributes to ROS production. (3) Oxidative damage including ROS activated TRPM2. (4) ROS-induced TRPM2 activation increased secondary zinc influx. (5) Increased translocated of zinc contributes to greater ROS production. (6) Zinc and ROS induces neuronal death. (1)–(6) Image shows the hypothesized cascade produced upon GCI-induced zinc influx and TRPM2 activation. (**B**) (7) Zinc translocated into the post-synaptic neurons via TRPM2 after GCI. (8) Cysteine supplied by NAC administration moves into post-synaptic neurons through excitatory amino acid carrier 1 (EAAC1). (9) Cysteine is converted to glutathione which has an anti-oxidant effect and inhibits ROS production. (10) Inhibition of ROS production leads to reduced TRPM2 activation. (11) Reduced TRPM2 activation leads to less secondary zinc influx. (12) Reduction of ROS production and secondary zinc influx reduces neuronal death. (7)–(12) Process shows possible neuroprotective cascade of NAC after GCI.

4. Materials and Methods

4.1. Ethics Statement and Experimental Animals

All animal care protocols and experimental procedures were approved by the Committee on Animal Use for Research at Hallym University (protocol # Hallym 2019-70, 21 February 2020). To test our hypothesis, experimental animal groups were divided as follows: sham (Vehicle, NAC) and GCI (Vehicle, NAC). All rats were housed in a consistently controlled environment (temperature: 22 ± 2 °C, humidity: 55 ± 5%, light regulation: 12-h light/dark cycle) and given water and standard feed by Purina (Gyeonggi-do, Korea) ad libitum. To minimize any suffering of experimental animals, we used 2~3% isoflurane anesthesia during all procedures. Additionally, this manuscript was written in accordance with the standards put forth in ARRIVE (Animals in Research: Reporting In Vivo Experiments) [69].

4.2. *Global Cerebral Ischemia Surgery*

The experimental disease model of global cerebral ischemia was performed as previously described and reported [70]. To explain again in detail, rats were deeply anesthetized with 2~3% isoflurane, which was ventilated using mixed 70% nitrous oxide and 30% oxygen and kept at a body temperature of 37 ± 1 °C using a homeothermic monitoring system (Harvard Apparatus, Holliston, MA, USA). To consistently monitor systemic arterial blood pressure and to remove blood as needed, a catheter filled with 10 units of heparin was inserted into the femoral artery. Then, common carotid arteries located beside the tracheal muscle were carefully isolated and transiently occluded. In this dissecting process, we used a surgical microscope (SZ61, Olympus, Shinjuku, Japan) to enhance surgical accuracy and avoid vagus nerve impairment. At the same time, to monitor the electroencephalograph (EEG), electrodes were placed in two bilateral burr holes. To induce the ischemic condition, we drained blood (8~10 cc) from the femoral artery and set systemic arterial blood pressure within the range of 40 ± 10 mmHg. The isolated bilateral common carotid arteries were occluded with a surgical clamp (Fine Science Tools, Foster city, CA, USA). When the systemic arterial blood pressure range was within 40 ± 10 mmHg and the electroencephalograph reached a sustained isoelectric point, we maintained these conditions for 7 min to induce the global cerebral ischemic condition. After occlusion, blood circulation to the brain was restored by unclamping the device and reperfusing the removed blood. During this period, the systemic arterial blood pressure and EEG signal were consistently monitored and vital signs of the experimental animal were periodically monitored and adjusted as required. Experimental animal groups were immediately administered NAC to the intraperitoneal space following restoration of blood perfusion and normal EEG activity; vehicle groups were given the same volume of 0.9% normal saline.

4.3. *Experimental Procedures and NAC Administration*

Planned experimental procedures were 3 days and 7 days. These time points mean the termination of GCI surgery. In the acute phase (3 days), GCI-induced neurodegenerative cascades were assessed using several immunostaining processes for histological evaluation. In the chronic phase (7 days), GCI-induced cognitive decline and neurological deficits were verified by behavior tests. Vehicle and NAC was administered daily during the acute and chronic phases. To investigate the effects of NAC post-administration to reduce GCI-induced hippocampal neurodegenerations, we used NAC (Sigma-Aldrich, St. Louis, MO, USA). NAC was dissolved with 0.9% normal saline and injected into the intraperitoneal space once per day for 3 days and 7 days at a dose of 150 mg/kg in the present study. Vehicle groups (sham and GCI) were administered the same volumes of 0.9% normal saline only.

4.4. *Sample Preparation*

Three and seven days after global cerebral ischemia, all experimental rats were deeply anesthetized with urethane (1.5 g/kg) dissolved in 0.9% normal saline to obtain brain samples. For removal of whole blood, deeply anesthetized experimental animals were intracardially perfused with 0.9% normal saline followed by 4% paraformaldehyde (PFA) dissolved in phosphate-buffered saline (PBS) for brain sample fixation. Terminated sample fixation occurred during perfusion, and the whole brain sample was obtained and was immersed in 4% PFA for one hour. After post-fixation, samples were moved into 30% sucrose for cryoprotection. Brain samples sank to the bottom of the tube, and the whole brain was coronally sectioned into thicknesses of 30 μm each using a cryostat microtome (CM1850, Leica, Wetzlar, Germany).

4.5. *Assessment of Neuronal Death*

Three or seven days after GCI, we estimated hippocampal neuronal death using Fluoro-Jade B (FJB, Histo-Chem, Jefferson, AR) staining method (as previously described in detail [12]). Approximately nine to ten coronal brain sections (based on 30-μm thickness, 270- to 300-μm intervals) were obtained from 3.00 to 4.68 mm caudal to bregma. These brain sections were mounted on gelatin-coated slides, and photographed using a fluorescence microscope (SZ61, Olympus, Shinjuku, Japan, FITC green fluorescence excitation-emission wavelength: 460–490 nm). To avoid experimenter bias, a blind observer counted the whole number of FJB-positive neurons in the hippocampal subiculum, cornu ammonis 1 (CA1), and CA2 regions. Collected data were used for statistical analysis.

4.6. Zinc Fluorescence Staining

To verify the alteration of intraneuronal free zinc concentrations under normal or ischemic conditions, fresh brain samples were obtained without transcardial perfusion process, immediately frozen, and stored in a freezer at a consistently maintained temperature of −80 °C. These samples were coronally sectioned with 10-μm thickness in cryostat and sectioned samples were stained with *N*-(6-methoxy-8-quinolyl)-para-toluenesulfonamide (TSQ; Molecular Probes, Eugene, OR, USA) [25]. In the present study, the concentration of TSQ solution contained 4.5 μM TSQ, 140 mM sodium barbital, and 140 mM sodium acetate. The TSQ-zinc binding fluorescence signal was verified using an Olympus fluorescence microscope (DAPI blue fluorescence excitation-emission wavelength: ~400 nm).

4.7. Histological Analysis

Before initiation of brain tissue immunostaining, blocking of endogenous peroxidase activity is important. The previously described activity was blocked by 1.2% hydrogen peroxide incubation for 20 min at room temperature. After incubation and washing in 0.01% phosphate buffered saline, sections were incubated with several antibodies to analyze our data. In this study, the antibodies used were as follows: 4HNE (diluted 1:500, Alpha Diagnostic Intl. Inc., San Antonio, TX, USA), GFAP (diluted 1:1000, Abcam, Cambridge, UK), Iba-1 (diluted 1:500, Abcam), TRPM2 (diluted 1:400, Abcam), and NeuN (diluted 1:500, Billerica, Millipore Co., Burlington, MA, USA).

4.8. Behavior Outcome Assessment

1. Adhesive removal test: to test whether NAC restores against GCI-induced sensorimotor deficit, all of the experimental groups were evaluated using the adhesive removal test method for 7 consecutive days after GCI. This behavior test was conducted with reference to previous descriptions [13,71]. To explain again in detail, the overall evaluation process was divided into the following steps. Before initiation, rats were acclimated to the transparent testing box (size: 45 × 35 × 20 cm) for 1 min. After acclimating, two pieces of adhesive tape (1 × 1 cm) were attached to the palm of each forepaw and the experimental animal's behavioral outcome for removal time in the testing box was observed (maximum time: 120 s). Removal time is defined as recognizing and detaching the adhesive tape on the bilateral forepaw. If the adhesive tape was detached by shaking its forepaw or bringing its forepaw to its mouth, time was recorded. This process was conducted for five trials with a minute between each trial. In the case that adhesive tapes could not be detached during the test period, removal time was considered the maximum.
2. Modified neurological severity score: to test whether NAC administration attenuated GCI-induced neurological deficits, we used the modified neurological severity score (mNSS) method [72]. The mNSS includes several evaluations of motor (muscle status, abnormal movement), sensory (visual, tactile, and proprioceptive), balance, and reflex functionality. The mNSS assessment criteria were graded from 0 (normal, no deficits) to 18 (maximum points). To explain in detail, this functional test is based on several criteria that include raising subject by the tail and observing flexion (3 points), walking on the floor (3 points), sensory test (2 points), maintaining balance on a beam (6 points), and absence of reflex/abnormal movements (4 points) [73]. This procedure was conducted consecutively for 7 days after GCI. A higher score means a more severe condition.

4.9. Statistical Analysis

All data analyses were conducted using a blind test to reduce researcher bias. All quantified results in the present study were displayed as the mean value ± standard error of mean (SEM), and statistically significant differences were considered at $p < 0.05$. Behavioral data were analyzed by analysis of variance (ANOVA) using Statistical Package for the Social Sciences (SPSS, Chicago, IL, USA). Comparisons between vehicle and NAC-treated groups were conducted with the Mann–Whitney U test, and other comparisons between 4 groups and the remaining data were analyzed by the Kruskal–Wallis test with post-hoc Bonferroni correction. Non-parametric tests were chosen because of the small sample size and lack of normally distributed data.

Author Contributions: D.K.H. researched the data, and wrote and edited the manuscript; A.R.K., S.H.L., J.H.J., B.S.K., D.H.K. and M.K.P. researched the data; K.-H.P., M.-S.L. reviewed and edited the manuscript. B.Y.C. and S.W.S. contributed to conceptualization and supervision of the study, and editing and writing of the manuscript. All authors read and approved the final manuscript.

References

1. Lo, E.H.; Dalkara, T.; Moskowitz, M.A. Mechanisms, challenges and opportunities in stroke. *Nat. Rev. Neurosci.* **2003**, *4*, 399–415. [CrossRef]
2. Cho, C.H.; Byun, H.R.; Jover-Mengual, T.; Pontarelli, F.; Dejesus, C.; Cho, A.R.; Zukin, R.S.; Hwang, J.Y. Gadd45b Acts as Neuroprotective Effector in Global Ischemia-Induced Neuronal Death. *Int. Neurourol. J.* **2019**, *23*, S11–S21. [CrossRef] [PubMed]
3. Tasca, C.I.; Dal-Cim, T.; Cimarosti, H. In vitro oxygen-glucose deprivation to study ischemic cell death. *Methods Mol. Biol.* **2015**, *1254*, 197–210. [CrossRef] [PubMed]
4. Mehta, S.L.; Pandi, G.; Vemuganti, R. Circular RNA Expression Profiles Alter Significantly in Mouse Brain After Transient Focal Ischemia. *Stroke* **2017**, *48*, 2541–2548. [CrossRef]
5. Zhou, L.; Lin, Q.; Wang, P.; Yao, L.; Leong, K.; Tan, Z.; Huang, Z. Enhanced neuroprotective efficacy of bone marrow mesenchymal stem cells co-overexpressing BDNF and VEGF in a rat model of cardiac arrest-induced global cerebral ischemia. *Cell Death Dis.* **2017**, *8*, e2774. [CrossRef]
6. Hu, H.J.; Song, M. Disrupted Ionic Homeostasis in Ischemic Stroke and New Therapeutic Targets. *J. Stroke Cereb. Dis.* **2017**, *26*, 2706–2719. [CrossRef] [PubMed]
7. Harukuni, I.; Bhardwaj, A. Mechanisms of brain injury after global cerebral ischemia. *Neurol. Clin.* **2006**, *24*, 1–21. [CrossRef]
8. Patel, A.R.; Ritzel, R.; McCullough, L.D.; Liu, F. Microglia and ischemic stroke: A double-edged sword. *Int. J. Physiol. Pathophysiol. Pharmacol.* **2013**, *5*, 73–90.
9. Barreto, G.; White, R.E.; Ouyang, Y.; Xu, L.; Giffard, R.G. Astrocytes: Targets for neuroprotection in stroke. *Cent. Nerv. Syst. Agents. Med. Chem.* **2011**, *11*, 164–173. [CrossRef]
10. Koh, J.Y.; Suh, S.W.; Gwag, B.J.; He, Y.Y.; Hsu, C.Y.; Choi, D.W. The role of zinc in selective neuronal death after transient global cerebral ischemia. *Science* **1996**, *272*, 1013–1016. [CrossRef]
11. Hong, D.K.; Kho, A.R.; Choi, B.Y.; Lee, S.H.; Jeong, J.H.; Lee, S.H.; Park, K.H.; Park, J.B.; Suh, S.W. Combined Treatment With Dichloroacetic Acid and Pyruvate Reduces Hippocampal Neuronal Death After Transient Cerebral Ischemia. *Front. Neurol.* **2018**, *9*, 137. [CrossRef] [PubMed]
12. Hong, D.K.; Choi, B.Y.; Kho, A.R.; Lee, S.H.; Jeong, J.H.; Kang, B.S.; Kang, D.H.; Park, K.H.; Suh, S.W. Carvacrol Attenuates Hippocampal Neuronal Death after Global Cerebral Ischemia via Inhibition of Transient Receptor Potential Melastatin 7. *Cells* **2018**, *7*, 231. [CrossRef] [PubMed]
13. Kho, A.R.; Choi, B.Y.; Lee, S.H.; Hong, D.K.; Lee, S.H.; Jeong, J.H.; Park, K.H.; Song, H.K.; Choi, H.C.; Suh, S.W. Effects of Protocatechuic Acid (PCA) on Global Cerebral Ischemia-Induced Hippocampal Neuronal Death. *Int. J. Mol. Sci.* **2018**, *19*, 1420. [CrossRef]

14. Petrovic-Djergovic, D.; Goonewardena, S.N.; Pinsky, D.J. Inflammatory Disequilibrium in Stroke. *Circ. Res.* **2016**, *119*, 142–158. [CrossRef] [PubMed]
15. Lee, S.Y.; Kim, J.H. Mechanisms underlying presynaptic Ca2+ transient and vesicular glutamate release at a CNS nerve terminal during in vitro ischaemia. *J. Physiol.* **2015**, *593*, 2793–2806. [CrossRef]
16. Bonaventura, A.; Liberale, L.; Vecchie, A.; Casula, M.; Carbone, F.; Dallegri, F.; Montecucco, F. Update on Inflammatory Biomarkers and Treatments in Ischemic Stroke. *Int. J. Mol. Sci.* **2016**, *17*, 1967. [CrossRef]
17. Shuttleworth, C.W.; Weiss, J.H. Zinc: New clues to diverse roles in brain ischemia. *Trends Pharmacol. Sci.* **2011**, *32*, 480–486. [CrossRef]
18. Weiss, J.H.; Sensi, S.L.; Koh, J.Y. Zn(2+): A novel ionic mediator of neural injury in brain disease. *Trends Pharmacol. Sci.* **2000**, *21*, 395–401. [CrossRef]
19. Kawahara, M.; Tanaka, K.I.; Kato-Negishi, M. Zinc, Carnosine, and Neurodegenerative Diseases. *Nutrients* **2018**, *10*, 147. [CrossRef]
20. Lee, S.R. Critical Role of Zinc as Either an Antioxidant or a Prooxidant in Cellular Systems. *Oxid. Med. Cell Longev.* **2018**, *2018*, 9156285. [CrossRef]
21. Portbury, S.D.; Adlard, P.A. Zinc Signal in Brain Diseases. *Int. J. Mol. Sci.* **2017**, *18*, 2506. [CrossRef] [PubMed]
22. Choi, B.Y.; Hong, D.K.; Jeong, J.H.; Lee, B.E.; Koh, J.Y.; Suh, S.W. Zinc transporter 3 modulates cell proliferation and neuronal differentiation in the adult hippocampus. *Stem. Cells* **2020**, *38*, 994–1006. [CrossRef] [PubMed]
23. McAllister, B.B.; Dyck, R.H. Zinc transporter 3 (ZnT3) and vesicular zinc in central nervous system function. *Neurosci. Biobehav. Rev.* **2017**, *80*, 329–350. [CrossRef]
24. Kho, A.R.; Choi, B.Y.; Kim, J.H.; Lee, S.H.; Hong, D.K.; Lee, S.H.; Jeong, J.H.; Sohn, M.; Suh, S.W. Prevention of hypoglycemia-induced hippocampal neuronal death by N-acetyl-L-cysteine (NAC). *Amino Acids* **2017**, *49*, 367–378. [CrossRef] [PubMed]
25. Choi, B.Y.; Lee, S.H.; Choi, H.C.; Lee, S.K.; Yoon, H.S.; Park, J.B.; Chung, W.S.; Suh, S.W. Alcohol dependence treating agent, acamprosate, prevents traumatic brain injury-induced neuron death through vesicular zinc depletion. *Transl. Res.* **2019**, *207*, 1–18. [CrossRef]
26. Higashi, Y.; Aratake, T.; Shimizu, S.; Shimizu, T.; Nakamura, K.; Tsuda, M.; Yawata, T.; Ueba, T.; Saito, M. Influence of extracellular zinc on M1 microglial activation. *Sci. Rep.* **2017**, *7*, 43778. [CrossRef]
27. Qi, Z.; Liang, J.; Pan, R.; Dong, W.; Shen, J.; Yang, Y.; Zhao, Y.; Shi, W.; Luo, Y.; Ji, X.; et al. Zinc contributes to acute cerebral ischemia-induced blood-brain barrier disruption. *Neurobiol. Dis.* **2016**, *95*, 12–21. [CrossRef]
28. Suh, S.W.; Hamby, A.M.; Gum, E.T.; Shin, B.S.; Won, S.J.; Sheline, C.T.; Chan, P.H.; Swanson, R.A. Sequential release of nitric oxide, zinc, and superoxide in hypoglycemic neuronal death. *J. Cereb. Blood. Flow. Metab.* **2008**, *28*, 1697–1706. [CrossRef]
29. Park, S.E.; Song, J.H.; Hong, C.; Kim, D.E.; Sul, J.W.; Kim, T.Y.; Seo, B.R.; So, I.; Kim, S.Y.; Bae, D.J.; et al. Contribution of Zinc-Dependent Delayed Calcium Influx via TRPC5 in Oxidative Neuronal Death and its Prevention by Novel TRPC Antagonist. *Mol. Neurobiol.* **2019**, *56*, 2822–2835. [CrossRef]
30. Sen, C.K. Antioxidant and redox regulation of cellular signaling: Introduction. *Med. Sci. Sports Exerc.* **2001**, *33*, 368–370. [CrossRef]
31. Kerksick, C.; Willoughby, D. The antioxidant role of glutathione and N-acetyl-cysteine supplements and exercise-induced oxidative stress. *J. Int. Soc. Sports Nutr.* **2005**, *2*, 38–44. [CrossRef] [PubMed]
32. Thanan, R.; Oikawa, S.; Hiraku, Y.; Ohnishi, S.; Ma, N.; Pinlaor, S.; Yongvanit, P.; Kawanishi, S.; Murata, M. Oxidative stress and its significant roles in neurodegenerative diseases and cancer. *Int. J. Mol. Sci.* **2014**, *16*, 193–217. [CrossRef] [PubMed]
33. Liu, Z.; Zhou, T.; Ziegler, A.C.; Dimitrion, P.; Zuo, L. Oxidative Stress in Neurodegenerative Diseases: From Molecular Mechanisms to Clinical Applications. *Oxid. Med. Cell Longev.* **2017**, *2017*, 2525967. [CrossRef] [PubMed]
34. Choi, B.Y.; Kim, I.Y.; Kim, J.H.; Lee, B.E.; Lee, S.H.; Kho, A.R.; Jung, H.J.; Sohn, M.; Song, H.K.; Suh, S.W. Decreased cysteine uptake by EAAC1 gene deletion exacerbates neuronal oxidative stress and neuronal death after traumatic brain injury. *Amino Acids* **2016**, *48*, 1619–1629. [CrossRef]
35. Rushworth, G.F.; Megson, I.L. Existing and potential therapeutic uses for N-acetylcysteine: The need for conversion to intracellular glutathione for antioxidant benefits. *Pharmacol. Ther.* **2014**, *141*, 150–159. [CrossRef]

36. Tardiolo, G.; Bramanti, P.; Mazzon, E. Overview on the Effects of N-Acetylcysteine in Neurodegenerative Diseases. *Molecules* **2018**, *23*, 3305. [CrossRef]
37. Jiang, L.H.; Yang, W.; Zou, J.; Beech, D.J. TRPM2 channel properties, functions and therapeutic potentials. *Expert Opin. Ther. Targets* **2010**, *14*, 973–988. [CrossRef]
38. Sita, G.; Hrelia, P.; Graziosi, A.; Ravegnini, G.; Morroni, F. TRPM2 in the Brain: Role in Health and Disease. *Cells* **2018**, *7*, 82. [CrossRef]
39. Turlova, E.; Feng, Z.P.; Sun, H.S. The role of TRPM2 channels in neurons, glial cells and the blood-brain barrier in cerebral ischemia and hypoxia. *Acta Pharmacol. Sin.* **2018**, *39*, 713–721. [CrossRef]
40. McHugh, D.; Flemming, R.; Xu, S.Z.; Perraud, A.L.; Beech, D.J. Critical intracellular Ca2+ dependence of transient receptor potential melastatin 2 (TRPM2) cation channel activation. *J. Biol. Chem.* **2003**, *278*, 11002–11006. [CrossRef]
41. Belrose, J.C.; Jackson, M.F. TRPM2: A candidate therapeutic target for treating neurological diseases. *Acta Pharmacol. Sin.* **2018**, *39*, 722–732. [CrossRef] [PubMed]
42. Zhu, T.; Zhao, Y.; Hu, H.; Zheng, Q.; Luo, X.; Ling, Y.; Ying, Y.; Shen, Z.; Jiang, P.; Shu, Q. TRPM2 channel regulates cytokines production in astrocytes and aggravates brain disorder during lipopolysaccharide-induced endotoxin sepsis. *Int. Immunopharmacol.* **2019**, *75*, 105836. [CrossRef] [PubMed]
43. Haraguchi, K.; Kawamoto, A.; Isami, K.; Maeda, S.; Kusano, A.; Asakura, K.; Shirakawa, H.; Mori, Y.; Nakagawa, T.; Kaneko, S. TRPM2 contributes to inflammatory and neuropathic pain through the aggravation of pronociceptive inflammatory responses in mice. *J. Neurosci.* **2012**, *32*, 3931–3941. [CrossRef] [PubMed]
44. Nilius, B.; Flockerzi, V. Mammalian transient receptor potential (TRP) cation channels. Preface. *Handb. Exp. Pharmacol.* **2014**, *223*, v–vi. [PubMed]
45. Yu, P.; Wang, Q.; Zhang, L.H.; Lee, H.C.; Zhang, L.; Yue, J. A cell permeable NPE caged ADP-ribose for studying TRPM2. *PLoS ONE* **2012**, *7*, e51028. [CrossRef] [PubMed]
46. Miller, B.A.; Cheung, J.Y. TRPM2 protects against tissue damage following oxidative stress and ischaemia-reperfusion. *J. Physiol.* **2016**, *594*, 4181–4191. [CrossRef]
47. Jang, B.G.; Won, S.J.; Kim, J.H.; Choi, B.Y.; Lee, M.W.; Sohn, M.; Song, H.K.; Suh, S.W. EAAC1 gene deletion alters zinc homeostasis and enhances cortical neuronal injury after transient cerebral ischemia in mice. *J. Trace Elem. Med. Biol.* **2012**, *26*, 85–88. [CrossRef]
48. Suh, S.W.; Garnier, P.; Aoyama, K.; Chen, Y.; Swanson, R.A. Zinc release contributes to hypoglycemia-induced neuronal death. *Neurobiol. Dis.* **2004**, *16*, 538–545. [CrossRef]
49. Suh, S.W.; Frederickson, C.J.; Danscher, G. Neurotoxic zinc translocation into hippocampal neurons is inhibited by hypothermia and is aggravated by hyperthermia after traumatic brain injury in rats. *J. Cereb. Blood Flow Metab.* **2006**, *26*, 161–169. [CrossRef]
50. Ye, M.; Yang, W.; Ainscough, J.F.; Hu, X.P.; Li, X.; Sedo, A.; Zhang, X.H.; Zhang, X.; Chen, Z.; Li, X.M.; et al. TRPM2 channel deficiency prevents delayed cytosolic Zn2+ accumulation and CA1 pyramidal neuronal death after transient global ischemia. *Cell Death Dis.* **2014**, *5*, e1541. [CrossRef]
51. Medvedeva, Y.V.; Ji, S.G.; Yin, H.Z.; Weiss, J.H. Differential Vulnerability of CA1 versus CA3 Pyramidal Neurons After Ischemia: Possible Relationship to Sources of Zn2+ Accumulation and Its Entry into and Prolonged Effects on Mitochondria. *J. Neurosci.* **2017**, *37*, 726–737. [CrossRef] [PubMed]
52. Hara, Y.; Wakamori, M.; Ishii, M.; Maeno, E.; Nishida, M.; Yoshida, T.; Yamada, H.; Shimizu, S.; Mori, E.; Kudoh, J.; et al. LTRPC2 Ca2+-permeable channel activated by changes in redox status confers susceptibility to cell death. *Mol. Cell* **2002**, *9*, 163–173. [CrossRef]
53. Takahashi, N.; Kozai, D.; Kobayashi, R.; Ebert, M.; Mori, Y. Roles of TRPM2 in oxidative stress. *Cell Calcium.* **2011**, *50*, 279–287. [CrossRef] [PubMed]
54. Berk, M.; Malhi, G.S.; Gray, L.J.; Dean, O.M. The promise of N-acetylcysteine in neuropsychiatry. *Trends Pharmacol. Sci.* **2013**, *34*, 167–177. [CrossRef] [PubMed]
55. Mandal, S.; Das, G.; Askari, H. Interactions of N-acetyl-l-cysteine with metals (Ni 2+, Cu 2+ and Zn 2+): An experimental and theoretical study. *Struct. Chem.* **2014**, *25*, 43–51. [CrossRef]
56. Allen, N.J.; Barres, B.A. Neuroscience: Glia-more than just brain glue. *Nature* **2009**, *457*, 675–677. [CrossRef]
57. Phatnani, H.; Maniatis, T. Astrocytes in neurodegenerative disease. *Cold Spring Harb. Perspect Biol.* **2015**, *7*. [CrossRef]
58. Lakhan, S.E.; Kirchgessner, A.; Hofer, M. Inflammatory mechanisms in ischemic stroke: Therapeutic approaches. *J. Transl. Med.* **2009**, *7*, 97. [CrossRef]

59. Kauppinen, T.M.; Higashi, Y.; Suh, S.W.; Escartin, C.; Nagasawa, K.; Swanson, R.A. Zinc triggers microglial activation. *J. Neurosci.* **2008**, *28*, 5827–5835. [CrossRef]
60. Malko, P.; Syed Mortadza, S.A.; McWilliam, J.; Jiang, L.H. TRPM2 Channel in Microglia as a New Player in Neuroinflammation Associated With a Spectrum of Central Nervous System Pathologies. *Front. Pharmacol.* **2019**, *10*, 239. [CrossRef]
61. Li, F.; Abuarab, N.; Sivaprasadarao, A. Reciprocal regulation of actin cytoskeleton remodelling and cell migration by Ca2+ and Zn2+: Role of TRPM2 channels. *J. Cell Sci.* **2016**, *129*, 2016–2029. [CrossRef] [PubMed]
62. Sensi, S.L.; Ton-That, D.; Sullivan, P.G.; Jonas, E.A.; Gee, K.R.; Kaczmarek, L.K.; Weiss, J.H. Modulation of mitochondrial function by endogenous Zn2+ pools. *Proc. Natl. Acad Sci. USA* **2003**, *100*, 6157–6162. [CrossRef] [PubMed]
63. Kim, Y.H.; Kim, E.Y.; Gwag, B.J.; Sohn, S.; Koh, J.Y. Zinc-induced cortical neuronal death with features of apoptosis and necrosis: Mediation by free radicals. *Neuroscience* **1999**, *89*, 175–182. [CrossRef]
64. Suh, S.W.; Gum, E.T.; Hamby, A.M.; Chan, P.H.; Swanson, R.A. Hypoglycemic neuronal death is triggered by glucose reperfusion and activation of neuronal NADPH oxidase. *J. Clin. Investig.* **2007**, *117*, 910–918. [CrossRef]
65. Noh, K.M.; Kim, Y.H.; Koh, J.Y. Mediation by membrane protein kinase C of zinc-induced oxidative neuronal injury in mouse cortical cultures. *J. Neurochem.* **1999**, *72*, 1609–1616. [CrossRef]
66. Li, X.; Jiang, L.H. A critical role of the transient receptor potential melastatin 2 channel in a positive feedback mechanism for reactive oxygen species-induced delayed cell death. *J. Cell Physiol.* **2019**, *234*, 3647–3660. [CrossRef]
67. Di, A.; Gao, X.P.; Qian, F.; Kawamura, T.; Han, J.; Hecquet, C.; Ye, R.D.; Vogel, S.M.; Malik, A.B. The redox-sensitive cation channel TRPM2 modulates phagocyte ROS production and inflammation. *Nat. Immunol.* **2011**, *13*, 29–34. [CrossRef] [PubMed]
68. Mortadza, S.S.; Sim, J.A.; Stacey, M.; Jiang, L.H. Signalling mechanisms mediating Zn(2+)-induced TRPM2 channel activation and cell death in microglial cells. *Sci. Rep.* **2017**, *7*, 45032. [CrossRef]
69. Kilkenny, C.; Browne, W.J.; Cuthill, I.C.; Emerson, M.; Altman, D.G. Improving bioscience research reporting: The ARRIVE guidelines for reporting animal research. *PLoS Biol.* **2010**, *8*, e1000412. [CrossRef]
70. Sanderson, T.H.; Wider, J.M. 2-vessel occlusion/hypotension: A rat model of global brain ischemia. *J. Vis. Exp.* **2013**. [CrossRef]
71. Bouet, V.; Boulouard, M.; Toutain, J.; Divoux, D.; Bernaudin, M.; Schumann-Bard, P.; Freret, T. The adhesive removal test: A sensitive method to assess sensorimotor deficits in mice. *Nat. Protoc.* **2009**, *4*, 1560–1564. [CrossRef] [PubMed]
72. Xing, Z.; Xia, Z.; Peng, W.; Li, J.; Zhang, C.; Fu, C.; Tang, T.; Luo, J.; Zou, Y.; Fan, R.; et al. Xuefu Zhuyu decoction, a traditional Chinese medicine, provides neuroprotection in a rat model of traumatic brain injury via an anti-inflammatory pathway. *Sci. Rep.* **2016**, *6*, 20040. [CrossRef] [PubMed]
73. Chen, J.; Sanberg, P.R.; Li, Y.; Wang, L.; Lu, M.; Willing, A.E.; Sanchez-Ramos, J.; Chopp, M. Intravenous administration of human umbilical cord blood reduces behavioral deficits after stroke in rats. *Stroke* **2001**, *32*, 2682–2688. [CrossRef] [PubMed]

8

Failed Neuroprotection of Combined Inhibition of L-Type and ASIC1a Calcium Channels with Nimodipine and Amiloride

Jonas Ort [1,*], Benedikt Kremer [1], Linda Grüßer [2], Romy Blaumeiser-Debarry [2], Hans Clusmann [1], Mark Coburn [3], Anke Höllig [1,†] and Ute Lindauer [1,†]

[1] Department of Neurosurgery, Medical Faculty, RWTH Aachen University, 52074 Aachen, Germany; bkremer@ukaachen.de (B.K.); hclusmann@ukaachen.de (H.C.); ahoellig@ukaachen.de (A.H.); ulindauer@ukaachen.de (U.L.)

[2] Department of Anaesthesiology, Medical Faculty, RWTH Aachen University, 52074 Aachen, Germany; lgruesser@ukaachen.de (L.G.); rblaumeiser-debarry@ukaachen.de (R.B.-D.)

[3] Department of Anaesthesiology and Intensive Care Medicine, University Hospital Bonn, 53127 Bonn, Germany; mark.coburn@ukbonn.de

* Correspondence: jort@ukaachen.de

† These authors have equal contributions.

Abstract: Effective pharmacological neuroprotection is one of the most desired aims in modern medicine. We postulated that a combination of two clinically used drugs—nimodipine (L-Type voltage-gated calcium channel blocker) and amiloride (acid-sensing ion channel inhibitor)—might act synergistically in an experimental model of ischaemia, targeting the intracellular rise in calcium as a pathway in neuronal cell death. We used organotypic hippocampal slices of mice pups and a well-established regimen of oxygen-glucose deprivation (OGD) to assess a possible neuroprotective effect. Neither nimodipine (at 10 or 20 μM) alone or in combination with amiloride (at 100 μM) showed any amelioration. Dissolved at 2.0 Vol.% dimethyl-sulfoxide (DMSO), the combination of both components even increased cell damage ($p = 0.0001$), an effect not observed with amiloride alone. We conclude that neither amiloride nor nimodipine do offer neuroprotection in an in vitro ischaemia model. On a technical note, the use of DMSO should be carefully evaluated in neuroprotective experiments, since it possibly alters cell damage.

Keywords: neuroprotection; neural injury; nimodipine; subarachnoid haemorrhage; acid-sensing ion channels; amiloride; oxygen-glucose deprivation

---

1. Introduction

Despite years of research pharmacological neuroprotection remains challenging. Neuronal cell death represents the smallest common denominator occurring within the pathophysiological cascade of acute cerebrovascular or traumatic brain diseases. For example, subarachnoid haemorrhage occurs with an incidence of 9/100,000 per year [1], while traumatic brain injury is one of the leading causes for death and disability in the young with reported incidences of 262/100,000 per year [2]. Considering the dreads of brain damage for patients and their dependants, therapeutic means of effective neuroprotection is possibly one of the most aimed-for means in modern medicine.

Although the pathomechanisms of neuronal cell death are yet to be fully understood, one of the first and most frequently investigated events is the elevation of intracellular calcium concentration. Elevated intracellular calcium represents a central part within the early phenomenon of excitotoxicity as well as all the pathways resulting in or from these raised ion concentrations [3–7]. Various drugs blocking the excitotoxicity-induced calcium influx have failed to show effective neuroprotection in the first place or failed in overcoming the translational roadblock from in vivo or animal in vitro experiments to actual clinical application (e.g., trials of glutamate-receptor antagonists) [8,9]. Beside calcium influx via glutamate receptor overactivation, calcium influx may also occur via voltage-gated calcium channels (VGCC) located within neuronal membranes. Additionally, VGCCs are also expressed by vascular smooth muscle cells responsible for intracellular calcium rise and vasoconstriction when activated.

The L-type calcium channel inhibitor nimodipine is well established as an oral agent for the management of delayed cerebral ischaemia (DCI) for patients after subarachnoid haemorrhage (SAH) [10–15]. Although nimodipine induces vascular smooth muscle relaxation [16] and hence is widely believed to reduce vasospasms, research has shown that the beneficial effects in SAH patients with DCI may not be primarily caused by this effect on larger cerebral vessels [12,17], but possibly by a direct neuroprotective effect. Experimental studies have been rather controversial with some arguing towards direct neuroprotection [18–21] and some against [22–25]. In brief, the inhibition of voltage-gated L-type calcium channels is believed to provide protection against raised intracellular calcium concentration once the cell depolarises in ischaemic conditions. However, it remains unclear whether this effect also counts for the observed beneficial effect of VGCC inhibitors in SAH.

Other possible drug targets regarding cerebral ischaemia are sodium- and (to a lesser extent) calcium-permeable acid-sensing ion channels (ASICs), with the ASIC1a subtype channel as the most prominent amongst them [26]. ASIC1a channels can be responsible for neuronal damage in acidosis and provide a neither voltage-gated nor glutamate-dependent mechanism for calcium influx. Amiloride can block this non-specifically [27–29]. Many experiments have already shown that neuroprotection can be achieved by blocking ASIC1a and thus targeting these channels might be promising [9,30,31]. Some studies point out connections between the affinity of ASIC for H^+ depending and the extracellular concentration of calcium [32,33], as it occurs in brain ischemia [34].

In our experiment, we investigated the possible neuroprotective effect of two clinically used drugs, which both block calcium channels: The L-type calcium channel inhibitor nimodipine and the acid-sensing ion channel (ASIC1a) blocker amiloride.

We hypothesised a possible synergistic neuroprotective effect of the two compounds being used in combination since ASIC channels are known to be influenced by external and internal calcium levels [32,33]. To assess our postulation, we used a well-established in vitro model of oxygen–glucose deprivation (OGD) in organotypic hippocampus slices of mice with propidium iodide (PI) staining for cell death assessment. Nimodipine was investigated for neuroprotective effects alone and in combination with amiloride to observe a possible synergistic interaction.

2. Results

2.1. OGD Damage

Comparing our control group (n = 102) with our OGD group (n = 96) a significant difference was seen ($p < 0.0001$, Mann–Whitney test), thus demonstrating significant and robust cell damage by our OGD regimen (Figure 1).

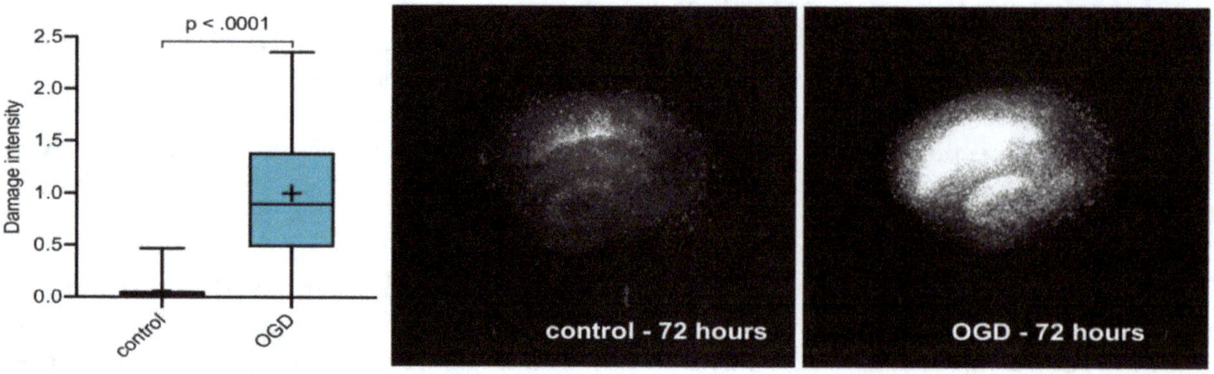

Figure 1. Damage intensity of the control group ($n = 101$) vs. oxygen–glucose deprivation (OGD) group ($n = 96$). Mann–Whitney U test was used to determine whether our OGD model caused adequate damage. Slice images shown are example slices for control and OGD groups, both at 72 h with typical means for the grey-scale value. Slice images are red-channel-filtered and contrast-enhanced.

2.2. Effect of DMSO as Vehicle on OGD-Induced Damage

To rule out possible effects of our vehicle, slices were incubated receiving dimethyl-sulfoxide (DMSO) without any drug in addition either as controls (Figure 2, left) or undergoing OGD (Figure 2, right) at levels of 0.1, 1.0, or 2.0 Vol.% DMSO. For pure vehicle control slices without OGD, there was a tendency towards a concentration dependent effect; however, with significant cell impairment observed only with the highest concentration of 2.0 Vol.% DMSO ($p = 0.0001$, Kruskal–Wallis with post hoc Dunn's test). Following OGD, there was a slight albeit far not significant tendendy towards a protective effect of DMSO (Figure 2, right: DMSO concentration of 1.0 Vol.%, $p = 0.2237$) compared with the OGD slices without vehicle or with other DMSO concentrations.

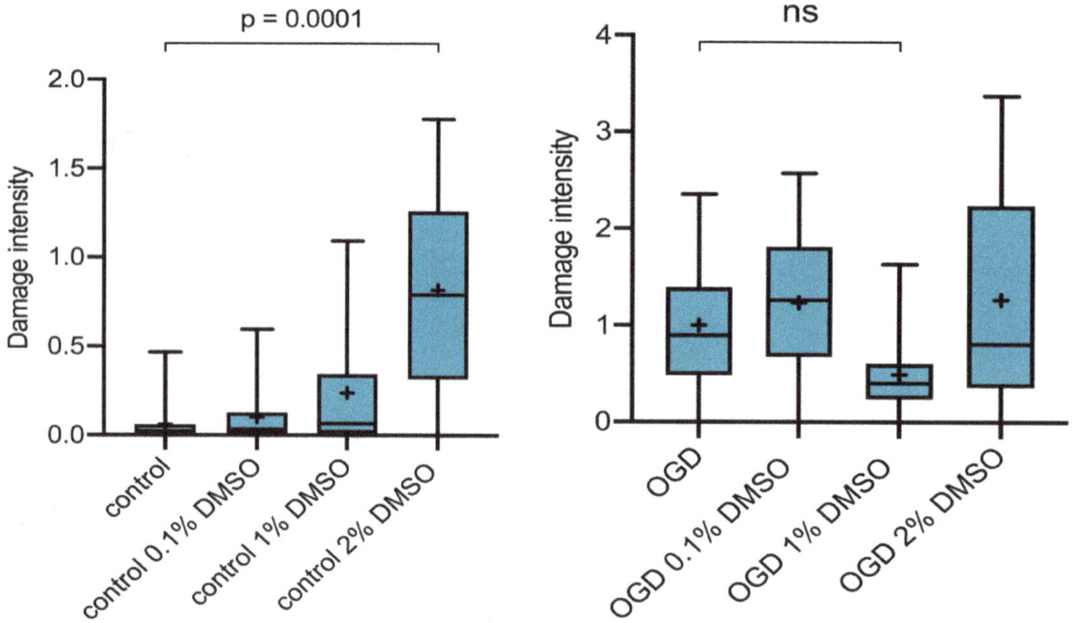

Figure 2. (**Left**): Slices receiving 2.0 Vol.% dimethyl-sulfoxide (DMSO) alone ($n = 20$) without undergoing OGD showed significantly ($p = 0.0001$) more cell damage. This effect can be observed for 0.1 ($n = 25$) and 1.0 Vol.% ($n = 12$) as well but at a much lower level without statistical significance. (**Right**): No significant effects of DMSO in slices undergoing OGD were observed for 0.1 ($n = 41$), 1.0 ($n = 19$) or 2.0 ($n = 45$) Vol.% DMSO compared to the OGD group without DMSO ($n = 96$). The figure depicts a tendency towards less cell damage at 1.0 Vol.% DMSO.

2.3. *Effect of Nimodipine at 10 or 20 μM Dissolved in Varying DMSO Concentrations*

L-type calcium channel blockage with nimodipine at either 10 or 20 μM dissolved in 0.1 or 1.0 Vol.% DMSO, respectively, did not show significant neuroprotection (Figure 3).

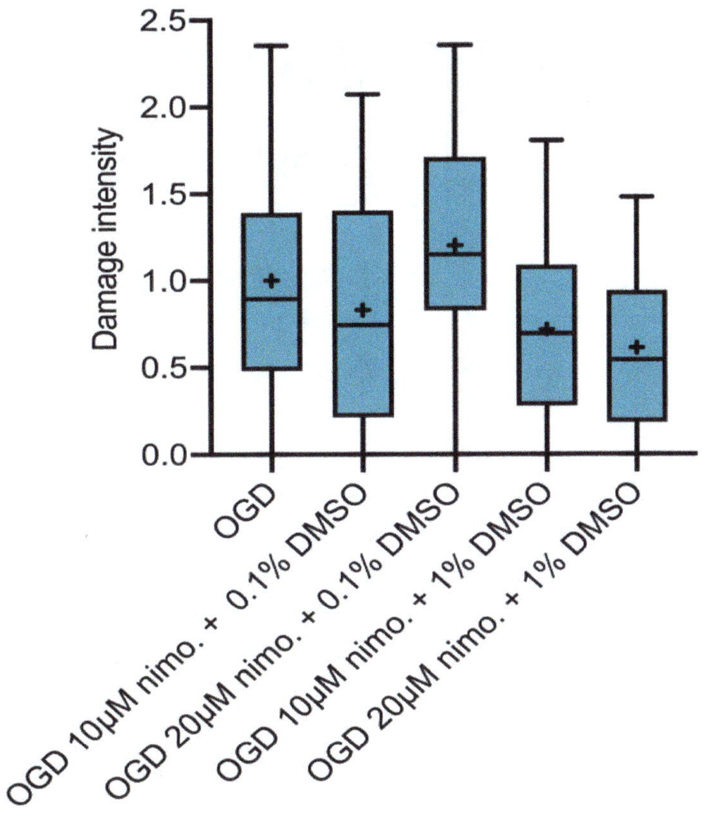

Figure 3. Slices undergoing OGD received nimodipine at either 10 or 20 μM dissolved in 0.1 or 1.0 Vol.% DMSO. No significant differences in cell damage were observed at 72 h after OGD (OGD n = 96; dissolved in 0.1 Vol.% DMSO: 10μM nimodipine n = 77, 20 μM nimodipine n = 64; dissolved in 1.0 Vol.% DMSO: 10 μM nimodipine n = 30, 20 μM nimodipine n = 25).

2.4. *Effect of Nimodipine at 10 or 20 μM in Combination with 100 μM Amiloride Dissolved in Varying DMSO Concentrations*

To observe a neuroprotective effect of combined blockage of L-type calcium channels and ASIC1a, a combination of 10 or 20 μM nimodipine and 100 μM amiloride dissolved in 1.1 Vol.% DMSO was applied. No significant effect for the combination of nimodipine and amiloride or amiloride alone at 1.0 Vol.% DMSO could be observed (Figure 4). Further, no significant difference was detected in slices receiving nimodipine at 10 or 20 μM in 1.0 Vol.% DMSO or with the vehicle alone. These slices showed a tendency towards less severe cell damage when compared to the OGD group and slices receiving regimens with 0.1 Vol.% DMSO (also Figure 4).

Lastly, treatment combination of 100 μM amiloride and either 10 or 20 μM nimodipine was investigated while using a final concentration of 2.0 Vol.% DMSO. No combination of nimodipine and amiloride or amiloride alone showed any significant neuroprotective effect. However, slices receiving the combination of 100 μM amiloride and 10μM (p = 0.0001, Kruskal–Wallis with post hoc Dunn's test, Cohen's d = 1.196243) or 20 μM (p = 0.0001, Kruskal–Wallis with post hoc Dunn's test, Cohen's d = 1.219638) nimodipine at 2.0 Vol.% DMSO displayed significantly higher levels of cell damage at 72 h after OGD compared to the OGD group without any treatment (Figure 5).

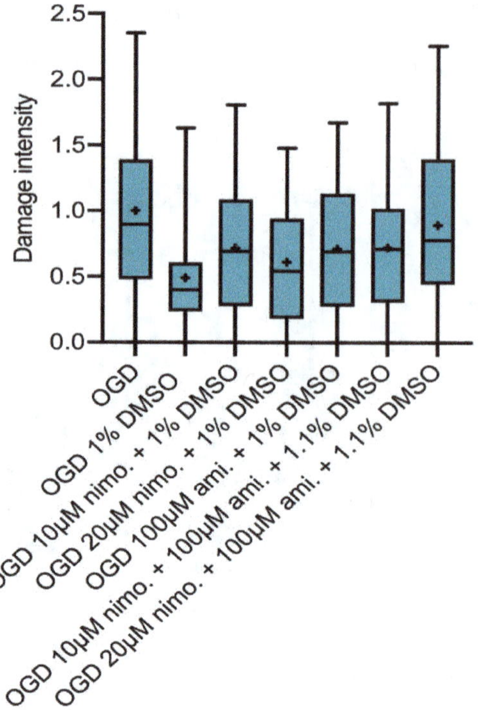

Figure 4. Slices receiving 10 ($n = 30$) or 20 µM ($n = 25$) nimodipine in 1.0 Vol.% DMSO compared to slices receiving 100 µM amiloride alone in 1 Vol.% DMSO ($n = 50$) or in combination with 10 ($n = 56$) or 20 µM ($n = 59$) nimodipine in 1.1 Vol.% DMSO. No significant difference in cell damage intensity was observed at 72 h after OGD.

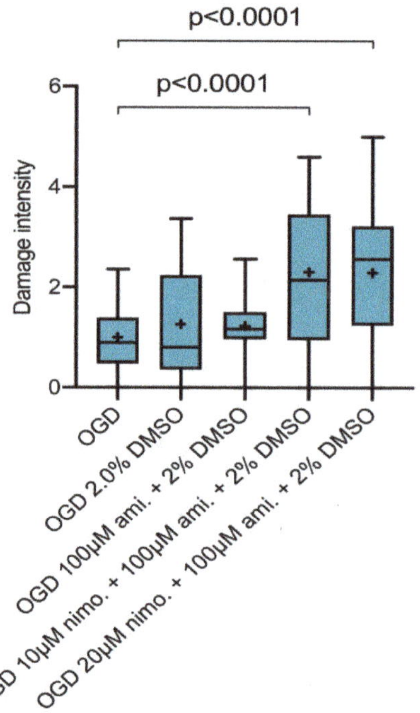

Figure 5. Slices receiving a combination of either 10 ($n = 47$) or 20 µM ($n = 46$) nimodipine with 100 µM amiloride in 2.0 Vol.% DMSO showed significant impairment of cell viability at 72 h (Kruskal–Wallis test with post hoc Dunn's test, $p < 0.0001$) compared to OGD slices ($n = 96$). This effect was not observed for slices receiving 100 µM amiloride in 2.0 Vol.% DMSO ($n = 43$) or 2.0 Vol.% DMSO alone ($n = 45$).

3. Discussion

In our study, we investigated the clinically commonly used drugs nimodipine and amiloride to test for neuroprotective effects in an in vitro model of brain ischemia using OGD. No protective effect could be observed for nimodipine or amiloride alone or in combination. Our model was already used in the past to prove neuroprotective effects of other drugs, such as the noble gas argon, which showed a protection of >80% in the best suited protocol [35]. DMSO, which was used as vehicle to dissolve both drugs, induced significant impairment of cell integrity at 2.0 Vol.% in our control slices (that did not undergo OGD) compared with the control group without DMSO. Paradoxically, this effect was not observed at the same concentration in slices undergoing OGD. There was even a tendency towards ameliorated levels of cell damage in OGD slices at 1.0 Vol.% DMSO (Figure 2, right). Interestingly, the combination of nimodipine and amiloride significantly increased cell damage when dissolved at 2.0 Vol.% DMSO. This effect was not apparent for 2.0 Vol.% DMSO alone or with the same concentration as vehicle for 100 μM amiloride. Nimodipine alone in 2.0 Vol.% DMSO was not investigated.

3.1. *The Role of Calcium for Cell Death and Failure to Provide Neuroprotection*

The exact mechanisms of neuronal cell death in ischemia are yet to be fully understood. Dirnagl et al. postulated in 1999 that there are several main mechanisms: excitotoxicity (i.e., damage through an overshooting release of neurotransmitters, mainly glutamate, followed by intracellular calcium overload), oxidative stress, cortical spreading depolarisations, inflammation, and apoptosis [36]. Calcium influx has long been labelled as "final common pathway" [3] of toxic cell death; however, this term might be misleading, since calcium itself activates a cascade of intracellular reactions and thus the possible mechanisms are manifold [37], e.g., a two-step model was suggested consisting of neuronal swelling in a first step and a delayed entrance of calcium in a second [23].

The main hypothesis of our study was that neuroprotection can be achieved by preventing the intracellular rise in calcium concentration by a combined blockade of two postulated calcium entry pathways, while blocking the L-Type calcium channel with nimodipine and the ASIC1a channel using amiloride.

Nimodipine has been reported to improve functional outcome in ischaemic and haemorrhagic stroke in in vivo animal experiments as well as in clinical trials [13,18,20,38,39] and is still the only therapeutic option in the treatment of DCI after SAH [40]. However, the effect of L-type channel inhibition might primarily be targeted to smooth muscle cell function to prevent large as well as small vessel contractions. A possible additional effect on neurons (and astrocytes) might be overrated. To separate direct neuroprotective from vascular effects, models without the dependency of blood circulation (such as cell culture or slice culture models) have been used to investigate this postulated effect of nimodipine and other VGCC inhibitors. Although there are data showing that nimodipine decreases membrane depolarization and thus calcium influx in OGD [21], Kass et al. for instance pointed out that it is rather the loss of calcium extrusion mechanisms (i.e., the dysfunction of the Ca^{2+}-ATPase and the Na^{+}-Ca^{2+}-Exchanger due to the loss of ATP in hypoxic condition [41]) and not an increased calcium influx that is responsible for cell damage [42]. In addition, the question remains how relevant the portion of the L-type channel for calcium overload within ischaemic damage is. Some data suggest Q-type and N-type channels are far more critical with regard to neuronal injury and that the L-type channel accounts for less than 10% of total damage [24]. Most of the intracellular calcium overload appears to be the result of excitotoxic activation of N-methyl-D-aspartate (NMDA) receptors that become permeable for the ion [41,43]. Moreover, only targeting calcium as single ion might be too simplistic. Goldberg and colleagues demonstrated in experiments that if only calcium is removed, the neuronal damage is enhanced. Only if calcium, sodium, and potassium are removed from the culture medium, protection is achieved. The group concluded that there are two phases to neuronal ischaemic damage pathways: the first one caused by acute swelling, the second one depending on the rise in intracellular calcium concentrations [23]. Thus, there are calcium-independent effects. Regarding these publications, it seems reasonable to conclude that nimodipine does play a role in the calcium metabolism of an ischaemia-exposed neuron; however, the L-type calcium channel alone is likely not central enough in the complex system of calcium-mediated cell death to act as a promising drug target. Our data show no evidence of a protective effect against OGD in our hippocampal slice culture model. This points towards a minor role for L-type calcium channels within the pathophysiological cascade of early ischaemic cell damage.

3.2. Amiloride and Combined L-Type Calcium Channel and ASICs Inhibition

ASICs have been identified to be accountable for increased levels of intracellular calcium in ischaemic conditions. Under acidic conditions, as it occurs during ischaemia, ASIC1a channels become permeable for calcium and provide a mechanism for calcium influx that is not dependent on depolarisation or excitotoxicity [29]. In our study, the ASIC channel inhibitor amiloride did not show any significant neuroprotective effect. This contrasts with other studies showing a protective effect of ASIC inhibition on brain injury [27]. Positive effects of ASIC inhibition were most prominent in a combined acidosis and OGD model. That may explain the insufficient protection of amiloride in our pure OGD model in which the OGD induced acidosis may be less pronounced. Besides, a combination of L-type calcium channel and ASIC inhibition by nimodipine plus amiloride did also not show a protective effect in our model. These findings point against a significant damaging role of calcium entry in parenchymal cells via VGCCs and ASICS during OGD in models not depending on an intact blood supply. In our study, the amount of damage was investigated 72 h after the insult. It can therefore not be ruled out that an early, only transient, and thus not sustained effect of calcium entry blockade via VGCCs and ASICs may have occurred.

Interestingly, in slices treated with regimes using the possibly harmful concentration of 2.0 Vol.% DMSO, we observed a significant further increase in cell damage only for slices where nimodipine and amiloride were applied in combination. DMSO at this high concentration already caused damage in our control slices without OGD. It is also known from the literature that DMSO higher than 5% may have harmful effects on biological tissue and cells [44,45]. Safe concentrations are described up to 3% in hippocampal neurons [44]. In combination with OGD, 2 Vol.% DMSO did not induce an increase in damage beyond the OGD induced damage. In addition, slices receiving DMSO at this high concentration with additional 100μM amiloride did not significantly differ from the OGD control group. We did not investigate nimodipine alone in a concentration of 2.0 Vol.% DMSO. Thus, we cannot draw conclusions whether this effect is caused by the combination of amiloride and nimodipine in 2.0 Vol.% DMSO, or whether nimodipine combined with high concentration of DMSO alone would have the same effect. The high DMSO concentration of 2 Vol.% may have affected the system in addition to OGD, inducing a setting of higher damage-susceptibility, where calcium channel inhibition (equal whether via nimodipine alone or in combination with amiloride) is even harmful instead of neuroprotective. If we assume a combined mechanism, impairment of regulatory systems responsible for ASIC function by the simultaneous L-type calcium channel inhibition with nimodipine might be the answer. This could either be caused by a reduction in intracellular calcium or by the missing reduction in extracellular calcium. Paukert et al., for example, showed that extracellular calcium influences ASIC function and can be competitively inhibited by calcium ions. Furthermore, they suggest that higher extracellular calcium shifts ASIC sensitivity to more acidic pH levels [33]. Admittedly, we would rather expect less ASIC activity and thus less damage if we follow this argumentation. A further explanation may be based on amiloride's unspecific effects. Amiloride does also interfere with other channels, e.g., Na^+/H^+- or Na^+/Ca^{2+}-exchangers and even T-type calcium channels [46]. As aforementioned, calcium extrusion mechanisms appear to be crucial for neuronal integrity. It could be imagined that unspecific blockage mechanisms in combination with L-type inhibition prevent calcium homeostasis mechanisms in the damaging environment of possible toxic effects of DMSO and OGD. Lastly, the concentration of 2.0 Vol.% DMSO is a comparably high choice for the solvent. We recommend avoiding this concentration if feasible.

3.3. Nimodipine—Most Important Effect on the Vasculature

Despite years of research, nimodipine is the only drug available that shows an improved functional outcome and positive effects on mortality after SAH. However, the exact underlying mechanism is still unclear [40]. As pointed out in this publication, a direct neuroprotective effect appears to be unlikely. After the CONSCIOUS-1 study [47], the scientific community changed their perspective on vasospasms of large vessels and DCI. The latter is now considered a complex condition with possible pathways in micro-thrombi [48,49], micro-vasculature spasms (mostly described in experiments and possibly a cause for the secondary development of micro-thrombi) [50–52], neuroinflammation [53,54], and cortical spreading depolarization [55]. Indeed, there is evidence from the literature that nimodipine interacts with several of the abovementioned mechanisms rather than directly acting on neurons, finally resulting in neuroprotection and better functional outcome. That explains a lack of neuroprotection in our model using organotypic slice cultures.

3.4. DMSO as Solvent

DMSO is a commonly used solvent in slice experiments similar to the one presented here. In healthy slices, DMSO applied for 72 h displayed significant damage to the slices at the highest concentration of 2 Vol.% tested. The lower concentrations only induced a concentration-dependent tendency towards slightly enhanced but not relevant damage. In contrast to this effect on slices without OGD, while applying DMSO following OGD, 1.0 Vol.% DMSO alone appears to induce a slight, although not statistically significant, reduction in cell damage. The highest concentration of 2 Vol.% DMSO did not show a protective effect but also did not significantly add to the OGD induced damage. This suggests identical damage pathways for DMSO at this high concentration and OGD. DMSO seems to have a U-shaped concentration-dependent effect on slices after OGD. Neuroprotective effects through DMSO have been described in different experimental designs and models [44,56,57], and thus, DMSO was even suggested as a treatment option for ischaemic brain conditions [58]. Lu and Mattson, e.g., report that DMSO inhibits the glutamate-induced (excitotoxic) calcium influx in hippocampal rat neurons at DMSO levels from 0.5 to 2.0% [44]. Suppression of excitotoxicity may thus also be a possible explanation for our observation of slightly protective effects at 1.0 Vol.%, since neuronal connections stay intact in organotypic hippocampal slices [59]. Another suggested explanation is DMSO's property as a scavenger for free oxygen radicals [58]. However, in our control slices, we observed a dose-depending increase in cell damage with significantly more damage for DMSO at 2.0 Vol.% compared to slices without DMSO or with 0.1 Vol.%. Contrary to the inhibiting effect on excitotoxicity, Galvao et al. have reported apoptosis-inducing effects in retinal cells using DMSO concentrations as low as 1% [60]. Zhang et al. confirmed these observations in experiments with neurons and astrocytes, reporting neuronal alterations at 0.5% DMSO [61]. In addition, even the smallest DMSO concentrations are described to have effects on cell metabolism, and the solvent possibly accumulates in brain slices [62]. From these diverse literature findings, a clear concentration-dependent effect—regardless of protective or harmful—cannot be identified. We consider it an important technical note to this paper that for brain slice experiments addressing mechanisms of neuroprotection, DMSO should be avoided if feasible. If DMSO is utilised, it should only be done so with the utmost caution and proper utilisation of vehicle controls.

3.5. Quality of Slices—Need for Defined Exclusion Criteria

In our group, we recognised that in many publications using organotypic hippocampus slices the inclusion criteria for slices are unclear or not exactly defined. Organotypic slice cultures are highly sensitive to external influences and can therefore be inhomogeneous with regard to cell damage [63]. We claim that a standardised inclusion pipeline would benefit further research conducted using this method. With the here-suggested pipeline (see Materials and Methods), we are confident that we enhanced the quality of data used for statistical analysis in our experiments.

3.6. Limitations

There are several limitations that may be considered given our conclusions:

Firstly, the described interactions of DMSO in the concentrations used may have interfered with the neuroprotective effects of both tested substances. However, this may only account for the highest concentration of 2.0 Vol.% of DMSO and not for the lower concentrations, not showing significant effects on the outcome in control as well as OGD. Secondly, we did not use a specific imaging technique to depict calcium concentrations. By applying well-established concentrations of nimodipine and amiloride, we are confident that an effective channel blockade was achieved, preventing calcium influx via these ion channels. Thirdly, we planned smaller groups for vehicle controls and control groups from the beginning to minimise the number of required animals. Thus, some control groups have limited sample size compared to treatment groups, and further power would be eligible regarding our observation of a possible neuroprotective effect of DMSO at a concentration of 1.0 Vol.%. Lastly, we did not investigate the effect of nimodipine in 2.0 Vol.% DMSO. Hence, it is not possible to draw specific conclusions from our observation of enhanced damage of combined treatment with nimodipine and amiloride at 2.0 Vol.% DMSO.

4. Materials and Methods

4.1. Mediums

Preparation medium (Gey's balanced salt solution (Sigma-Aldrich, Munich, Germany), 5 mg/mL D-(+)Glucose (Roth, Karlsruhe, Germany)) [63] was used for initial slice manufacturing. The growth medium used for slice culturing consisted of 50% Eagle minimal essential medium with Earle's salts (Sigma-Aldrich), 25% Hank's balanced salt solution (Sigma-Aldrich), 25% heat inactive horse serum (Sigma-Aldrich) with additional 5 mg/mL D-(+)Glucose (Roth, Karlsruhe, Germany), 1 Vol.% antibiotic/antimycotic solution [penicillin G GIBCO™, 10,000 units/mL, streptomycin sulphate 10 mg/mL, amphotericin B 25 µg/mL] (Thermo Fisher Scientific, Waltham, MA, USA), 5 µL/mL medium L-Glutamine solution (Sigma-Aldrich) and 10 µL/mL HEPES buffer solution (Sigma-Aldrich) [63]. For experiments, the experimental medium (75% Eagle minimal essential medium with Earle's salts (Sigma-Aldrich), 25% Hank's balanced salt solution (Sigma-Aldrich) with additional, 5 mg/mL D-(+)Glucose (Roth, Karlsruhe, Germany), 1 Vol.% antibiotic/antimycotic solution [penicillin G GIBCO™, 10,000 units/mL, streptomycin sulphate 10 mg/mL, amphotericin B 25 µg/mL] (Thermo Fisher Scientific, Waltham, MA, USA), 5 µL/mL L-Glutamine solution (Sigma-Aldrich) and 10 µL/mL HEPES buffer solution (Sigma-Aldrich)) or OGD medium (75% Eagle minimal essential medium with Earle's salts (Sigma-Aldrich), 25% Hank's balanced salt solution (Sigma-Aldrich) with additional 1 Vol.% antibiotic/antimycotic solution [penicillin G GIBCO™, 10,000 units/mL, streptomycin sulphate 10 mg/mL, amphotericin B 25 µg/mL] (Thermo Fisher Scientific, Waltham, MA, USA), 5 µL/mL L-Glutamine solution (Sigma-Aldrich) and 10 µL/mL HEPES buffer solution (Sigma-Aldrich)) were used, respectively. In essence, OGD medium is simply experimental medium without D-(+)Glucose.

4.2. Slice Preparation and Cultivation

The experiments in this article were strictly conducted according to institutional and governmental guidelines (TierSchG) with institutional permission by the animal protection representative of the Institute of Animal Research at the RWTH Aachen University Hospital and the local institutional committee (LANUV North Rhine-Westphalia, TV-11141A4). After decapitation of 4–7-day-old mice pups (C57BL/6N from Charles Rivers Laboratories, Sulzfeld, Germany and from Janvier Labs, La Rochelle, France, $n = 138$), their brains were extracted and instantaneously immersed into ice-cold preparation medium. The hippocampus slices were prepared using an already established method [58,63]. In brief, the brains were sagittally divided in half, and the frontal pole, as well as the cerebellum, was resected. Using a McIlwain Tissue Chopper (The Mickle Laboratory Engineering Co. ltd. [Now: Cavey Laboratory Engineering Co. ltd], Gomshall, UK), the brains were sliced into

400 μM thick slices from which the hippocampus was then carefully dissected. The hippocampus slices were then transferred onto MilliCell tissue culture inserts (MilliCell-CM, Millipore Corporation, Billerica, MA, USA) placed in 1 mL growth medium. Slices were cultivated at 37 °C and 5% CO2 for 14 days with the growth medium exchanged one day after the preparation and every following third day. On average, 9.1 slices per pup were prepared. Slices of one animal were allocated in two wells, which were then randomly allocated to the experimental groups to avoid allocation of slices of the same animal to only one experimental group. Overview in Figure 6a.

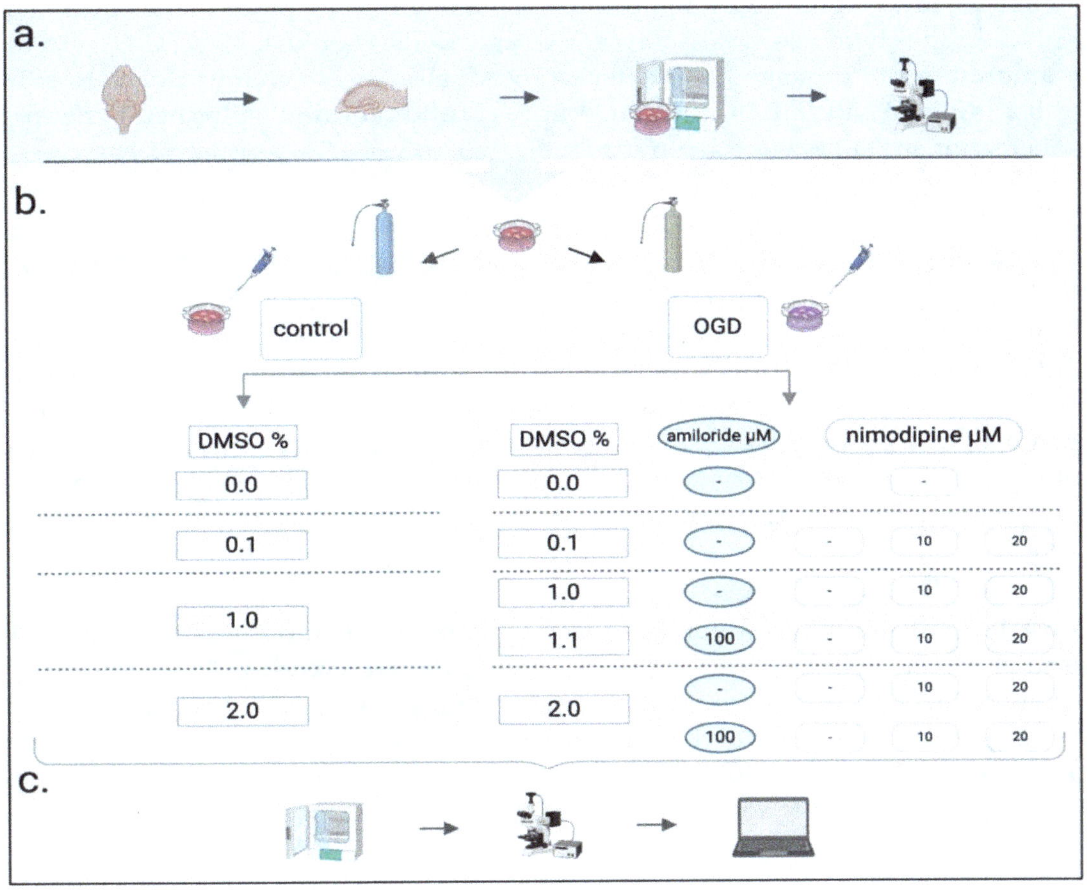

Figure 6. Experimental design. (**a**) Slice preparation, culturing for 14 days and baseline propidium iodide (PI) imaging. (**b**) OGD experiments with overview of experimental groups. (**c**) Incubation for 72 h after OGD, PI imaging for cell death assessment at 72 h, analysis of experimental groups. Created with BioRender.com.

4.3. Imaging

To obtain baseline images, immediately before the OGD experiment growth medium was exchanged for the experimental medium with additional 3 μL/mL propidium iodide (PI) and then incubated again for a minimum of 30 min at 37 °C and 5% CO_2. Propidium iodide stains DNA of cells with impaired cell membrane and was used to assess the number of cells damaged [64] using a fluorescence microscope (Zeiss Axioplan, Carl Zeiss MicroImaging GmbH, Jena, Germany) (exposure time was calculated for every imaging session and typically ranged between 15.500 and 16.500 milliseconds) and MetaVue software (MetaVue, Molecular Devices, Sunnyvale, CA, USA). Imaging was performed at baseline for all slices and 72 h after experiments. Imaging is depicted in Figure 6a,c.

4.4. Oxygen–Glucose Deprivation (OGD)

For OGD (Figure 6b), first OGD medium was aerated with 95% N_2, 5% CO_2 for 30 min using a Spectron flowmeter FLM-32 (Spectron Gas Control Systems GmbH, Frankfurt, Germany) at a rate of 15% at 0.2 bar to desaturate the OGD medium from oxygen and warmed up afterwards. The medium was quickly exchanged with OGD medium for the OGD groups and normal experimental medium for control groups, respectively, before immediately being transferred into air-tight experimental chambers (750 mL volume). Chambers containing OGD slices were then flushed with 95% N_2, 5% CO_2 at a rate of 100% at 0.5 bar for 6 min (resulting in a flow of 2.73 L/min) to guarantee a sufficiently hypoxic environment [35]. The chambers were then sealed, and OGD was sustained for 60 min to receive a reasonable amount of cell damage [23]. After OGD, all slices were changed back to experimental medium with additional 3 μL/mL propidium iodide (PI) and randomly allocated to neuroprotective protocols. Thereafter, the slices were again incubated at 37 °C and 5% CO_2 for 72 h.

4.5. Neuroprotective Protocols

Neuroprotective drugs were dissolved using dimethyl-sulfoxide (DMSO) (Sigma-Aldrich, St. Louis, MO, USA) [65]. Vehicle controls were performed for OGD and control groups for 0.1 Vol.%, 1.0 Vol.% and 2.0 Vol.% DMSO. For OGD groups, nimodipine was applied at 10 or 20 μM dissolved in either 0.1 Vol.% or 1.0 Vol.% DMSO and in combination with amiloride at 100 μM [27] again at 10 or 20 μM with 1.1 Vol.% or 2.0 Vol.% DMSO, respectively. Finally, we applied amiloride at 100 μM alone with either 1.0 Vol.% or 2.0 Vol.% DMSO. All agents remained within the medium for 72 h after OGD or time control, ending the experiments with the final imaging. An overview of all protective protocols can be seen in Figure 6b and in Appendix A.

4.6. Cell Death Assessment

PI resulted in red staining of damaged cells. To assess the amount of cell death within each slice, we used python to split channels for each picture into red, green, and blue and then created a corresponding picture in grey values for the red channel only. Again, using python, histograms were created for each picture depicting the corresponding grey-scale values from 0 to 255. A threshold for pixels below a grey-scale value of 100 was used to filter background fluorescence [35,63,66]. Finally, all pixel values were summed to resulting in one value per pixel representing the total damage for each slice.

4.7. Pre-Statistical Image Processing

To further process the slices for total damage analysis, the following exclusion criteria were defined. Every slice was excluded when [1.] more than one slice was shown on the corresponding images at 72 h (n = 6 excluded), when [2.] the dentate gyrus was not reliably identifiable (n = 57 excluded), when [3.] the CA1-region was not reliably identifiable (n = 28 excluded), when [4.] we identified unexplained dark spots in the picture (n = 31 excluded), when [5.] PI clots were observed on the image (n = 18 excluded), when [6.] slices were not plane but exhibited "wrinkling" that likely occurred in the cultivation process (n = 78 excluded), or when [7.] slices presented an inhomogeneous margin, likely due to inadequate preparation technique (n = 67 excluded). In total, 227 slices were excluded, and 1032 slices were used for further analysis. It should be noted that several slices showed more than one of the abovementioned features. We provide examples and possible explanations for our observations in the Appendix B.

In addition, to only include slices showing no preparation and cultivation induced damage already before OGD, we specified a maximal pre-damage threshold at the mean plus one standard deviation of all 1032 slices so far identified as useful. Seventy-four slices at 0 h presented a level of pre-experimental damage that was above that threshold. Finally, we defined a further threshold for the slices at 72 h after OGD to obviate extreme outliers in each of the experimental groups. For each of our 20 experimental groups, we established an individual threshold of the mean plus two times the standard deviation as a maximal damage plausibly caused by our OGD method (this excluded 33 slices at 72 h). By applying these criteria, comparability between slices was enhanced, as pre-damaged slices were restrained from entering the experiment and unrealistic outliers were excluded. The experimenter applied all exclusion criteria blinded to the slice allocation to the experimental groups. In total, 334 slices were eliminated, and 925 slices were included in our final analysis.

4.8. Statistical Analysis

Statistical Analysis was performed using GraphPad Prism version 8.2.0 for Windows (GraphPad Software, San Diego, CA, USA). Our data were normalised with the mean of the untreated OGD group as reference. Using a Kolmogorov–Smirnov test, we concluded that the assumption of a normal distribution was not met by our data. A two-tailed Mann–Whitney test between our control and our OGD group was used to verify our OGD model caused adequate damage. We used the Kruskal–Wallis test comparing the mean of rank of each group with every other group between the 72 h data of all OGD groups and for our control groups, respectively. Dunn's test was used to correct for multiple comparisons. For all statistical analysis, a p-value <0.05 was considered significant. To calculate Cohen's D, a short Python script was used.

5. Conclusions

The cellular mechanisms of neuronal ischaemic damage are incredibly complex and effective neuroprotection is—as desired as it might be for all professionals working in that field—still a long way down the road. The idea of only targeting one of the mechanisms, while ischemia activates a symphony of potentially harmful pathways, is probably too simplistic. Nevertheless, the role of calcium is crucial, and the interplay of different calcium channels and their respective effect on cell injury needs further research efforts. Nimodipine remains a hot topic in SAH research mainly due to its vascular effect. Based on encouraging recent findings of a possible calcium-independent effect of nimodipine on microglia [67], we suggest to additionally add a perspective of possible neuro-regeneration to the list of experimental questions, as well as further observing effects on the microvasculature.

We again want to stress that in vitro experiments using DMSO as a solvent should be evaluated critically, since the popular drug vehicle interacts with neuronal damage mechanisms.

Author Contributions: Conceptualization, J.O., U.L., M.C., and A.H.; methodology, J.O., B.K., L.G., U.L., and M.C.; software, J.O.; validation, J.O., U.L., and A.H.; formal analysis, J.O.; investigation, J.O.; resources, H.C. and M.C.; data curation, J.O.; writing—original draft preparation, J.O.; writing—review and editing, all.; visualization, J.O.; supervision, U.L., R.B.-D., and A.H.; project administration, U.L.; funding acquisition, H.C., U.L., and A.H. All authors have read and agreed to the published version of the manuscript.

Acknowledgments: The authors want to thank Joachim Weis and the Institute of Neuropathology, RWTH Aachen University for their support especially regarding the use of laboratory infrastructure. In addition, we thank Tamara Fechter and Lisa Liebenstund for their support in laboratory work and maintenance. Lastly, the first author wants to thank Patrick Emonts for his tutoring in python and the help in the initial scripts used for the data analysis.

Abbreviations

ASIC	Acid-sensing ion channel
DCI	Delayed cerebral ischaemia
DMSO	Dimethyl-sulfoxide
OGD	Oxygen–glucose deprivation
PI	Propidium iodide
SAH	Subarachnoid haemorrhage

Appendix A

Table A1. Overview of all experimental regimes.

OGD/Control	Vol.% DMSO	Nimodipine Concentration in µM	Amiloride Concentration in µM	n Slices	Median	95% CI (Lower–Upper)
Control	-	-	-	101	0.02308	0.01774–0.03227
Control	0.1	-	-	25	0.03409	0.01500–0.05189
Control	1.0	-	-	12	0.06632	0.01006–0.3592
Control	1.0	-	100	63	0.1470	0.09480–0.1877
Control	2.0	-	-	20	0.7912	0.3633–1.253
Control	2.0	-	100	6	0.02141	0.000–0.1145
OGD	-	-	-	96	0.8978	0.8099–1.118
OGD	0.1	-	-	41	1.261	0.8406–1.697
OGD	0.1	10	-	77	0.7449	0.4920–1.027
OGD	0.1	20	-	64	1.152	0.9478–1.471
OGD	1.0	-	-	19	0.4013	0.2374–0.6065
OGD	1.0	10	-	30	0.6925	0.3331–1.012
OGD	1.0	20	-	25	0.5422	0.2462–0.8696
OGD	1.0	-	100	50	0.6901	0.4543–0.8942
OGD	1.1	10	100	56	0.7106	0.4539–0.8876
OGD	1.1	20	100	59	0.7777	0.5228–1.001
OGD	2.0	-	-	45	0.8082	0.5730–1.515
OGD	2.0	-	100	43	1.172	1.067–1.353
OGD	2.0	10	100	47	2.147	1.775–3.085
OGD	2.0	20	100	46	2.563	1.526–2.939

Appendix B

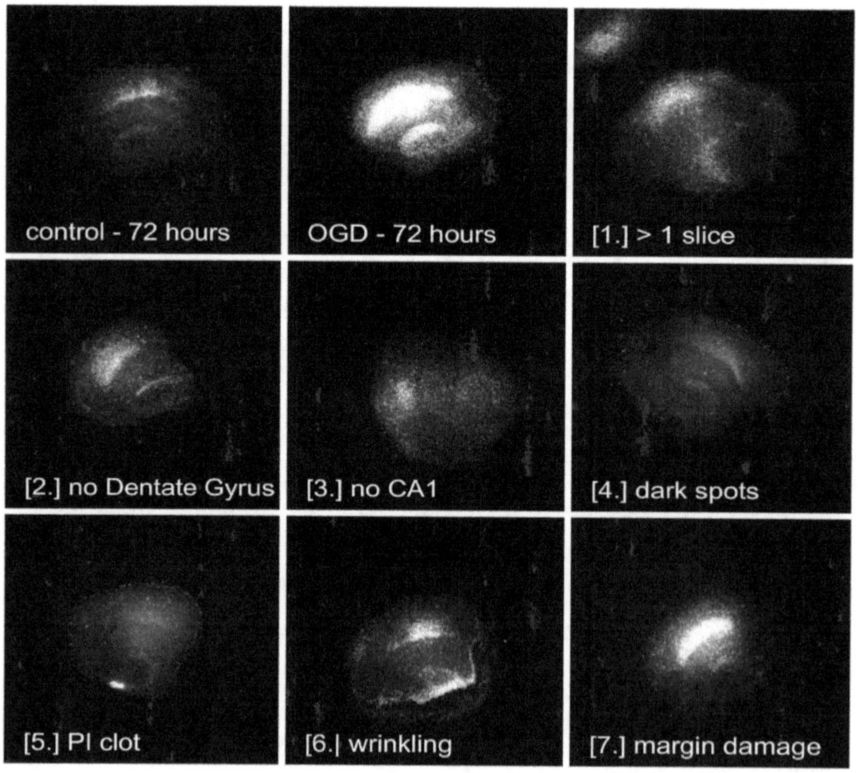

Figure A1. Example slices for our exclusion criteria. Upper left and middle picture show normal slices at 72 h after OGD or control, respectively. [1.] Image files with more than one slice were excluded. If the dentate gyrus [2.] or the CA1 region [3.] were not or only unreliably identifiable, slices were excluded. [4.] Dark spots and [7.] inhomogeneous margins are likely due to imprecise preparation technique, while [6.] wrinkling is most likely caused by problems in the culturing process. Lastly, [5.] on a few slices, PI clots were present. Again, slice images are red-channel-filtered and contrast-enhanced. Contrast enhancement does not change grey scale values and is purely performed to ensure a more comfortable visual evaluation of slice images.

The python scripts can be found at https://github.com/jonasort/OGD-analysis-scripts-in-Python. All questions may be asked to the corresponding author.

References

1. De Rooij, N.K.; Linn, F.H.; van der Plas, J.A.; Algra, A.; Rinkel, G.J. Incidence of subarachnoid haemorrhage: A systematic review with emphasis on region, age, gender and time trends. *J. Neurol. Neurosurg. Psychiatry* **2007**, *78*, 1365–1372. [CrossRef] [PubMed]
2. Peeters, W.; van den Brande, R.; Polinder, S.; Brazinova, A.; Steyerberg, E.W.; Lingsma, H.F.; Maas, A.I. Epidemiology of traumatic brain injury in Europe. *Acta Neurochir.* **2015**, *157*, 1683–1696. [CrossRef] [PubMed]
3. Schanne, F.A.; Kane, A.B.; Young, E.E.; Farber, J.L. Calcium dependence of toxic cell death: A final common pathway. *Science* **1979**, *206*, 700–702. [CrossRef] [PubMed]
4. Siesjo, B.K. Calcium and cell death. *Magnesium* **1989**, *8*, 223–237. [PubMed]
5. Siesjo, B.K.; Bengtsson, F.; Grampp, W.; Theander, S. Calcium, excitotoxins, and neuronal death in the brain. *Ann. N. Y. Acad. Sci.* **1989**, *568*, 234–251. [CrossRef]
6. Dubinsky, J.M. Examination of the role of calcium in neuronal death. *Ann. N. Y. Acad. Sci.* **1993**, *679*, 34–42. [CrossRef]
7. Dubinsky, J.M. Intracellular calcium levels during the period of delayed excitotoxicity. *J. Neurosci.* **1993**, *13*, 623–631. [CrossRef]
8. Wahlgren, N.G.; Ahmed, N. Neuroprotection in cerebral ischaemia: Facts and fancies–the need for new approaches. *Cerebrovasc. Dis.* **2004**, 153–166. [CrossRef]
9. O'Bryant, Z.; Vann, K.T.; Xiong, Z.G. Translational strategies for neuroprotection in ischemic stroke–focusing on acid-sensing ion channel 1a. *Transl. Stroke Res.* **2014**, *5*, 59–68. [CrossRef]
10. D'Souza, S. Aneurysmal Subarachnoid Hemorrhage. *J. Neurosurg. Anesthesiol.* **2015**, *27*, 222–240. [CrossRef]
11. Pala, A.; Schick, J.; Klein, M.; Mayer, B.; Schmitz, B.; Wirtz, C.R.; Konig, R.; Kapapa, T. The influence of nimodipine and vasopressors on outcome in patients with delayed cerebral ischemia after spontaneous subarachnoid hemorrhage. *J. Neurosurg.* **2019**. [CrossRef]
12. Lawton, M.T.; Vates, G.E. Subarachnoid Hemorrhage. *N. Eng. J. Med.* **2017**, *377*, 257–266. [CrossRef] [PubMed]
13. Dorhout Mees, S.M.; Rinkel, G.J.; Feigin, V.L.; Algra, A.; van den Bergh, W.M.; Vermeulen, M.; van Gijn, J. Calcium antagonists for aneurysmal subarachnoid haemorrhage. *Cochrane Database Syst. Rev.* **2007**. [CrossRef] [PubMed]
14. Pickard, J.D.; Murray, G.D.; Illingworth, R.; Shaw, M.D.; Teasdale, G.M.; Foy, P.M.; Humphrey, P.R.; Lang, D.A.; Nelson, R.; Richards, P.; et al. Effect of oral nimodipine on cerebral infarction and outcome after subarachnoid haemorrhage: British aneurysm nimodipine trial. *BMJ* **1989**, *298*, 636–642. [CrossRef] [PubMed]
15. Ohman, J.; Heiskanen, O. Effect of nimodipine on the outcome of patients after aneurysmal subarachnoid hemorrhage and surgery. *J. Neurosurg.* **1988**, *69*, 683–686. [CrossRef] [PubMed]
16. Towart, R.; Kazda, S. The cellular mechanism of action of nimodipine (BAY e 9736), a new calcium antagonist. *Br. J. Pharmacol.* **1979**, *67*, 409P–410P. [CrossRef] [PubMed]
17. Petruk, K.C.; West, M.; Mohr, G.; Weir, B.K.; Benoit, B.G.; Gentili, F.; Disney, L.B.; Khan, M.I.; Grace, M.; Holness, R.O.; et al. Nimodipine treatment in poor-grade aneurysm patients. Results of a multicenter double-blind placebo-controlled trial. *J. Neurosurg.* **1988**, *68*, 505–517. [CrossRef]
18. Uematsu, D.; Greenberg, J.H.; Hickey, W.F.; Reivich, M. Nimodipine attenuates both increase in cytosolic free calcium and histologic damage following focal cerebral ischemia and reperfusion in cats. *Stroke* **1989**, *20*, 1531–1537. [CrossRef]

19. Greiner, C.; Schmidinger, A.; Hulsmann, S.; Moskopp, D.; Wolfer, J.; Kohling, R.; Speckmann, E.J.; Wassmann, H. Acute protective effect of nimodipine and dimethyl sulfoxide against hypoxic and ischemic damage in brain slices. *Brain Res.* **2000**, *887*, 316–322. [CrossRef]
20. Krieglstein, J.; Lippert, K.; Poch, G. Apparent independent action of nimodipine and glutamate antagonists to protect cultured neurons against glutamate-induced damage. *Neuropharmacology* **1996**, *35*, 1737–1742. [CrossRef]
21. Pisani, A.; Calabresi, P.; Tozzi, A.; D'Angelo, V.; Bernardi, G. L-type Ca2+ channel blockers attenuate electrical changes and Ca2+ rise induced by oxygen/glucose deprivation in cortical neurons. *Stroke* **1998**, *29*, 196–201; discussion 202. [CrossRef] [PubMed]
22. Kass, I.S.; Cottrell, J.E.; Chambers, G. Magnesium and cobalt, not nimodipine, protect neurons against anoxic damage in the rat hippocampal slice. *Anesthesiology* **1988**, *69*, 710–715. [CrossRef] [PubMed]
23. Goldberg, M.P.; Choi, D.W. Combined oxygen and glucose deprivation in cortical cell culture: Calcium-dependent and calcium-independent mechanisms of neuronal injury. *J. Neurosci* **1993**, *13*, 3510–3524. [CrossRef] [PubMed]
24. Small, D.L.; Monette, R.; Buchan, A.M.; Morley, P. Identification of calcium channels involved in neuronal injury in rat hippocampal slices subjected to oxygen and glucose deprivation. *Brain Res.* **1997**, *753*, 209–218. [CrossRef]
25. Martinez-Sanchez, M.; Striggow, F.; Schroder, U.H.; Kahlert, S.; Reymann, K.G.; Reiser, G. Na(+) and Ca(2+) homeostasis pathways, cell death and protection after oxygen-glucose-deprivation in organotypic hippocampal slice cultures. *Neuroscience* **2004**, *128*, 729–740. [CrossRef]
26. Waldmann, R.; Champigny, G.; Bassilana, F.; Heurteaux, C.; Lazdunski, M. A proton-gated cation channel involved in acid-sensing. *Nature* **1997**, *386*, 173–177. [CrossRef]
27. Xiong, Z.G.; Zhu, X.M.; Chu, X.P.; Minami, M.; Hey, J.; Wei, W.L.; MacDonald, J.F.; Wemmie, J.A.; Price, M.P.; Welsh, M.J.; et al. Neuroprotection in ischemia: Blocking calcium-permeable acid-sensing ion channels. *Cell* **2004**, *118*, 687–698. [CrossRef]
28. Xiong, Z.G.; Chu, X.P.; Simon, R.P. Ca2+ -permeable acid-sensing ion channels and ischemic brain injury. *J. Membr. Biol* **2006**, *209*, 59–68. [CrossRef]
29. Yermolaieva, O.; Leonard, A.S.; Schnizler, M.K.; Abboud, F.M.; Welsh, M.J. Extracellular acidosis increases neuronal cell calcium by activating acid-sensing ion channel 1a. *Proc. Natl. Acad. Sci. USA* **2004**, *101*, 6752–6757. [CrossRef]
30. Pignataro, G.; Simon, R.P.; Xiong, Z.G. Prolonged activation of ASIC1a and the time window for neuroprotection in cerebral ischaemia. *Brain* **2007**, *130*, 151–158. [CrossRef]
31. Osmakov, D.I.; Andreev, Y.A.; Kozlov, S.A. Acid-sensing ion channels and their modulators. *Biochemistry* **2014**, *79*, 1528–1545. [CrossRef] [PubMed]
32. Paukert, M.; Babini, E.; Pusch, M.; Grunder, S. Identification of the Ca2+ blocking site of acid-sensing ion channel (ASIC) 1: Implications for channel gating. *J. Gen. Physiol.* **2004**, *124*, 383–394. [CrossRef] [PubMed]
33. Babini, E.; Paukert, M.; Geisler, H.S.; Grunder, S. Alternative splicing and interaction with di- and polyvalent cations control the dynamic range of acid-sensing ion channel 1 (ASIC1). *J. Biol. Chem.* **2002**, *277*, 41597–41603. [CrossRef] [PubMed]
34. Harris, R.J.; Symon, L.; Branston, N.M.; Bayhan, M. Changes in extracellular calcium activity in cerebral ischaemia. *J. Cereb. Blood Flow Metab.* **1981**, *1*, 203–209. [CrossRef] [PubMed]
35. Loetscher, P.D.; Rossaint, J.; Rossaint, R.; Weis, J.; Fries, M.; Fahlenkamp, A.; Ryang, Y.M.; Grottke, O.; Coburn, M. Argon: Neuroprotection in in vitro models of cerebral ischemia and traumatic brain injury. *Crit. Care* **2009**, *13*, R206. [CrossRef] [PubMed]
36. Dirnagl, U.; Iadecola, C.; Moskowitz, M.A. Pathobiology of ischaemic stroke: An integrated view. *Trends Neurosci.* **1999**, *22*, 391–397. [CrossRef]
37. Ogawa, S.; Kitao, Y.; Hori, O. Ischemia-induced neuronal cell death and stress response. *Antioxid. Redox. Signal.* **2007**, *9*, 573–587. [CrossRef]
38. Gelmers, H.J.; Gorter, K.; de Weerdt, C.J.; Wiezer, H.J. A controlled trial of nimodipine in acute ischemic stroke. *N. Engl. J. Med.* **1988**, *318*, 203–207. [CrossRef]
39. Lee, K.S.; Lee, K.C.; Choi, J.U. Clinical trial of a calcium channel blocker in patients with aneurysmal subarachnoid hemorrhage–prevention of delayed ischemic deficits. *Yonsei Med. J.* **1987**, *28*, 126–130. [CrossRef]

40. Rowland, M.J.; Hadjipavlou, G.; Kelly, M.; Westbrook, J.; Pattinson, K.T. Delayed cerebral ischaemia after subarachnoid haemorrhage: Looking beyond vasospasm. *Br. J. Anaesth.* **2012**, *109*, 315–329. [CrossRef]
41. Won, S.J.; Kim, D.Y.; Gwag, B.J. Cellular and molecular pathways of ischemic neuronal death. *J. Biochem. Mol. Biol.* **2002**, *35*, 67–86. [CrossRef] [PubMed]
42. Kass, I.S.; Lipton, P. Calcium and long-term transmission damage following anoxia in dentate gyrus and CA1 regions of the rat hippocampal slice. *J. Physiol.* **1986**, *378*, 313–334. [CrossRef] [PubMed]
43. Benveniste, H.; Jorgensen, M.B.; Diemer, N.H.; Hansen, A.J. Calcium accumulation by glutamate receptor activation is involved in hippocampal cell damage after ischemia. *Acta Neurol. Scand.* **1988**, *78*, 529–536. [CrossRef] [PubMed]
44. Lu, C.; Mattson, M.P. Dimethyl sulfoxide suppresses NMDA- and AMPA-induced ion currents and calcium influx and protects against excitotoxic death in hippocampal neurons. *Exp. Neurol.* **2001**, *170*, 180–185. [CrossRef] [PubMed]
45. Yuan, C.; Gao, J.Y.; Guo, J.C.; Bai, L.; Marshall, C.; Cai, Z.Y.; Wang, L.M.; Xiao, M. Dimethyl Sulfoxide Damages Mitochondrial Integrity and Membrane Potential in Cultured Astrocytes. *PLoS ONE* **2014**, *9*. [CrossRef] [PubMed]
46. Xiong, Z.G.; Pignataro, G.; Li, M.; Chang, S.Y.; Simon, R.P. Acid-sensing ion channels (ASICs) as pharmacological targets for neurodegenerative diseases. *Curr. Opin. Pharmacol.* **2008**, *8*, 25–32. [CrossRef] [PubMed]
47. Macdonald, R.L.; Kassell, N.F.; Mayer, S.; Ruefenacht, D.; Schmiedek, P.; Weidauer, S.; Frey, A.; Roux, S.; Pasqualin, A.; CONSCIOUS-1 Investigators. Clazosentan to overcome neurological ischemia and infarction occurring after subarachnoid hemorrhage (CONSCIOUS-1): Randomized, double-blind, placebo-controlled phase 2 dose-finding trial. *Stroke* **2008**, *39*, 3015–3021. [CrossRef]
48. Vergouwen, M.D.; Vermeulen, M.; Coert, B.A.; Stroes, E.S.; Roos, Y.B. Microthrombosis after aneurysmal subarachnoid hemorrhage: An additional explanation for delayed cerebral ischemia. *J. Cereb. Blood Flow Metab.* **2008**, *28*, 1761–1770. [CrossRef]
49. Suzuki, S.; Kimura, M.; Souma, M.; Ohkima, H.; Shimizu, T.; Iwabuchi, T. Cerebral microthrombosis in symptomatic cerebral vasospasm–a quantitative histological study in autopsy cases. *Neurol. Med. Chir.* **1990**, *30*, 309–316. [CrossRef]
50. Friedrich, B.; Muller, F.; Feiler, S.; Scholler, K.; Plesnila, N. Experimental subarachnoid hemorrhage causes early and long-lasting microarterial constriction and microthrombosis: An in-vivo microscopy study. *J. Cereb. Blood Flow Metab.* **2012**, *32*, 447–455. [CrossRef]
51. Wellman, G.C.; Koide, M. Impact of subarachnoid hemorrhage on parenchymal arteriolar function. *Acta Neurochir. Suppl.* **2013**, *115*, 173–177. [CrossRef] [PubMed]
52. Budohoski, K.P.; Guilfoyle, M.; Helmy, A.; Huuskonen, T.; Czosnyka, M.; Kirollos, R.; Menon, D.K.; Pickard, J.D.; Kirkpatrick, P.J. The pathophysiology and treatment of delayed cerebral ischaemia following subarachnoid haemorrhage. *J. Neurol. Neurosurg. Psychiatry* **2014**, *85*, 1343–1353. [CrossRef] [PubMed]
53. Lucke-Wold, B.P.; Logsdon, A.F.; Manoranjan, B.; Turner, R.C.; McConnell, E.; Vates, G.E.; Huber, J.D.; Rosen, C.L.; Simard, J.M. Aneurysmal Subarachnoid Hemorrhage and Neuroinflammation: A Comprehensive Review. *Int. J. Mol. Sci.* **2016**, *17*, 497. [CrossRef] [PubMed]
54. de Oliveira Manoel, A.L.; Macdonald, R.L. Neuroinflammation as a Target for Intervention in Subarachnoid Hemorrhage. *Front. Neurol.* **2018**, *9*, 292. [CrossRef]
55. Dreier, J.P.; Major, S.; Manning, A.; Woitzik, J.; Drenckhahn, C.; Steinbrink, J.; Tolias, C.; Oliveira-Ferreira, A.I.; Fabricius, M.; Hartings, J.A.; et al. Cortical spreading ischaemia is a novel process involved in ischaemic damage in patients with aneurysmal subarachnoid haemorrhage. *Brain* **2009**, *132*, 1866–1881. [CrossRef]
56. Di Giorgio, A.M.; Hou, Y.; Zhao, X.; Zhang, B.; Lyeth, B.G.; Russell, M.J. Dimethyl sulfoxide provides neuroprotection in a traumatic brain injury model. *Restor. Neurol. Neurosci.* **2008**, *26*, 501–507.
57. Shimizu, S.; Simon, R.P.; Graham, S.H. Dimethylsulfoxide (DMSO) treatment reduces infarction volume after permanent focal cerebral ischemia in rats. *Neurosci. Lett.* **1997**, *239*, 125–127. [CrossRef]
58. Phillis, J.W.; Estevez, A.Y.; O'Regan, M.H. Protective effects of the free radical scavengers, dimethyl sulfoxide and ethanol, in cerebral ischemia in gerbils. *Neurosci. Lett.* **1998**, *244*, 109–111. [CrossRef]
59. Stoppini, L.; Buchs, P.-A.; Muller, D. A simple method for organotypic cultures of nervous tissue. *J. Neurosci. Methods* **1991**, *37*, 173–182. [CrossRef]

60. Galvao, J.; Davis, B.; Tilley, M.; Normando, E.; Duchen, M.R.; Cordeiro, M.F. Unexpected low-dose toxicity of the universal solvent DMSO. *FASEB J.* **2014**, *28*, 1317–1330. [CrossRef]
61. Zhang, C.; Deng, Y.; Dai, H.; Zhou, W.; Tian, J.; Bing, G.; Zhao, L. Effects of dimethyl sulfoxide on the morphology and viability of primary cultured neurons and astrocytes. *Brain Res. Bull.* **2017**, *128*, 34–39. [CrossRef] [PubMed]
62. Nasrallah, F.A.; Garner, B.; Ball, G.E.; Rae, C. Modulation of brain metabolism by very low concentrations of the commonly used drug delivery vehicle dimethyl sulfoxide (DMSO). *J. Neurosci. Res.* **2008**, *86*, 208–214. [CrossRef] [PubMed]
63. Grüßer, L.; Blaumeiser-Debarry, R.; Krings, M.; Kremer, B.; Höllig, A.; Rossaint, R.; Coburn, M. Argon attenuates the emergence of secondary injury after traumatic brain injury within a 2-hour incubation period compared to desflurane: An in vitro study. *Med. Gas. Res.* **2017**, *7*, 93–100. [CrossRef] [PubMed]
64. Macklis, J.D.; Madison, R.D. Progressive incorporation of propidium iodide in cultured mouse neurons correlates with declining electrophysiological status: A fluorescence scale of membrane integrity. *J. Neurosci. Methods* **1990**, *31*, 43–46. [CrossRef]
65. Brayton, C.F. Dimethyl sulfoxide (DMSO): A review. *Cornell Vet.* **1986**, *76*, 61–90. [PubMed]
66. Krings, M.; Höllig, A.; Liu, J.; Grüßer, L.; Rossaint, R.; Coburn, M. Desflurane impairs outcome of organotypic hippocampal slices in an in vitro model of traumatic brain injury. *Med. Gas. Res.* **2016**, *6*, 3–9. [CrossRef]
67. Schampel, A.; Volovitch, O.; Koeniger, T.; Scholz, C.J.; Jorg, S.; Linker, R.A.; Wischmeyer, E.; Wunsch, M.; Hell, J.W.; Ergun, S.; et al. Nimodipine fosters remyelination in a mouse model of multiple sclerosis and induces microglia-specific apoptosis. *Proc. Natl. Acad. Sci. USA* **2017**, *114*, E3295–E3304. [CrossRef]

9

Neurotrophic Factor BDNF, Physiological Functions and Therapeutic Potential in Depression, Neurodegeneration and Brain Cancer

Luca Colucci-D'Amato [1,2,*], Luisa Speranza [3] and Floriana Volpicelli [4]

1 Department of Environmental, Biological and Pharmaceutical Sciences and Technologies, University of Campania "Luigi Vanvitelli", 81100 Caserta, Italy
2 InterUniversity Center for Research in Neurosciences (CIRN), University of Campania "Luigi Vanvitelli", 80131 Naples, Italy
3 Department of Neuroscience, Albert Einstein College of Medicine, New York, NY 10461, USA; luisa.speranza@einsteinmed.org
4 Department of Pharmacy, School of Medicine and Surgery, University of Naples Federico II, 80131 Naples, Italy; floriana.volpicelli@unina.it
* Correspondence: luca.colucci@unicampania.it

Abstract: Brain-derived neurotrophic factor (BDNF) is one of the most distributed and extensively studied neurotrophins in the mammalian brain. BDNF signals through the tropomycin receptor kinase B (TrkB) and the low affinity p75 neurotrophin receptor (p75NTR). BDNF plays an important role in proper growth, development, and plasticity of glutamatergic and GABAergic synapses and through modulation of neuronal differentiation, it influences serotonergic and dopaminergic neurotransmission. BDNF acts as paracrine and autocrine factor, on both pre-synaptic and post-synaptic target sites. It is crucial in the transformation of synaptic activity into long-term synaptic memories. BDNF is considered an instructive mediator of functional and structural plasticity in the central nervous system (CNS), influencing dendritic spines and, at least in the hippocampus, the adult neurogenesis. Changes in the rate of adult neurogenesis and in spine density can influence several forms of learning and memory and can contribute to depression-like behaviors. The possible roles of BDNF in neuronal plasticity highlighted in this review focus on the effect of antidepressant therapies on BDNF-mediated plasticity. Moreover, we will review data that illustrate the role of BDNF as a potent protective factor that is able to confer protection against neurodegeneration, in particular in Alzheimer's disease. Finally, we will give evidence of how the involvement of BDNF in the pathogenesis of brain glioblastoma has emerged, thus opening new avenues for the treatment of this deadly cancer.

Keywords: BDNF; miRNAs; neurogenesis; synaptic plasticity; depression; neurodegeneration; glioblastoma

---

1. Introduction

The neurotrophin BDNF is one of the most studied and well characterized neurotrophic factors in the CNS. It regulates many different cellular processes involved in the development and maintenance of normal brain function by binding and activating the TrkB, a member of the larger family of Trk receptors. In the brain, BDNF is expressed by glutamatergic neurons [1], glial cells, such as astrocytes isolated from the cortex and hippocampus, but not from the striatum [2], and microglia [3]. During embryogenesis, BDNF–TrkB signaling promotes the differentiation of cortical progenitor cells and later promotes differentiation of cortical progenitor cells into neurons (i.e., neurogenesis) [4]. Several lines of evidence also suggest that the BDNF/TrkB signaling is involved in adult neurogenesis in the hippocampus with differing effects in the dentate gyrus (DG) and subventricular zone (SVZ) [5].

Adult neurogenesis in the dentate gyrus is enhanced by voluntary exercise, exposure to an enriched environment, and chronic antidepressant administration. Recently, it has also been proposed that caloric restriction and intermittent fasting in particular, appears to positively modulate hippocampal neurogenesis and BDNF [6]. The connection between BDNF and the modulation of hippocampal neurogenesis by external stimuli is a topic that has been extensively studied in recent years [7]. It has been demonstrated that voluntary physical exercise, like an enriched environment, increases expression of BDNF in the hippocampus [8], as well as hippocampal neurogenesis [9]. Physical exercise is one particularly effective strategy for increasing circulating levels of BDNF [10,11] and improving brain function [12–14].

In addition, studies also show that BDNF is an important regulator of synaptic transmission and long-term potentiation (LTP) in the hippocampus and in other brain regions. The effects of BDNF on LTP are mediated by the TrkB receptor. Especially in the hippocampus, this neurotrophin is thought to act on both the pre- and post-synaptic compartments, modulating synaptic efficacy, either by changing the pre-synaptic transmitter release, or by increasing post-synaptic transmitter sensitivity [15,16] to induce a long-lasting increase in synaptic plasticity. Additionally, converging data now suggest a role for BDNF in the pathophysiology of brain-associated illnesses. Deficits in BDNF signaling are reported to contribute to the pathogenesis of several major diseases, such as Huntington's disease, Alzheimer's disease (AD), depression, schizophrenia, bipolar, and anxiety disorders. Thus, manipulating the BDNF signaling may present a viable approach to treat a variety of neurological and psychiatric disorders. BDNF protein is also detectable outside of the nervous system in several non-neuronal tissues, such as in endothelial cells [17,18], cardiomyocytes [19], vascular smooth muscle cells [17], leukocytes [20], platelets [21,22], and megakaryocytes [19]. Therefore, it may also be involved in cancer, angiogenesis, reduction of glucose production from the liver [23], and in the uptake of glucose in peripheral tissues (see [24] for review). In addition, BDNF promotes the development of neuromuscular synapses and is required for fiber-type specification, suggesting a potential role as a therapeutic target in muscle diseases [25]. In this review, first we examine the currently known mechanisms of BDNF signaling, information essential for the creation of BDNF-based therapeutics. Next, we focus on the effects of antidepressants on BDNF-mediated plasticity. Additionally, we highlight the function of BDNF as a potent factor capable of conferring protection against neurodegeneration. Finally, we touch on the newly emerging role of BDNF in the pathogenesis of brain gliomas.

2. The Human BDNF Gene: Transcripts and Variants

2.1. BDNF Transcripts

The *BDNF* gene codes for a neurotrophin that is highly expressed in the CNS [26]. At the beginning of 2000s, the only data available about the structure and regulation of the *BDNF* gene were from Timmusk and colleagues, which identified in rats four 5′ exons linked to separate promoters and one 3′ exon encoding the preproBDNF protein [27–29]. These four *BDNF* promoters owned multiple points of *BDNF* mRNA regulation and suggested an activity-dependent regulation [28–31]. Further studies, published in 2007, clarified that *BDNF* has a complex gene structure with 11 different exons in humans, nine different exons in rodents, and nine alternative promoters for both groups [32,33]. Despite this complexity, the coding sequence is located in exon IX in both human and rodents. The latter includes the common sequence that encodes for the proBDNF protein. All other exons are untranslated regions with a start codon present in exons I, VII, VIII, and IX of the human *BDNF* gene. Exon IX is present in all BDNF mRNA isoforms. It is supposed that the nine alternative promoters can regulate the complex spatio-temporal expression of *BDNF* gene and allow BDNF to respond to a greater variety of stimuli. For instance, in human brain tissues, all exons are expressed, but to different degrees and in different brain structures [33]. Human heart tissue, instead, expresses high levels of *BDNF* isoforms containing exon IV and exon IX [33].

Currently, two *BDNF* promoters, promoter I and promoter IV, have been well characterized for their response after the activation of the L-type voltage gated calcium channel (L-VGCC) or the n-methyl-d-aspartate (NMDA) receptor. Activation of L-VGCC and NMDA receptors mediate intracellular Ca^{2+}-signaling and regulate several aspects of brain functions (for review [34,35]). Promoter I is more responsive to neuronal activity and induces activity-dependent expression of BDNF in vitro and in vivo. It contains calcium-responsive elements (CaREs) and cyclic adenosine monophosphate (cAMP)/calcium response element (CRE) [29,36–38]. Deletion of CRE or overexpression of dominant negative of CREB (cAMP-response element-binding protein) significantly impairs rat BDNF promoter I response to neuronal depolarization [38]. Human BDNF promoter I is similar to rat promoter, since an orthologous CRE-like element is also present [39]. However, mutation of this site did not affect human *BDNF* promoter I response to depolarization [39]. Human BDNF promoter I also contains an activator protein 1 (AP1) -like element and an asymmetric E-box-like element [39]. Mutation in E-box-like element reduces human *BDNF* promoter I induction, impairing the response to neuronal depolarization [39].

Another highly characterized *BDNF* promoter is the *BDNF* promoter IV that contributes significantly to activity-dependent *BDNF* transcription. Human and rat *BDNF* promoter IV are similar. In this promoter, three CaREs and three other regulatory elements involved in regulating rat *BDNF* promoter response to NMDA receptor activation have been identified [40]. NMDA receptor activation is capable of triggering *BDNF* exon IV transcription through a protein-signaling cascade requiring extracellular signal-regulated kinase (ERK), Ca^{2+}/calmodulin-dependent protein kinase (CaMK) II/IV, phosphoinositide 3-kinases (PI3K), and phospholipase C (PLC). *BDNF* exon IV expression also seems capable of further stimulating its own expression through TrkB activation [41]. Additionally to the CaREs, two positive regulators have been identified: the NF-kB (nuclear factor kappa-light-chain-enhancer of activated B cells) [42] and NFAT (nuclear factor of activated T-cells) binding sites [30,43]. In contrast to these positive regulators, *BDNF* promoter IV also contains a negative regulatory element, the class B E-box. This is a binding site for a basic helix-loop-helix protein, BHLHB2, a suppressor of the bHLH gene superfamily [43,44]. NMDA treatment is able to remove BHLHB2 binding to the E-box and to increase rat *BDNF* promoter IV activity [43,44]. Disruption of *BDNF* promoter IV in mice significantly reduced the number of parvalbumin GABAergic neurons in the prefrontal cortex and impaired GABAergic activity [45]. These mice displayed depression-like behavior such as anhedonia-like behavior and increased latency to escape in the learned helplessness test [45]. Further evidence suggests a relationship between stress exposure and epigenetic regulation of *BDNF* promoter IV with the development of psychiatric disorders. Specifically, changes in *BDNF* promoter IV methylation levels are implicated in depression [46,47]. Preliminary evidence has demonstrated that patients with major depressive disorder (MDD) present a hypomethylation of the CpG-87 site of the promoter IV region of *BDNF* gene and are less likely to benefit from antidepressants [47,48]. In addition, *BDNF* disruption from promoter IV-derived transcripts impairs fear expression in mice, suggesting that cells expressing *BDNF* from promoter IV critically regulate hippocampal-prefrontal plasticity during fear memory [49,50].

2.2. miRNAs and BDNF

MicroRNAs (miRNAs) are a class of evolutionary conserved small non-coding single-strand RNA molecules, 18–25 nucleotide long, able to bind to 3′ untranslated regions (3′ UTR) of target mRNAs and promote their degradation or suppress their translation into proteins. MiRNAs are expressed abundantly within the nervous system in a tissue-specific manner and are crucial players in several biological processes, including neurogenesis, neuronal maturation, synapse formation, axon guidance, neurite outgrowth and neuronal plasticity [51–53]. Accumulating data indicate that synthesis of BDNF may be affected by miRNAs, indeed, a regulatory negative feedback loop between BDNF and miRNAs exists. That is, while BDNF treatment stimulates neuronal miRNAs expression, miRNAs generally inhibit the expression of BDNF [54]. This negative feedback loop is maintained in a state of equilibrium in normal cells. Alterations in miRNAs or in BDNF contribute to the pathogenic mechanisms involved in neurodegenerative diseases or neuropsychiatric disorders.

A number of recent studies, obtained from high throughput sequencing screening of different brain regions or from neurological disorders, have identified seven miRNAs (miR-15a, miR-206, miR-155-5p, miR-16, miR-103-3p, miR-330-3p, Let-7a-3p) correlated with BDNF [55]. Previous data published by Schratt et al. reported the involvement of miR-134 in BDNF-regulated dendritic spine size in hippocampal neurons. They demonstrate that miR-134 negatively regulates the spine size via repressing the translation of LIM kinase 1, which is known to regulate dendritic structures. BDNF is able to relieve the inhibition of LIM kinase 1 translation, and in this manner contribute to synaptic development, maturation and/or plasticity [56]. Recently, Baby et al. [57] found that miR-134 mediates post-transcriptional regulation of CREB1 and BDNF, as previously described by Gao et al. [58], who demonstrated that mutant mice lacking Sirtuin 1 (SIRT1) catalytic activity shows reduction in both CREB and BDNF proteins and upregulation of miR-134. Thus, higher levels of miR-134 negatively regulate synaptic plasticity [58]. MiR-134-mediated post-transcriptional regulation of CREB1 and BDNF prevents cognitive deficits in chronic unpredicted mild stress model (CUMS) [59]. At the same time, data published by Xin and coworkers [60] demonstrate that miR-202-3p silencing reduces the damage to hippocampal nerve in CUMS rats through the upregulation of BNDF expression. miRNAs could be an effective target also for the treatment of depression. Recent data demonstrate that miR-124-mediated post-transcriptional regulation of CREB1 and BDNF can improve depression-like behavior in a rat model [61]. Instead, miR-153 through the inhibition of activation of the JAK-STAT signaling pathway improves BDNF expression and influences the proliferative ability of hippocampal neurons in autistic mice [62].

In vitro studies have also allowed analysis of the effect of neurotoxins or anesthetic agents on miRNAs expression and in turn, on BDNF expression. For instance, differentiated PC12 cells, treated with 1-methyl-4-phenylpyridinium (MPP), show upregulation of miR-34a, miR-141, and miR-9, suggesting that perturbed expression of them may contribute to Parkinson's disease (PD)-related pathogenic processes, probably by affecting the expression of B-cell lymphoma 2 (BCL2), BDNF, and SIRT1 as potential targets [63].

Instead, studies in vitro on embryonic stem cell-derived neurons demonstrated that inhibition of miR-375 and miR-107 ameliorates ketamine-induced neurotoxicity via inverse regulation of the BDNF gene [64,65].

In summary, understanding the different functions of the various BDNF transcripts, the modulation of the expression of specific exons, and investigating the function of the BDNF-related miRNAs may represent a promising strategy to restore enduring changes in gene expression in response, for example, to environmental insults. This, in turn, might open new therapeutic perspectives for the treatment of neurodegenerative and neuropsychiatric disorders.

2.3. *Biology of BDNF*

Synthesis and maturation of BDNF is a multistage process, involving the formation of several precursor isoforms. The BDNF protein, discovered in 1982 [66], is a highly conserved protein of 247 amino acids, synthesized and folded in the endoplasmic reticulum as preproBDNF (32–35 kDa). Upon translocation to the Golgi apparatus, the signal sequence of the preregion is rapidly cleaved, and the isoform proBDNF (28–32 kDa) is generated [67]. The proBDNF is further cleaved to reach the mature isoform (mBDNF, 13 kDa) [67,68]. Intracellular proteolytic cleavage of proBDNF may occur by the subtilisin-kexin family of endoproteases such as furin, or in intracellular vesicles by convertases [69,70] (Figure 1).

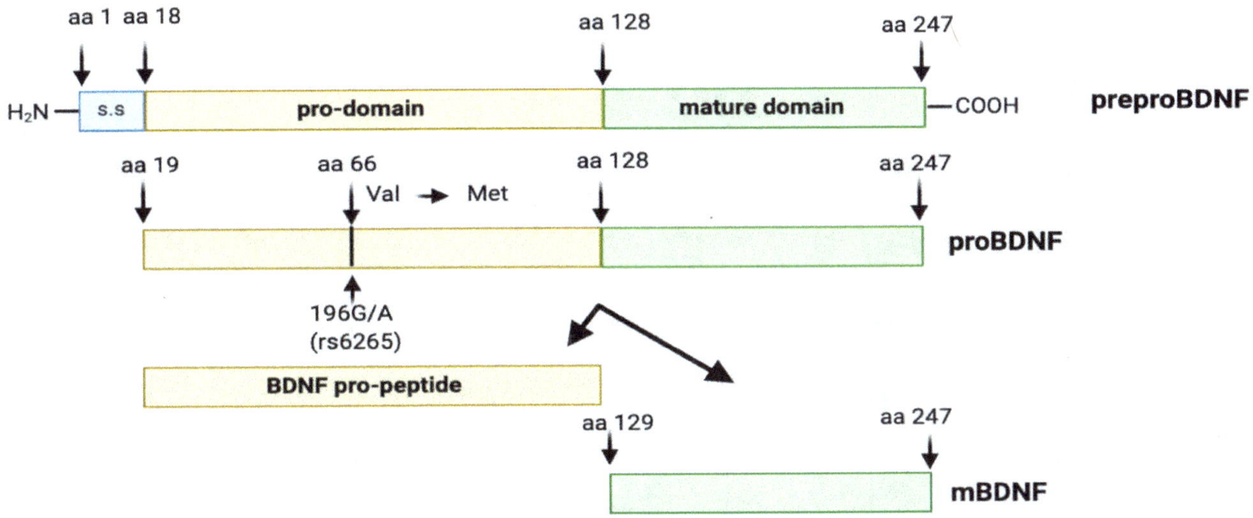

Figure 1. Brain-derived neurotrophic factor (BDNF) protein structure. The preproBDNF consists of three sequences: signal sequence (s.s), pro-domain, and mature domain. The intra- or extracellular cleavage of preproBDNF generates functionally active isoforms: BDNF pro-peptide and mature BDNF (mBDNF), each of which exhibits a characteristic affinity to a specific type of receptor. Arrowheads indicate known protease cleavage sites involved in the processing of mature BDNF. The position of the single nucleotide polymorphism (rs6265, Val66Met) and the substitution of valine (Val) in methionine (Met) at codon (aa) 66 in the human BDNF gene is indicated by an arrow.

Extracellular cleavage of proBDNF is determined by plasmin [71] and matrix metalloproteases 2 and 9 (MMP2 and MMP9) [72,73]. Depending on the cell type, BDNF can be secreted in a constitutive or activity-dependent manner [74]. In neuronal cells, both proBDNF and mBDNF are released following cell membrane depolarization [75–77]. The balance of proBDNF and mBDNF depends on the particular stages of brain development and regions. In the early postnatal period, the concentration of proBDNF is higher and may be considered as an important factor modulating brain function; while mBDNF prevails in adulthood and is important for processes occurring in adulthood, such as neuroprotection and synaptic plasticity [78]. Both proBDNF and mBDNF are active, eliciting opposing effects via the p75 neurotrophin receptor (p75NTR), a member of the tumor necrosis factor (TNF) receptor family and TrkB receptor, respectively. In resting form, both types of receptor are located in the membrane of intracellular vesicles. Stimulation with cAMP, Ca^{2+}, or electrical impulse initiates their transfer and fusion with the cellular membrane [79,80].

The mature domain of proBDNF interacts preferentially with p75NTR, mediating synaptic pruning in the prenatal brain [81]. ProBDNF, through its pro-domain, can also interact with the sortilin receptor or other vacuolar protein sorting 10 protein (Vps10p) (Figure 2). Thus, proBDNF binding to specific receptors triggers signaling pathways, which can determine neuronal fate via promoting their death or survival [82,83]. The proBDNF/p75NTR/sortilin binding complex initiates signaling cascades leading to the activation of c-Jun amino terminal kinase (JNK). This pathway is involved in neuronal apoptosis [82,83]. High levels of p75NTR expression are detected during brain development and post-traumatic recovery [84]. When mature domain of BDNF binds to p75NTR, the RIP2 (serine/threonine-protein kinase 2)/TRAF6 (tumor necrosis factor receptor associated factor 6)-mediated pathway is initiated, which leads to NF-kB activation [82,85]. The activation of NF-kB promotes neuronal survival and maintenance during brain development [85]. In addition, p75NTR interacts also with the Ras homologous (Rho) protein family. This pathway is reported to regulate neuronal growth cone development and motility [85].

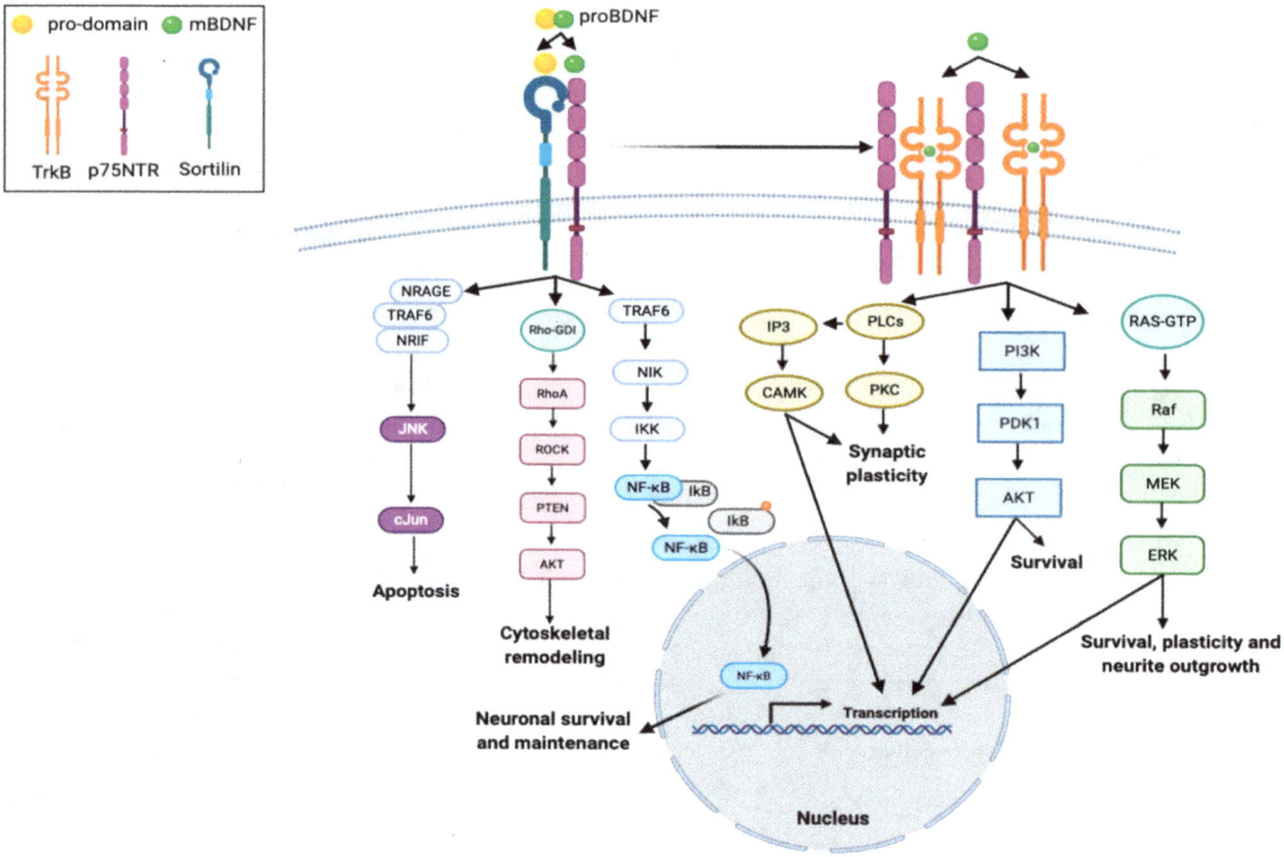

Figure 2. Intracellular signaling cascades activated by interaction of BDNF isoforms with its receptors. proBDNF and mBDNF bind to different receptors, respectively. The mBDNF isoform exhibits highest affinity for the tyrosine kinase B receptor (TrkB) receptor, which when stimulated undergoes homodimerization and autophosphorylation, but also binds the low affinity neurotrophin receptor p75NTR. The interaction between the TrkB receptor and the p75NTR receptor in a complex increases the ligand binding affinity to BDNF. Sortilin is considered a co-receptor for p75NTR. The proBDNF isoform, consisting of two sequences (pro-domain and mature domain), interacts with specific receptors, sortilin and p75NTR, respectively. The binding of proBDNF to a p75NTR/sortilin-complex induces signaling pathways that are specific for proBDNF. The binding of proBDNF in combination with sortilin causes the involvement of neurotrophin receptor-interacting factor (NRIF), tumor necrosis factor receptor-associated factor 6 (TRAF6), and neurotrophin receptor-interacting MAGE homologue (NRAGE) proteins. This pathway activates the JNK-associated pathway that promotes programmed cell death, or the receptor-interacting serine/threonine-protein kinase 2 (RIP2) /TRAF6-mediated pathway is initiated. Multi-subunit IκB kinase (IKK) phosphorylates (orange dot) the inhibitor of kB (IkB) protein, which results in dissociation of IkB from NF-κB. The activated nuclear factor kappa B (NF-kB) is then translocated into the nucleus where it binds to specific sequences of DNA and promotes neuronal survival and maintenance. In addition, p75NTR interacts with the Rho family of proteins, whose activation mediates the activity of Rho-associated protein kinase (ROCK), which subsequently leads to activation of the AKT pathway, involved in cytoskeletal remodeling. The mBDNF/TrkB receptor complex triggers signaling pathways associated with activation of phosphatidylinositol 3-kinase (PI3K), phospholipase C gamma (PLC-γ), and GTP-ases of the Rho family, involved in survival, plasticity and neurite outgrowth, transcription regulation, and synaptic plasticity.

mBDNF binds with the high-affinity TrkB receptor, the receptor dimerizes, and the intracellular tyrosine residues are autophosphorylated [86]. Phosphorylated-TrkB activates several enzymes: PI3K, mitogen-activated protein kinase (MAPK), PLC-γ, and guanosine triphosphate hydrolases (GTP-ases) of the Rho gene family [87–89]. mBDNF-TrkB-signaling pathways regulate multiple events, such as apoptosis and survival of neurons [90–92], dendritic growth [93–96], spine maturation and stabilization, development of synapses [96–98], learning- and memory-processes-dependent synaptic plasticity [99,100].

PI3K/Akt-related pathway exerts antiapoptotic and pro-survival activity and modulates NMDA receptor-dependent synaptic plasticity [101–103]. The PI3K/Akt/mTOR cascade enhances dendritic growth and branching through regulation of protein synthesis and cytoskeleton development [104,105].

The MAPK/Ras-signaling cascade regulates protein synthesis during neuronal differentiation [85] and is also required for the activation of ERK 1/2 and CREB [106,107]. This pathway is crucial not only for early response gene expression (e.g., c-Fos), but also for cytoskeleton protein synthesis (e.g., Arc and cypin) [87], as well as dendritic growth and branching in hippocampal neurons [94,108].

The PLC-γ-dependent pathway evokes activation of CAM kinase and protein kinase C (PKC), which subsequently increases the 1,2-diacylglycerol (DAG) and Ca^{2+} ion concentrations [89]. The PKC-dependent pathway is reported to enhance synaptic plasticity [85] (Figure 2).

In summary, the specific role of BDNF in the regulation of numerous brain physiological processes depends on the interaction of its isoforms with different types of receptors. This, in turn, elicits the activation of signaling pathways that are critical for processes of brain development, synaptic plasticity, and protection and/or regeneration after damage. Perturbation of the BDNF synthesis, resulting in dysfunctions of its signaling cascades, may be responsible for triggering several pathological processes.

2.4. The Human BDNF Variant Val66Met

BDNF level in the peripheral tissues, brain, and blood may be also affected by gene polymorphism. The pro-domain of BDNF is the locus of a functional human BDNF polymorphism (SNPs) Val66Met, also known as rs6265 or G196Apolymorphism [109]. This point mutation causes a substitution of Valine (Val) to Methionine (Met) at codon 66 (Val66Met) in the pro-domain of *BDNF* (Figure 1). The Val66Met polymorphism does not exist in the mouse or other model organisms. Thus, multiple studies aim to mimic the function of BDNF Val66Met in cellular models or in genetically engineered mouse models. The BDNF Val66Met variant was first identified in the late 1990s and in 2002 the first two genetic studies investigating the BDNF Val66Met polymorphism in the pathogenesis of neurodegenerative disease were published [110,111]. The functionality of BDNF Val66Met variant was only confirmed in 2003 [112], where BDNF Val66Met polymorphism was shown to disrupt the episodic memory in humans. In addition, Egan et al. [112] also demonstrated that in hippocampal cultures BDNF Val66Met polymorphism did not alter BDNF expression per se, but the perisomatic localization of BDNF. Then, in 2005 it was discovered that the BDNF Val66Met substitution also disrupts the sortilin-binding site, impairing activity-mediated secretion of BDNF [113]. Likewise, the BDNF Val66Met substitution also disrupts the translin-binding site, which impairs dendritic targeting of BDNF mRNA [114]. Thus, the principle molecular mechanism associated with the BDNF Val66Met polymorphism is the deficient activity-dependent release of BDNF, which consequently impacts the efficiency of BDNF-TrkB signaling [113]. Following the demonstration that this SNP was functionally relevant over the past 18 years, more than 1700 studies have investigated the effects of this polymorphism on brain function in health, as well as in diseases, particularly in neuropsychiatric disorders [115,116]. The BDNF Val66Met polymorphism has been associated with cerebral cortex plasticity [117,118], with gray matter structures [119,120], or white matter integrities and structural networks [121,122]. More specifically, BDNF Val66Met polymorphism is associated with cognitive processes [112,123–127], and cognitive impairment in neurodegenerative disease, such as Parkinson's disease (PD) [128,129] and AD [130,131], and even more with several brain disorders, including MDD and bipolar disorder [132–137], epilepsy [138–140], schizophrenia [125,141–144], aging and dementia [145] and stroke [117,146,147]. Met66, but not Val66, BDNF pro-domain can induce the growth cone retraction in young hippocampal neurons [148]. Although many studies have demonstrated the possible genetic effects of this BDNF polymorphism in diseases or brain function, other articles have failed to replicate the findings. The discrepancies of BDNF Val66Met genetic studies may result from many factors such as environmental factors, ethnicity, age, and sex.

3. Neuroplasticity in MDD: The Effects of Antidepressant Therapies

3.1. Major Depressive Disorder

Major depressive disorder is one of the most prevalent and debilitating psychiatric disorders with high impact on the quality of life and negative effects on mood, behavior, and cognition [149]. Over the past few decades, several mechanisms have been investigated in the pathophysiology of MDD, including altered serotonergic, noradrenergic, dopaminergic, and glutamatergic systems, increased inflammation, hypothalamic-pituitary-adrenal axis abnormalities, vascular changes, and decreased neurogenesis and neuroplasticity. In particular, a decrease in serotonergic neurotransmission is regarded as the main etiopathogenetic mechanism occurring in depressed patients. Thus, the most common drugs used to treat MDD are serotonin reuptake inhibitor (SSRI) that block SERT and thus increase serotonin in the raphe nucleus at post-synapse. Therefore, a misbalance in the serotonin production and/or release is believed to play a central role in determining MDD. This led to finding, by means of genetic, proteomic and pharmacological tools, molecules able to increase the expression of serotonin in neurons by modulating neural genes or proteins [150–152]. Among these molecules, TPH2, the rate-limiting enzyme responsible for brain serotonin biosynthesis, plays a crucial role and is amenable of genetic and pharmacological manipulation [153,154]. Nevertheless, in 1997 Duman and Nestler formulated the neurotrophin hypothesis of depression [155]. This theory is now supported by studies demonstrating a decrease in BDNF mRNA and protein levels in postmortem critical regions, such as the hippocampus, prefrontal cortex and amygdala, in patients with MDD compared to controls.

3.2. BDNF and Neuronal Plasticity

Brain development occurs through coordinated processes of neuro- and gliogenesis, formation of neuronal projections and synaptogenesis, and programmed cell death and elimination of improperly formed connections, together resulting in the formation of the functionally and morphologically adjusted structure of the adult brain [156,157]. Neuroplasticity or brain plasticity is the ability of the nervous system to reorganize its structure, function, and connections in response to extrinsic or intrinsic stimuli [158]. Neuronal plasticity in rodents has been well-documented during the last decades, whereas neuroplasticity in the human brain largely remains indirect, mostly because of methodological limitations as well as ethical constraints. Neuronal plasticity includes different mechanisms excellently reviewed by Castren [159]. One of these is the neurogenesis, i.e., the formation of newborn neurons in proliferative areas. There is solid evidence that neurogenesis occurs in the adult mammalian brain. In rodent adult brains, neurogenesis is mainly restricted to the subventricular zone and the subgranular zone of the dentate gyrus in the hippocampus and olfactory bulbs [156]. An accumulating body of evidence indicates that BDNF is involved in the regulation of migration of neuronal progenitors along the rostral migratory stream and neuronal settlement in the olfactory bulb [160] and also acts during the later stages of neurogenesis [161,162].

Neuronal plasticity is extensively studied during critical periods, a time window during the early phase of brain development, when neuronal circuits are noticeably sensitive to being shaped by external stimuli and experience, producing permanent and large-scale changes to neural circuits. The same circuits can be shaped by experience later in life, but to a lesser degree. After the ending of critical periods, neuronal plasticity and changes in network structure are more restricted. However, recent data indicate that several drugs used for the treatment of neuropsychiatric disorders can directly induce plasticity and reactivate a critical period-like plasticity in the adult brain. The first functional evidence for the role of neurotrophins in plasticity was obtained in the visual cortex. The observation that BDNF synthesis in the visual cortex is regulated by visual stimulation made BDNF the prime candidate for this activity-dependent regulated factor [163–165]. In transgenic mice with early overexpression of

BDNF, an accelerated onset and end of the critical period and precocious maturation of inhibitory circuits was observed. Conversely, mice raised in the dark and resulting in lower levels of BDNF showed a delayed visual plasticity [166,167]. In addition, a disruption in the binding between promoter regions of BDNF exon IV and cAMP response element-binding protein (CREB) results in decreased inhibitory input [168], which impairs the critical period plasticity.

3.3. BDNF and Synaptic Plasticity

Another mechanism involved in neuronal plasticity is the modification of mature neuronal morphology, involving axonal and dendritic arborization and pruning, an increase in spine density, and synaptogenesis [169]. Epigenetic mechanisms involved in the transcriptional regulation of genes also can contribute to synaptic plasticity. Several in vitro and in vivo studies analyzed the effects of BDNF on plasticity. Cazorla et al. proved that 48 h of BDNF stimulation in PC12 cells, transfected with TrkB, increased neurite outgrowth compared to the non-treated cells [170]. Interestingly, BDNF stimulation was able to promote dendritic outgrowth and spine formation [171,172] in primary hippocampal cells grown in B27-deprived medium. This neuroplastic effect is probably achieved through the activation of intracellular-signaling cascades [173,174]. Recent data suggest that intracellular overexpression of BDNF in hippocampal developing neurons induces maturation of excitatory and inhibitory synapses, with respect to exogenous application of BDNF [175]. BDNF mice lacking BDNF die during the second postnatal week [176] and BDNF deficit causes inhibition of dendritic arborization [92, 177] and reduction of expression of genes functionally related to vesicular trafficking and synaptic communication [178]. Instead, heterozygous BDNF mice survive into adulthood and BDNF is required for several forms of LTP, the main mechanism mediating plasticity [179]. At morphological level, these mice display a specific hippocampal volume reduction [180] similar to that observed in heterozygous TrkB mice [181,182], but in contrast to p75NTR-deficient mice [183]. These findings suggest a link between hippocampal volume and BDNF-mediated TrkB signaling [181,182]. Over the last years, BDNF has been extensively studied as an important regulator of synaptic transmission and LTP in the hippocampus and in other brain regions. The effects of BDNF in LTP are mediated by TrkB receptors. In particular, in the hippocampus the neurotrophin is thought to act at pre- and post-synaptic levels, modulating synaptic efficacy either by changes in pre-synaptic transmitter release, or by increased post-synaptic transmitter sensitivity (see e.g., [15,16]) to induce a long-lasting increase in synaptic plasticity. This depends on individual circumstances. Thus, BDNF can be: (i) either, a mediator or a modulator of synaptic plasticity, (ii) both, a neurotransmitter that acts both at pre- and post-synaptic level simultaneously at the same individual synapse. Recent data published from Lin et al. revealed that in CA3 or CA1 regions anterograde BDNF-TrkB signaling is involved in LTP induction, while anterograde and retrograde BDNF-TrkB signaling contributes to LTP maintenance. BDNF in both pre-synaptic and post-synaptic terminals modulate basal neurotransmission and pre-synaptic TrkB, probably regulating pre-synaptic release [184]. In addition, it has also been shown that BDNF regulates the transport of mRNAs along dendrites and their translation at the synapse. These processes occur by modulating the initiation and elongation phases of protein synthesis, and by acting on specific miRNAs [100]. Local protein synthesis responds with rapid and subtle modulation of the proteome to remodel the synaptic regions in response to stimuli [185]. Protein turnover is required for synaptic plasticity, and BDNF-signaling has been also described as a crucial regulator for maintaining the baseline autophagic activity in the brain. BDNF deficiency causes an uncontrolled rise in autophagic degradation [186].

BDNF is one of the most studied synaptic molecules that efficiently modify synaptic strength and can act as a mediator, modulator, or instructor of synaptic plasticity. Specific changes in dendritic spines, as well as in adult hippocampal neurogenesis, can be correlated to several forms of learning and memory. BDNF is one of the most inspiring molecules to better understand the disadvantageous synaptic learning underlying the etiology of depression, accompanied by declines in the rate of adult neurogenesis and in spine densities [181].

3.4. BDNF in Depressed Patients

BDNF protein and TrkB receptor are detectable in several non-neuronal tissues, including endothelial cells [17,18], cardiomyocytes [19], vascular smooth muscle cells [17], leukocytes [20], megakaryocytes [19], and platelets [21,22]. Serum BDNF has been clearly demonstrated to originate from the progenitors of platelets [21]. Platelets are the major source of peripheral BDNF and are important for storing the BDNF secreted from other tissues [187]. Over the last years, there has been a great interest in peripheral BDNF measures in relation to psychiatric illness. It has been studied as biomarker reflecting these disorders [188,189]. However, there is no evidence that serum BDNF is related to brain BDNF and neuroplasticity. Nevertheless, the low serum concentration of BDNF has often been associated with the pathophysiology of MDD [190–192]. An aspect to consider is if the serum BDNF levels are dependent on the release of BDNF from platelets [193]. The significance of the lower BDNF levels in depression is currently unclear. The temporal correlation between serum BDNF levels and the antidepressant effect seems to be indirect: ketamine and electroconvulsive shock treatment increase serum BDNF levels only gradually, while their antidepressant effect appears quickly [194]. There are two studies that directly observed a reduction of BDNF levels in platelets of patients with MDD [195,196]. Another study showed that BDNF levels of platelet were significantly decreased compared to the controls. In this study, the BDNF levels were normalized compared to control with SSRIs treatment [197]. Taken together, these studies strongly suggest that changes in serum BDNF levels reflect altered BDNF release from blood platelets. Thus, given the similarities in the regulation of BDNF synthesis between megakaryocytes and neurons, there may be parallels between the brain, BDNF in serum, and release. Nevertheless, within the CNS a reduction in BDNF and TrkB expression has been reported in the hippocampus and prefrontal cortex of post-mortem brain tissues of suicide victims [198,199]. In addition, several meta-analyses data confirm the association of the Val66Met polymorphism with an increase of susceptibility to develop mood disorders [200–202]. Finally, a recent paper showed that subjects with the Met allele of the BDNF gene are more likely to develop depression [134].

A disruption in serotonin signaling in the brain is also believed to be involved in the pathophysiology of depression. Changes in synaptic serotonin levels and receptor levels are coupled with altered synaptic plasticity and neurogenesis [203,204]. It has been proposed that chronic treatment with conventional antidepressants, such as SSRIs, but not acute administration increases neurogenesis [205–207] and selective SSRIs might reactivate serotonin's ability to mediate developmental plasticity. BDNF acts as a modulator of the 5-HT system and vice versa, acting as the link between the antidepressant drug and the neuroplastic changes. Close molecular connections between serotonin receptors and neurotrophic proteins such as BDNF and intracellular signaling cascades are responsible for cytoskeletal rearrangement [169,208–211]. Thus, dysregulation in 5-HT–BDNF interaction may be responsible for the development of neuropsychiatric and behavioral abnormalities [212].

Understanding the function of the members of the BDNF system in response to the challenges of the environment and the interaction with different 5-HT receptors in health and disease will lead to new classes of drugs that could be used in therapy for psychiatric and neurodegenerative disorders.

3.5. Effect of Antidepressant Therapies on Plasticity BDNF-Mediated

3.5.1. BDNF and Antidepressant Treatments

Multiple lines of evidence suggest that antidepressant treatments increase BDNF mRNA and protein levels in the cerebral cortex and hippocampus (for review see [213,214]). This increase is partly due to a reduction of histone acetylation in the *BDNF* promoter regions. The involvement of BDNF in the efficacy of antidepressant treatments has mainly been demonstrated in rodent models. It has been demonstrated that all pharmacological classes of clinical antidepressants increase TrkB autophosphorylation and signaling in the hippocampus and forebrain, effects observed within hours after the administration of the drug [203,215]. Similar results in BDNF mRNA and TrkB phosphorylation have been observed after acute treatment with ketamine [216–219]. In rodents, injection of BDNF in the hippocampus reduces depression-like behavior [220], in contrast injection of BDNF into the nucleus accumbens or ventral tegmental area promotes depressive effects [221], demonstrating the network-dependent effect of BDNF in mood regulation. Interestingly, conditional knockout of BDNF in forebrain regions increases depressive behavior in females, but not in male mice [222], and blocks the effects of antidepressants desipramine or ketamine [216,223]. Similarly, conditional deletion of TrkB in dentate gyrus or inhibition of TrkB signaling by a dominant-negative TrkB receptor blocks the effects of antidepressants [224,225]. In addition, mice with Val66Met polymorphism are insensitive to antidepressants [226]. Recent evidence demonstrates that the antidepressant effects of GLYX-13, a novel glutamatergic compound that acts as an NMDA modulator with glycine-like partial agonist properties, are blocked by intra-medial prefrontal cortex infusion of an anti-BDNF antibody or in mice with a knock-in of the BDNF Val66Met allele. Pharmacological inhibition of BDNF-TrkB signaling or L-type voltage-dependent Ca^{2+} channels (VDCCs) blocks the antidepressant behavioral actions of GLYX-13 [227].

Taken together, these data suggest that BDNF serves as a transducer, acting as the link between the antidepressant drug and the neuroplastic changes that result in the improvement of depressive symptoms.

3.5.2. Beneficial Effects of Exercise on Plasticity: The Role of BDNF

Several lines of evidence suggest that exercise has beneficial effects on plasticity and BDNF could be a link between plasticity and physical activity. Although it has been proven that exercise in MDD patients reduced depressive symptoms [228–230], neuroplasticity per se has not yet been monitored in these patients. However, voluntary physical exercise, like an enriched environment, increases expression of BDNF in the hippocampus [8], as well as hippocampal neurogenesis [9] and this could improve brain function by enhancing plasticity, cognition, learning, and memory [12–14]. Physical exercise is one particularly effective strategy for increasing circulating levels of BDNF [10,11]. It has repeatedly been demonstrated that an acute bout of aerobic exercise transiently increases both serum and plasma BDNF in an intensity-dependent manner [10,11]. Exercise increases the release of BDNF from the human brain [231,232] suggesting that exercise also mediates central BDNF production in humans. It has been suggested that miR-34a potentially can also mediate changes in BDNF expression and may reflect the decrease in performance after overtraining [233].

Multiple studies suggest that BDNF has a dominant role in mediating the effects of physical activity on cognitive changes [234]. It has been shown that three months of aerobic exercise training increases hippocampal volume in healthy individuals and in patients with schizophrenia by 12% and 16%, respectively [235]. The question whether exercise regulates muscle-derived circulating factors that can pass through the blood–brain barrier and stimulate BDNF production in the brain remains unclear. In 2016, Moon et al. show that the myokine cathepsin B (Ctsb) might be involved in mediating the exercise-induced improvement in hippocampal neurogenesis, memory, and learning [236]. Mice lacking Ctsb showed depression-like symptoms when they were forced to swim [236].

Other papers have demonstrated that exercise induces upregulation in skeletal muscle of PGC1α, a transcriptional co-activator of mitochondrial biogenesis and oxidative metabolism in brown adipose tissue and muscle. In muscle, the increase of PGC1α expression stimulates an upregulation of FNDC5, a membrane protein that is cleaved and secreted into the circulation as the myokine irisin [237]. FNDC5 cross the blood–brain barrier inducing BDNF expression in the hippocampus, in this way BDNF plays a role in neurogenesis and reward-related learning and motivation [238]. Current research has also shown that high intensity exercise increases peripheral lactate and BDNF levels; at the same time lactate infusion at rest can increase peripheral and central BDNF levels. Lactate and BDNF can induce neuroplasticity [239]. In addition, acute elevation of BDNF did not compensate for hypoxia-induced cognition impairment [240].

The identification of exercise-related factors that have a direct or indirect effect on brain function has the potential to highlight novel therapeutic targets for neurodegenerative diseases.

4. The Protective Role of BDNF on Neurodegeneration

Neurodegenerative diseases comprise a wide range of neurological diseases such as AD, PD, Huntington's disease, and amyotrophic lateral sclerosis (ALS), characterized by the deterioration and then the death of selective nuclei of neurons in the brain or the spinal cord. They are chronic and progressive diseases, currently incurable and highly debilitating, causing a tremendous emotional and economic burden on patients, their families, and society. AD, the most frequent among neurodegenerative diseases, accounts for about 70% of dementia cases all over the world, that is about 35 million people. It is estimated to cost more than 480 billion euros each year throughout the world (Sources: OMS, EBC (European Brain Council)). Currently, no pharmacological treatment is available to cure or even significantly slow down the course of neurodegenerative diseases. For these reasons, experimental findings showing that physical exercise, exposure to an enriched environment, metabolic changes and nutritional and/or cognitive intervention, may exert a protective role on neurodegeneration either by delaying the onset and/or curbing the course of the disease, raise hope that these new tools might be useful also in clinical practice. BDNF appears to be crucial or, in some cases even essential, to mediate the neuroprotective effects of the above-mentioned environmental stimuli (Figure 3). In particular, as discussed above, it is well established that BDNF accounts for the hippocampal adult neurogenesis, which, in turn, can be stimulated by a number of conditions such as physical exercise, enriched environment, hormonal balance (i.e., steroid hormones such a cortisol and testosterone) and nutritional intervention (i.e., fasting, low-calorie intake, low-carb diet, selective nutrient intakes), capable of increasing the BDNF level [241].

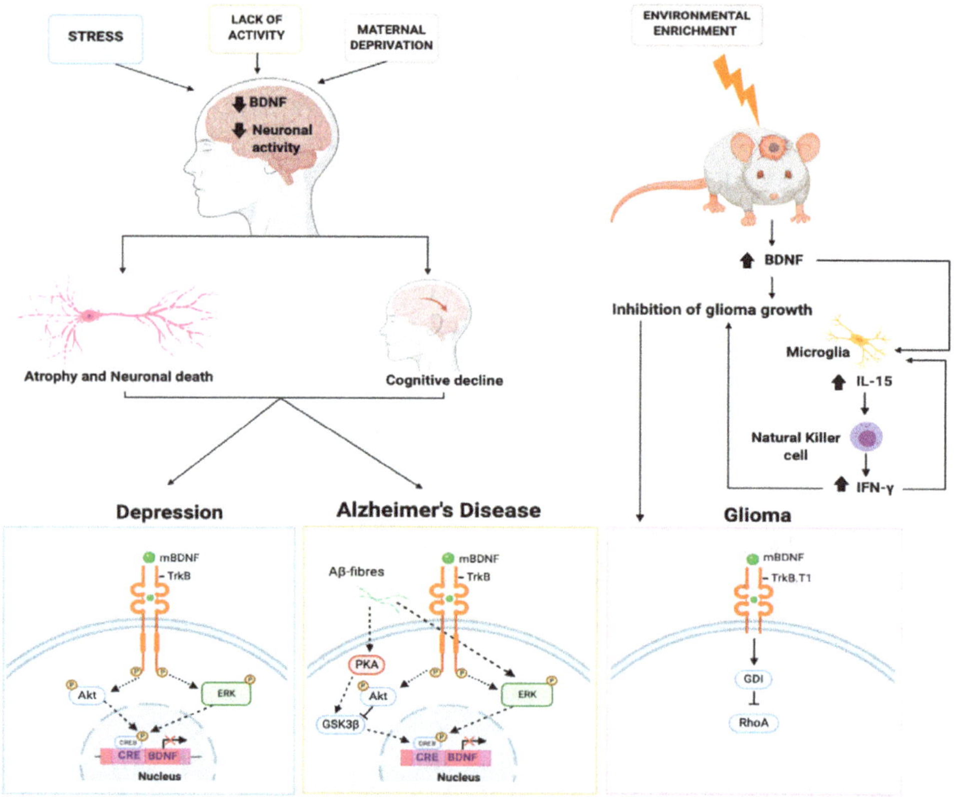

Figure 3. The molecular mechanisms mediated by BDNF involved in depression, Alzheimer's disease, and glioma. External stimuli (stress, maternal deprivation, or lack of activity) causing epigenetic regulation processes can induce a reduction in BDNF expression level and in neuronal activity.

This results in atrophy, neuronal death, and cognitive decline, which may contribute to depression or Alzheimer's disease. In these pathologies the BDNF/TrkB signaling, which activates the downstream Akt and ERK signaling, is altered. Thus, such alterations cause an impairment of CREB signaling resulting in BDNF downregulation. The alteration of phosphorylation (P) inhibits (red X) the transcriptional machinery. In the mouse brain, environmental enrichment induces an increase of BDNF. BDNF, binding the truncated form of TrkB receptor (TrkB.T1), signals directly to the Rho protein dissociation inhibitor (GDI). The latter detaches from TrkB.T1 and binds to the small G protein RhoA, leading to an inhibition of glioma cell migration. BDNF stimulates also indirectly the production of IL-15 in microglia, which in turn stimulates the natural killer cells to produce IFN-γ. IFN-γ contributes to reducing glioma growth.

4.1. The Protective Role of BDNF on Alzheimer's Disease

A reduced level of BDNF has been found in patients affected by neurodegenerative diseases such as Parkinson's, Huntington's and Alzheimer's disease as well as in mild cognitive impairment, the latter being a prodromal stage of AD, characterized by a slight decline of cognitive abilities including memory, thinking and judging skills [242–245]. In some instances, the levels of BDNF even correlate with the severity of the diseases, pointing towards a pathogenetic link between BDNF and AD [246]. Although there are some papers reporting an increase of BDNF in serum or in the post-mortem brain, this might be due either to compensatory mechanisms or its release from immune cells or pharmacological treatments known to raise BDNF (i.e., antidepressants) [241].

Recently, a very complex study explored the role of physical activity in a genetic mouse model of AD. This study provided the most compelling evidence of the relationship between physical activity, adult hippocampal neurogenesis, BDNF, and AD. This study elegantly confirms that adult hippocampal neurogenesis plays a pivotal role in brain resilience to AD. They manipulated with pharmacological and genetic tool neurogenesis as well as BDNF, clearly showing that physical exercise needs neurogenesis to protect the brain from AD and that BDNF is essential for such a protection. In addition, it provides evidence that adult hippocampal neurogenesis can counteract AD memory impairment, only in combination with BDNF, whereas if neurogenesis is experimentally blocked, BDNF does not exert beneficial effects. Finally, pharmacological increase of BDNF further ameliorates AD pathology [247]. Thus, agents that promote both BDNF signaling and neurogenesis might be the key to preventing or curing AD. As far as metabolism is concerned, it has been shown that intermitting fasting, by causing a transition from utilization of carbohydrate and glucose to a fatty acid and ketones source of energy (refer to as "G-K shift") generates a number of beneficial cognitive, metabolic, and cardiovagal effects. BDNF is increased upon intermitting fasting and mediates at least part of these effects. Its increase is stimulated by the ketone body, β-hydroxybutyrate that inhibits histone deacetylases that repress BDNF promoters [248]. Recently, the role of BDNF and neuroprotection in the context of metabolism and fasting has been nicely reviewed by Mattson et al. [6].

4.2. BDNF and Ras-ERK-CREB Signaling in Alzheimer's Disease

BDNF, as also discussed above, causes the activation of the Ras-ERK signaling cascade leading to the phosphorylation of CREB. Such a pathway exerts a well-known trophic and protective role on neuronal cells both in vitro and in vivo in a variety of neurodegenerative models, including AD, PD, and Huntington's diseases. Nevertheless, it has become clear that the Ras-ERK pathway may also foster neurodegeneration or hamper the action of neurotrophic factors when activated by noxious stimuli as occurs for instance in PD and AD [249]. In particular, it has been shown in a number of different cellular models such as primary cortical rat neurons, rat B103 neuroblastoma cells, and A1 mouse mesencephalic cells, that APP and/or Aβ42 oligomer induces the activation of Ras-ERK and GSK-3 signaling, that, in turn, causes hyperphosphorylation of tau and APP at Thr668. The involvement of these molecular events in the pathogenesis AD is corroborated by the finding that activation of Ras-ERK and GSK-3 correlates with Aβ levels in the brain of AD patients [250,251]. Aberrant stimulation of Ras-ERK signaling forces neurons to enter the cell cycle as shown by the expression and nuclear accumulation of cyclin D1 and the subsequent G1/S progression. Since neurons lack functional cell cycle machinery, these events lead to cell death (i.e., mitotic catastrophe) instead of cell division. Interestingly, as clearly shown in the mouse model of familial AD APPswe/PS1ΔE9 mice, although ERK phosphorylation is enhanced compared to the wild type counterpart, it does not result in normal CREB phosphorylation. The impairment in CREB signaling parallels to impairment in a number of cognitive tests [252]. Therefore, in AD, BDNF downregulation is mediated by the impairment of CREB signaling caused by amyloid β [253] (Figure 3).

5. BDNF and Brain Cancer: An Unexpected Role. An Oncogene or a Tumor Suppressor?

The role of BDNF and its cognate receptor TrkB in cancer, including brain cancer, has been recognized for a long time [254]. In many types of cancers, BDNF and/or TrkB have been found expressed or in some cases over-expressed [255]. This is not surprising since growth factors, including neurotrophic factors, and their tyrosine kinase receptors have long been involved in tumors with different cell-dependent mechanisms, fostering proliferation, enhancing anti-apoptotic signaling, and making cells unresponsive to anti-proliferative stimuli [256]. The direct oncogenic activity of TrkB might also be due to the crosstalk with EGF receptors that together with its ligand is well-known to promote cell transformation. BDNF administration not only does phosphorylate TrkB but also EGFR [257]. In line with these observations, it has been recently shown that BDNF produced by glioblastoma (GBM) differentiated cells acts on GBM stem cells, fostering their growth through paracrine signaling [258].

However, recently another study showed that exposing mice to an enriched environment is able to decrease the growth of intracranial glioma, decreasing proliferation and invasion, and improving overall survival. Such an effect is achieved by means of both indirect and direct mechanisms. The former acts via natural killer cells of the innate immune system, whereas the latter utilizes BDNF stimulation of its truncated receptor TrkB.T1 on glioma cancer cells. BDNF binding the TrkB.T1 receptor signals to the Rho protein dissociation inhibitor (RhoGDI), the latter detaches from TrkB.T1 and binds to the small G protein RhoA, leading to its inhibition. The authors found that an enriched environment causes the synthesis of IL-15 and BDNF. When mice bearing the glioma and not housed in enriched environments were infused with BDNF, they reduced tumor size and macrophage infiltration. Thus, showing that at least in part, BDNF accounts for the oncolytic effect elicited by the enriched environment [259]. In a more recent study, the same group delved deeper into the mechanisms, finding that enriched environment changes glioma-associated myeloid cells. BDNF plays a central role by stimulating the production of IL-15 in microglia, which in turn stimulates the natural killer cells to produce IFN-γ. Natural killer cells were responsible for the switch to an oncolytic environment [260] (Figure 3).

Taken together, a scenario emerges where BDNF, acting on different cells is able to reorganize the brain microenvironment in such a way that it becomes resilient to neurodegeneration or oncolytic for tumors. In this regard, although supported by much more preliminary data, it seems that also other compounds might share these properties [261,262].

6. Conclusions

In this review, we discussed the role of BDNF in neurogenesis, differentiation, survival, synaptic plasticity, and transmission to reorganize the brain microenvironment. All BDNF gene products, such as proBDNF, mature BDNF, and even the isolated proBDNF domain, are known to exert functional activity. One of the most important features of BDNF is that it can act as a local, paracrine and/or autocrine factor, on both pre-synaptic and post-synaptic target sites. Here, we presented the contribution of altered BDNF signaling in the pathophysiology of brain diseases, including mental disorders (i.e., depression), neurodegenerative diseases, (i.e., Alzheimer's disease), and brain tumor (i.e., glioblastoma). BDNF is one of the best-studied synaptic molecules that efficiently modify synaptic strength and it can act as a mediator, modulator, or instructor of synaptic plasticity. In neurons, the cellular processes that regulate the amount of both BDNF mRNA and protein, the changes in the efficiency of secretion, and transport of BDNF protein may affect synaptic function and cell survival. BDNF is one of the most inspiring molecules to better understand the disadvantageous synaptic learning underlying the etiology of depression, accompanied by the decline in the rate of adult neurogenesis and in spine densities. Furthermore, BDNF appears to exert a potent role in neuroprotection and/or brain regeneration by modulating signaling pathways such Ras-ERK-CREB, thus rendering neuronal cells resilient to neurodegeneration. Finally, BDNF appears to be crucial in the pathogenesis and development of brain tumors such as glioblastoma by reorganizing its microenvironment. Thus, understanding the physiologic and pathologic BDNF signaling and finding tools to modulate its expression (mRNA and/or protein) is a prerequisite for a potential BDNF-based therapy.

Author Contributions: Original draft preparation, writing and editing, L.C.-D., L.S.; original draft preparation, writing and review, F.V. All authors have read and agreed to the published version of the manuscript.

Abbreviations

AD	Alzheimer's Disease
AP1	Activator Protein 1
BCL2	B-cell lymphoma 2
BDNF	Brain-Derived Neurotrophic Factor
BHLHB2	Helix-loop-helix protein
CaMK	Ca^{2+}/calmodulin-dependent protein kinase
cAMP/CRE	Cyclic adenosine monophosphate calcium response element
CaREs	Calcium-responsive elements
CREB	CREB
Ctsb	Myokine cathepsin B
CUMS	Chronic Unpredicted Mild Stress model
DAG	1,2-diacylglycerol
ERK	Extracellular signal-regulated kinase
GTP-ases	guanosine triphosphate hydrolases
JNK	c-Jun amino terminal kinase
IKK	Multi-subunit IκB kinase
IkB	Inhibitor of kB
L-VGCC	L-type voltage gated calcium channel
LTP	Long-Term Potentiation
MAPK	Mitogen-activated protein kinase
MDD	Major depressive disorder
Met	Methionine
miRNAs	microRNAs
MMP	Matrix Metalloproteases
MPP	1-methyl-4-phenylpyridinium
NF-kB	Nuclear Factor kappa-light-chain-enhancer of activated B cells
NMDA	N-Methyl-D-Aspartate
NRAGE	Neurotrophin receptor-interacting MAGE homologue
NRIF	Neurotrophin receptor interacting factor
PD	Parkinson's disease
p75NTR	p75 neurotrophin receptor
PI3K	Phosphoinositide 3-kinases
PKC	Protein kinase C
PLC	Phospholipase C
Rho	Ras homolog

ROCK	Rho-associated protein kinase
SIRT1	Sirtuin 1
SNPs	Polymorphism
SSRIs	Serotonin reuptake inhibitor
TRAF6	Tumor necrosis factor receptor associated factor 6
TrkB	Tropomycin receptor kinase B
Val	Valine
VDCCs	L-type voltage-dependent Ca^{2+} channels
Vps10p	Vacuolar protein sorting 10 protein

References

1. Andreska, T.; Aufmkolk, S.; Sauer, M.; Blum, R. High abundance of BDNF within glutamatergic presynapses of cultured hippocampal neurons. *Front. Cell Neurosci.* **2014**, *8*, 107. [CrossRef]
2. Clarke, L.E.; Liddelow, S.A.; Chakraborty, C.; Münch, A.E.; Heiman, M.; Barres, B.A. Normal aging induces A1-like astrocyte reactivity. *Proc. Natl. Acad. Sci. USA* **2018**, *115*, E1896–E1905. [CrossRef]
3. Parkhurst, C.N.; Yang, G.; Ninan, I.; Savas, J.N.; Yates, J.R.; Lafaille, J.J.; Hempstead, B.L.; Littman, D.R.; Gan, W.B. Microglia promote learning-dependent synapse formation through brain-derived neurotrophic factor. *Cell* **2013**, *155*, 1596–1609. [CrossRef]
4. Bartkowska, K.; Paquin, A.; Gauthier, A.S.; Kaplan, D.R.; Miller, F.D. Trk signaling regulates neural precursor cell proliferation and differentiation during cortical development. *Development* **2007**, *134*, 4369–4380. [CrossRef]
5. Vilar, M.; Mira, H. Regulation of Neurogenesis by Neurotrophins during Adulthood: Expected and Unexpected Roles. *Front. Neurosci.* **2016**, *10*, 26. [CrossRef]
6. Mattson, M.P.; Moehl, K.; Ghena, N.; Schmaedick, M.; Cheng, A. Intermittent metabolic switching, neuroplasticity and brain health. *Nat. Rev. Neurosci.* **2018**, *19*, 63–80. [CrossRef]
7. Numakawa, T.; Odaka, H.; Adachi, N. Actions of Brain-Derived Neurotrophin Factor in the Neurogenesis and Neuronal Function, and Its Involvement in the Pathophysiology of Brain Diseases. *Int. J. Mol. Sci.* **2018**, *19*, 3650. [CrossRef]
8. Loprinzi, P.D.; Day, S.; Deming, R. Acute Exercise Intensity and Memory Function: Evaluation of the Transient Hypofrontality Hypothesis. *Medicina (Kaunas)* **2019**, *55*, 445. [CrossRef]
9. Fabel, K.; Wolf, S.A.; Ehninger, D.; Babu, H.; Leal-Galicia, P.; Kempermann, G. Additive effects of physical exercise and environmental enrichment on adult hippocampal neurogenesis in mice. *Front. Neurosci.* **2009**, *3*, 50. [CrossRef]
10. Knaepen, K.; Goekint, M.; Heyman, E.M.; Meeusen, R. Neuroplasticity-exercise-induced response of peripheral brain-derived neurotrophic factor: A systematic review of experimental studies in human subjects. *Sports Med.* **2010**, *40*, 765–801. [CrossRef]
11. Szuhany, K.L.; Bugatti, M.; Otto, M.W. A meta-analytic review of the effects of exercise on brain-derived neurotrophic factor. *J. Psychiatr. Res.* **2015**, *60*, 56–64. [CrossRef] [PubMed]
12. van Praag, H.; Shubert, T.; Zhao, C.; Gage, F.H. Exercise enhances learning and hippocampal neurogenesis in aged mice. *J. Neurosci.* **2005**, *25*, 8680–8685. [CrossRef] [PubMed]
13. Tuon, T.; Souza, P.S.; Santos, M.F.; Pereira, F.T.; Pedroso, G.S.; Luciano, T.F.; De Souza, C.T.; Dutra, R.C.; Silveira, P.C.; Pinho, R.A. Physical Training Regulates Mitochondrial Parameters and Neuroinflammatory Mechanisms in an Experimental Model of Parkinson's Disease. *Oxid. Med. Cell. Longev.* **2015**, *2015*, 261809. [CrossRef] [PubMed]
14. Vilela, T.C.; Muller, A.P.; Damiani, A.P.; Macan, T.P.; da Silva, S.; Canteiro, P.B.; de Sena Casagrande, A.; Pedroso, G.D.S.; Nesi, R.T.; de Andrade, V.M.; et al. Strength and Aerobic Exercises Improve Spatial Memory in Aging Rats Through Stimulating Distinct Neuroplasticity Mechanisms. *Mol. Neurobiol.* **2017**, *54*, 7928–7937. [CrossRef]
15. Itami, C.; Kimura, F.; Kohno, T.; Matsuoka, M.; Ichikawa, M.; Tsumoto, T.; Nakamura, S. Brain-derived neurotrophic factor-dependent unmasking of "silent" synapses in the developing mouse barrel cortex. *Proc. Natl. Acad. Sci. USA* **2003**, *100*, 13069–13074. [CrossRef]

16. Edelmann, E.; Lessmann, V.; Brigadski, T. Pre-and postsynaptic twists in BDNF secretion and action in synaptic plasticity. *Neuropharmacology* **2014**, *76 Pt C*, 610–627. [CrossRef]
17. Nakahashi, T.; Fujimura, H.; Altar, C.A.; Li, J.; Kambayashi, J.; Tandon, N.N.; Sun, B. Vascular endothelial cells synthesize and secrete brain-derived neurotrophic factor. *FEBS Lett.* **2000**, *470*, 113–117. [CrossRef]
18. Wang, H.; Ward, N.; Boswell, M.; Katz, D.M. Secretion of brain-derived neurotrophic factor from brain microvascular endothelial cells. *Eur. J. Neurosci.* **2006**, *23*, 1665–1670. [CrossRef]
19. Pius-Sadowska, E.; Machaliński, B. BDNF-A key player in cardiovascular system. *J. Mol. Cell. Cardiol.* **2017**, *110*, 54–60. [CrossRef]
20. Anders, Q.S.; Ferreira, L.V.B.; Rodrigues, L.C.M.; Nakamura-Palacios, E.M. BDNF mRNA Expression in Leukocytes and Frontal Cortex Function in Drug Use Disorder. *Front. Psychiatry* **2020**, *11*, 469. [CrossRef]
21. Chacón-Fernández, P.; Säuberli, K.; Colzani, M.; Moreau, T.; Ghevaert, C.; Barde, Y.A. Brain-derived Neurotrophic Factor in Megakaryocytes. *J. Biol. Chem.* **2016**, *291*, 9872–9881. [CrossRef] [PubMed]
22. Amadio, P.; Sandrini, L.; Ieraci, A.; Tremoli, E.; Barbieri, S.S. Effect of Clotting Duration and Temperature on BDNF Measurement in Human Serum. *Int. J. Mol. Sci.* **2017**, *18*, 1987. [CrossRef] [PubMed]
23. Meek, T.H.; Wisse, B.E.; Thaler, J.P.; Guyenet, S.J.; Matsen, M.E.; Fischer, J.D.; Taborsky, G.J.; Schwartz, M.W.; Morton, G.J. BDNF action in the brain attenuates diabetic hyperglycemia via insulin-independent inhibition of hepatic glucose production. *Diabetes* **2013**, *62*, 1512–1518. [CrossRef] [PubMed]
24. Marosi, K.; Mattson, M.P. BDNF mediates adaptive brain and body responses to energetic challenges. *Trends Endocrinol. Metab.* **2014**, *25*, 89–98. [CrossRef] [PubMed]
25. Delezie, J.; Weihrauch, M.; Maier, G.; Tejero, R.; Ham, D.J.; Gill, J.F.; Karrer-Cardel, B.; Rüegg, M.A.; Tabares, L.; Handschin, C. BDNF is a mediator of glycolytic fiber-type specification in mouse skeletal muscle. *Proc. Natl. Acad. Sci. USA* **2019**, *116*, 16111–16120. [CrossRef]
26. Tettamanti, G.; Cattaneo, A.G.; Gornati, R.; de Eguileor, M.; Bernardini, G.; Binelli, G. Phylogenesis of brain-derived neurotrophic factor (BDNF) in vertebrates. *Gene* **2010**, *450*, 85–93. [CrossRef]
27. Metsis, M.; Timmusk, T.; Arenas, E.; Persson, H. Differential usage of multiple brain-derived neurotrophic factor promoters in the rat brain following neuronal activation. *Proc. Natl. Acad. Sci. USA* **1993**, *90*, 8802–8806. [CrossRef]
28. Timmusk, T.; Lendahl, U.; Funakoshi, H.; Arenas, E.; Persson, H.; Metsis, M. Identification of brain-derived neurotrophic factor promoter regions mediating tissue-specific, axotomy-, and neuronal activity-induced expression in transgenic mice. *J. Cell Biol.* **1995**, *128*, 185–199. [CrossRef]
29. Timmusk, T.; Palm, K.; Metsis, M.; Reintam, T.; Paalme, V.; Saarma, M.; Persson, H. Multiple promoters direct tissue-specific expression of the rat BDNF gene. *Neuron* **1993**, *10*, 475–489. [CrossRef]
30. Vashishta, A.; Habas, A.; Pruunsild, P.; Zheng, J.J.; Timmusk, T.; Hetman, M. Nuclear factor of activated T-cells isoform c4 (NFATc4/NFAT3) as a mediator of antiapoptotic transcription in NMDA receptor-stimulated cortical neurons. *J. Neurosci.* **2009**, *29*, 15331–15340. [CrossRef]
31. Volpicelli, F.; Caiazzo, M.; Greco, D.; Consales, C.; Leone, L.; Perrone-Capano, C.; Colucci D'Amato, L.; di Porzio, U. Bdnf gene is a downstream target of Nurr1 transcription factor in rat midbrain neurons in vitro. *J. Neurochem.* **2007**, *102*, 441–453. [CrossRef] [PubMed]
32. Aid, T.; Kazantseva, A.; Piirsoo, M.; Palm, K.; Timmusk, T. Mouse and rat BDNF gene structure and expression revisited. *J. Neurosci. Res.* **2007**, *85*, 525–535. [CrossRef] [PubMed]
33. Pruunsild, P.; Kazantseva, A.; Aid, T.; Palm, K.; Timmusk, T. Dissecting the human BDNF locus: Bidirectional transcription, complex splicing, and multiple promoters. *Genomics* **2007**, *90*, 397–406. [CrossRef] [PubMed]
34. Paoletti, P.; Bellone, C.; Zhou, Q. NMDA receptor subunit diversity: Impact on receptor properties, synaptic plasticity and disease. *Nat. Rev. Neurosci.* **2013**, *14*, 383–400. [CrossRef] [PubMed]
35. Simms, B.A.; Zamponi, G.W. Neuronal voltage-gated calcium channels: Structure, function, and dysfunction. *Neuron* **2014**, *82*, 24–45. [CrossRef]
36. Shieh, P.B.; Hu, S.C.; Bobb, K.; Timmusk, T.; Ghosh, A. Identification of a signaling pathway involved in calcium regulation of BDNF expression. *Neuron* **1998**, *20*, 727–740. [CrossRef]
37. Tao, X.; Finkbeiner, S.; Arnold, D.B.; Shaywitz, A.J.; Greenberg, M.E. Ca2+ influx regulates BDNF transcription by a CREB family transcription factor-dependent mechanism. *Neuron* **1998**, *20*, 709–726. [CrossRef]
38. Tabuchi, A.; Sakaya, H.; Kisukeda, T.; Fushiki, H.; Tsuda, M. Involvement of an upstream stimulatory factor as well as cAMP-responsive element-binding protein in the activation of brain-derived neurotrophic factor gene promoter I. *J. Biol. Chem.* **2002**, *277*, 35920–35931. [CrossRef]

39. Pruunsild, P.; Sepp, M.; Orav, E.; Koppel, I.; Timmusk, T. Identification of cis-elements and transcription factors regulating neuronal activity-dependent transcription of human BDNF gene. *J. Neurosci.* **2011**, *31*, 3295–3308. [CrossRef]
40. Tao, X.; West, A.E.; Chen, W.G.; Corfas, G.; Greenberg, M.E. A calcium-responsive transcription factor, CaRF, that regulates neuronal activity-dependent expression of BDNF. *Neuron* **2002**, *33*, 383–395. [CrossRef]
41. Zheng, F.; Wang, H. NMDA-mediated and self-induced bdnf exon IV transcriptions are differentially regulated in cultured cortical neurons. *Neurochem. Int.* **2009**, *54*, 385–392. [CrossRef] [PubMed]
42. Lipsky, R.H.; Xu, K.; Zhu, D.; Kelly, C.; Terhakopian, A.; Novelli, A.; Marini, A.M. Nuclear factor kappaB is a critical determinant in N-methyl-D-aspartate receptor-mediated neuroprotection. *J. Neurochem.* **2001**, *78*, 254–264. [CrossRef] [PubMed]
43. Zheng, F.; Zhou, X.; Moon, C.; Wang, H. Regulation of brain-derived neurotrophic factor expression in neurons. *Int. J. Physiol. Pathophysiol. Pharmacol.* **2012**, *4*, 188–200. [PubMed]
44. Jiang, X.; Tian, F.; Du, Y.; Copeland, N.G.; Jenkins, N.A.; Tessarollo, L.; Wu, X.; Pan, H.; Hu, X.Z.; Xu, K.; et al. BHLHB2 controls Bdnf promoter 4 activity and neuronal excitability. *J. Neurosci.* **2008**, *28*, 1118–1130. [CrossRef]
45. Sakata, K.; Woo, N.H.; Martinowich, K.; Greene, J.S.; Schloesser, R.J.; Shen, L.; Lu, B. Critical role of promoter IV-driven BDNF transcription in GABAergic transmission and synaptic plasticity in the prefrontal cortex. *Proc. Natl. Acad. Sci. USA* **2009**, *106*, 5942–5947. [CrossRef]
46. Keller, S.; Sarchiapone, M.; Zarrilli, F.; Videtic, A.; Ferraro, A.; Carli, V.; Sacchetti, S.; Lembo, F.; Angiolillo, A.; Jovanovic, N.; et al. Increased BDNF promoter methylation in the Wernicke area of suicide subjects. *Arch. Gen. Psychiatry* **2010**, *67*, 258–267. [CrossRef]
47. Tadić, A.; Müller-Engling, L.; Schlicht, K.F.; Kotsiari, A.; Dreimüller, N.; Kleimann, A.; Bleich, S.; Lieb, K.; Frieling, H. Methylation of the promoter of brain-derived neurotrophic factor exon IV and antidepressant response in major depression. *Mol. Psychiatry* **2014**, *19*, 281–283. [CrossRef]
48. Lieb, K.; Dreimüller, N.; Wagner, S.; Schlicht, K.; Falter, T.; Neyazi, A.; Müller-Engling, L.; Bleich, S.; Tadić, A.; Frieling, H. BDNF Plasma Levels and BDNF Exon IV Promoter Methylation as Predictors for Antidepressant Treatment Response. *Front. Psychiatry* **2018**, *9*, 511. [CrossRef]
49. Sakata, K.; Duke, S.M. Lack of BDNF expression through promoter IV disturbs expression of monoamine genes in the frontal cortex and hippocampus. *Neuroscience* **2014**, *260*, 265–275. [CrossRef]
50. Hill, J.L.; Hardy, N.F.; Jimenez, D.V.; Maynard, K.R.; Kardian, A.S.; Pollock, C.J.; Schloesser, R.J.; Martinowich, K. Loss of promoter IV-driven BDNF expression impacts oscillatory activity during sleep, sensory information processing and fear regulation. *Transl. Psychiatry* **2016**, *6*, e873. [CrossRef]
51. Volpicelli, F.; Speranza, L.; Pulcrano, S.; De Gregorio, R.; Crispino, M.; De Sanctis, C.; Leopoldo, M.; Lacivita, E.; di Porzio, U.; Bellenchi, G.C.; et al. The microRNA-29a Modulates Serotonin 5-HT7 Receptor Expression and Its Effects on Hippocampal Neuronal Morphology. *Mol. Neurobiol.* **2019**, *56*, 8617–8627. [CrossRef] [PubMed]
52. De Gregorio, R.; Pulcrano, S.; De Sanctis, C.; Volpicelli, F.; Guatteo, E.; von Oerthel, L.; Latagliata, E.C.; Esposito, R.; Piscitelli, R.M.; Perrone-Capano, C.; et al. miR-34b/c Regulates Wnt1 and Enhances Mesencephalic Dopaminergic Neuron Differentiation. *Stem Cell Rep.* **2018**, *10*, 1237–1250. [CrossRef] [PubMed]
53. McNeill, E.; Van Vactor, D. MicroRNAs shape the neuronal landscape. *Neuron* **2012**, *75*, 363–379. [CrossRef] [PubMed]
54. Keifer, J.; Zheng, Z.; Ambigapathy, G. A MicroRNA-BDNF Negative Feedback Signaling Loop in Brain: Implications for Alzheimer's Disease. *Microrna* **2015**, *4*, 101–108. [CrossRef] [PubMed]
55. Khani-Habibabadi, F.; Askari, S.; Zahiri, J.; Javan, M.; Behmanesh, M. Novel BDNF-regulatory microRNAs in neurodegenerative disorders pathogenesis: An in silico study. *Comput. Biol. Chem.* **2019**, *83*, 107153. [CrossRef] [PubMed]
56. Schratt, G.M.; Tuebing, F.; Nigh, E.A.; Kane, C.G.; Sabatini, M.E.; Kiebler, M.; Greenberg, M.E. A brain-specific microRNA regulates dendritic spine development. *Nature* **2006**, *439*, 283–289. [CrossRef]
57. Baby, N.; Alagappan, N.; Dheen, S.T.; Sajikumar, S. MicroRNA-134-5p inhibition rescues long-term plasticity and synaptic tagging/capture in an Aβ(1-42)-induced model of Alzheimer's disease. *Aging Cell* **2020**, *19*, e13046. [CrossRef]

58. Gao, J.; Wang, W.Y.; Mao, Y.W.; Gräff, J.; Guan, J.S.; Pan, L.; Mak, G.; Kim, D.; Su, S.C.; Tsai, L.H. A novel pathway regulates memory and plasticity via SIRT1 and miR-134. *Nature* **2010**, *466*, 1105–1109. [CrossRef]
59. Shen, J.; Xu, L.; Qu, C.; Sun, H.; Zhang, J. Resveratrol prevents cognitive deficits induced by chronic unpredictable mild stress: Sirt1/miR-134 signalling pathway regulates CREB/BDNF expression in hippocampus in vivo and in vitro. *Behav. Brain Res.* **2018**, *349*, 1–7. [CrossRef]
60. Xin, C.; Xia, J.; Liu, Y.; Zhang, Y. MicroRNA-202-3p Targets Brain-Derived Neurotrophic Factor and Is Involved in Depression-Like Behaviors. *Neuropsychiatr. Dis. Treat.* **2020**, *16*, 1073–1083. [CrossRef]
61. Yang, C.R.; Zhang, X.Y.; Liu, Y.; Du, J.Y.; Liang, R.; Yu, M.; Zhang, F.Q.; Mu, X.F.; Li, F.; Zhou, L.; et al. Antidepressant Drugs Correct the Imbalance Between proBDNF/p75NTR/Sortilin and Mature BDNF/TrkB in the Brain of Mice with Chronic Stress. *Neurotox. Res.* **2020**, *37*, 171–182. [CrossRef] [PubMed]
62. You, Y.H.; Qin, Z.Q.; Zhang, H.L.; Yuan, Z.H.; Yu, X. MicroRNA-153 promotes brain-derived neurotrophic factor and hippocampal neuron proliferation to alleviate autism symptoms through inhibition of JAK-STAT pathway by LEPR. *Biosci. Rep.* **2019**, *39*. [CrossRef]
63. Rostamian Delavar, M.; Baghi, M.; Safaeinejad, Z.; Kiani-Esfahani, A.; Ghaedi, K.; Nasr-Esfahani, M.H. Differential expression of miR-34a, miR-141, and miR-9 in MPP+-treated differentiated PC12 cells as a model of Parkinson's disease. *Gene* **2018**, *662*, 54–65. [CrossRef] [PubMed]
64. Zhao, X.; Shu, F.; Wang, X.; Wang, F.; Wu, L.; Li, L.; Lv, H. Inhibition of microRNA-375 ameliorated ketamine-induced neurotoxicity in human embryonic stem cell derived neurons. *Eur. J. Pharmacol.* **2019**, *844*, 56–64. [CrossRef] [PubMed]
65. Jiang, J.D.; Zheng, X.C.; Huang, F.Y.; Gao, F.; You, M.Z.; Zheng, T. MicroRNA-107 regulates anesthesia-induced neural injury in embryonic stem cell derived neurons. *IUBMB Life* **2019**, *71*, 20–27. [CrossRef] [PubMed]
66. Barde, Y.A.; Edgar, D.; Thoenen, H. Purification of a new neurotrophic factor from mammalian brain. *EMBO J.* **1982**, *1*, 549–553. [CrossRef]
67. Foltran, R.B.; Diaz, S.L. BDNF isoforms: A round trip ticket between neurogenesis and serotonin? *J. Neurochem.* **2016**, *138*, 204–221. [CrossRef]
68. Mizui, T.; Ishikawa, Y.; Kumanogoh, H.; Kojima, M. Neurobiological actions by three distinct subtypes of brain-derived neurotrophic factor: Multi-ligand model of growth factor signaling. *Pharmacol. Res.* **2016**, *105*, 93–98. [CrossRef]
69. Lu, J.; Wu, Y.; Sousa, N.; Almeida, O.F. SMAD pathway mediation of BDNF and TGF beta 2 regulation of proliferation and differentiation of hippocampal granule neurons. *Development* **2005**, *132*, 3231–3242. [CrossRef]
70. Kowiański, P.; Lietzau, G.; Czuba, E.; Waśkow, M.; Steliga, A.; Moryś, J. BDNF: A Key Factor with Multipotent Impact on Brain Signaling and Synaptic Plasticity. *Cell Mol. Neurobiol.* **2018**, *38*, 579–593. [CrossRef]
71. Pang, P.T.; Teng, H.K.; Zaitsev, E.; Woo, N.T.; Sakata, K.; Zhen, S.; Teng, K.K.; Yung, W.H.; Hempstead, B.L.; Lu, B. Cleavage of proBDNF by tPA/plasmin is essential for long-term hippocampal plasticity. *Science* **2004**, *306*, 487–491. [CrossRef]
72. Mizoguchi, H.; Nakade, J.; Tachibana, M.; Ibi, D.; Someya, E.; Koike, H.; Kamei, H.; Nabeshima, T.; Itohara, S.; Takuma, K.; et al. Matrix metalloproteinase-9 contributes to kindled seizure development in pentylenetetrazole-treated mice by converting pro-BDNF to mature BDNF in the hippocampus. *J. Neurosci.* **2011**, *31*, 12963–12971. [CrossRef]
73. Vafadari, B.; Salamian, A.; Kaczmarek, L. MMP-9 in translation: From molecule to brain physiology, pathology, and therapy. *J. Neurochem.* **2016**, *139* (Suppl. S2), 91–114. [CrossRef]
74. Mowla, S.J.; Farhadi, H.F.; Pareek, S.; Atwal, J.K.; Morris, S.J.; Seidah, N.G.; Murphy, R.A. Biosynthesis and post-translational processing of the precursor to brain-derived neurotrophic factor. *J. Biol. Chem.* **2001**, *276*, 12660–12666. [CrossRef] [PubMed]
75. Conner, J.M.; Lauterborn, J.C.; Yan, Q.; Gall, C.M.; Varon, S. Distribution of brain-derived neurotrophic factor (BDNF) protein and mRNA in the normal adult rat CNS: Evidence for anterograde axonal transport. *J. Neurosci.* **1997**, *17*, 2295–2313. [CrossRef]
76. Dieni, S.; Matsumoto, T.; Dekkers, M.; Rauskolb, S.; Ionescu, M.S.; Deogracias, R.; Gundelfinger, E.D.; Kojima, M.; Nestel, S.; Frotscher, M.; et al. BDNF and its pro-peptide are stored in presynaptic dense core vesicles in brain neurons. *J. Cell Biol.* **2012**, *196*, 775–788. [CrossRef] [PubMed]
77. Yang, J.; Siao, C.J.; Nagappan, G.; Marinic, T.; Jing, D.; McGrath, K.; Chen, Z.Y.; Mark, W.; Tessarollo, L.; Lee, F.S.; et al. Neuronal release of proBDNF. *Nat. Neurosci.* **2009**, *12*, 113–115. [CrossRef]

78. Yang, J.L.; Lin, Y.T.; Chuang, P.C.; Bohr, V.A.; Mattson, M.P. BDNF and exercise enhance neuronal DNA repair by stimulating CREB-mediated production of apurinic/apyrimidinic endonuclease 1. *Neuromolecular Med.* **2014**, *16*, 161–174. [CrossRef]
79. Du, J.; Feng, L.; Yang, F.; Lu, B. Activity- and Ca(2+)-dependent modulation of surface expression of brain-derived neurotrophic factor receptors in hippocampal neurons. *J. Cell Biol.* **2000**, *150*, 1423–1434. [CrossRef] [PubMed]
80. Meyer-Franke, A.; Wilkinson, G.A.; Kruttgen, A.; Hu, M.; Munro, E.; Hanson, M.G.; Reichardt, L.F.; Barres, B.A. Depolarization and cAMP elevation rapidly recruit TrkB to the plasma membrane of CNS neurons. *Neuron* **1998**, *21*, 681–693. [CrossRef]
81. Deinhardt, K.; Chao, M.V. Shaping neurons: Long and short range effects of mature and proBDNF signalling upon neuronal structure. *Neuropharmacology* **2014**, *76 Pt C*, 603–609. [CrossRef]
82. Anastasia, A.; Deinhardt, K.; Chao, M.V.; Will, N.E.; Irmady, K.; Lee, F.S.; Hempstead, B.L.; Bracken, C. Val66Met polymorphism of BDNF alters prodomain structure to induce neuronal growth cone retraction. *Nat. Commun.* **2013**, *4*, 2490. [CrossRef]
83. Teng, H.K.; Teng, K.K.; Lee, R.; Wright, S.; Tevar, S.; Almeida, R.D.; Kermani, P.; Torkin, R.; Chen, Z.Y.; Lee, F.S.; et al. ProBDNF induces neuronal apoptosis via activation of a receptor complex of p75NTR and sortilin. *J. Neurosci.* **2005**, *25*, 5455–5463. [CrossRef] [PubMed]
84. Roux, P.P.; Colicos, M.A.; Barker, P.A.; Kennedy, T.E. p75 neurotrophin receptor expression is induced in apoptotic neurons after seizure. *J. Neurosci.* **1999**, *19*, 6887–6896. [CrossRef] [PubMed]
85. Reichardt, L.F. Neurotrophin-regulated signalling pathways. *Philos. Trans. R. Soc. Lond. B Biol. Sci.* **2006**, *361*, 1545–1564. [CrossRef]
86. Kaplan, D.R.; Miller, F.D. Neurotrophin signal transduction in the nervous system. *Curr. Opin. Neurobiol.* **2000**, *10*, 381–391. [CrossRef]
87. Gonzalez, A.; Moya-Alvarado, G.; Gonzalez-Billaut, C.; Bronfman, F.C. Cellular and molecular mechanisms regulating neuronal growth by brain-derived neurotrophic factor. *Cytoskeleton (Hoboken)* **2016**, *73*, 612–628. [CrossRef]
88. Huang, E.J.; Reichardt, L.F. Trk receptors: Roles in neuronal signal transduction. *Annu. Rev. Biochem.* **2003**, *72*, 609–642. [CrossRef]
89. Minichiello, L. TrkB signalling pathways in LTP and learning. *Nat. Rev. Neurosci.* **2009**, *10*, 850–860. [CrossRef]
90. Patel, A.V.; Krimm, R.F. BDNF is required for the survival of differentiated geniculate ganglion neurons. *Dev. Biol.* **2010**, *340*, 419–429. [CrossRef]
91. Chen, J.; Shehadah, A.; Pal, A.; Zacharek, A.; Cui, X.; Cui, Y.; Roberts, C.; Lu, M.; Zeitlin, A.; Hariri, R.; et al. Neuroprotective effect of human placenta-derived cell treatment of stroke in rats. *Cell Transplant.* **2013**, *22*, 871–879. [CrossRef] [PubMed]
92. Wu, Y.; Wang, R.; Wang, Y.; Gao, J.; Feng, L.; Yang, Z. Distinct Impacts of Fullerene on Cognitive Functions of Dementia vs. Non-dementia Mice. *Neurotox. Res.* **2019**, *36*, 736–745. [CrossRef] [PubMed]
93. Gorski, J.A.; Zeiler, S.R.; Tamowski, S.; Jones, K.R. Brain-derived neurotrophic factor is required for the maintenance of cortical dendrites. *J. Neurosci.* **2003**, *23*, 6856–6865. [CrossRef] [PubMed]
94. Kwon, M.; Fernández, J.R.; Zegarek, G.F.; Lo, S.B.; Firestein, B.L. BDNF-promoted increases in proximal dendrites occur via CREB-dependent transcriptional regulation of cypin. *J. Neurosci.* **2011**, *31*, 9735–9745. [CrossRef]
95. Orefice, L.L.; Waterhouse, E.G.; Partridge, J.G.; Lalchandani, R.R.; Vicini, S.; Xu, B. Distinct roles for somatically and dendritically synthesized brain-derived neurotrophic factor in morphogenesis of dendritic spines. *J. Neurosci.* **2013**, *33*, 11618–11632. [CrossRef]
96. Zagrebelsky, M.; Tacke, C.; Korte, M. BDNF signaling during the lifetime of dendritic spines. *Cell Tissue Res.* **2020**. [CrossRef]
97. Yoshii, A.; Constantine-Paton, M. Postsynaptic localization of PSD-95 is regulated by all three pathways downstream of TrkB signaling. *Front. Synaptic Neurosci.* **2014**, *6*, 6. [CrossRef]
98. Chen, S.D.; Wu, C.L.; Hwang, W.C.; Yang, D.I. More Insight into BDNF against Neurodegeneration: Anti-Apoptosis, Anti-Oxidation, and Suppression of Autophagy. *Int. J. Mol. Sci.* **2017**, *18*, 545. [CrossRef]

99. Opazo, P.; Watabe, A.M.; Grant, S.G.; O'Dell, T.J. Phosphatidylinositol 3-kinase regulates the induction of long-term potentiation through extracellular signal-related kinase-independent mechanisms. *J. Neurosci.* **2003**, *23*, 3679–3688. [CrossRef]
100. Leal, G.; Bramham, C.R.; Duarte, C.B. BDNF and Hippocampal Synaptic Plasticity. *Vitam. Horm.* **2017**, *104*, 153–195. [CrossRef]
101. Baydyuk, M.; Xu, B. BDNF signaling and survival of striatal neurons. *Front. Cell. Neurosci.* **2014**, *8*, 254. [CrossRef]
102. Waterhouse, E.G.; An, J.J.; Orefice, L.L.; Baydyuk, M.; Liao, G.Y.; Zheng, K.; Lu, B.; Xu, B. BDNF promotes differentiation and maturation of adult-born neurons through GABAergic transmission. *J. Neurosci.* **2012**, *32*, 14318–14330. [CrossRef] [PubMed]
103. Park, H.; Poo, M.M. Neurotrophin regulation of neural circuit development and function. *Nat. Rev. Neurosci.* **2013**, *14*, 7–23. [CrossRef]
104. Jaworski, J.; Spangler, S.; Seeburg, D.P.; Hoogenraad, C.C.; Sheng, M. Control of dendritic arborization by the phosphoinositide-3'-kinase-Akt-mammalian target of rapamycin pathway. *J. Neurosci.* **2005**, *25*, 11300–11312. [CrossRef] [PubMed]
105. Kumar, V.; Zhang, M.X.; Swank, M.W.; Kunz, J.; Wu, G.Y. Regulation of dendritic morphogenesis by Ras-PI3K-Akt-mTOR and Ras-MAPK signaling pathways. *J. Neurosci.* **2005**, *25*, 11288–11299. [CrossRef] [PubMed]
106. Finkbeiner, S.; Tavazoie, S.F.; Maloratsky, A.; Jacobs, K.M.; Harris, K.M.; Greenberg, M.E. CREB: A major mediator of neuronal neurotrophin responses. *Neuron* **1997**, *19*, 1031–1047. [CrossRef]
107. Xing, J.; Kornhauser, J.M.; Xia, Z.; Thiele, E.A.; Greenberg, M.E. Nerve growth factor activates extracellular signal-regulated kinase and p38 mitogen-activated protein kinase pathways to stimulate CREB serine 133 phosphorylation. *Mol. Cell. Biol.* **1998**, *18*, 1946–1955. [CrossRef]
108. Segal, M.; Kreher, U.; Greenberger, V.; Braun, K. Is fragile X mental retardation protein involved in activity-induced plasticity of dendritic spines? *Brain Res.* **2003**, *972*, 9–15. [CrossRef]
109. Petryshen, T.L.; Sabeti, P.C.; Aldinger, K.A.; Fry, B.; Fan, J.B.; Schaffner, S.F.; Waggoner, S.G.; Tahl, A.R.; Sklar, P. Population genetic study of the brain-derived neurotrophic factor (BDNF) gene. *Mol. Psychiatry* **2010**, *15*, 810–815. [CrossRef]
110. Momose, Y.; Murata, M.; Kobayashi, K.; Tachikawa, M.; Nakabayashi, Y.; Kanazawa, I.; Toda, T. Association studies of multiple candidate genes for Parkinson's disease using single nucleotide polymorphisms. *Ann. Neurol.* **2002**, *51*, 133–136. [CrossRef]
111. Ventriglia, M.; Bocchio Chiavetto, L.; Benussi, L.; Binetti, G.; Zanetti, O.; Riva, M.A.; Gennarelli, M. Association between the BDNF 196 A/G polymorphism and sporadic Alzheimer's disease. *Mol. Psychiatry* **2002**, *7*, 136–137. [CrossRef]
112. Egan, M.F.; Kojima, M.; Callicott, J.H.; Goldberg, T.E.; Kolachana, B.S.; Bertolino, A.; Zaitsev, E.; Gold, B.; Goldman, D.; Dean, M.; et al. The BDNF val66met polymorphism affects activity-dependent secretion of BDNF and human memory and hippocampal function. *Cell* **2003**, *112*, 257–269. [CrossRef]
113. Chen, Z.Y.; Patel, P.D.; Sant, G.; Meng, C.X.; Teng, K.K.; Hempstead, B.L.; Lee, F.S. Variant brain-derived neurotrophic factor (BDNF) (Met66) alters the intracellular trafficking and activity-dependent secretion of wild-type BDNF in neurosecretory cells and cortical neurons. *J. Neurosci.* **2004**, *24*, 4401–4411. [CrossRef] [PubMed]
114. Chiaruttini, C.; Vicario, A.; Li, Z.; Baj, G.; Braiuca, P.; Wu, Y.; Lee, F.S.; Gardossi, L.; Baraban, J.M.; Tongiorgi, E. Dendritic trafficking of BDNF mRNA is mediated by translin and blocked by the G196A (Val66Met) mutation. *Proc. Natl. Acad. Sci. USA* **2009**, *106*, 16481–16486. [CrossRef] [PubMed]
115. Tsai, S.J. Salivary gland low-intensity pulsed ultrasound (LIPUS) stimulation as a potential treatment for various BDNF-implicated neuropsychiatric disorders. *Med. Hypotheses* **2020**, *137*, 109560. [CrossRef] [PubMed]
116. Lin, C.C.; Huang, T.L. Brain-derived neurotrophic factor and mental disorders. *Biomed. J.* **2020**, *43*, 134–142. [CrossRef] [PubMed]
117. Di Lazzaro, V.; Pellegrino, G.; Di Pino, G.; Corbetto, M.; Ranieri, F.; Brunelli, N.; Paolucci, M.; Bucossi, S.; Ventriglia, M.C.; Brown, P.; et al. Val66Met BDNF gene polymorphism influences human motor cortex plasticity in acute stroke. *Brain Stimul.* **2015**, *8*, 92–96. [CrossRef]

118. Morin-Moncet, O.; Latulipe-Loiselle, A.; Therrien-Blanchet, J.M.; Theoret, H. BDNF Val66Met polymorphism is associated with altered activity-dependent modulation of short-interval intracortical inhibition in bilateral M1. *PLoS ONE* **2018**, *13*, e0197505. [CrossRef]
119. Hashimoto, T.; Fukui, K.; Takeuchi, H.; Yokota, S.; Kikuchi, Y.; Tomita, H.; Taki, Y.; Kawashima, R. Effects of the BDNF Val66Met Polymorphism on Gray Matter Volume in Typically Developing Children and Adolescents. *Cereb. Cortex* **2016**, *26*, 1795–1803. [CrossRef]
120. Meng, W.D.; Sun, S.J.; Yang, J.; Chu, R.X.; Tu, W.; Liu, Q. Elevated Serum Brain-Derived Neurotrophic Factor (BDNF) but not BDNF Gene Val66Met Polymorphism Is Associated with Autism Spectrum Disorders. *Mol. Neurobiol.* **2017**, *54*, 1167–1172. [CrossRef]
121. Montag, C.; Basten, U.; Stelzel, C.; Fiebach, C.J.; Reuter, M. The BDNF Val66Met polymorphism and anxiety: Support for animal knock-in studies from a genetic association study in humans. *Psychiatry Res.* **2010**, *179*, 86–90. [CrossRef] [PubMed]
122. Park, C.H.; Kim, J.; Namgung, E.; Lee, D.W.; Kim, G.H.; Kim, M.; Kim, N.; Kim, T.D.; Kim, S.; Lyoo, I.K.; et al. The BDNF Val66Met Polymorphism Affects the Vulnerability of the Brain Structural Network. *Front. Hum. Neurosci.* **2017**, *11*, 400. [CrossRef] [PubMed]
123. Hariri, A.R.; Goldberg, T.E.; Mattay, V.S.; Kolachana, B.S.; Callicott, J.H.; Egan, M.F.; Weinberger, D.R. Brain-derived neurotrophic factor val66met polymorphism affects human memory-related hippocampal activity and predicts memory performance. *J. Neurosci.* **2003**, *23*, 6690–6694. [CrossRef] [PubMed]
124. Pezawas, L.; Verchinski, B.A.; Mattay, V.S.; Callicott, J.H.; Kolachana, B.S.; Straub, R.E.; Egan, M.F.; Meyer-Lindenberg, A.; Weinberger, D.R. The brain-derived neurotrophic factor val66met polymorphism and variation in human cortical morphology. *J. Neurosci.* **2004**, *24*, 10099–10102. [CrossRef] [PubMed]
125. Ho, B.C.; Milev, P.; O'Leary, D.S.; Librant, A.; Andreasen, N.C.; Wassink, T.H. Cognitive and magnetic resonance imaging brain morphometric correlates of brain-derived neurotrophic factor Val66Met gene polymorphism in patients with schizophrenia and healthy volunteers. *Arch. Gen. Psychiatry* **2006**, *63*, 731–740. [CrossRef] [PubMed]
126. Montag, C.; Weber, B.; Fliessbach, K.; Elger, C.; Reuter, M. The BDNF Val66Met polymorphism impacts parahippocampal and amygdala volume in healthy humans: Incremental support for a genetic risk factor for depression. *Psychol. Med.* **2009**, *39*, 1831–1839. [CrossRef] [PubMed]
127. Xia, H.; Du, X.; Yin, G.; Zhang, Y.; Li, X.; Cai, J.; Huang, X.; Ning, Y.; Soares, J.C.; Wu, F.; et al. Effects of smoking on cognition and BDNF levels in a male Chinese population: Relationship with BDNF Val66Met polymorphism. *Sci. Rep.* **2019**, *9*, 217. [CrossRef]
128. Altmann, V.; Schumacher-Schuh, A.F.; Rieck, M.; Callegari-Jacques, S.M.; Rieder, C.R.; Hutz, M.H. Val66Met BDNF polymorphism is associated with Parkinson's disease cognitive impairment. *Neurosci. Lett.* **2016**, *615*, 88–91. [CrossRef]
129. Wang, Q.; Liu, J.; Guo, Y.; Dong, G.; Zou, W.; Chen, Z. Association between BDNF G196A (Val66Met) polymorphism and cognitive impairment in patients with Parkinson's disease: A meta-analysis. *Braz. J. Med. Biol. Res.* **2019**, *52*, e8443. [CrossRef]
130. Franzmeier, N.; Ren, J.; Damm, A.; Monté-Rubio, G.; Boada, M.; Ruiz, A.; Ramirez, A.; Jessen, F.; Düzel, E.; Rodríguez Gómez, O.; et al. The BDNF. *Mol. Psychiatry* **2019**. [CrossRef]
131. Yin, Y.; Su, X.; Pan, L.; Li, C. BDNF Val66Met polymorphism and cognitive impairment in Parkinson's disease-a meta-analysis. *Neurol. Sci.* **2019**, *40*, 1901–1907. [CrossRef] [PubMed]
132. Dalby, R.B.; Elfving, B.; Poulsen, P.H.; Foldager, L.; Frandsen, J.; Videbech, P.; Rosenberg, R. Plasma brain-derived neurotrophic factor and prefrontal white matter integrity in late-onset depression and normal aging. *Acta Psychiatr. Scand.* **2013**, *128*, 387–396. [CrossRef] [PubMed]
133. Choi, S.; Han, K.M.; Won, E.; Yoon, B.J.; Lee, M.S.; Ham, B.J. Association of brain-derived neurotrophic factor DNA methylation and reduced white matter integrity in the anterior corona radiata in major depression. *J. Affect. Disord.* **2015**, *172*, 74–80. [CrossRef]
134. Youssef, M.M.; Underwood, M.D.; Huang, Y.Y.; Hsiung, S.C.; Liu, Y.; Simpson, N.R.; Bakalian, M.J.; Rosoklija, G.B.; Dwork, A.J.; Arango, V.; et al. Association of BDNF Val66Met Polymorphism and Brain BDNF Levels with Major Depression and Suicide. *Int. J. Neuropsychopharmacol.* **2018**, *21*, 528–538. [CrossRef]
135. Caldieraro, M.A.; McKee, M.; Leistner-Segal, S.; Vares, E.A.; Kubaski, F.; Spanemberg, L.; Brusius-Facchin, A.C.; Fleck, M.P.; Mischoulon, D. Val66Met polymorphism association with serum BDNF and inflammatory biomarkers in major depression. *World J. Biol. Psychiatry* **2018**, *19*, 402–409. [CrossRef]

136. Rong, C.; Park, C.; Rosenblat, J.D.; Subramaniapillai, M.; Zuckerman, H.; Fus, D.; Lee, Y.L.; Pan, Z.; Brietzke, E.; Mansur, R.B.; et al. Predictors of Response to Ketamine in Treatment Resistant Major Depressive Disorder and Bipolar Disorder. *Int. J. Environ. Res. Public Health* **2018**, *15*, 771. [CrossRef]
137. Mandolini, G.M.; Lazzaretti, M.; Pigoni, A.; Delvecchio, G.; Soares, J.C.; Brambilla, P. The impact of BDNF Val66Met polymorphism on cognition in Bipolar Disorder: A review: Special Section on "Translational and Neuroscience Studies in Affective Disorders"Section Editor, Maria Nobile MD, PhD. This Section of JAD focuses on the relevance of translational and neuroscience studies in providing a better understanding of the neural basis of affective disorders. The main aim is to briefly summaries relevant research findings in clinical neuroscience with particular regards to specific innovative topics in mood and anxiety disorders. *J. Affect. Disord.* **2019**, *243*, 552–558. [CrossRef]
138. Chen, N.C.; Chuang, Y.C.; Huang, C.W.; Lui, C.C.; Lee, C.C.; Hsu, S.W.; Lin, P.H.; Lu, Y.T.; Chang, Y.T.; Hsu, C.W.; et al. Interictal serum brain-derived neurotrophic factor level reflects white matter integrity, epilepsy severity, and cognitive dysfunction in chronic temporal lobe epilepsy. *Epilepsy Behav.* **2016**, *59*, 147–154. [CrossRef] [PubMed]
139. Sidhu, M.K.; Thompson, P.J.; Wandschneider, B.; Foulkes, A.; de Tisi, J.; Stretton, J.; Perona, M.; Thom, M.; Bonelli, S.B.; Burdett, J.; et al. The impact of brain-derived neurotrophic factor Val66Met polymorphism on cognition and functional brain networks in patients with intractable partial epilepsy. *CNS Neurosci. Ther.* **2019**, *25*, 223–232. [CrossRef] [PubMed]
140. Doherty, C.; Hogue, O.; Floden, D.P.; Altemus, J.B.; Najm, I.M.; Eng, C.; Busch, R.M. BDNF and COMT, but not APOE, alleles are associated with psychiatric symptoms in refractory epilepsy. *Epilepsy Behav.* **2019**, *94*, 131–136. [CrossRef]
141. Kheirollahi, M.; Kazemi, E.; Ashouri, S. Brain-Derived Neurotrophic Factor Gene Val66Met Polymorphism and Risk of Schizophrenia: A Meta-analysis of Case-Control Studies. *Cell. Mol. Neurobiol.* **2016**, *36*, 1–10. [CrossRef] [PubMed]
142. Xia, H.; Zhang, G.; Du, X.; Zhang, Y.; Yin, G.; Dai, J.; He, M.X.; Soares, J.C.; Li, X.; Zhang, X.Y. Suicide attempt, clinical correlates, and BDNF Val66Met polymorphism in chronic patients with schizophrenia. *Neuropsychology* **2018**, *32*, 199–205. [CrossRef]
143. Huang, E.; Hettige, N.C.; Zai, G.; Tomasi, J.; Huang, J.; Zai, C.C.; Pivac, N.; Nikolac Perkovic, M.; Tiwari, A.K.; Kennedy, J.L. BDNF Val66Met polymorphism and clinical response to antipsychotic treatment in schizophrenia and schizoaffective disorder patients: A meta-analysis. *Pharmacogenomics J.* **2019**, *19*, 269–276. [CrossRef] [PubMed]
144. Han, M.; Deng, C. BDNF as a pharmacogenetic target for antipsychotic treatment of schizophrenia. *Neurosci. Lett.* **2020**, *726*, 133870. [CrossRef] [PubMed]
145. Brown, A.; Machan, J.T.; Hayes, L.; Zervas, M. Molecular organization and timing of Wnt1 expression define cohorts of midbrain dopamine neuron progenitors in vivo. *J. Comp. Neurol.* **2011**, *519*, 2978–3000. [CrossRef]
146. Ramos-Cejudo, J.; Gutiérrez-Fernández, M.; Otero-Ortega, L.; Rodríguez-Frutos, B.; Fuentes, B.; Vallejo-Cremades, M.T.; Hernanz, T.N.; Cerdán, S.; Díez-Tejedor, E. Brain-derived neurotrophic factor administration mediated oligodendrocyte differentiation and myelin formation in subcortical ischemic stroke. *Stroke* **2015**, *46*, 221–228. [CrossRef]
147. Balkaya, M.; Cho, S. Genetics of stroke recovery: BDNF val66met polymorphism in stroke recovery and its interaction with aging. *Neurobiol. Dis.* **2019**, *126*, 36–46. [CrossRef]
148. Lohia, R.; Salari, R.; Brannigan, G. Sequence specificity despite intrinsic disorder: How a disease-associated Val/Met polymorphism rearranges tertiary interactions in a long disordered protein. *PLoS Comput. Biol.* **2019**, *15*, e1007390. [CrossRef]
149. Rock, P.L.; Roiser, J.P.; Riedel, W.J.; Blackwell, A.D. Cognitive impairment in depression: A systematic review and meta-analysis. *Psychol. Med.* **2014**, *44*, 2029–2040. [CrossRef]
150. Severino, V.; Farina, A.; Colucci-D'Amato, L.; Reccia, M.G.; Volpicelli, F.; Parente, A.; Chambery, A. Secretome profiling of differentiated neural mes-c-myc A1 cell line endowed with stem cell properties. *Biochim. Biophys. Acta* **2013**, *1834*, 2385–2395. [CrossRef]
151. Colucci-D'Amato, L.; Farina, A.; Vissers, J.P.; Chambery, A. Quantitative neuroproteomics: Classical and novel tools for studying neural differentiation and function. *Stem Cell Rev. Rep.* **2011**, *7*, 77–93. [CrossRef]

152. Di Lieto, A.; Leo, D.; Volpicelli, F.; di Porzio, U.; Colucci-D'Amato, L. FLUOXETINE modifies the expression of serotonergic markers in a differentiation-dependent fashion in the mesencephalic neural cell line A1 mes c-myc. *Brain Res.* **2007**, *1143*, 1–10. [CrossRef] [PubMed]
153. Nawa, Y.; Kaneko, H.; Oda, M.; Tsubonoya, M.; Hiroi, T.; Gentile, M.T.; Colucci-D'Amato, L.; Takahashi, R.; Matsui, H. Functional characterization of the neuron-restrictive silencer element in the human tryptophan hydroxylase 2 gene expression. *J. Neurochem.* **2017**, *142*, 827–840. [CrossRef] [PubMed]
154. Gentile, M.T.; Nawa, Y.; Lunardi, G.; Florio, T.; Matsui, H.; Colucci-D'Amato, L. Tryptophan hydroxylase 2 (TPH2) in a neuronal cell line: Modulation by cell differentiation and NRSF/rest activity. *J. Neurochem.* **2012**, *123*, 963–970. [CrossRef] [PubMed]
155. Duman, R.S.; Heninger, G.R.; Nestler, E.J. A molecular and cellular theory of depression. *Arch. Gen. Psychiatry* **1997**, *54*, 597–606. [CrossRef] [PubMed]
156. Colucci-D'Amato, L.; di Porzio, U. Neurogenesis in adult CNS: From denial to opportunities and challenges for therapy. *Bioessays* **2008**, *30*, 135–145. [CrossRef] [PubMed]
157. Colucci-D'Amato, L.; Bonavita, V.; di Porzio, U. The end of the central dogma of neurobiology: Stem cells and neurogenesis in adult CNS. *Neurol. Sci.* **2006**, *27*, 266–270. [CrossRef] [PubMed]
158. Cramer, S.C.; Sur, M.; Dobkin, B.H.; O'Brien, C.; Sanger, T.D.; Trojanowski, J.Q.; Rumsey, J.M.; Hicks, R.; Cameron, J.; Chen, D.; et al. Harnessing neuroplasticity for clinical applications. *Brain* **2011**, *134*, 1591–1609. [CrossRef]
159. Castrén, E. Neuronal network plasticity and recovery from depression. *JAMA Psychiatry* **2013**, *70*, 983–989. [CrossRef]
160. Snapyan, M.; Lemasson, M.; Brill, M.S.; Blais, M.; Massouh, M.; Ninkovic, J.; Gravel, C.; Berthod, F.; Götz, M.; Barker, P.A.; et al. Vasculature guides migrating neuronal precursors in the adult mammalian forebrain via brain-derived neurotrophic factor signaling. *J. Neurosci.* **2009**, *29*, 4172–4188. [CrossRef]
161. Bergami, M.; Rimondini, R.; Santi, S.; Blum, R.; Götz, M.; Canossa, M. Deletion of TrkB in adult progenitors alters newborn neuron integration into hippocampal circuits and increases anxiety-like behavior. *Proc. Natl. Acad. Sci. USA* **2008**, *105*, 15570–15575. [CrossRef] [PubMed]
162. Chan, K.L.; Tong, K.Y.; Yip, S.P. Relationship of serum brain-derived neurotrophic factor (BDNF) and health-related lifestyle in healthy human subjects. *Neurosci. Lett.* **2008**, *447*, 124–128. [CrossRef]
163. Zafra, F.; Lindholm, D.; Castrén, E.; Hartikka, J.; Thoenen, H. Regulation of brain-derived neurotrophic factor and nerve growth factor mRNA in primary cultures of hippocampal neurons and astrocytes. *J. Neurosci.* **1992**, *12*, 4793–4799. [CrossRef] [PubMed]
164. Castrén, E.; Antila, H. Neuronal plasticity and neurotrophic factors in drug responses. *Mol. Psychiatry* **2017**, *22*, 1085–1095. [CrossRef] [PubMed]
165. Castrén, E.; Zafra, F.; Thoenen, H.; Lindholm, D. Light regulates expression of brain-derived neurotrophic factor mRNA in rat visual cortex. *Proc. Natl. Acad. Sci. USA* **1992**, *89*, 9444–9448. [CrossRef] [PubMed]
166. Gianfranceschi, L.; Siciliano, R.; Walls, J.; Morales, B.; Kirkwood, A.; Huang, Z.J.; Tonegawa, S.; Maffei, L. Visual cortex is rescued from the effects of dark rearing by overexpression of BDNF. *Proc. Natl. Acad. Sci. USA* **2003**, *100*, 12486–12491. [CrossRef]
167. Hensch, T.K.; Bilimoria, P.M. Re-opening Windows: Manipulating Critical Periods for Brain Development. *Cerebrum* **2012**, *2012*, 11.
168. Hong, E.J.; McCord, A.E.; Greenberg, M.E. A biological function for the neuronal activity-dependent component of Bdnf transcription in the development of cortical inhibition. *Neuron* **2008**, *60*, 610–624. [CrossRef]
169. Volpicelli, F.; Speranza, L.; di Porzio, U.; Crispino, M.; Perrone-Capano, C. The serotonin receptor 7 and the structural plasticity of brain circuits. *Front. Behav. Neurosci.* **2014**, *8*, 318. [CrossRef]
170. Cazorla, M.; Arrang, J.M.; Prémont, J. Pharmacological characterization of six trkB antibodies reveals a novel class of functional agents for the study of the BDNF receptor. *Br. J. Pharmacol.* **2011**, *162*, 947–960. [CrossRef]
171. Park, S.W.; Nhu, l.H.; Cho, H.Y.; Seo, M.K.; Lee, C.H.; Ly, N.N.; Choi, C.M.; Lee, B.J.; Kim, G.M.; Seol, W.; et al. p11 mediates the BDNF-protective effects in dendritic outgrowth and spine formation in B27-deprived primary hippocampal cells. *J. Affect. Disord.* **2016**, *196*, 1–10. [CrossRef]
172. Katoh-Semba, R.; Asano, T.; Ueda, H.; Morishita, R.; Takeuchi, I.K.; Inaguma, Y.; Kato, K. Riluzole enhances expression of brain-derived neurotrophic factor with consequent proliferation of granule precursor cells in the rat hippocampus. *FASEB J.* **2002**, *16*, 1328–1330. [CrossRef]

173. Cavanaugh, J.E.; Ham, J.; Hetman, M.; Poser, S.; Yan, C.; Xia, Z. Differential regulation of mitogen-activated protein kinases ERK1/2 and ERK5 by neurotrophins, neuronal activity, and cAMP in neurons. *J. Neurosci.* **2001**, *21*, 434–443. [CrossRef]
174. Lin, E.; Cavanaugh, J.E.; Leak, R.K.; Perez, R.G.; Zigmond, M.J. Rapid activation of ERK by 6-hydroxydopamine promotes survival of dopaminergic cells. *J. Neurosci. Res.* **2008**, *86*, 108–117. [CrossRef] [PubMed]
175. Rauti, R.; Cellot, G.; D'Andrea, P.; Colliva, A.; Scaini, D.; Tongiorgi, E.; Ballerini, L. BDNF impact on synaptic dynamics: Extra or intracellular long-term release differently regulates cultured hippocampal synapses. *Mol. Brain* **2020**, *13*, 43. [CrossRef] [PubMed]
176. Ernfors, P.; Lee, K.F.; Jaenisch, R. Mice lacking brain-derived neurotrophic factor develop with sensory deficits. *Nature* **1994**, *368*, 147–150. [CrossRef]
177. Gao, X.; Smith, G.M.; Chen, J. Impaired dendritic development and synaptic formation of postnatal-born dentate gyrus granular neurons in the absence of brain-derived neurotrophic factor signaling. *Exp. Neurol.* **2009**, *215*, 178–190. [CrossRef]
178. Mariga, A.; Zavadil, J.; Ginsberg, S.D.; Chao, M.V. Withdrawal of BDNF from hippocampal cultures leads to changes in genes involved in synaptic function. *Dev. Neurobiol.* **2015**, *75*, 173–192. [CrossRef]
179. Aarse, J.; Herlitze, S.; Manahan-Vaughan, D. The requirement of BDNF for hippocampal synaptic plasticity is experience-dependent. *Hippocampus* **2016**, *26*, 739–751. [CrossRef]
180. Magariños, A.M.; Li, C.J.; Gal Toth, J.; Bath, K.G.; Jing, D.; Lee, F.S.; McEwen, B.S. Effect of brain-derived neurotrophic factor haploinsufficiency on stress-induced remodeling of hippocampal neurons. *Hippocampus* **2011**, *21*, 253–264. [CrossRef]
181. von Bohlen Und Halbach, O.; von Bohlen Und Halbach, V. BDNF effects on dendritic spine morphology and hippocampal function. *Cell Tissue Res.* **2018**, *373*, 729–741. [CrossRef]
182. von Bohlen und Halbach, O.; Minichiello, L.; Unsicker, K. TrkB but not trkC receptors are necessary for postnatal maintenance of hippocampal spines. *Neurobiol. Aging* **2008**, *29*, 1247–1255. [CrossRef]
183. Dokter, M.; Busch, R.; Poser, R.; Vogt, M.A.; von Bohlen Und Halbach, V.; Gass, P.; Unsicker, K.; von Bohlen Und Halbach, O. Implications of p75NTR for dentate gyrus morphology and hippocampus-related behavior revisited. *Brain Struct. Funct.* **2015**, *220*, 1449–1462. [CrossRef]
184. Lin, P.Y.; Kavalali, E.T.; Monteggia, L.M. Genetic Dissection of Presynaptic and Postsynaptic BDNF-TrkB Signaling in Synaptic Efficacy of CA3-CA1 Synapses. *Cell Rep.* **2018**, *24*, 1550–1561. [CrossRef]
185. Eyman, M.; Cefaliello, C.; Mandile, P.; Piscopo, S.; Crispino, M.; Giuditta, A. Training old rats selectively modulates synaptosomal protein synthesis. *J. Neurosci. Res.* **2013**, *91*, 20–29. [CrossRef]
186. Nikoletopoulou, V.; Sidiropoulou, K.; Kallergi, E.; Dalezios, Y.; Tavernarakis, N. Modulation of Autophagy by BDNF Underlies Synaptic Plasticity. *Cell Metab.* **2017**, *26*, 230–242. [CrossRef]
187. Fujimura, H.; Altar, C.A.; Chen, R.; Nakamura, T.; Nakahashi, T.; Kambayashi, J.; Sun, B.; Tandon, N.N. Brain-derived neurotrophic factor is stored in human platelets and released by agonist stimulation. *Thromb. Haemost.* **2002**, *87*, 728–734. [CrossRef]
188. Klein, A.B.; Williamson, R.; Santini, M.A.; Clemmensen, C.; Ettrup, A.; Rios, M.; Knudsen, G.M.; Aznar, S. Blood BDNF concentrations reflect brain-tissue BDNF levels across species. *Int. J. Neuropsychopharmacol.* **2011**, *14*, 347–353. [CrossRef]
189. Mondal, A.C.; Fatima, M. Direct and indirect evidences of BDNF and NGF as key modulators in depression: Role of antidepressants treatment. *Int. J. Neurosci.* **2019**, *129*, 283–296. [CrossRef]
190. Molendijk, M.L.; Spinhoven, P.; Polak, M.; Bus, B.A.; Penninx, B.W.; Elzinga, B.M. Serum BDNF concentrations as peripheral manifestations of depression: Evidence from a systematic review and meta-analyses on 179 associations (N=9484). *Mol. Psychiatry* **2014**, *19*, 791–800. [CrossRef]
191. Polyakova, M.; Stuke, K.; Schuemberg, K.; Mueller, K.; Schoenknecht, P.; Schroeter, M.L. BDNF as a biomarker for successful treatment of mood disorders: A systematic & quantitative meta-analysis. *J. Affect. Disord.* **2015**, *174*, 432–440. [CrossRef] [PubMed]
192. Kishi, T.; Yoshimura, R.; Ikuta, T.; Iwata, N. Brain-Derived Neurotrophic Factor and Major Depressive Disorder: Evidence from Meta-Analyses. *Front. Psychiatry* **2017**, *8*, 308. [CrossRef] [PubMed]
193. Serra-Millàs, M. Are the changes in the peripheral brain-derived neurotrophic factor levels due to platelet activation? *World J. Psychiatry* **2016**, *6*, 84–101. [CrossRef] [PubMed]

194. Allen, A.P.; Naughton, M.; Dowling, J.; Walsh, A.; Ismail, F.; Shorten, G.; Scott, L.; McLoughlin, D.M.; Cryan, J.F.; Dinan, T.G.; et al. Serum BDNF as a peripheral biomarker of treatment-resistant depression and the rapid antidepressant response: A comparison of ketamine and ECT. *J. Affect. Disord.* **2015**, *186*, 306–311. [CrossRef]
195. Lee, B.H.; Kim, Y.K. Reduced platelet BDNF level in patients with major depression. *Prog. Neuropsychopharmacol. Biol. Psychiatry* **2009**, *33*, 849–853. [CrossRef]
196. Pandey, G.N.; Dwivedi, Y.; Rizavi, H.S.; Ren, X.; Zhang, H.; Pavuluri, M.N. Brain-derived neurotrophic factor gene and protein expression in pediatric and adult depressed subjects. *Prog. Neuropsychopharmacol. Biol. Psychiatry* **2010**, *34*, 645–651. [CrossRef]
197. Serra-Millàs, M.; López-Vílchez, I.; Navarro, V.; Galán, A.M.; Escolar, G.; Penadés, R.; Catalán, R.; Fañanás, L.; Arias, B.; Gastó, C. Changes in plasma and platelet BDNF levels induced by S-citalopram in major depression. *Psychopharmacology* **2011**, *216*, 1–8. [CrossRef]
198. Dwivedi, Y. *The Neurobiological Basis of Suicide*; CRC Press: Boca Raton, FL, USA, 2012.
199. Pandey, G.N.; Ren, X.; Rizavi, H.S.; Conley, R.R.; Roberts, R.C.; Dwivedi, Y. Brain-derived neurotrophic factor and tyrosine kinase B receptor signalling in post-mortem brain of teenage suicide victims. *Int. J. Neuropsychopharmacol.* **2008**, *11*, 1047–1061. [CrossRef]
200. Hosang, G.M.; Shiles, C.; Tansey, K.E.; McGuffin, P.; Uher, R. Interaction between stress and the BDNF Val66Met polymorphism in depression: A systematic review and meta-analysis. *BMC Med.* **2014**, *12*, 7. [CrossRef]
201. Li, M.; Du, W.; Shao, F.; Wang, W. Cognitive dysfunction and epigenetic alterations of the BDNF gene are induced by social isolation during early adolescence. *Behav. Brain Res.* **2016**, *313*, 177–183. [CrossRef]
202. Yan, T.; Wang, L.; Kuang, W.; Xu, J.; Li, S.; Chen, J.; Yang, Y. Brain-derived neurotrophic factor Val66Met polymorphism association with antidepressant efficacy: A systematic review and meta-analysis. *Asia Pac. Psychiatry* **2014**, *6*, 241–251. [CrossRef]
203. Castrén, E.; Rantamäki, T. The role of BDNF and its receptors in depression and antidepressant drug action: Reactivation of developmental plasticity. *Dev. Neurobiol.* **2010**, *70*, 289–297. [CrossRef] [PubMed]
204. Crispino, M.; Volpicelli, F.; Perrone-Capano, C. Role of the Serotonin Receptor 7 in Brain Plasticity: From Development to Disease. *Int. J. Mol. Sci.* **2020**, *21*, 505. [CrossRef] [PubMed]
205. Alenina, N.; Klempin, F. The role of serotonin in adult hippocampal neurogenesis. *Behav. Brain Res.* **2015**, *277*, 49–57. [CrossRef] [PubMed]
206. Malberg, J.E.; Eisch, A.J.; Nestler, E.J.; Duman, R.S. Chronic antidepressant treatment increases neurogenesis in adult rat hippocampus. *J. Neurosci.* **2000**, *20*, 9104–9110. [CrossRef] [PubMed]
207. Santarelli, L.; Saxe, M.; Gross, C.; Surget, A.; Battaglia, F.; Dulawa, S.; Weisstaub, N.; Lee, J.; Duman, R.; Arancio, O.; et al. Requirement of hippocampal neurogenesis for the behavioral effects of antidepressants. *Science* **2003**, *301*, 805–809. [CrossRef]
208. Rantamäki, T.; Castrén, E. Targeting TrkB neurotrophin receptor to treat depression. *Expert Opin. Ther. Targets* **2008**, *12*, 705–715. [CrossRef] [PubMed]
209. Speranza, L.; Labus, J.; Volpicelli, F.; Guseva, D.; Lacivita, E.; Leopoldo, M.; Bellenchi, G.C.; di Porzio, U.; Bijata, M.; Perrone-Capano, C.; et al. Serotonin 5-HT7 receptor increases the density of dendritic spines and facilitates synaptogenesis in forebrain neurons. *J. Neurochem.* **2017**, *141*, 647–661. [CrossRef]
210. Speranza, L.; Giuliano, T.; Volpicelli, F.; De Stefano, M.E.; Lombardi, L.; Chambery, A.; Lacivita, E.; Leopoldo, M.; Bellenchi, G.C.; di Porzio, U.; et al. Activation of 5-HT7 receptor stimulates neurite elongation through mTOR, Cdc42 and actin filaments dynamics. *Front. Behav. Neurosci.* **2015**, *9*, 62. [CrossRef]
211. Speranza, L.; Chambery, A.; Di Domenico, M.; Crispino, M.; Severino, V.; Volpicelli, F.; Leopoldo, M.; Bellenchi, G.C.; di Porzio, U.; Perrone-Capano, C. The serotonin receptor 7 promotes neurite outgrowth via ERK and Cdk5 signaling pathways. *Neuropharmacology* **2013**, *67*, 155–167. [CrossRef]
212. Popova, N.K.; Naumenko, V.S. Neuronal and behavioral plasticity: The role of serotonin and BDNF systems tandem. *Expert Opin. Ther. Targets* **2019**, *23*, 227–239. [CrossRef] [PubMed]
213. Castrén, E. Neurotrophins and psychiatric disorders. *Handb. Exp. Pharmacol.* **2014**, *220*, 461–479. [CrossRef] [PubMed]
214. Castrén, E.; Kojima, M. Brain-derived neurotrophic factor in mood disorders and antidepressant treatments. *Neurobiol. Dis.* **2017**, *97*, 119–126. [CrossRef] [PubMed]

215. Castrén, E.; Rantamäki, T. Role of brain-derived neurotrophic factor in the aetiology of depression: Implications for pharmacological treatment. *CNS Drugs* **2010**, *24*, 1–7. [CrossRef]
216. Lepack, A.E.; Fuchikami, M.; Dwyer, J.M.; Banasr, M.; Duman, R.S. BDNF release is required for the behavioral actions of ketamine. *Int. J. Neuropsychopharmacol.* **2014**, *18*. [CrossRef]
217. Abdallah, C.G.; Sanacora, G.; Duman, R.S.; Krystal, J.H. Ketamine and rapid-acting antidepressants: A window into a new neurobiology for mood disorder therapeutics. *Annu. Rev. Med.* **2015**, *66*, 509–523. [CrossRef] [PubMed]
218. Monteggia, L.M.; Zarate, C. Antidepressant actions of ketamine: From molecular mechanisms to clinical practice. *Curr. Opin. Neurobiol.* **2015**, *30*, 139–143. [CrossRef] [PubMed]
219. Björkholm, C.; Monteggia, L.M. BDNF-a key transducer of antidepressant effects. *Neuropharmacology* **2016**, *102*, 72–79. [CrossRef] [PubMed]
220. Hoshaw, B.A.; Malberg, J.E.; Lucki, I. Central administration of IGF-I and BDNF leads to long-lasting antidepressant-like effects. *Brain Res.* **2005**, *1037*, 204–208. [CrossRef]
221. Eisch, A.J.; Bolaños, C.A.; de Wit, J.; Simonak, R.D.; Pudiak, C.M.; Barrot, M.; Verhaagen, J.; Nestler, E.J. Brain-derived neurotrophic factor in the ventral midbrain-nucleus accumbens pathway: A role in depression. *Biol. Psychiatry* **2003**, *54*, 994–1005. [CrossRef]
222. Monteggia, L.M.; Luikart, B.; Barrot, M.; Theobold, D.; Malkovska, I.; Nef, S.; Parada, L.F.; Nestler, E.J. Brain-derived neurotrophic factor conditional knockouts show gender differences in depression-related behaviors. *Biol. Psychiatry* **2007**, *61*, 187–197. [CrossRef] [PubMed]
223. Monteggia, L.M.; Barrot, M.; Powell, C.M.; Berton, O.; Galanis, V.; Gemelli, T.; Meuth, S.; Nagy, A.; Greene, R.W.; Nestler, E.J. Essential role of brain-derived neurotrophic factor in adult hippocampal function. *Proc. Natl. Acad. Sci. USA* **2004**, *101*, 10827–10832. [CrossRef] [PubMed]
224. Saarelainen, T.; Hendolin, P.; Lucas, G.; Koponen, E.; Sairanen, M.; MacDonald, E.; Agerman, K.; Haapasalo, A.; Nawa, H.; Aloyz, R.; et al. Activation of the TrkB neurotrophin receptor is induced by antidepressant drugs and is required for antidepressant-induced behavioral effects. *J. Neurosci.* **2003**, *23*, 349–357. [CrossRef] [PubMed]
225. Li, Y.; Luikart, B.W.; Birnbaum, S.; Chen, J.; Kwon, C.H.; Kernie, S.G.; Bassel-Duby, R.; Parada, L.F. TrkB regulates hippocampal neurogenesis and governs sensitivity to antidepressive treatment. *Neuron* **2008**, *59*, 399–412. [CrossRef]
226. Liu, R.J.; Lee, F.S.; Li, X.Y.; Bambico, F.; Duman, R.S.; Aghajanian, G.K. Brain-derived neurotrophic factor Val66Met allele impairs basal and ketamine-stimulated synaptogenesis in prefrontal cortex. *Biol. Psychiatry* **2012**, *71*, 996–1005. [CrossRef]
227. Kato, T.; Fogaça, M.V.; Deyama, S.; Li, X.Y.; Fukumoto, K.; Duman, R.S. BDNF release and signaling are required for the antidepressant actions of GLYX-13. *Mol. Psychiatry* **2018**, *23*, 2007–2017. [CrossRef]
228. Herring, M.P.; Puetz, T.W.; O'Connor, P.J.; Dishman, R.K. Effect of exercise training on depressive symptoms among patients with a chronic illness: A systematic review and meta-analysis of randomized controlled trials. *Arch. Intern. Med.* **2012**, *172*, 101–111. [CrossRef]
229. Ota, K.T.; Duman, R.S. Environmental and pharmacological modulations of cellular plasticity: Role in the pathophysiology and treatment of depression. *Neurobiol. Dis.* **2013**, *57*, 28–37. [CrossRef]
230. Schuch, F.B.; Vancampfort, D.; Richards, J.; Rosenbaum, S.; Ward, P.B.; Stubbs, B. Exercise as a treatment for depression: A meta-analysis adjusting for publication bias. *J. Psychiatr. Res.* **2016**, *77*, 42–51. [CrossRef]
231. Rasmussen, P.; Brassard, P.; Adser, H.; Pedersen, M.V.; Leick, L.; Hart, E.; Secher, N.H.; Pedersen, B.K.; Pilegaard, H. Evidence for a release of brain-derived neurotrophic factor from the brain during exercise. *Exp. Physiol.* **2009**, *94*, 1062–1069. [CrossRef]
232. Seifert, T.; Brassard, P.; Wissenberg, M.; Rasmussen, P.; Nordby, P.; Stallknecht, B.; Adser, H.; Jakobsen, A.H.; Pilegaard, H.; Nielsen, H.B.; et al. Endurance training enhances BDNF release from the human brain. *Am. J. Physiol. Regul. Integr. Comp. Physiol.* **2010**, *298*, R372–R377. [CrossRef] [PubMed]
233. Xu, L.; Zheng, Y.L.; Yin, X.; Xu, S.J.; Tian, D.; Zhang, C.Y.; Wang, S.; Ma, J.Z. Excessive Treadmill Training Enhances Brain-Specific MicroRNA-34a in the Mouse Hippocampus. *Front. Mol. Neurosci.* **2020**, *13*, 7. [CrossRef] [PubMed]
234. de Assis, G.G.; de Almondes, K.M. Exercise-dependent BDNF as a Modulatory Factor for the Executive Processing of Individuals in Course of Cognitive Decline. A Systematic Review. *Front. Psychol.* **2017**, *8*, 584. [CrossRef] [PubMed]

235. Pajonk, F.G.; Wobrock, T.; Gruber, O.; Scherk, H.; Berner, D.; Kaizl, I.; Kierer, A.; Müller, S.; Oest, M.; Meyer, T.; et al. Hippocampal plasticity in response to exercise in schizophrenia. *Arch. Gen. Psychiatry* **2010**, *67*, 133–143. [CrossRef] [PubMed]
236. Moon, H.Y.; Becke, A.; Berron, D.; Becker, B.; Sah, N.; Benoni, G.; Janke, E.; Lubejko, S.T.; Greig, N.H.; Mattison, J.A.; et al. Running-Induced Systemic Cathepsin B Secretion Is Associated with Memory Function. *Cell Metab.* **2016**, *24*, 332–340. [CrossRef] [PubMed]
237. Boström, P.; Wu, J.; Jedrychowski, M.P.; Korde, A.; Ye, L.; Lo, J.C.; Rasbach, K.A.; Boström, E.A.; Choi, J.H.; Long, J.Z.; et al. A PGC1-α-dependent myokine that drives brown-fat-like development of white fat and thermogenesis. *Nature* **2012**, *481*, 463–468. [CrossRef]
238. Wrann, C.D.; White, J.P.; Salogiannnis, J.; Laznik-Bogoslavski, D.; Wu, J.; Ma, D.; Lin, J.D.; Greenberg, M.E.; Spiegelman, B.M. Exercise induces hippocampal BDNF through a PGC-1α/FNDC5 pathway. *Cell Metab.* **2013**, *18*, 649–659. [CrossRef]
239. Müller, P.; Duderstadt, Y.; Lessmann, V.; Müller, N.G. Lactate and BDNF: Key Mediators of Exercise Induced Neuroplasticity? *J. Clin. Med.* **2020**, *9*, 1136. [CrossRef]
240. Piotrowicz, Z.; Chalimoniuk, M.; Płoszczyca, K.; Czuba, M.; Langfort, J. Exercise-Induced Elevated BDNF Level Does Not Prevent Cognitive Impairment Due to Acute Exposure to Moderate Hypoxia in Well-Trained Athletes. *Int. J. Mol. Sci.* **2020**, *21*, 5569. [CrossRef]
241. Miranda, M.; Morici, J.F.; Zanoni, M.B.; Bekinschtein, P. Brain-Derived Neurotrophic Factor: A Key Molecule for Memory in the Healthy and the Pathological Brain. *Front. Cell Neurosci.* **2019**, *13*, 363. [CrossRef]
242. Hock, C.; Heese, K.; Hulette, C.; Rosenberg, C.; Otten, U. Region-specific neurotrophin imbalances in Alzheimer disease: Decreased levels of brain-derived neurotrophic factor and increased levels of nerve growth factor in hippocampus and cortical areas. *Arch. Neurol.* **2000**, *57*, 846–851. [CrossRef]
243. Zuccato, C.; Marullo, M.; Conforti, P.; MacDonald, M.E.; Tartari, M.; Cattaneo, E. Systematic assessment of BDNF and its receptor levels in human cortices affected by Huntington's disease. *Brain Pathol.* **2008**, *18*, 225–238. [CrossRef] [PubMed]
244. Narisawa-Saito, M.; Wakabayashi, K.; Tsuji, S.; Takahashi, H.; Nawa, H. Regional specificity of alterations in NGF, BDNF and NT-3 levels in Alzheimer's disease. *Neuroreport* **1996**, *7*, 2925–2928. [CrossRef]
245. Hoxha, E.; Lippiello, P.; Zurlo, F.; Balbo, I.; Santamaria, R.; Tempia, F.; Miniaci, M.C. The Emerging Role of Altered Cerebellar Synaptic Processing in Alzheimer's Disease. *Front. Aging Neurosci.* **2018**, *10*, 396. [CrossRef] [PubMed]
246. Peng, S.; Wuu, J.; Mufson, E.J.; Fahnestock, M. Precursor form of brain-derived neurotrophic factor and mature brain-derived neurotrophic factor are decreased in the pre-clinical stages of Alzheimer's disease. *J. Neurochem.* **2005**, *93*, 1412–1421. [CrossRef] [PubMed]
247. Choi, S.H.; Bylykbashi, E.; Chatila, Z.K.; Lee, S.W.; Pulli, B.; Clemenson, G.D.; Kim, E.; Rompala, A.; Oram, M.K.; Asselin, C.; et al. Combined adult neurogenesis and BDNF mimic exercise effects on cognition in an Alzheimer's mouse model. *Science* **2018**, *361*. [CrossRef] [PubMed]
248. Sleiman, S.F.; Henry, J.; Al-Haddad, R.; El Hayek, L.; Abou Haidar, E.; Stringer, T.; Ulja, D.; Karuppagounder, S.S.; Holson, E.B.; Ratan, R.R.; et al. Exercise promotes the expression of brain derived neurotrophic factor (BDNF) through the action of the ketone body β-hydroxybutyrate. *Elife* **2016**, *5*. [CrossRef] [PubMed]
249. Colucci-D'Amato, L.; Perrone-Capano, C.; di Porzio, U. Chronic activation of ERK and neurodegenerative diseases. *Bioessays* **2003**, *25*, 1085–1095. [CrossRef] [PubMed]
250. Kirouac, L.; Rajic, A.J.; Cribbs, D.H.; Padmanabhan, J. Activation of Ras-ERK Signaling and GSK-3 by Amyloid Precursor Protein and Amyloid Beta Facilitates Neurodegeneration in Alzheimer's Disease. *eNeuro* **2017**, *4*. [CrossRef]
251. Nizzari, M.; Barbieri, F.; Gentile, M.T.; Passarella, D.; Caorsi, C.; Diaspro, A.; Taglialatela, M.; Pagano, A.; Colucci-D'Amato, L.; Florio, T.; et al. Amyloid-β protein precursor regulates phosphorylation and cellular compartmentalization of microtubule associated protein tau. *J. Alzheimers Dis.* **2012**, *29*, 211–227. [CrossRef]
252. Bartolotti, N.; Segura, L.; Lazarov, O. Diminished CRE-Induced Plasticity is Linked to Memory Deficits in Familial Alzheimer's Disease Mice. *J. Alzheimers Dis.* **2016**, *50*, 477–489. [CrossRef] [PubMed]
253. Rosa, E.; Fahnestock, M. CREB expression mediates amyloid β-induced basal BDNF downregulation. *Neurobiol. Aging* **2015**, *36*, 2406–2413. [CrossRef] [PubMed]

254. Thiele, C.J.; Li, Z.; McKee, A.E. On Trk–the TrkB signal transduction pathway is an increasingly important target in cancer biology. *Clin. Cancer Res.* **2009**, *15*, 5962–5967. [CrossRef] [PubMed]
255. Xiong, J.; Zhou, L.I.; Lim, Y.; Yang, M.; Zhu, Y.H.; Li, Z.W.; Fu, D.L.; Zhou, X.F. Mature brain-derived neurotrophic factor and its receptor TrkB are upregulated in human glioma tissues. *Oncol. Lett.* **2015**, *10*, 223–227. [CrossRef] [PubMed]
256. Colucci-D'Amato, G.L.; D'Alessio, A.; Califano, D.; Cali, G.; Rizzo, C.; Nitsch, L.; Santelli, G.; de Franciscis, V. Abrogation of nerve growth factor-induced terminal differentiation by ret oncogene involves perturbation of nuclear translocation of ERK. *J. Biol. Chem.* **2000**, *275*, 19306–19314. [CrossRef]
257. Radin, D.P.; Patel, P. BDNF: An Oncogene or Tumor Suppressor? *Anticancer. Res.* **2017**, *37*, 3983–3990. [CrossRef]
258. Wang, X.; Prager, B.C.; Wu, Q.; Kim, L.J.Y.; Gimple, R.C.; Shi, Y.; Yang, K.; Morton, A.R.; Zhou, W.; Zhu, Z.; et al. Reciprocal Signaling between Glioblastoma Stem Cells and Differentiated Tumor Cells Promotes Malignant Progression. *Cell Stem Cell* **2018**, *22*, 514–528. [CrossRef]
259. Garofalo, S.; D'Alessandro, G.; Chece, G.; Brau, F.; Maggi, L.; Rosa, A.; Porzia, A.; Mainiero, F.; Esposito, V.; Lauro, C.; et al. Enriched environment reduces glioma growth through immune and non-immune mechanisms in mice. *Nat. Commun.* **2015**, *6*, 6623. [CrossRef]
260. Garofalo, S.; Porzia, A.; Mainiero, F.; Di Angelantonio, S.; Cortese, B.; Basilico, B.; Pagani, F.; Cignitti, G.; Chece, G.; Maggio, R.; et al. Environmental stimuli shape microglial plasticity in glioma. *Elife* **2017**, *6*. [CrossRef]
261. Colucci-D'Amato, L.; Cimaglia, G. As a potential source of neuroactive compounds to promote and restore neural functions. *J. Tradit. Complement. Med.* **2020**, *10*, 309–314. [CrossRef]
262. Gentile, M.T.; Ciniglia, C.; Reccia, M.G.; Volpicelli, F.; Gatti, M.; Thellung, S.; Florio, T.; Melone, M.A.; Colucci-D'Amato, L. Ruta graveolens L. induces death of glioblastoma cells and neural progenitors, but not of neurons, via ERK 1/2 and AKT activation. *PLoS ONE* **2015**, *10*, e0118864. [CrossRef] [PubMed]

10

GPR4 Knockout Improves the Neurotoxin-Induced, Caspase-Dependent Mitochondrial Apoptosis of the Dopaminergic Neuronal Cell

Md Ezazul Haque [1], Mahbuba Akther [1], Shofiul Azam [1], Dong-Kug Choi [1,2] and In-Su Kim [2,*]

1 Department of Applied Life Science, Graduate School, Konkuk University, Chungju 27478, Korea; mdezazulhaque@yahoo.com (M.E.H.); smritymahbuba@gmail.com (M.A.); shofiul_azam@hotmail.com (S.A.); choidk@kku.ac.kr (D.-K.C.)

2 Department of Biotechnology, Research Institute of Inflammatory Disease (RID), College of Biomedical and Health Science, Konkuk University, Chungju 27478, Korea

* Correspondence: kis5497@kku.ac.kr

Abstract: In Parkinson's disease, mitochondrial oxidative stress-mediated apoptosis is a major cause of dopaminergic neuronal loss in the substantia nigra (SN). G protein-coupled receptor 4 (GPR4), previously recognised as an orphan G protein coupled-receptor (GPCR), has recently been claimed as a member of the group of proton-activated GPCRs. Its activity in neuronal apoptosis, however, remains undefined. In this study, we investigated the role of GPR4 in the 1-methyl-4-phenylpyridinium ion (MPP^+) and hydrogen peroxide (H_2O_2)-treated apoptotic cell death of stably GPR4-overexpressing and stably GPR4-knockout human neuroblastoma SH-SY5Y cells. In GPR4-OE cells, MPP^+ and H_2O_2 were found to significantly increase the expression levels of both mRNA and proteins of the pro-apoptotic Bcl-2-associated X protein (Bax) genes, while they decreased the anti-apoptotic B-cell lymphoma 2 (Bcl-2) genes. In addition, MPP^+ treatment activated Caspase-3, leading to the cleavage of poly (ADP-ribose) polymerase (PARP) and decreasing the mitochondrial membrane potential ($\Delta\Psi m$) in GPR4-OE cells. In contrast, H_2O_2 treatment significantly increased the intracellular calcium ions (Ca^{2+}) and reactive oxygen species (ROS) in GPR4-OE cells. Further, chemical inhibition by NE52-QQ57, a selective antagonist of GPR4, and knockout of GPR4 by clustered regularly interspaced short palindromic repeats (CRISPR)/Cas9 decreased the Bax/Bcl-2 ratio and ROS generation, and stabilised the $\Delta\Psi m$, thus protecting the SH-SY5Y cells from MPP^+- or H_2O_2-induced apoptotic cell death. Moreover, the knockout of GPR4 decreased the proteolytic degradation of phosphatidylinositol biphosphate (PIP_2) and subsequent release of the endoplasmic reticulum (ER)-stored Ca^{2+} in the cytosol. Our results suggest that the pharmacological inhibition or genetic deletion of GPR4 improves the neurotoxin-induced caspase-dependent mitochondrial apoptotic pathway, possibly through the modulation of PIP_2 degradation-mediated calcium signalling. Therefore, GPR4 presents a potential therapeutic target for neurodegenerative disorders such as Parkinson's disease.

Keywords: apoptosis; neurodegeneration; GPR4 receptor; MPP^+; Parkinson's disease; CRISPR/cas9

---

1. Introduction

Parkinson's disease (PD) is a neurodegenerative disorder characterised by dopamine deficiency. An important pathological basis of PD is the loss of dopaminergic neurons due to apoptotic cell death in the substantia nigra (SN) of the brain [1]. An array of evidence suggests that reactive oxygen species (ROS)-induced oxidative stress is a major cause of the dopaminergic neuronal loss in the SN [2]. Mitochondria are key players in apoptosis during this neurodegeneration. In a cell undergoing apoptosis, mitochondria increase the production of oxyradicals and open the pores of its membranes, leading to the depolarisation of its transmembrane potential ($\Delta\psi m$) and the release of cytochrome C [3,4]. The B-cell lymphoma 2 (Bcl-2) family of proteins, which includes anti-apoptotic Bcl-2 and pro-apoptotic Bcl-2-associated X protein (Bax) members, plays a critical role in the initiation of the apoptotic pathway. When anti-apoptotic Bcl-2 localises in the mitochondrial inner membrane from the outer membrane, the intermembrane space protein, cytochrome C, is released. This binds to apoptotic peptidase activating factor 1 (APAF1) and forms a heptameric structure, known as the apoptosome. Apoptosomes recruit caspase 9 and activate a series of events, eventually activating Caspase-3 as a result [5]. Surprisingly, poly (ADP-ribose) polymerase (PARP), a nuclear protein involved in DNA repair that is specifically cleaved to a signature 89-kDa fragment, has been implicated as an early marker for apoptotic cell death in neurons [6]. The characteristic hallmarks of the mitochondrial oxidative damage-induced apoptosis pathway can be considered to be the opening of the mitochondrial permeability transition pore (mPTP), the collapse of the mitochondrial membrane potential ($\Delta\Psi m$), the release of cytochrome C, the activation of Caspase-3, and proteolytic degradation of PARP [7,8]. Surprisingly, the endoplasmic reticulum (ER) acts as a reservoir of calcium ions (Ca^{2+}). The ER can release Ca^{2+} through either its ryanodine (RYR) or inositol trisphosphate (IP3) receptors. Ca^{2+}, once released from the ER, is taken up by the mitochondrial Ca^{2+} uniporter (MCU) located in the mitochondrial inner membrane [9]. An increase in mitochondrial Ca^{2+} is associated with an increase of the mPTP opening and ROS generation, a decrease in $\Delta\Psi m$, and release of cytochrome C, as well as excitotoxicity and apoptosis [10–12]. Recent findings suggest that an increase in the Ca^{2+} released from the ER can increase the mitochondrial oxidant stress of the substantia nigra pars compacta (SNc) dopaminergic (DA) neurons [10,13]. Alteration of the intracellular calcium homeostasis PD cybrids has also been reported [14].

1-methyl-4-phenylpyridinium ion (MPP^+) and hydrogen peroxide (H_2O_2) are the most widely employed neurotoxins, due to their ability to mimic a PD-like syndrome with apoptotic cell death through mitochondrial oxidative damage, in both cellular and animal models of PD [15–17]. MPP^+, the active metabolite of 1-methyl-4-phenyl-1,2,3,6-tetrahydropyridine (MPTP), generates 5–7 times more ROS by selectively inhibiting mitochondrial complex I, thus initiating pro-apoptotic Bax/Bcl-2-dependent apoptotic cell death [15]. Besides, MPP^+- and H_2O_2-mediated oxidative stress have also been reported to cause mitochondrial oxidative stress-mediated apoptotic cell death [18]. Moreover, MPP^+- and H_2O_2-mediated cell death are associated with the alteration of intracellular Ca^{2+} homeostasis. An increase in intracellular Ca^{2+} due to ER stress also potentiates a decrease in $\Delta\Psi m$, the release of cytochrome C, and the induction of apoptosis [12,19–21]. Therefore, the inhibition of pro-apoptotic signalling, or the decrease of intracellular ROS and Ca^{2+}, may be beneficial for the protection of dopaminergic neuronal loss in PD.

G protein-coupled receptor 4 (GPR4), a proton-sensing receptor, is highly sensitive to the alteration of extracellular proton concentration [22]. It belongs to a small G protein-coupled proton-sensing receptor family that includes ovarian cancer G protein-coupled receptor 1 (OGR1), also referred to as GPR68, G2A, also termed GPR132, and T-cell death-associated gene 8 (TDAG8), also known as GPR65. These receptors signal through either to phosphoinositide mediated increase in intracellular Ca^{2+} or through modulating adenylate cyclase activity [23,24]. Information regarding the distribution and biology of GPR4 in the brain of an individual with PD is limited. An abundant level of GPR4 expression was observed in the retro-trapezoidal nucleus locus coeruleus, the cerebrovascular endothelium, the neurons of the dorsal raphe, and the lateral septum of a GPR4-knock-in mouse model [25]. Recently, the role of GPR4 in inflammation during ER stress pathway-mediated apoptotic cell death has been reported. In human umbilical vein endothelial cells (HUVEC) and other disease models, such as that of myocardial ischemic mice, knocking out GPR4 has been found to reduce cardiomyocyte apoptosis and improve cardiac function [26–28]. However, no study has yet to elucidate the role of GPR4 on apoptotic cell death in neurodegenerative disorders. Therefore, this work aims to forge an understanding of the role of GPR4 in neurotoxin-induced, mitochondrial oxidative stress-mediated apoptosis in a PD model. In particular, through our study of the overexpression and genetic deletion of GPR4, we investigate the role of GPR4 in the mitochondrial apoptosis pathway.

2. Results

2.1. Expression of GPR4 Is Upregulated in Neurotoxin-Stimulated Apoptosis in SH-SY5Y Cells

To investigate the concentrations of MPP^+ and H_2O_2 that precipitated a cell death of nearly 50% in the SH-SY5Y cells, 24 h serum-starved SH-SY5Y cells were treated with MPP^+ (0.25, 0.5, and 1 mM) or H_2O_2 (50, 75, and 125 μM) for 24 h. As is shown in Figure 1A, when treated with the various concentrations of MPP^+ (1 mM; 56.511 ± 1.55%) and H_2O_2 (125 μM; 53.12 ± 2.34%), half of the cell population in the MTT assay died. Furthermore, the mRNA and protein expressions of GPR4 in SH-SY5Y cells in both MPP^+- (1 mM) and H_2O_2- (125 μM) treated serum-free media gradually increased in a time-dependent manner (3–24 h; Figure 1B).

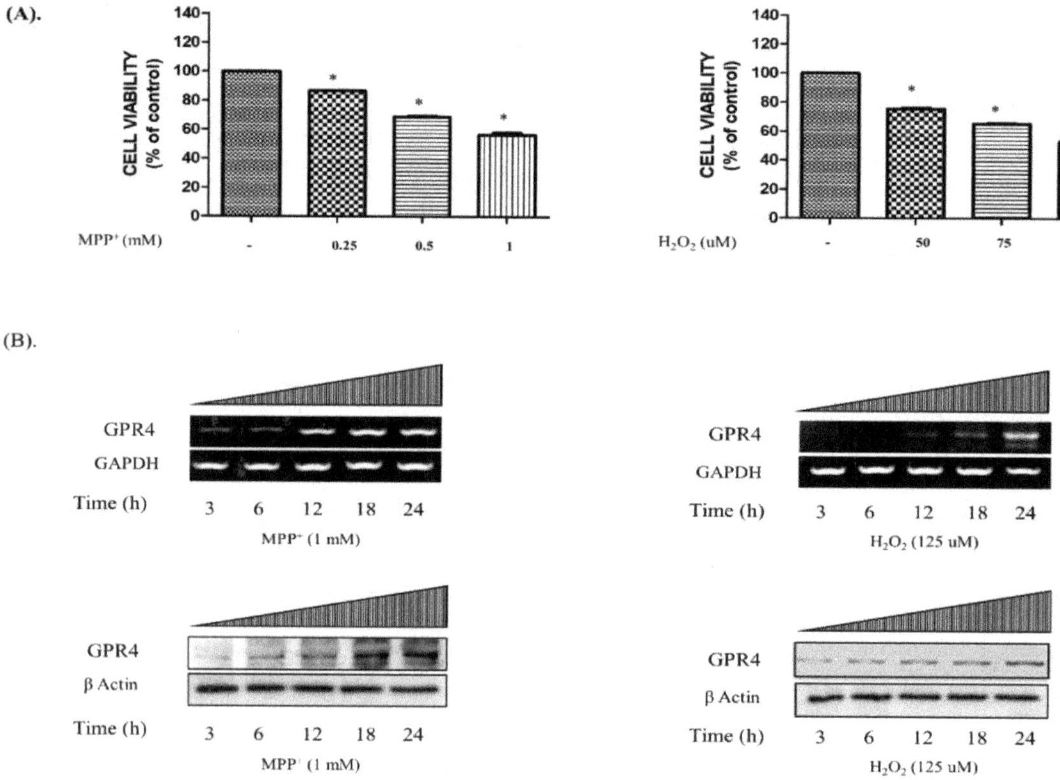

Figure 1. The cellular viability and the mRNA and protein expressions of GPR4 in MPP^+- and H_2O_2-treated SH-SY5Y cells. 24 h serum-starved SH-SY5Y cells were treated with different concentrations of MPP^+ (0.25, 0.5, and 1 mM) and H_2O_2 (50, 75, and 125 μM) for 24 h in serum-free culture media. (**A**) The cellular viability of the SH-SY5Y cell after treatment with different concentrations of MPP^+ and H_2O_2 in serum-free media for 24 h. (**B**) Reverse transcription-polymerase chain reaction (RT-PCR) and immunoblotting demonstrate the mRNA and protein expressions of GPR4 in SH-SY5Y cells at different time points (3, 6, 12, 18, and 24 h) after stimulation with MPP^+ (1 mM) and H_2O_2 (125 μM) in serum-free media. Glyceraldehyde-3-phosphate dehydrogenase (GAPDH) and β-actin were utilised as the internal controls. Mean ± standard error of the mean (SEM; $n = 3$) was employed to express the data. Tukey's multiple comparison test was performed using a one-way analysis of variance (ANOVA). Each * $p < 0.05$ refers to the other sample concentrations compared with the control cells.

2.2. Knockout of GPR4 Protects SH-SY5Y Cells from Neurotoxin-Stimulated Apoptosis in SH-SY5Y Cells

To assess the effect of GPR4 overexpression and knockout on MPP^+-induced apoptotic cell death, 24 h serum-starved SH-SY5Y cells were treated with MPP^+ (1 mM) for 24 h in serum-free media

(Figure 2). Following the MPP^+ (1 mM) treatment for 24 h in serum-free media, the number of SH-SY5Y viable cells decreased. Furthermore, the cells became rounded, displayed an increased neurite retraction, and were found to be loosely attached to the plate. Under bright-field optics, the GPR4-OE cells treated with MPP^+ (1 mM) exhibited less cell viability, with increased rounded cells, increased neurite retraction, and loose attachment to the surface. In contrast, the GPR4-KO cells treated with MPP^+ (1 mM) were more viable, strongly attached, neuronal shaped, and demonstrated less neuronal retraction than both the control and the GPR4-OE cells (Figure 2A).

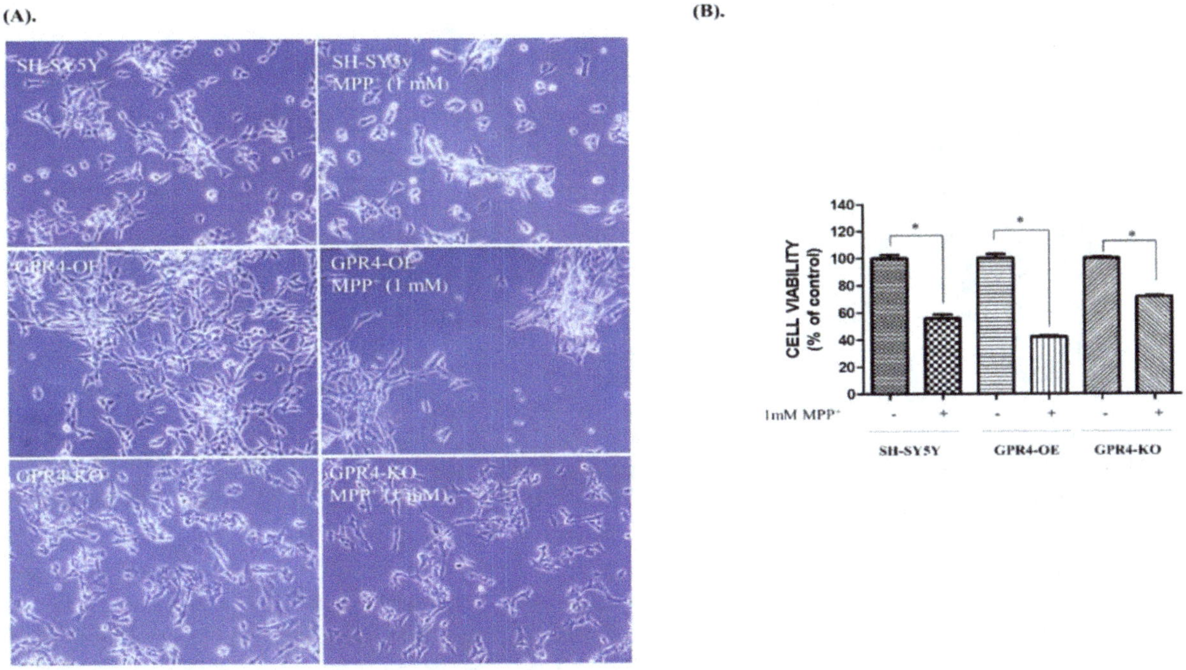

Figure 2. The cellular viability and morphology of MPP^+-treated SH-SY5Y cells that were stably GPR4-overexpressing (GPR4-OE) or GPR4-knockout (GPR4-KO). 24 h serum-starved SH-SY5Y cells were treated with MPP^+ (1 mM) for 24 h in serum-free culture media. (**A**) The morphology of SH-SY5Y GPR4-OE and GPR4-KO cells was observed through bright-field microscopy. (**B**) Cell viability was evaluated using an MTT assay. Mean ± SEM ($n = 3$) was employed to express the data. Tukey's multiple comparison test was performed using a one-way ANOVA. Each * $p < 0.05$ refers to the other sample concentrations compared with the control cells.

Cell viability was assessed with an MTT assay. The control SH-SY5Y cells presented a 55.67 ± 5.22% cell survival rate, whereas only 42.00 ± 2.01% of the GPR4-OE cells treated with MPP^+ (1 mM) survived. In contrast, the MPP^+-treated GPR4-KO cells had a significantly higher cell survival rate (71.63 ± 3.54%), at 15% higher than for the MPP^+-treated control SH-SY5Y cells and almost 30% higher than for the MPP^+-treated GPR4-OE cells (Figure 2B).

2.3. *Knockout of GPR4 Decreases the Bax/Bcl-2 mRNA Ratio during Neurotoxin-Induced Apoptosis in SH-SY5Y Cells*

To determine the role of GPR4 in both MPP^+- (1 mM) and H_2O_2- (125 μM) stimulated apoptotic cell death, we investigated the expression levels of the Bcl-2 family proteins (Bax and Bcl-2). Many studies suggest that the Bcl-2 family plays a critical role in the mitochondrial apoptotic pathway. Bax enhances the release of cytochrome C from the space of the mitochondrial intermembrane to the cytosol, resulting in apoptosis. In contrast, Bcl-2 prevents apoptosis through its prevention of cytochrome C release, thereby maintaining mitochondrial cellular integrity [29,30]. In this study, an RT-PCR was employed to assess the mRNA expression levels of GPR4, Bax, and Bcl-2 in 24 h serum-starved SH-SY5Y cells treated with either MPP^+ (1 mM) or H_2O_2 (125 μM; Figure 3A).

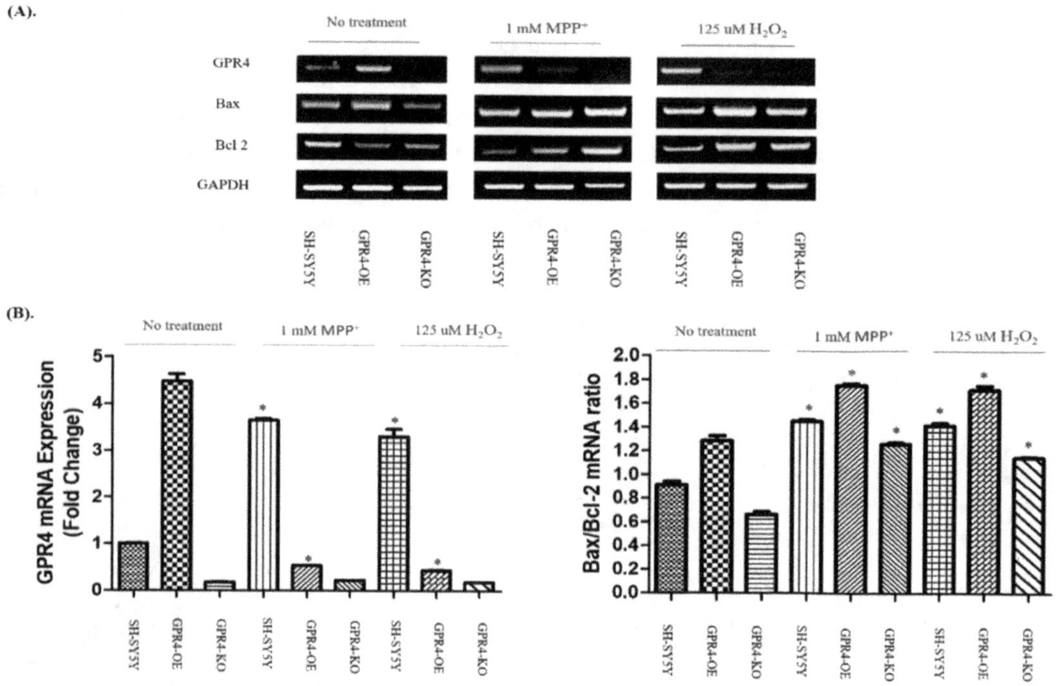

Figure 3. The measurement of GPR4 mRNA expression and the Bax/Bcl-2 mRNA ratio in MPP^+- and H_2O_2-treated SH-SY5Y cells that were stably GPR4-OE or GPR4-KO. (**A**) An RT-PCR illustrating the mRNA expression of pro-apoptotic Bax, anti-apoptotic Bcl-2, and GAPDH in SH-SY5Y, GPR4-OE, and GPR4-KO cells after stimulation with MPP^+ (1 mM) and H_2O_2 (125 μM) in serum-free media for 24 h. (**B**) A semi-quantification of the GPR4 mRNA and Bax/Bcl-2 mRNA expressions relative to GAPDH. This semi-quantification of the respective mRNA expression levels was performed on ImageJ software; GAPDH was utilised as an internal control. Mean ± SEM (n = 3) was employed to express the data. Tukey's multiple comparison test was performed using a one-way ANOVA. Each * $p < 0.05$ refers to the sample concentration compared with the same group of non-treated cells.

A semiquantitative analysis (Figure 3B) of the RT-PCR bands highlighted a more than 4-fold increase in the expression of GPR4 in the GPR4-OE cells without any treatment, compared with the non-treated SH-SY5Y cells. In comparison with the non-treated SH-SY5Y cells, neurotoxins increased the expression of GPR4 in the GPR4-OE cells by 3–4-fold (MPP^+, 3.65 ± 0.03; H_2O_2, 3.31 ± 0.17), whereas no significant difference in the GPR4 expression of the GPR4-OE cells (MPP^+, 0.53 ± 0.003; H_2O_2, 0.04 ± 0.003) was observed.

Interestingly, the ratio of Bax/Bcl-2 mRNA expression for non-treated GPR4-OE cells was slightly higher (1.40 ± 0.08) than that for the control SH-SY5Y cells, whereas the Bax/Bcl-2 mRNA ratio was slightly lower (0.73 ± 0.904) in the non-treated GPR4-KO group than that for the control SH-SY5Y cells. For the SHSY-5Y cells, treatment with MPP^+ or H_2O_2 significantly increased the ratio of Bax/Bcl-2 mRNA expression (MPP^+, 1.59 ± 0.02; H_2O_2, 1.55 ± 0.04). Yet, the ratio of Bax/Bcl-2 mRNA expression in MPP^+- and H_2O_2-stimulated GPR4-OE cells was significantly higher (MPP^+, 1.92 ± 0.03; H_2O_2, 1.88 ± 0.07) than the neurotoxin-treated SH-SY5Y and non-treated GPR4-OE cells. Meanwhile, the ratio of Bax/Bcl-2 mRNA expression in both MPP^+- and H_2O_2-stimulated GPR4-KO cells was significantly lower (MPP^+, 1.38 ± 0.02; H_2O_2, 1.25 ± 0.02) than both the neurotoxin-treated SH-SY5Y and GPR4-OE cells.

2.4. Effect of a GPR4 Antagonist on the Cellular Morphology and GPR4 mRNA Expression of SH-SY5Y Cells

To investigate the effect of the pharmacological inhibition of GPR4, we adopted a GPR4 antagonist, NE52-QQ57. At the physiological pH, NE 52-QQ57 has been reported to effectively block the cAMP that is released by GPR4 activation (IC_{50} 26.8 nM) in HEK293 cells [3]. In this study, the impact of GPR4 antagonist, NE52-QQ57, on the cellular morphology and mRNA expression of GPR4 in MPP^+- (1 mM) treated, 24 h serum-starved SH-SY5Y cells was assessed (Figure 4). The SH-SY5Y cells were treated with NE52-QQ57 (1 μM) at pH 7.4 and incubated for 24 h in serum-free culture media, to evaluate the effect of NE52-QQ57 on cell morphology and viability. However, no morphological alteration or cellular toxicity was observed in the control SH-SY5Y, GPR4-OE, or GPR4-KO cells (Figure 4A).

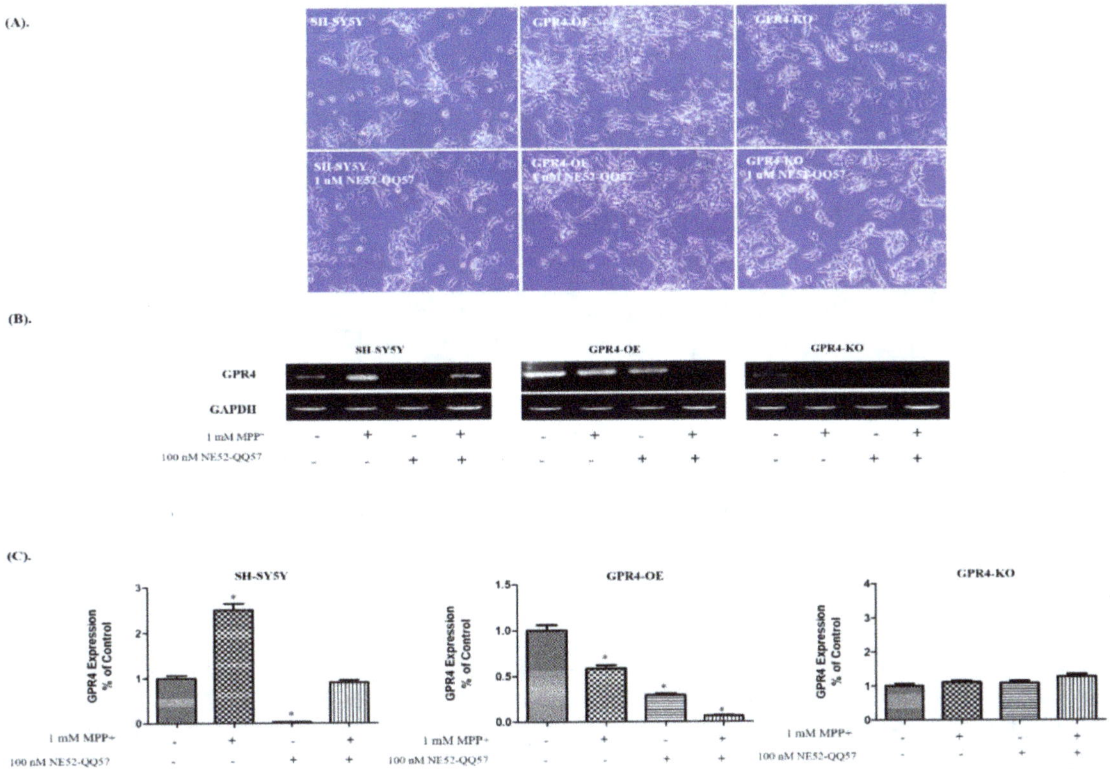

Figure 4. The effect of GPR4 antagonist, NE52-QQ57, on the cellular morphology and on GPR4 mRNA expression in MPP^+-treated SH-SY5Y cells that were stably GPR4-OE or GPR4-KO. 24 h serum-starved SH-SY5Y cells were treated for 1 h with NE52-QQ57 followed by either a 24 h incubation or MPP^+ (1 mM) stimulation for 24 h in serum-free culture media. (**A**) The cell viability and morphology of SH-SY5Y, GPR4-OE, and GPR4-KO cells that were pre-treated for 1 h with NE52-QQ57. (**B**) An RT-PCR highlighting the mRNA expression of GPR4 and GAPDH in SH-SY5Y, GPR4-OE, and GPR4-KO cells pre-treated for 1 h with NE52-QQ57. (**C**) A semi-quantification of GPR4 mRNA expression relative to GAPDH. This semi-quantification of the respective mRNA expression levels was performed on ImageJ software; GAPDH was utilised as an internal control. Mean ± SEM ($n = 3$) was employed to express the data. Tukey's multiple comparison test was performed using a one-way ANOVA. Each * $p < 0.05$ refers to the sample concentration compared with the same group of non-treated cells.

For an RT-PCR, RNA was isolated from the cells pre-treated with NE52-QQ57 (1 μM) at pH 7.4; this was incubated for an additional 24 h in serum-free media, with or without MPP^+ (1 mM) stimulation. The resulting levels of GPR4 mRNA expression illustrated that the NE52-QQ5 (100 nM) had effectively blocked the expression of GPR4 on the control SH-SY5Y and the GPR4-OE cells, similar to genetically GPR4-KO cells (Figure 4B).

A semi-quantitative analysis (Figure 4C) of the RT-PCR bands demonstrated that the NE52-QQ5 significantly reduced GPR4 expression in the SH-SY5Y (0.02 ± 0.001 folds) and the GPR4-OE cells (0.29 ± 0.02 folds), compared with the nontreated SH-SY5Y and GPR4-OE cells, respectively. Moreover, treatment with NE52-QQ5 (100 nM) decreased GPR4 mRNA expression in the MPP^+ (1 mM) treated SH-SY5Y (0.9 ± 0.06 folds) and GPR4-OE cells (0.06 ± 0.004 folds), compared with the MPP^+-stimulated SH-SY5Y and GPR4-OE cells, respectively.

2.5. *Knockout of GPR4 Decreases the Bax/Bcl-2 Protein Ratio and the Cleavage of PARP Expression in Neurotoxin-Stimulated SH-SY5Y Cells*

MPP^+-treated SH-SY5Y cells were assessed with immunoblotting to evaluate the effect of GPR4 antagonist, NE52-QQ57, on GPR4; the pro-apoptotic proteins, Bax and Bcl-2; and cleaved PARP expression (Figure 5). The SH-SY5Y cells were pre-treated with NE52-QQ57 (100 nM) at pH 7.4. This was followed by 24 h incubation, or MPP^+ (1 mM) stimulation for 24 h in serum-free media.

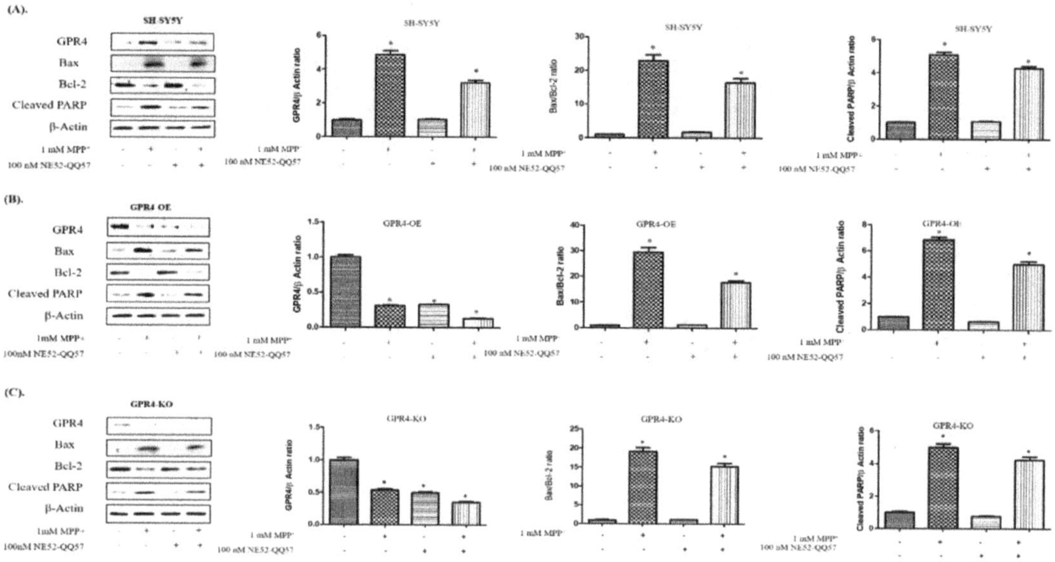

Figure 5. The effect of GPR4 antagonist, NE52-QQ57, on the GPR4 and pro-apoptotic protein expressions in MPP^+-treated SH-SY5Y cells that were stably GPR4-OE or GPR4-KO. 24 h serum-starved SH-SY5Y cells were pre-treated for 1 h with NE52-QQ57 (100 μM); this was followed by MPP^+ (1 mM) stimulation for 24 h in serum-free culture media. (**A**) An immunoblot and semi-quantification of the respective protein expressions of GPR4, Bax, Bcl-2, Cleaved PARP, and β-Actin in SH-SY5Y cells. (**B**) An immunoblot and semi-quantification of the respective protein expressions of GPR4, Bax, Bcl-2, cleaved PARP, and β-Actin in GPR4-OE cells. (**C**) An immunoblot and semi-quantification of the respective protein expressions of GPR4, Bax, Bcl-2, cleaved PARP, and β-Actin in GPR4-KO cells. β-Actin was utilised as an internal control. Mean ± SEM ($n = 3$) was employed to express the data. Tukey's multiple comparison test was performed using a one-way ANOVA. Each * $p < 0.05$ refers to the sample concentration compared with the same group of non-treated cells.

For the control SH-SY5Y cells, MPP^+ stimulation significantly increased the Bax/Bcl-2 ratio (22.94 ± 2.02 folds) and the cleaved PARP (5.09 ± 0.18 folds), in comparison with the non-treated control SH-SY5Y cells. Pre-treatment with the NE52-QQ57 (100 nM) significantly lowered the GPR4 expression (3.21 ± 0.18 folds), Bax/Bcl-2 ratio (16.47 ± 1.45 folds), and cleavage of PARP (4.29 ± 0.15 folds) in the MPP^+-stimulated cells, in comparison with the SH-SY5Y cells that were only MPP^+-treated (Figure 5A). For GPR4-OE cells, MPP^+ stimulation significantly increased the Bax/Bcl-2 ratio (29.49 ± 2.06 folds) and the cleaved PARP (6.85 ± 0.23 folds), in comparison with the non-treated GPR4-OE cells. Similar to the RT-PCR results, pre-treatment with NE52-QQ57 (100 nM) significantly lowered the GPR4 expression (0.13 ± 0.003 folds), Bax/Bcl-2 ratio (17.81 ± 0.86 folds), and cleavage of PARP (4.98 ± 0.26 folds) in the MPP^+- and NE52-QQ57-treated cells, in comparison with the GPR4-OE cells that were only treated with MPP^+ (Figure 5B). In the GPR4-KO cells, MPP^+ increased the Bax/Bcl-2 ratio (19.15 ± 1.45 folds) and cleaved PARP (4.99 ± 0.27 folds), in comparison with non-treated GPR4-KO cells. In contrast, MPP^+-stimulated GPR4-KO cells that were pre-treated with NE52-QQ57 (100 nM) demonstrated only a minor increase in Bax/Bcl-2 ratio (15.24 ± 0.91 folds) and cleavage of PARP (4.23 ± 0.22 folds), in comparison with GPR4-KO cells that were only MPP^+-treated (Figure 5C). Overall, the GPR4-KO cells displayed a lesser increase in the Bax/Bcl-2 ratio (19.15 ± 1.45 folds) and a decrease in the PARP cleavage (4.99 ± 0.27 folds), in comparison with both the MPP^+-stimulated SHSY-5Y (Bax/Bcl-2, 22.94 ± 2.02 folds; cleaved PARP, 5.09 ± 0.18 folds) and GPR4-OE cells (Bax/Bcl-2, 29.49 ± 2.06 folds; cleaved PARP, 6.85 ± 0.23 folds). Thus, less apoptotic cell death was induced by MPP^+.

2.6. Knockout of GPR4 Decreases the Caspase-3 Activity and Lowers the ROS Generation in Neurotoxin-Stimulated SH-SY5Y Cells

Caspases are important factors that trigger apoptosis. Caspase-3, in particular, is a crucial biomarker and executor of neuronal apoptosis [31]. To evaluate Caspase-3 activity, immunoblotting and a caspase activity assay were performed (Figure 6). SH-SY5Y cells were treated with MPP^+ (1 mM) for 24 h in serum-free media, while cell lysates were analysed through a western blot and a caspase activity assay. MPP^+-treated GPR4-OE cells demonstrated a significant increase in their cleaved Caspase-3 protein levels, whereas knockout of GPR4 prevented an MPP^+ stimulated increase in the level of cleaved Caspase-3 (Figure 6A).

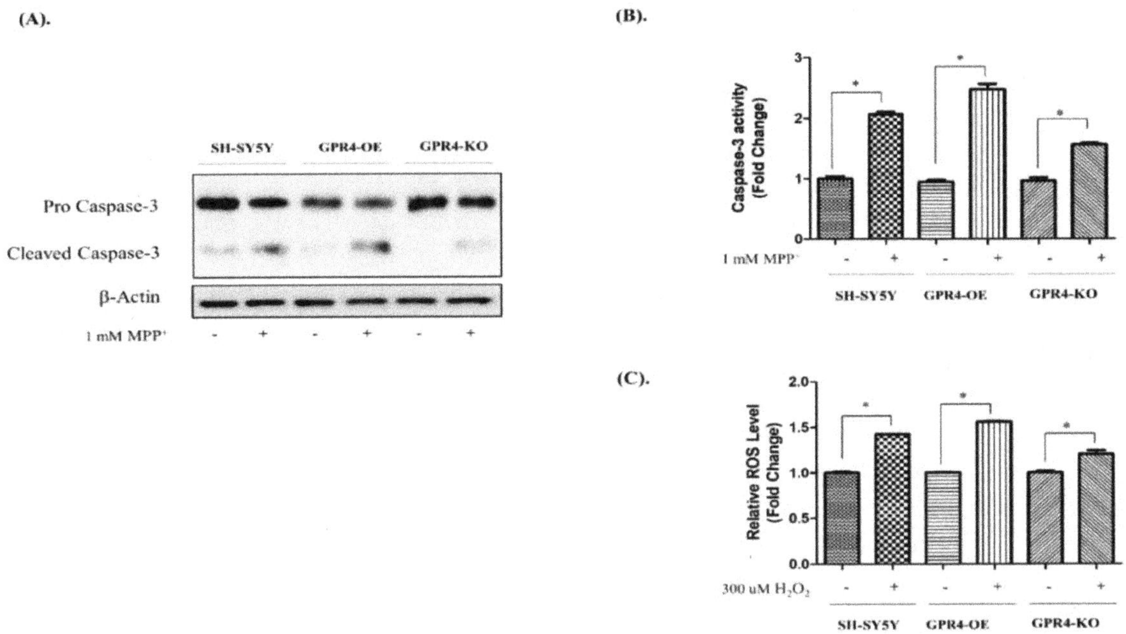

Figure 6. The Caspase-3 activity and intracellular ROS generation in MPP^+- and H_2O_2-treated SH-SY5Y cells that were stably GPR4-OE or GPR4-KO. 24 h serum-starved SH-SY5Y cells were treated with MPP^+ (1 mM) for 24 h in serum-free culture media for an immunoblot and a caspase activity assay. SH-SY5Y, GPR4-OE, and GPR4-KO cells were treated with H_2O_2 (300 μM) for 1 h in serum-free culture media for a 2′,7′-dichlorofluorescein diacetate (DCFDA) assay. (**A**) An immunoblot of the pro caspase & cleaved Caspase-3 and β-Actin. (**B**) Caspase-3 activity was measured using a colorimetric assay kit (Sigma, CAS No. CASP-3-C) in MPP^+-induced apoptotic cells. (**C**) The relative intracellular ROS level after 1 h of H_2O_2 (300 μM) treatment of 24 h serum-starved SH-SY5Y, GPR4-OE, and GPR4-KO cells. β-Actin was utilised as an internal control. Mean ± SEM ($n = 3$) was employed to express the data. Tukey's multiple comparison test was performed using a one-way ANOVA. Each * $p < 0.05$ refers to the sample concentration compared with the same group of non-treated cells.

The Caspase-3 activity assay results were in complete agreement with the Caspase-3 activity demonstrated in the immunoblot data (Figure 6B). MPP^+-treated GPR4-KO cells presented a lower level of caspase activity (1.55 ± 0.03 folds) than the MPP^+-treated SHSY-5Y (2.06 ± 0.04 folds) and GPR4-OE cells (2.47 ± 0.011 folds; Figure 6B).

We evaluated the effects of GPR4 overexpression and knockout on H_2O_2-induced intracellular ROS generation in SH-SY5Y cells [19]. In our study, the protective effect of the knockout of GPR4 against H_2O_2 resulted in lower intracellular ROS levels measured in the SH-SY5Y cells. DCFDA, a fluorescent dye that in the presence of ROS is oxidised to fluorescent DCF, was utilised for the detection of intracellular ROS levels. Treatment of the SH-SY5Y cells with H_2O_2 (300 μM) for 1 h led to a marked increase in their intracellular ROS levels. In H_2O_2-treated GPR4-OE cells, the level of intracellular ROS generation was 1.56 ± 0.01 folds higher than that of the non-treated GPR4-OE cells, whereas the H_2O_2-treated GPR4-KO cells demonstrated a lower level of ROS generation (1.20 ± 0.04 folds) in comparison with both the H_2O_2-treated control SH-SY5Y (1.42 ± 0.001 folds) and the H_2O_2-treated GPR4-OE cells (1.56 ± 0.01 folds; Figure 6B).

2.7. Knockout of GPR4 Increases the Mitochondrial Membrane Potential (MMP) in Neurotoxin-Stimulated SH-SY5Y Cells

Excess intracellular ROS leads to swelling of the mitochondrial matrix and rupture of the outer membrane, which opens up the mitochondrial permeability transition pores (mPTPs). As a result, the mitochondrial membrane potential (MMP) is disrupted and mitochondrial oxidative stress-mediated apoptosis is initiated [4].

In this study, to measure the MMP, 24 h serum-starved SH-SY5Y cells were treated with MPP^+ (1 mM) for 24 h in serum-free culture media. MMP was then determined through a JC-10 fluorescence quantitative assay. Similarly, in a separate experiment in a 6-well plate, cells were utilised for JC-10 fluorescence microscopy to visualise the red and green fluorescence.

Aggregated JC-10 is an indicator of MMP; the greater the ratio of red/green fluorescence, the higher the level of MMP. In a quantitative JC-10 fluorescence microplate assay, the MPP^+-treated SHSY-5Y cells presented a lower red/green fluorescence ratio (44.75 ± 0.82%) than the untreated SH-SY5Y cells (Figure 7A). The MPP^+-treated GPR4-OE cells, meanwhile, displayed the lowest red/green fluorescence ratio of all the samples (39.44 ± 0.39%), indicating a loss of MMP. In contrast, GPR4 knockout prevented the loss of MMP for the MPP^+-treated GPR4-KO cells, as indicated by a higher red/green fluorescence ratio (65.44 ± 0.99%). Therefore, the MPP^+-stimulated GPR4-KO cells demonstrated a higher level of MMP than either the MPP^+-stimulated SH-SY5Y (44.75 ± 0.82%) or the GPR-OE (39.44 ± 0.39%) cells.

In this study, the aggregated JC-10 created red fluorescence in the polarised mitochondrial membrane. When the MMP collapsed in apoptotic cells, the JC-10 retained its monomeric form, which is characterised by green fluorescence. An increase in the red/green fluorescence intensity ratio indicated intact mitochondria. In a separate experiment, to visualise the JC-10 fluorescence dye in the MPP^+-treated cells, JC-10 fluorescence microscopy was employed. In the control SHSY-5Y cells, both red and green fluorescence was observed, with a high level of red fluorescence and low level of green fluorescence. In contrast, the level of green fluorescence was higher and the red fluorescence remarkably lower in both the MPP^+-treated SHSY-5Y and GPR4-OE cells, when compared with the control SHSY-5Y cells. In the MPP^+-treated GPR4-KO cells, the red fluorescence was restored close to that of the control SHSY-5Y cells, while the level of green fluorescence was decreased (Figure 7B). These results suggest that GPR4 knockout restores the MPP^+-induced a loss of MMP in dopaminergic neurons.

2.8. Knockout of GPR4 Decreases the Intracellular Calcium in Neurotoxin-Stimulated SH-SY5Y Cells

Increases in intracellular Ca^{2+} in association with MPP^+- or H_2O_2-mediated apoptotic cell death have been previously reported [32]. Several studies have suggested that an increase in the intracellular Ca^{2+} released from the ER store by the inositol trisphosphate receptor (IP_3R) is directly responsible for mitochondrial Ca^{2+} overload [33,34]. However, the exact mechanism by which MPP^+ or H_2O_2 stimulation increases the intracellular calcium is not clearly understood. Interestingly, several studies have demonstrated that H_2O_2-/MPP^+-mediated mitochondrial oxidative stress is associated with an intracellular Ca^{2+} spike, which increases the Bax/Bcl-2 ratio, the release of cytochrome C, mitochondrial depolarisation, and the Caspase-3 activity in neuronal cells [19,32].

Previous reports have suggested that many G protein coupled-receptors (GPCRs), such as GPR4, which releases $G_{\beta\gamma}$ and activates G_i, are capable of Ca^{2+} signalling. Few GPCRs, however, harness $G_{\beta\gamma}$-dependent activation of PLC_{β} to release ER-stored Ca^{2+} into the cytoplasm through PIP_2 degradation [35,36]. In this study, the MPP^+-treated GPR4-OE cells demonstrated an increased proteolytic degradation of PIP_2, in comparison with the SH-SY5Y cells treated with MPP^+. Contrastingly, the MPP^+-stimulated GPR4-KO cells presented a particularly low degradation of PIP_2 compared with both the MPP^+-stimulated SH-SY5Y and GPR4-OE cells (Figure 8A).

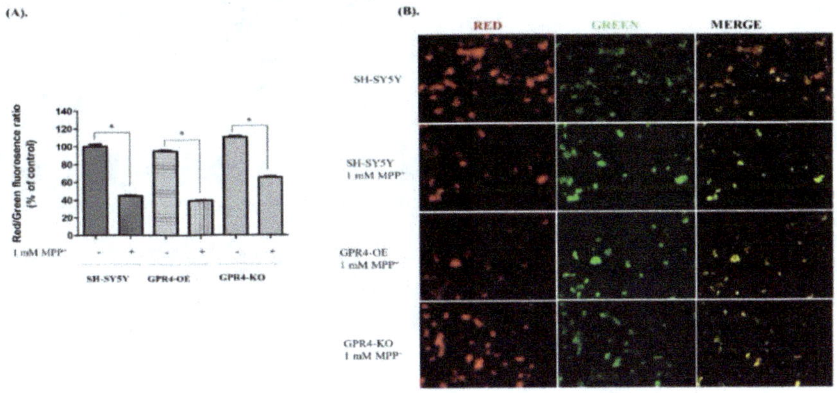

Figure 7. The measurement of mitochondrial membrane potential (MMP) in MPP^+-treated SH-SY5Y cells that were stably GPR4-OE or GPR4-GPR4-KO. 24 h serum-starved SH-SY5Y cells were treated with MPP^+ (1 mM) for 24 h in serum-free culture media; a JC-10 fluorescence quantitative assay (according to the manufacturer's instructions) and fluorescence microscopy were then employed to measure their MMP. (**A**) The percentage ratios of J-aggregates (red) and J-monomers (green). (**B**) MMP changes were monitored with a JC-10 dye that is detectable through fluorescence microscopy. Mean ± SEM ($n = 3$) was employed to express the data. Tukey's multiple comparison test was performed using a one-way ANOVA. Each * $p < 0.05$ refers to the sample concentration compared with the same group of non-treated cells.

To evaluate whether GPR4 overexpression increased intracellular calcium through $G_{\beta\gamma}$ modulation of the PLC_{β}-PIP_2 pathway, SH-SY5Y cells were treated with MPP^+ (1 mM) for 24 h in serum-free media. Cell lysates were analysed through western blotting to determine the degradation of PIP_2. The SH-SY5Y cells were treated with H_2O_2 (200 μM) for 2 h 30 min to determine their relative intracellular Ca^{2+}, utilising a Fluo-4 AM calcium indicator in a fluorescence microplate assay. Similarly, in a separate 6-well plate, cells stained with a Fluo-4 AM calcium indicator were observed under a fluorescence microscope.

The quantitative analysis of intracellular Ca^{2+}, as indicated by the Fluo-4 AM microplate assay, found levels of intracellular Ca^{2+} for the H_2O_2-treated GPR4-OE cells that were 369.58 ± 24.75% higher than those for the non-treated GPR4-OE cells. In contrast, the H_2O_2-treated GPR4-KO cells presented significantly lower levels of intracellular Ca^{2+} (181.28 ± 0.85%), in comparison with the H_2O_2-treated SH-SY5Y (243.25 ± 7.81%) and H_2O_2-treated GPR4-OE cells (369.58 ± 24.75%; Figure 8B).

In a separate experiment to visualise intracellular Ca^{2+} levels in the H_2O_2-treated cells, Fluo-4 AM fluorescence microscopy was employed. This round of microscopy demonstrated similar results to those obtained from the quantitative microplate assay. H_2O_2-treated GPR4-OE cells displayed the highest levels of green Fluo-4 AM fluorescence, while H_2O_2-treated GPR4-KO cells produced lower levels of green Fluo-4 AM fluorescence than both the H_2O_2-treated SH-SY5Y and GPR4-KO cells (Figure 8C). Overall, these data suggest that the increase in intracellular calcium associated with H_2O_2- or MPP^+-mediated mitochondrial oxidative stress is exaggerated by GPR4 overexpression, whereas GPR4 knockout prevents an increase in intracellular Ca^{2+} through the decrease of PIP_2 degradation, and thus restricts the release of Ca^{2+} from the ER by preventing the degradation of

PIP$_2$. Therefore, GPR4-PLC$_β$-PIP$_2$ signalling may act as a key factor through which GPR4 increases intracellular calcium and potentiates mitochondrial oxidative stress-mediated apoptosis.

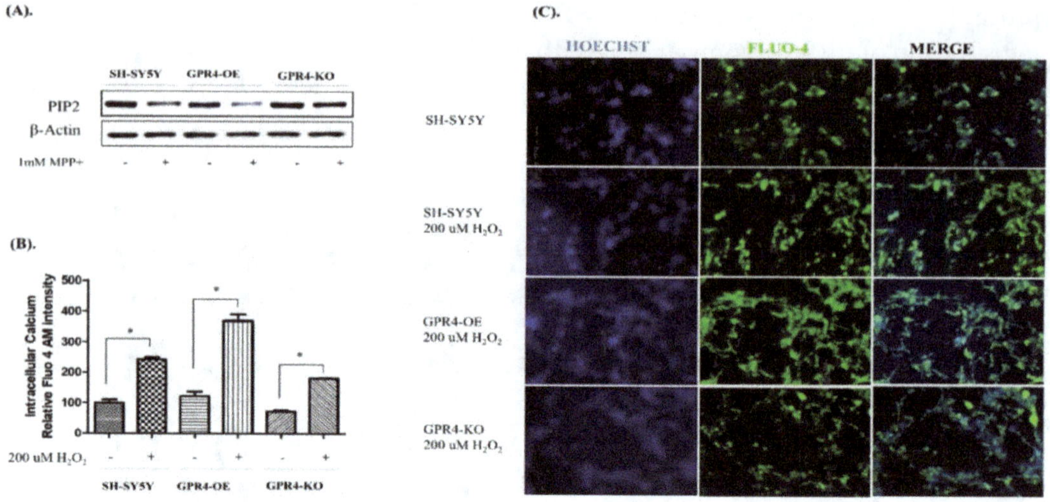

Figure 8. Phosphatidylinositol biphosphate (PIP$_2$) calcium signalling and intracellular calcium levels in MPP$^+$-treated SH-SY5Y cells that were stably GPR4-OE or GPR4-KO. 24 h serum-starved SH-SY5Y cells were treated with MPP$^+$ (1 mM) for 24 h in serum-free culture media for the purpose of immunoblotting. The SH-SY5Y cells were then treated with H_2O_2 (200 μM) for 2 h 30 min in serum-free culture media and subjected to a Fluo-4 AM fluorescence assay and fluorescence microscopy. Detection of the Fluo-4 AM fluorescence intensity and related imaging were carried out according to the manufacturer's instructions. Cells were counter-stained with Hoechst dye. (**A**) An immunoblot of the PIP$_2$ and β-Actin. (**B**) A quantitative analysis of the Fluo-4 AM fluorescence intensity in H_2O_2- (200 μM) treated cells. (**C**) Fluo-4 AM calcium imaging of the intracellular calcium level. Mean ± SEM (n = 3) was employed to express the data. Tukey's multiple comparison test was performed using a one-way ANOVA. Each * $p < 0.05$ refers to the sample concentration compared with the same group of non-treated cells.

3. Discussion

In this study, we investigated the roles of GPR4 overexpression, pharmacological inhibition, and genetic knockout in the mitochondrial oxidative stress-induced apoptotic cell death that is associated with PD. Although many studies have reported the activation of GPR4 at the physiological pH range (7.0–7.4), overexpression of GPR4 showed relatively high GPR4 activity at neutral pH 7.4 [37]. In transiently GPR4-overexpressing HEK293 cells, GPR4 is inactive at pHs higher than 8.0, whereas it is highly active at the physiological pH, 7.4, and substantially less active at pHs down to 6.8 (plausible in the range of physiological acidification) [38]. The pH sensitivity of GPR4 has been reported to vary for different cells, though potentially due to the methods employed in different laboratories [25]. In the natively GPR4-expressing cell, HUVEC, pHs from 7.4 to 7.0 have been shown to result in a 1.5-fold activation of GPR4 [25]. In this study, we found an increase in GPR4 mRNA expression at pH 7.4 in both SH-SY5Y and stably GPR4-OE cells in serum-starved media (data not added). A very slight increase in the expression of GPR4 was observed at pH 6.4. Therefore, to maintain consistency, we conducted all the experiments at a pH ~7.4. This was also the pH of the culture media that we employed.

Human-derived neuroblastoma SH-SY5Y cells are widely used in neuroscientific research as an in vitro model for the investigation of neuronal differentiation and neuroprotective events. Stimulation with several neurotoxins, such as MPP$^+$, MPTP, rotenone, 6-OHDA, and H_2O_2, has been utilised to induce oxidative stress-mediated apoptotic death, thereby mimicking neurodegenerative diseases, including PD and aging [39–41]. To determine the final concentration of H_2O_2 and MPP$^+$, SH-SY5Y cells were treated with H_2O_2 at different concentrations, ranging from 75 μM to 125 μM, for 24 h, as well as with MPP^+, ranging from 250 μM to 1 mM. H_2O_2 and MPP^+ both decreased the cell viability in a concentration-dependent manner, with optimum cytotoxicity being observed at concentrations of 125 μM for H_2O_2 and 1 mM for MPP^+; these concentrations were selected for further experiments to determine their cytotoxicity in the serum-free SH-SY5Y cell line. In our study, GPR4 mRNA and protein expressions were increased in a time-dependent manner for 24 h in both MPP^+- and H_2O_2-treated SH-SY5Y cells. Hence, GPR4 is directly linked with MPP^+- and H_2O_2-induced apoptotic cell death.

Both the pro-apoptotic protein, Bax, and the anti-apoptotic protein, Bcl-2, are members of the Bcl-2 family and are directly involved in apoptotic cell death. The balance between these two proteins of the Bcl-2 family, or an increase in the Bax/Bcl-2 ratio, indicates the early phases of an apoptotic cascade [29,30]. Significant increases in ROS, or the Bax/Bcl-2 ratio, result in the collapse of the mitochondrial membrane potential, the release of cytochrome C, the activation of Caspase-3, the cleavage of PARP, and, subsequently, apoptotic cell death [6,7]. Both MPP^+- and H_2O_2-induced apoptotic cell deaths bear the characteristic hallmarks of an increase in the Bax/Bcl-2 ratio, the release of cytochrome-C, and the activation of the proteolytic enzyme, Caspase-3, which cleaves PARP and induces apoptotic cell death [7,8]. In our study, the overexpression of GPR4 in SH-SY5Y cells significantly increased the effect of either MPP^+ or H_2O_2 and increased the Bax/Bcl-2 ratio, as was seen in both the immunoblot and RT-PCR. As a result, this significantly increased the protein level of the cleaved Caspase-3, the Caspase-3 mediated cleavage of PARP, and the Caspase-3 activity. On the contrary, the CRISPR/Cas9 knockout of GPR4 was found to result in a lesser increase in the Bax/Bcl-2 mRNA and protein ratio in both MPP^+- and H_2O_2-treated cells. Knockout of GPR4 was also shown to reduce the cleavage of PARP after MPP^+ treatment. NE52-QQ57, a selective antagonist of GPR4, demonstrated a similar level of the inhibition of GPR4 expression, as was determined through both our immunoblots and RT-PCR.

We further investigated the effect of GPR4 on mitochondrial oxidative stress-induced increases in intracellular ROS generation and MMP. Surprisingly, GPR4-OE was found to significantly increase tricellular ROS generation in SH-SY5Y cells, whereas GPR4-KO generated a lower level of intracellular ROS accumulation, after a high concentration of H_2O_2 treatment. Similarly, through both a JC-10 assay and fluorescence microscopy, the knockout of GPR4 was found to decrease mitochondrial membrane depolarisation. In JC-10-tagged fluorescence microscopy, knockout of GPR4 was seen to prevent MPP^+ stimulated decrease red fluorescence and increase green fluorescence. The latter was highly increased in the case of GPR4-OE as membrane depolarisation occurs 24 h after MPP^+ treatment.

Besides mitochondrial dysfunction, abnormal protein aggregation and dysregulated Ca^{2+} homeostasis are other factors that may be involved in the neurodegeneration observed in individuals with PD [42]. Recent findings suggest that increases in cytosolic Ca^{2+} occur at both early and late stages of the apoptotic pathway. In both cases, ER Ca^{2+} channels are linked with the release of Ca^{2+} to the cytoplasm [33,34]. However, the exact mechanism by which intracellular Ca^{2+} modulates mitochondrial oxidative stress-mediated apoptosis remains elusive. Many studies have suggested that MPP^+- and H_2O_2-induced apoptosis are associated with an increase in intracellular calcium levels [43]. For example, Sing et al. (2016) demonstrated that the administration of Nimodipine, an L-type calcium channel blocker, protected from MPTP-induced dopaminergic neuronal death in an animal model of PD. More importantly, providing evidence for Nimodipine as a means to improve mitochondrial integrity and function. In the study, Nimodipine attenuated the MPTP-induced loss of tyrosine hydroxylase-positive dopaminergic neurons in the SN. It also improved mitochondrial oxygen consumption and inhibited ROS production, as well as improving mitochondrial integrity and function in striatal mitochondria [43]. These findings provide evidence in support of the notion that calcium signalling is linked with neurotoxin-induced mitochondrial dysfunction and neurodegeneration. GPR4 is a G_s-coupled receptor that signals through adenylate cyclase and also via G proteins G_{13} and $G_{q/11}$. GPR4 is well known for its ability to recognise phospholipase C β (PLC_β) as its canonical target [44]. G_q class α subunits, or $G_{\beta\gamma}$ released by GPCR, activate Ca^{2+} signalling through $G_{\beta\gamma}$-dependent activation of PLC_β. Upon activation, PLC_β hydrolyses PIP_2 to generate IP_3. IP_3 binds to the ER-resident IP_3 receptors, which act as Ca^{2+} release channels to release ER-stored Ca^{2+} into the cytoplasm [35]. In this study, overexpression of GPR4 significantly increased the intracellular calcium level in both MPP^+- and H_2O_2-treated cells (MPP^+ data not given), whereas knockout generated very little change in the intracellular calcium. These findings were also observed in our study when employing the Fluo-4 AM indicator. To determine how GPR4 can modulate the intracellular calcium level, we investigated GPCR-mediated calcium signalling. We found that GPR4 knockout decreases the breakdown of PIP_2, which is a critical step in Ca^{2+} release from the ER to the cytoplasm. Therefore, decreased intracellular Ca^{2+} may be responsible for GPR4-mediated neuroprotection against MPP^+- or H_2O_2-induced apoptotic cell death. Our study, for the first time, demonstrated that the knockout of GPR4 protects SH-SY5Y cells from both MPP^+- and H_2O_2-stimulated mitochondrial apoptotic cell death, in association with a decrease in intracellular Ca^{2+}.

In summary, our study suggests that overexpression of GPR4 potentiates neurotoxin-induced mitochondrial oxidative stress, whereas a knockout or pharmacological inhibition of GPR4 improves the neurotoxin-induced, caspase-dependent mitochondrial apoptosis of dopaminergic neuronal cells. This study has also found that GPR4 can increase intracellular Ca^{2+} through the degradation of PIP_2. Further investigation is required to determine how GPR4-mediated calcium signalling can mitigate the neuronal cell death seen in neurodegenerative disorders, including PD.

4. Materials and Methods

4.1. Reagents and Antibodies

1-methyl-4-phenylpyridinium ion MPP^+, H_2O_2, and 3-(3,4-dimehylthiazol-2-yl)-2,5-diphenyl-tetrazolium bromide (MTT) were obtained from Sigma-Aldrich (St. Louis, MO, USA). 96-well tissue culture plates, along with six-well and 100 mm culture dishes, were obtained from Nunc Inc. (North Aurora Road, Naperville, IL, USA). Foetal bovine serum (FBS) and Dulbecco's modified Eagle's medium (DMEM/F12) were purchased from Gibco-BRL Technologies (Gaithersburg, MD, USA). RIPA buffer (10×) was purchased from Millipore (Milford, MA, USA). Tween 80 was obtained from Calbiochem (Gibbstown, NJ, USA). All other chemicals utilised in this research were of analytical grade and were purchased, unless otherwise noted, from Sigma-Aldrich.

4.2. Cell Culture and Transfection

The human dopaminergic neuroblastoma SH-SY5Y cell line was acquired from the American Type Culture Collection (ATCC; Manassas, VA, USA). SH-SY5Y cells were cultured in DMEM/F12 with or without phenol red and HEPES, supplemented with 100 U/mL penicillin/streptomycin and 10% (v/v) inactivated foetal bovine serum. The SH-SY5Y cells were maintained in a 5% CO_2 and 95% humidified air incubator at 37 °C for the time indicated in the experiments. MPP^+ and H_2O_2 were dissolved in three-times distilled water (3DW).

To overexpress and knockout the human GPR4 gene, a GPR4 lentiviral vector (CMV; pLenti-GIII-CMV-C-term-HA) and a GPR4 sgRNA CRISPR/Cas9 lentiviral vector (pLenti-U6-sgRNA-SFFV-Cas9-2A-Puro) were designed, to generate stable GPR4-overexpressing (GPR4-OE) and stable GPR4-knockout (GPR4-KO) SH-SY5Y lines. Briefly, the SH-SY5Y cells were transferred into 60 mm plates at a density of 5×10^4 cells/mL to achieve ~70% confluence at the time of transfection. The cells were transfected using the Lipofectamine® 3000 transfection reagent (ThermoFisher, Langenselbold Germany; #L3000015), according to the manufacturer's protocol. Both the GPR4-overexpression and knockout-silencing genes were designed to carry puromycin-resistance genes and were produced using the Lentivector Expression System (Applied Biological Materials Inc. (ABM), Canada). Stable single clones were selected following 3–5 weeks of puromycin treatment (1 μg/μL). GPR4 overexpression and knockout in the stably infected clones were assessed through RT-PCR and western blotting. A sequence analysis of the GPR4 insert was also employed.

4.3. Measurement of Cell Viability

The cytotoxicity of the MPP^+- and H_2O_2-treated SH-SY5Y cells was measured with an MTT assay, involving the reduction of formazan crystals [41]. SH-SY5Y cells (2.2×10^4 cells/mL) were pre-treated in 24-well plates with NE 52-QQ57 (100 nM) and left in serum-free cell culture media for 1 h; this was followed by stimulation with or without MPP^+ (1 mM) or H_2O_2 for 24 h. After MPP^+ or H_2O_2 stimulation, the medium was replaced with 0.5 mg/mL MTT solution, before the plates were incubated for 3 h at 37 °C. The supernatant was carefully removed and the formazan crystals were dissolved in dimethyl sulfoxide (DMSO) by gentle shaking for 10 min. A microplate reader (Molecular device, Sunnyvale, CA, USA) was utilised to measure the absorbance at 550 nm.

4.4. Total RNA Isolation for RT-PCR

SH-SY5Y cells (2.2×10^4 cells/mL) were pre-treated in 60 mm cell culture dishes with NE 52-QQ57 (100 nM), then left in serum-free cell culture media for 1 h, followed by stimulation with or without MPP^+ (1 mM) or H_2O_2 for 18 h, once again in serum-free media. TRIzol (Invitrogen; Burlington, ON, Canada) was employed to extract the total RNA from the cells. 2.5 µg total RNA from each group was reverse-transcribed using a first-strand cDNA synthesis kit (Invitrogen). The following primers were utilised for PCR: GPR4 sense, 5′-CCGTTGTCAAGACCGGGG-3′; GPR4 anti-sense, 5′-TCCTAGGACCCCCAGAAAGCA-3′; Bax sense, 5′-CACCAAGGTGCCGGAACTGA-3′; Bax anti-sense, 5′-AATGCCCATGTCCCCCAATC-3′; Bcl-2 sense, 5′-ACGACTTCTCCCGCCGCTAC-3′; Bcl-2 anti-sense, 5′-CCCAGCCTCCGTTATCCTGG-3′; GAPDH sense, 5′-GCAGTGGCAAAGTGGAGATTG-3′; and GAPDH anti-sense, 5′-TGCAGGATGCATTGCTGACA-3′. Then, adopting the previously mentioned primers, the cDNA was amplified through PCR [45]. GAPDH was employed as an internal control to evaluate the relative levels of expression of other genes. PCR products were analysed on 1.0–1.2% agarose gels stained with GelRed (Sigma-Aldrich; St. Louis, MO, USA). The gels were photographed and, utilising ImageJ (NIH) software, the pixel intensity for each band in the photographs was measured and normalised to the band intensity of the GAPDH mRNA, to quantify its relative expression.

4.5. Immunoblot Analysis

SH-SY5Y cells (2.2×10^4 cells/mL) were pre-treated in 60 mm cell culture dishes with NE 52-QQ57 (100 nM) and left in serum-free media for 1 h. They were then stimulated with or without MPP^+ (1 mM) or H_2O_2 for 24 h, again in a serum-free media. Next, the cells were washed two times with PBS and lysed for 10 min at 4 °C using an RIPA lysis buffer (with protease and phosphatase inhibitors). Supernatants were collected for further investigation after the cell lysates were centrifuged at 14,000 rpm, at 4 °C. The protein concentration of each sample was measured and normalised using a DC Protein Assay kit (Bio-Rad). Equal amounts of proteins (20–30 µg) were loaded and separated electrophoretically in 8, 10, and 12% sodium dodecyl sulphate-polyacrylamide gels; these were then transferred to polyvinylidene difluoride membranes (Millipore; Bedford, MA, USA). The membranes were incubated overnight at 4 °C, with corresponding primary antibodies, GPR4 (1:500) from Novus Biologicals (Centennial, CO, USA), BCL-2 (1:1000), Caspase-3 (1:1000), cleaved Caspase-3 (1:1000), cleaved PARP (1:1000) from Santa Cruz Biotechnology (Santa Cruz, CA, USA), Bax (1:1000) from Cell Signaling Co. (Boston, MA, USA), PIP_2 (1:500) from Abcam (Cambridge, United Kingdom), and β-Actin (1:2000) from Sigma-Aldrich (St. Louis, MO, USA), followed by 1 h incubation with horseradish peroxidase (HRP)-conjugated secondary antibodies (1:2000; Cell signalling, MA, USA). The blots were visualised using a Biorad-ECL (Bio-Rad Laboratories; Hercules, CA, USA) and photographed. Using ImageJ (NIH) software, the pixel intensity for each band in the photographs was measured and normalised to the band intensity of β-Actin, to quantify its relative expression.

4.6. Detection of Intracellular ROS

The ROS-sensitive fluorescent dye, 2′,7′-dichlorofluorescein diacetate (DCFDA; Sigma-Aldrich), was utilised to measure the intracellular ROS levels. SH-SY5Y cells (2.2×10^4 cells/mL) were cultured in black 96-well plates in DMEM/F12 without phenol red. Then, 60–70% confluence cells were stimulated with H_2O_2 (300 μM) for 1 h in serum-free media and then washed twice with PBS, followed by a 30 min incubation with DCFDA (10 μM) in PBS. The cells were then rinsed with PBS twice. Finally, 200 μL PBS was added, and fluorescence was measured using 485 nm excitation and 535 nm in a fluorescence microplate reader (Molecular Device; Sunnyvale, CA, USA).

4.7. Assessment of Caspase-3 Activity

Caspase-3 activity was measured using a Colorimetric Caspase-3 Assay Kit (Sigma-Aldrich; St. Louis, MO, USA), as described previously [41]. The reaction mixture (total volume, 200 μL) was distributed in 96-well plates and incubated at 37 °C for 90 min. Absorbance values were measured at wavelengths of 405 nm in a Tecan Microplate Reader (Meilen; Zurich, Switzerland).

4.8. Assessment of Mitochondrial Membrane Potential (MMP)

A JC-10-based Mitochondrial Membrane Potential Assay Kit (Abcam; Cambridge, United Kingdom) was employed to assess MMP, while a fluorescence microscope was utilised to visualise the JC-10 staining, according to the manufacturer's instructions. In brief, SH-SY5Y cells (2.2×10^4 cells/mL) were cultured in black, 96-well plates for quantification and in 6-well plates for imaging in DMEM/F12 without phenol red. Then, 60–70% confluence cells were stimulated with MPP^+ (1 mM) for 24 h in serum-free media. The cells were incubated with a JC-10 dye loading solution at 37 °C for 1 h and protected from the light. For the 96-well plates, their fluorescence intensities ($\lambda_{ex} = 490/\lambda_{em} = 525$ nm) and ($\lambda_{ex} = 540/\lambda_{em} = 590$ nm) the red-green fluorescence ratios were measured using a fluorescence microplate reader (Molecular Device; Sunnyvale, CA, USA), while confocal images were acquired with a Nikon Eclipse Ts2-FL diascopic and epi-fluorescence illumination microscope.

4.9. Detection of Intracellular Calcium

Intracellular calcium was assessed with a Fluo-4 AM dye (Abcam; Cambridge, United Kingdom) and confocal microscopy, following the manufacturer's instructions. Fluo-4 AM was diluted in DMSO containing 2 mM probenecid and 0.02% pluronic F-127. In brief, the SH-SY5Y cells (2.2×10^4 cells/mL) were cultured in black, 96-well plates for quantification and in 6-well plates for imaging in DMEM/F12 without phenol red. Then, 60–70% confluence cells were stimulated with H_2O_2 (200 μM) for 2 h 30 min in serum-free media. The cells were washed with PBS containing probenecid (2 mM) at room temperature. The cells were incubated with the Fluo-4 AM (2 μM) dye loading solution at 37 °C for 30 min and protected from light, then washed with PBS containing probenecid (2 mM) at room temperature for 30 min. For the 96-well plates, the fluorescence intensities ($\lambda_{ex} = 488/\lambda_{em} = 515$ nm) were measured using a fluorescence microplate reader (Molecular Device; Sunnyvale, CA, USA), and confocal images were acquired with a Nikon Eclipse Ts2-FL diascopic and epi-fluorescence illumination microscope.

4.10. Statistical Analyses

Statistical analyses were performed using GraphPad Prism software, version 5 (GraphPad, La Jolla, CA, USA). Data are expressed as means ± standard error (SEM) of at least three independent experiments. One-way analysis of variance (ANOVA) followed by Tukey's post hoc analysis were performed to determine the significant differences between the groups. p-values < 0.05 were considered statistically significant.

Author Contributions: M.E.H., D.-K.C., and I.-S.K. conceptualized and designed the study; I.-S.K. supervised and corresponded; M.E.H. conducted the experiments and wrote the manuscript; M.E.H. and M.A. analyzed the data; M.A. and S.A. have reviewed the literature and proof read the manuscript. All authors have read and agreed

Acknowledgments: Authors especially like to thank Md Jakaria for his support during the whole research.

Abbreviations

MPTP	1-Methyl-4-Phenyl-1,2,3,6-Tetrahydropyridine
MPP^+	1-Methyl-4-Phenylpyridinium Ion
MTT	3-(3,4-Dimehylthiazol-2-Yl)-2,5-Diphenyl-Tetrazolium Bromide
DCF-DA	7′-Dichlorofluorescein Diacetate
DMEM	Dulbecco's Modified Eagle's Medium
ER	Endoplasmic Reticulum
FBS	Fetal Bovine Serum
HUVEC	Human Umbilical Vein Endothelial Cells
MMP	Mitochondrial Membrane Potential
Mptp	Mitochondrial Permeability Transition Pore
PIP2	Phosphatidylinositol Biphosphate
PARP	Poly (ADP-Ribose) Polymerase
SN	Substantia Nigra
TDAG8	T-Cell Death-Associated Gene 8
OGR1	The Ovarian Cancer G Protein-Coupled Receptor 1

References

1. Zhang, Q.; Hu, C.; Huang, J.; Liu, W.; Lai, W.; Leng, F.; Tang, Q.; Liu, Y.; Wang, Q.; Zhou, M.; et al. ROCK1 induces dopaminergic nerve cell apoptosis via the activation of Drp1-mediated aberrant mitochondrial fission in Parkinson's disease. *Exp. Mol. Med.* **2019**, *51*, 1–13. [CrossRef] [PubMed]
2. Henchcliffe, C.; Beal, M.F. Mitochondrial biology and oxidative stress in Parkinson disease pathogenesis. *Nat. Clin. Pract. Neurol.* **2008**, *4*, 600–609. [CrossRef]
3. Mattson, M.P. Apoptosis in neurodegenerative disorders. *Nat. Rev. Mol. Cell Biol.* **2000**, *1*, 120–130. [CrossRef]
4. Ly, J.D.; Grubb, D.R.; Lawen, A.J.A. The mitochondrial membrane potential ($\Delta\psi$ m) in apoptosis; an update. *Apoptosis* **2003**, *8*, 115–128. [PubMed]
5. Prenek, L.; Boldizsár, F.; Kugyelka, R.; Ugor, E.; Berta, G.; Németh, P.; Berki, T. The regulation of the mitochondrial apoptotic pathway by glucocorticoid receptor in collaboration with Bcl-2 family proteins in developing T cells. *Apoptosis* **2017**, *22*, 239–253. [CrossRef] [PubMed]
6. Gerace, E.; Masi, A.; Resta, F.; Felici, R.; Landucci, E.; Mello, T.; Pellegrini-Giampietro, D.; Mannaioni, G.; Moroni, F. PARP-1 activation causes neuronal death in the hippocampal CA1 region by increasing the expression of Ca^{2+}-permeable AMPA receptors. *Neurobiol. Dis.* **2014**, *70*, 43–52. [CrossRef] [PubMed]
7. Chaitanya, G.V.; Alexander, J.S.; Babu, P.P. PARP-1 cleavage fragments: Signatures of cell-death proteases in neurodegeneration. *Cell Commun. Signal.* **2010**, *8*, 31. [CrossRef]
8. More, S.V.; Choi, D.-K. Atractylenolide-I Protects Human SH-SY5Y Cells from 1-Methyl-4-Phenylpyridinium-Induced Apoptotic Cell Death. *Int. J. Mol. Sci.* **2017**, *18*, 1012. [CrossRef]
9. Kirichok, Y.; Krapivinsky, G.; Clapham, D.E. The mitochondrial calcium uniporter is a highly selective ion channel. *Nat. Cell Biol.* **2004**, *427*, 360–364. [CrossRef]
10. Surmeier, D.J.; Guzman, J.N.; Sanchez-Pandila, J.; Schumacker, P.T. The role of calcium and mitochondrial oxidant stress in the loss of substantia nigra pars compacta dopaminergic neurons in Parkinson's disease. *Neuroscience* **2011**, *198*, 221–231.
11. Gunter, T.E.; Gunter, K.K. Uptake of Calcium by Mitochondria: Transport and Possible Function. *IUBMB Life* **2001**, *52*, 197–204. [CrossRef]

12. Haupt, S.; Raghu, D.; Haupt, Y. p53 Calls upon CIA (Calcium Induced Apoptosis) to Counter Stress. *Front. Oncol.* **2015**, *5*, 57. [CrossRef] [PubMed]
13. Mosharov, E.V.; Larsen, K.E.; Kanter, E.; Phillips, K.A.; Wilson, K.; Schmitz, Y.; Krantz, D.E.; Kobayashi, K.; Edwards, R.H.; Sulzer, D. Interplay between Cytosolic Dopamine, Calcium, and α-Synuclein Causes Selective Death of Substantia Nigra Neurons. *Neuron* **2009**, *62*, 218–229. [CrossRef] [PubMed]
14. Sheehan, J.P.; Swerdlow, R.H.; Parker, W.D.; Miller, S.W.; Davis, R.E.; Tuttle, J.B. Altered calcium homeostasis in cells transformed by mitochondria from individuals with Parkinson's disease. *J. Neurochem.* **1997**, *68*, 1221–1233. [CrossRef] [PubMed]
15. Singer, T.P.; Ramsay, R.R. Mechanism of the neurotoxicity of MPTP. *FEBS Lett.* **1990**, *274*, 1–8. [CrossRef]
16. Przedborski, S.; Jackson-Lewis, V. Mechanisms of MPTP toxicity. *Mov. Disord.* **1998**, *13*, 35–38.
17. Dumont, A.; Hehner, S.P.; Hofmann, T.G.; Ueffing, M.; Dröge, W.; Schmitz, M.L. Hydrogen peroxide-induced apoptosis is CD95-independent, requires the release of mitochondria-derived reactive oxygen species and the activation of NF-κB. *Oncogene* **1999**, *18*, 747–757. [CrossRef]
18. Wang, C.; Youle, R.J. The role of mitochondria in apoptosis. *Annu. Rev. Genet.* **2009**, *43*, 95–118. [CrossRef]
19. Uğuz, A.C.; Öz, A.; Nazıroğlu, M. Curcumin inhibits apoptosis by regulating intracellular calcium release, reactive oxygen species and mitochondrial depolarization levels in SH-SY5Y neuronal cells. *J. Recept. Signal Transduct.* **2016**, *36*, 395–401. [CrossRef]
20. Knaryan, V.H.; Samantaray, S.; Park, S.; Azuma, M.; Inoue, J.; Banik, N.L.; Sookyoung, P. SNJ-1945, a calpain inhibitor, protects SH-SY5Y cells against MPP^+ and rotenone. *J. Neurochem.* **2014**, *130*, 280–290. [CrossRef]
21. Meyer, T.N.; Gloy, J.; Hug, M.J.; Greger, R.; Schollmeyer, P.; Pavenstädt, H. Hydrogen peroxide increases the intracellular calcium activity in rat mesangial cells in primary culture. *Kidney Int.* **1996**, *49*, 388–395. [CrossRef] [PubMed]
22. Ludwig, M.-G.; Vanek, M.; Guerini, D.; Gasser, J.A.; Jones, C.E.; Junker, U.; Hofstetter, H.; Wolf, R.M.; Seuwen, K. Proton-sensing G-protein-coupled receptors. *Nat. Cell Biol.* **2003**, *425*, 93–98. [CrossRef] [PubMed]
23. Ishii, S.; Kihara, Y.; Shimizu, T. Identification of T Cell Death-associated Gene 8 (TDAG8) as a Novel Acid Sensing G-protein-coupled Receptor. *J. Biol. Chem.* **2005**, *280*, 9083–9087. [CrossRef] [PubMed]
24. Justus, C.R.; Dong, L.; Yang, L.V. Acidic tumor microenvironment and pH-sensing G protein-coupled receptors. *Front. Physiol.* **2013**, *4*, 354. [CrossRef]
25. Hosford, P.; Mosienko, V.; Kishi, K.; Jurisic, G.; Seuwen, K.; Kinzel, B.; Ludwig, M.; Wells, J.; Christie, I.; Koolen, L.; et al. CNS distribution, signalling properties and central effects of G-protein coupled receptor 4. *Neuropharmacology* **2018**, *138*, 381–392. [CrossRef]
26. Dong, B.; Zhang, X.; Fan, Y.; Cao, S.; Zhang, Y. Acidosis promotes cell apoptosis through the G protein-coupled receptor 4/CCAAT/enhancer-binding protein homologous protein pathway. *Oncol. Lett.* **2018**, *16*, 6735–6741. [CrossRef]
27. Krewson, E.A.; Sanderlin, E.J.; Marie, M.A.; Akhtar, S.N.; Velcicky, J.; Loetscher, P.; Yang, L.V. The Proton-Sensing GPR4 Receptor Regulates Paracellular Gap Formation and Permeability of Vascular Endothelial Cells. *iScience* **2020**, *23*, 100848. [CrossRef]
28. Dong, B.; Zhou, H.; Han, C.; Yao, J.; Xu, L.; Zhang, M.; Fu, Y.; Xia, Q. Ischemia/Reperfusion-Induced CHOP Expression Promotes Apoptosis and Impairs Renal Function Recovery: The Role of Acidosis and GPR4. *PLoS ONE* **2014**, *9*, e110944. [CrossRef]
29. Mortadza, S.S.; Sim, J.A.; Stacey, M.; Jiang, L.-H. Signalling mechanisms mediating Zn^{2+}-induced TRPM2 channel activation and cell death in microglial cells. *Sci. Rep.* **2017**, *7*, srep45032. [CrossRef]
30. Gross, A.; McDonnell, J.M.; Korsmeyer, S.J. BCL-2 family members and the mitochondria in apoptosis. *Genes Dev.* **1999**, *13*, 1899–1911. [CrossRef]
31. Hartmann, A.; Hunot, S.; Michel, P.P.; Muriel, M.-P.; Vyas, S.; Faucheux, B.A.; Mouatt-Prigent, A.; Turmel, H.; Srinivasan, A.; Ruberg, M.; et al. Caspase-3: A vulnerability factor and final effector in apoptotic death of dopaminergic neurons in Parkinson's disease. *Proc. Natl. Acad. Sci. USA* **2000**, *97*, 2875–2880. [CrossRef] [PubMed]
32. Jung, S.; Chung, Y.; Lee, Y.; Lee, Y.; Cho, J.W.; Shin, E.-J.; Kim, H.-C.; Oh, Y.J. Buffering of cytosolic calcium plays a neuroprotective role by preserving the autophagy-lysosome pathway during MPP^+-induced neuronal death. *Cell Death Discov.* **2019**, *5*, 130. [CrossRef] [PubMed]

33. Kruman, I.; Guo, Q.; Mattson, M.P. Calcium and reactive oxygen species mediate staurosporine-induced mitochondrial dysfunction and apoptosis in PC12 cells. *J. Neurosci. Res.* **1998**, *51*, 293–308. [CrossRef]
34. Lynch, K.; Fernández, G.; Pappalardo, A.; Peluso, J.J. Basic Fibroblast Growth Factor Inhibits Apoptosis of Spontaneously Immortalized Granulosa Cells by Regulating Intracellular Free Calcium Levels through a Protein Kinase Cδ-Dependent Pathway. *Endocrinol.* **2000**, *141*, 4209–4217. [CrossRef]
35. Kiselyov, K.; Shin, D.M.; Muallem, S. Signalling specificity in GPCR-dependent Ca^{2+} signalling. *Cell. Signal.* **2003**, *15*, 243–253. [CrossRef]
36. Frick, K.K.; Krieger, N.S.; Nehrke, K.; Bushinsky, A.D. Metabolic Acidosis Increases Intracellular Calcium in Bone Cells Through Activation of the Proton Receptor OGR1. *J. Bone Miner. Res.* **2009**, *24*, 305–313. [CrossRef] [PubMed]
37. Tobo, M.; Tomura, H.; Mogi, C.; Wang, J.-Q.; Liu, J.-P.; Komachi, M.; Damirin, A.; Kimura, T.; Murata, N.; Kurose, H.; et al. Previously postulated "ligand-independent" signaling of GPR4 is mediated through proton-sensing mechanisms. *Cell. Signal.* **2007**, *19*, 1745–1753. [CrossRef] [PubMed]
38. Kumar, N.N.; Velic, A.; Soliz, J.; Shi, Y.; Li, K.; Wang, S.; Weaver, J.L.; Sen, J.; Abbott, S.B.; Lazarenko, R.M.; et al. Regulation of breathing by CO_2 requires the proton-activated receptor GPR4 in retrotrapezoid nucleus neurons. *Science* **2015**, *348*, 1255–1260. [CrossRef]
39. Wang, X.; Wang, W.; Li, L.; Perry, G.; Lee, H.-G.; Zhu, X. Oxidative stress and mitochondrial dysfunction in Alzheimer's disease. *Biochim. Biophys. Acta (BBA) Mol. Basis Dis.* **2014**, *1842*, 1240–1247. [CrossRef]
40. Fall, C.P.; Bennett, J.P. Characterization and time course of MPP^+ -induced apoptosis in human SH-SY5Y neuroblastoma cells. *J. Neurosci. Res.* **1999**, *55*, 620–628. [CrossRef]
41. Kim, I.-S.; Ganesan, P.; Choi, D.-K. Cx43 Mediates Resistance against MPP^+-Induced Apoptosis in SH-SY5Y Neuroblastoma Cells via Modulating the Mitochondrial Apoptosis Pathway. *Int. J. Mol. Sci.* **2016**, *17*, 1819. [CrossRef] [PubMed]
42. Dauer, W.; Przedborski, S.J.N. Parkinson's disease: Mechanisms and models. *Neuron* **2003**, *39*, 889–909.
43. Singh, A.; Verma, P.; Balaji, G.; Samantaray, S.; Mohanakumar, K.P. Nimodipine, an L-type calcium channel blocker attenuates mitochondrial dysfunctions to protect against 1-methyl-4-phenyl-1,2,3,6-tetrahydropyridine-induced Parkinsonism in mice. *Neurochem. Int.* **2016**, *99*, 221–232. [CrossRef] [PubMed]
44. Liu, J.-P.; Nakakura, T.; Tomura, H.; Tobo, M.; Mogi, C.; Wang, J.-Q.; He, X.-D.; Takano, M.; Damirin, A.; Komachi, M.; et al. Each one of certain histidine residues in G-protein-coupled receptor GPR4 is critical for extracellular proton-induced stimulation of multiple G-protein-signaling pathways. *Pharmacol. Res.* **2010**, *61*, 499–505. [CrossRef]
45. Karthivashan, G.; Park, S.-Y.; Kweon, M.-H.; Kim, J.; Haque, E.; Cho, D.-Y.; Kim, I.-S.; Cho, E.-A.; Ganesan, P.; Choi, D.-K. Ameliorative potential of desalted Salicornia europaea *L. extract* in multifaceted Alzheimer's-like scopolamine-induced amnesic mice model. *Sci. Rep.* **2018**, *8*, 7174. [CrossRef] [PubMed]

11

Liver Growth Factor "LGF" as a Therapeutic Agent for Alzheimer's Disease

Rafael Gonzalo-Gobernado [1,2,†], Juan Perucho [1,†], Manuela Vallejo-Muñoz [1,†], Maria José Casarejos [1], Diana Reimers [1], Adriano Jiménez-Escrig [1,3], Ana Gómez [1], Gonzalo M. Ulzurrun de Asanza [1] and Eulalia Bazán [1,*]

1 Servicio de Neurobiología, Instituto Ramón y Cajal de Investigación Sanitaria (IRYCIS), 28034 Madrid, Spain; rd.gonzalo@cnb.csic.es (R.G.-G.); juan.perucho@outlook.com (J.P.); manuela.vmqm@gmail.com (M.V.-M.); m.jose.casarejos@hrc.es (M.J.C.); diana.reimers@hrc.es (D.R.); adriano.jimenez@hrc.es (A.J.E.); go.s6506@hotmail.com (A.G.); gonzalo.munoz@hrc.es (G.M.U.d.A.)
2 National Centre for Biotechnology (CNB), CSIC, 28049 Madrid, Spain
3 Servicio de Neurología, Hospital Ramón y Cajal, 28034 Madrid, Spain
* Correspondence: eulalia.bazan@hrc.es
† These authors contributed equally to this work.

Abstract: Alzheimer's disease (AD) is a progressive degenerative disorder and the most common cause of dementia in aging populations. Although the pathological hallmarks of AD are well defined, currently no effective therapy exists. Liver growth factor (LGF) is a hepatic albumin–bilirubin complex with activity as a tissue regenerating factor in several neurodegenerative disorders such as Parkinson's disease and Friedreich's ataxia. Our aim here was to analyze the potential therapeutic effect of LGF on the APPswe mouse model of AD. Twenty-month-old mice received intraperitoneal (i.p.) injections of 1.6 μg LGF or saline, twice a week during three weeks. Mice were sacrificed one week later, and the hippocampus and dorsal cortex were prepared for immunohistochemical and biochemical studies. LGF treatment reduced amyloid-β (Aβ) content, phospho-Tau/Tau ratio and the number of Aβ plaques with diameter larger than 25 μm. LGF administration also modulated protein ubiquitination and HSP70 protein levels, reduced glial reactivity and inflammation, and the expression of the pro-apoptotic protein Bax. Because the administration of this factor also restored cognitive damage in APPswe mice, we propose LGF as a novel therapeutic tool that may be useful for the treatment of AD.

Keywords: liver growth factor; Alzheimer's disease; inflammation; neuroprotection; microglia; Tg2576 transgenic mice; amyloid-beta

---

1. Introduction

Alzheimer's disease (AD), the most common cause of dementia, was discovered by Alois Alzheimer in 1901. The prevalence of AD is about 1% in individuals aged 60–64, but shows an exponential increase with age, so that in people aged 85 years or older the prevalence is between 24–33% in the Western World. The hallmarks of the disease are extracellular deposits of plaques composed of amyloid-β (Aβ) and intracellular neurofibrillary tangles, composed of hyperphosphorylated tau (phospho-tau), a normal axonal protein that binds to microtubules [1]. The relationship among Aβ deposits, tangle formation and neurodegeneration, and cell death is not clear at present. The areas more vulnerable for the neurodegeneration processes are the cortex and the hippocampus, affecting mechanisms of spatial, semantic and episodic memories [2]. Other processes implicated in the pathological pathways in AD are cholinergic dysfunction, neuroinflammation, calcium channels, oxidation, iron chelation, abnormalities in the mitochondrial DNA and lipid metabolism, among others [3].

Therapeutic strategies in AD trying to ameliorate or eliminate its main disturbances, include the elimination of Aβ deposits, vaccination and immunization against Aβ, inhibitors of β or γ-secretases (enzymes excising Aβ from APP), antifibrillisation agents, statins (inhibitors of cholesterol synthesis), neuroprotectors, antioxidants and anti-inflammatory drugs, among others (reviewed in [4]). However, although the pathological hallmarks of AD are well defined, no effective therapy exists currently.

Liver growth factor (LGF) is a hepatic mitogen purified in 1986 by Dr. Diaz-Gil's group [5]. This 64 kDa factor is an albumin–bilirubin complex that stimulates the proliferation of different cell types, and promotes regeneration of damaged tissues including the brain (reviewed in [6]). Thus, administration of LGF was able to stimulate axonal growth in the striatum, to increase the number of dopaminergic neurons in the damaged substantia nigra, and to improve rotational behavior stimulated by apomorphine in experimental Parkinson's disease [7,8]. LGF also promoted the proliferation and migration of neural progenitors from the forebrain subventricular zone [9], and improved the viability, differentiation and integration of stem cell grafts into the host tissue [10]. Besides, our previous studies have reported the remarkable anti-inflammatory and antioxidant activities of LGF in extracerebral tissues [11–13], and in several experimental models of neurodegeneration where its main cellular target in the brain appears to be microglia [7,9,14,15]. Both effects are considered to be closely related with Alzheimer's disease pathology [16,17].

To analyze the potential therapeutic effectiveness of LGF in AD, we have used Tg2576 transgenic mice (from now APPswe mice) that over-express the Swedish APP mutation (K670N/M671L) on a C57Bl/6 9 SJL background [18]. From 12 months onwards, these mice show Aβ plaque depositions in the hippocampus and cerebral cortex, reactive gliosis, inflammation and cognitive impairment that are neuropathological features of AD [19]. Chronic LGF administration to a 20–21-month-old APPswe mouse, significantly reduces Aβ and phospho-Tau protein levels and modulates protein ubiquitination and the expression of the heat shock protein 70 (Hsp70) that is involved in Aβ clearance. LGF also reduces microglia activation, astrogliosis and the expression of the apoptosis-associated speck-like protein containing a CARD (ASC), which is a component of the inflammatory response and cognitive impairment in AD pathology. Moreover, LGF up-regulates the expression of the Nuclear factor erythroid 2-related factor 2 (Nrf2), which plays an important role against oxidative stress. Because these beneficial effects correlate with a better cognitive outcome in APPswe mice, we may propose LGF as a potential novel therapeutic tool that may be useful for the treatment of AD.

2. Results

2.1. LGF Improves Behavioral Working Memory in APPswe Mice

The alternance index in the Y-maze, a parameter considered as an indicator of mnemonic function, was significantly reduced in the APPswe mice with respect to WT (Figure 1A). This important marker of working memory was recovered in APP-LGF treated mice (Figure 1A). APP mice also exhibited a reduced number of entries in comparison with WT mice, indicating a low general locomotor activity (18.8 ± 0.9 ($n = 10$) and 11 ± 1.8* ($n = 11$) in WT and APP mice, respectively * $p \leq 0.05$ vs. WT). Instead, no significant differences were observed in the number of entries after LGF treatment in comparison with APP mice (APP-LGF: 13 ± 1.7 ($n = 12$)).

The marble-burying test is a useful model of neophobia, anxiety, and obsessive-compulsive behavior. As shown in Figure 1B, the marble burying test index was significantly reduced in APPswe aged mice, and LGF recovered this index of potential hippocampal affection.

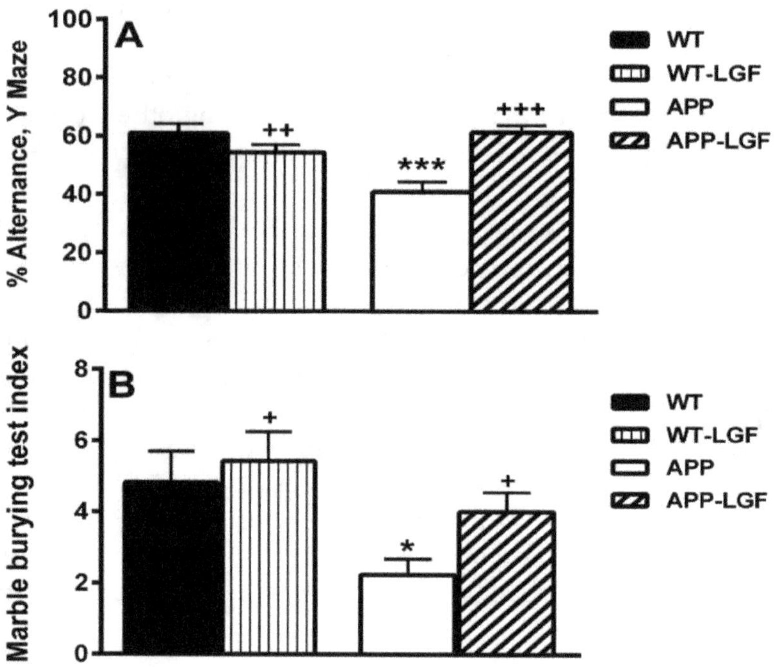

Figure 1. Liver growth factor (LGF) improves cognitive behavior in APPswe mice. Panel (**A**) shows how the alternance index in the Y-maze is significantly reduced in APP mice, and how LGF treatment recovers this important marker of working memory. As shown in panel (**B**), the marble burying test index is significantly reduced in APP mice, and LGF recovers this potential index of hippocampal and cortical affection. Results represent the mean ± SEM of 11 to 16 independent mice. The statistical analysis was performed by one-way ANOVA followed by Newman–Keuls test. * $p \leq 0.05$, *** $p \leq 0.001$ vs. wild type (WT). + $p \leq 0.01$, ++ $p \leq 0.01$, +++ $p \leq 0.001$ vs. APP mice.

2.2. LGF Modulatesβ-Amyloid Protein Expression in Hippocampus and Cerebral Cortex of APPswe Mice

β-amyloid protein accumulation in the Central Nervous System (CNS) is the most important feature of the experimental model of AD used in this study. As shown in Figure 2A, APPswe mice expressed the APP 695 human protein, and several Aβ peptides of different molecular weight lower than 60 kDa which expression was up-regulated in the hippocampus and cerebral cortex, in comparison with WT mice (Figure 2B). The immunohistochemical analysis also revealed the presence of Aβ-positive plaques in the hippocampus (40 ± 7 (n = 5) Aβ-positive plaques/mm^2) and cerebral cortex (38 ± 6 (n = 5) Aβ-positive plaques/mm^2) of APPswe mice. These plaques had different sizes with a 78 ± 9% of them showing a diameter lower than 25 μm in both brain structures (Figure 2C). In the APP-LGF experimental group, the total number of plaques was not significantly different to that observed in APPswe mice (54.6 ± 3.2 (n = 4) and 44 ± 3.5 (n = 4) Aβ-positive plaques/mm^{2}in the hippocampus and cerebral cortex, respectively). However, LGF treatment significantly reduced Aβ protein levels (Figure 2B), and the number of plaques with a diameter higher than 25 μm compared to APPswe mice treated with the vehicle (Figure 2D). Besides, LGF slightly augmented, but not significantly, augmented the percentage of plaques with a diameter lower than 25 μm by 1.5 ± 0.1-fold and 1.3 ± 0.14-fold in the hippocampus and cerebral cortex, respectively.

2.3. Effects of LGF in Tau Phosphorylation and Protein Ubiquitination

A neuropathological feature of AD is the accumulation of Tau and ubiquitin in the neurofibrillary tangles (NFT). At 20 months of age, phospho-Tau/Tau ratio was increased by 2.5-fold in the hippocampus of APPswe mice, and LGF administration partially reduced this parameter to similar values of those observed in WT mice (Figure 3A,D). Phospho-Tau/Tau ratio was similar in the cerebral cortex of

APPswe and WT mice, but LGF treatment significantly reduced this ratio below WT levels (Figure 3A). A similar effect was observed in the cerebral cortex of WT-LGF treated mice (Figure 3A).

Protein ubiquitination is essential in an important number of processes including protein degradation by the proteosome. Accumulation of polyubiquitinated proteins was observed in the hippocampus and cerebral cortex of APPswe mice, and LGF administration reduced this parameter in both structures (Figure 3B,D).

HSP-70 is a chaperone that allows the correct folding of mis-folded proteins that could lead to their aggregation. As shown in Figure 3C, the hippocampus of APP-LGF treated mice showed significantly higher levels of HSP-70 than WT or APPswe mice. HSP-70 protein expression was down-regulated in the cerebral cortex of APPswe mice, and LGF treatment restored its levels to control values (Figure 3C,D).

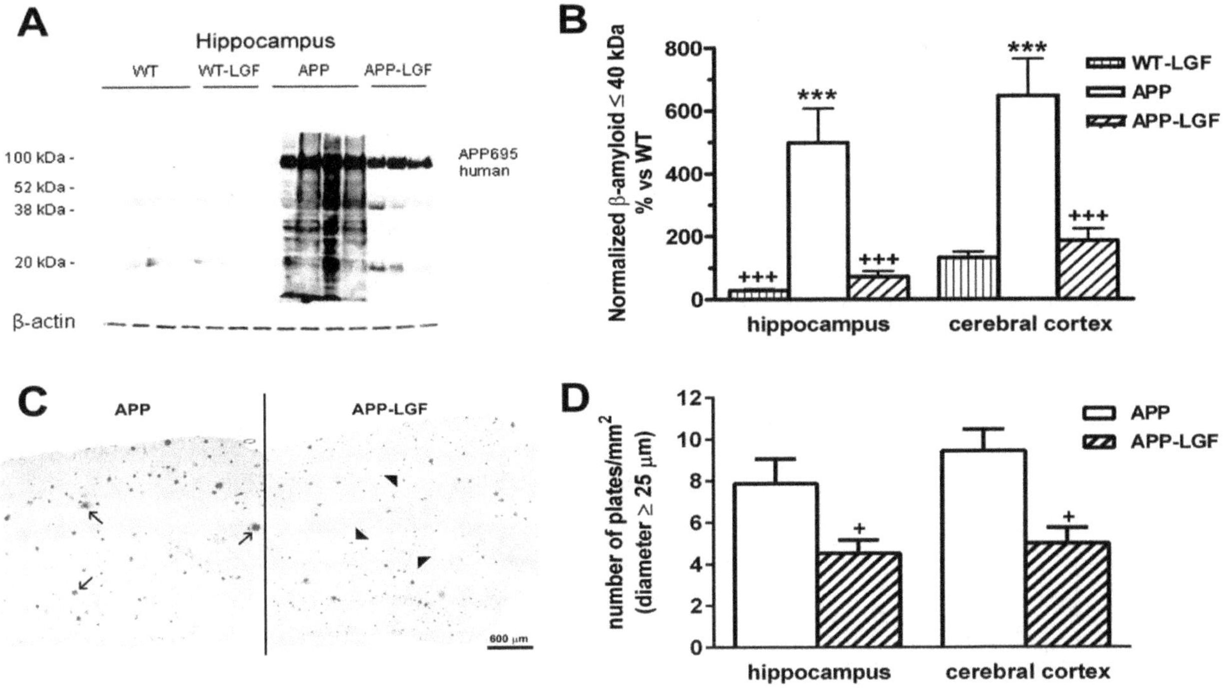

Figure 2. LGF reduces amyloid-β accumulation and the size of amyloid-β positive plaques in the hippocampus and cerebral cortex of APPswe mice. Panels (**A**,**B**) show a Western blot representative image of Aβ aggregates in the hippocampus (**A**) and the quantification of Aβ-aggregates ≤40 kDa in the hippocampus and cerebral cortex (**B**). Note that Aβ protein levels are up-regulatedin the hippocampus and cerebral cortex of APPswe mice and that LGF treatment significantly reduces its expression in both structures. Panel (**C**) shows a representative image of Aβ-positive plaques of large (**C**, black arrows) and small size (**C**, black arrowheads) in one hemisphere of APP mice brain (scale bar: 600 μm). Note that in APP-LGF mice, large plaques are reduced, while small plaques increase. Panel (**D**) shows how LGF treatment significantly reduces the number of plaques with a diameter higher than 25 μm in the hippocampus and cerebral cortex. Results represent the mean ± SEM of 7 to 8 (**B**) and 4 to 5 (**D**) independent mice in each experimental group. The statistical analysis was performed by one-way ANOVA followed by Newman–Keuls test. *** $p \leq 0.001$ vs. WT. + $p \leq 0.05$, +++ $p \leq 0.001$ vs. APP mice.

2.4. LGF Modulates Microglia Activation and Reduces Inflammation in APPswe Mice

Recent reports suggest that microglia play an important role in the evolution of AD. The immunohistochemical analysis of the hippocampus and cerebral cortex of APPswe mice showed that the number of microglial cells that expressed the Ionized Calcium Binding Protein-1 (Iba1) was significantly higher than in WT control mice (Figure 4A). Most of the Iba1-positive cells associated with the plaques were located around them (Figure 4B), and a few showed Iba1-positive processes penetrating into the plaques (Figure 4C). Iba1 protein levels were also up-regulated in both structures (Figure 4D,H), suggesting the presence of activated microglia in these mice. Increased proliferation has also been associated with microglia activation. As shown in Figure 4E, the expression of PCNA was significantly increased in the hippocampus and cerebral cortex of APPswe mice. Similar to this finding, BrdU incorporation was higher in these mice than in the WT group in both structures (Figure 4F), and more than 61 ± 4% ($n = 8$) of the proliferating cells were Iba1-positive microglia (Figure 4G).

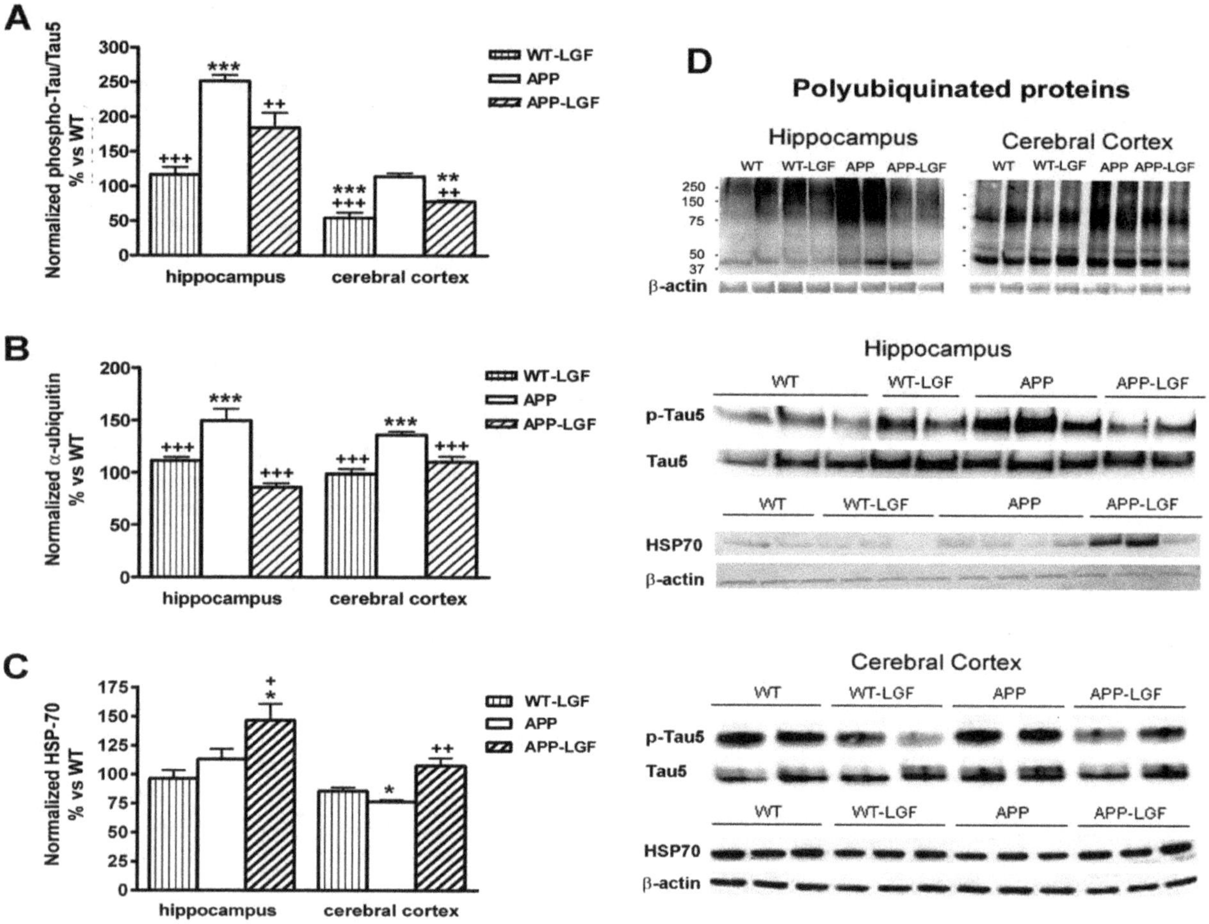

Figure 3. Effects of LGF in tau pathology, ubiquitinated protein levels and HSP70 heat shock protein expression. Panel (**A**), shows the relative optical density of phospho-tau/tau ratio analyzed by Western blot and expressed as % vs. WT. Note how LGF treatment reduces the expression of phosphorylated tau in the hippocampus and cerebral cortex in APP mice. Panels (**B**,**C**) show the quantification of accumulated ubiquitinated proteins (**B**) and HSP-70 (**C**) in the hippocampus and cerebral cortex of APPswe mice. Note how LGF reduces the accumulation of ubiquitinated proteins (**B**) and increases HSP70 expression (**C**). Panel (**D**) shows representative Western blot images of phospho-tau, total tau, Hsp-70 and β-actin as charge control. Results represent the mean ± SEM of 4 to 8 independent mice. The statistical analysis was performed by one-way ANOVA followed by Newman–Keuls test. * $p \leq 0.05$, ** $p \leq 0.01$, *** $p \leq 0.001$ vs. WT. + $p \leq 0.05$, ++ $p \leq 0.01$, +++ $p \leq 0.001$ vs. APPswe mice.

The APP-LGF group of animals showed a significant reduction in Iba1 (Figure 4D,H) and PCNA protein expression (Figure 4E,H), and a slight but reduced number of BrdU-positive cells in comparison with APPswe mice (Figure 4F). Besides, LGF treatment increased from 6 ± 2.9 ($n = 3$) to 19 ± 11 ($n = 4$) the percentage of Iba1-positive cells, which prolongations penetrated profoundly in the plaques in the hippocampus.

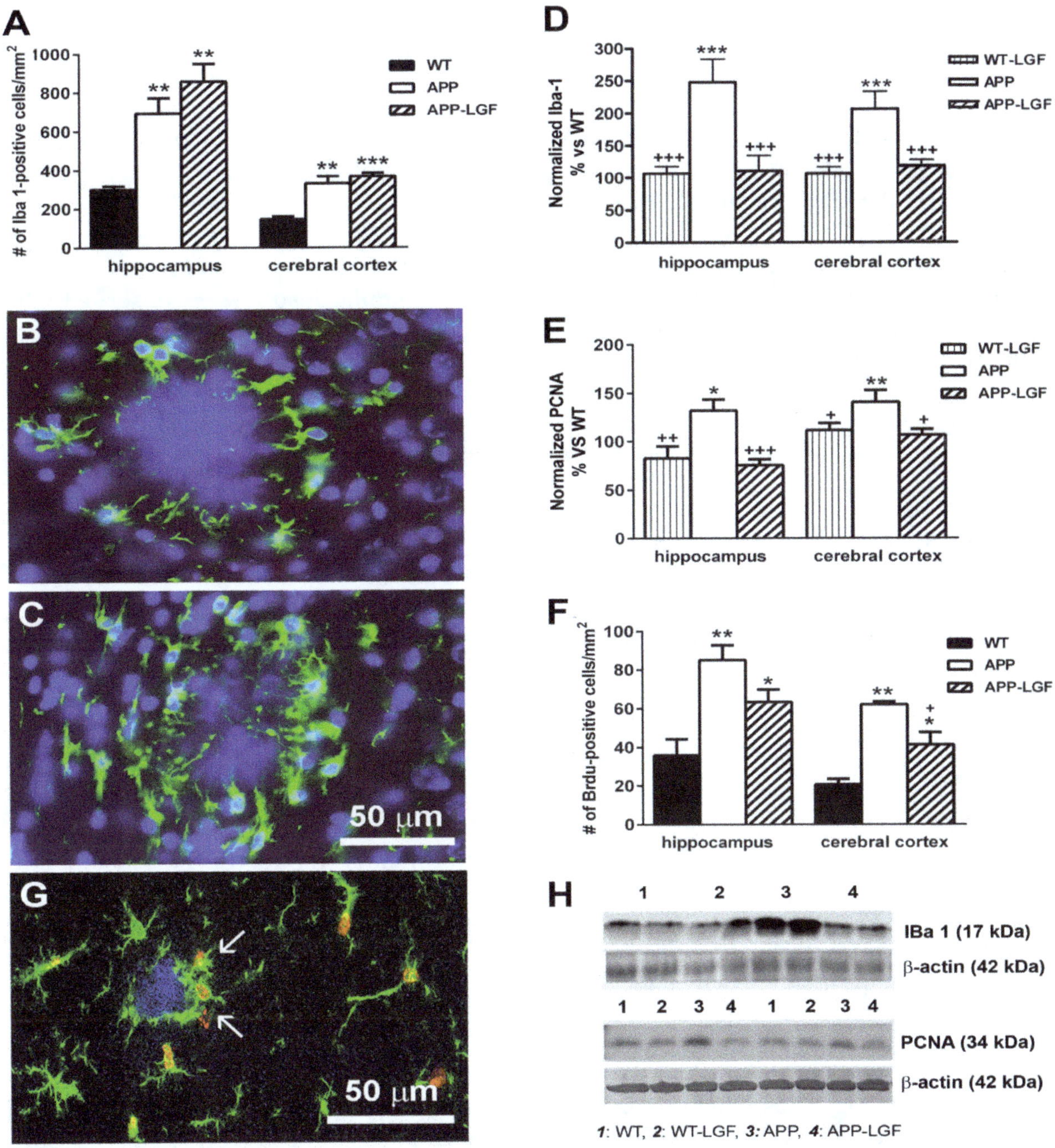

Figure 4. Liver growth factor modulates microglia cell activity in the hippocampus and cerebral cortex of APPswe mice. Panel (**A**) shows the quantification of Iba1-positive microglia cells in APPswe mice. Panels (**B**,**C**) show different responses of Iba1-positive cells: in (**B**) microglial prolongations do not penetrate inside the deposit, while in (**C**) they actively phagocytize the plaque (scale bar: 50 μm). Panels (**D**,**E**) show quantitative Western blot analysis of Iba1 (**D**) and PCNA (**E**) protein expression. Note how LGF administration significantly reduces the over-expression of Iba1 (**D**) and PCNA (**E**) in the hippocampus and cerebral cortex. LGF also reduces BrdU cell incorporation (**F**) as an index of cellular proliferation. Note how BrdU (**G**, red) is associated with Iba1-positive cells (**G**, green, white arrows). Panel (**H**) show representative Western blots of Iba1 and PCNA and their respective β-actin as charge control. The results represent the mean ± SEM of 4 (**A**,**F**) and 8 to 10 (**D**,**E**). independent mice. The statistical analysis was performed by one-way ANOVA followed by Newman–Keuls test. * $p \leq 0.05$, ** $p \leq 0.01$, *** $p \leq 0.001$ vs. WT. + $p \leq 0.05$, ++ $p \leq 0.01$, +++ $p \leq 0.001$ vs. APPswe mice.

GFAP is a protein expressed by astrocytes for which up-regulation has been associated with inflammatory states in chronic processes as AD and aging. As shown in Figure 5A, GFAP was over-expressed in the hippocampus and cerebral cortex of APPswe mice, and LGF treatment significantly reduced its levels in both structures. On the other hand, LGF decreased ASC protein levels that were up-regulated in the hippocampus and the cerebral cortex of APPswe aged mice (Figure 5B,D). ASC is involved in the production of Interleukin-1beta (Il-1beta) but, neither APP nor APP-LGF treated mice showed any significant change in the levels of this pro-inflammatory cytokine in the hippocampus (113 ± 6 (n = 6) and 101 ± 7 (n = 6) % of IL-1beta expression vs. WT in APP and APP-LGF treated mice, respectively) and the cerebral cortex (102 ± 11 (n = 5) and 92 ± 12 (n = 6) % of IL-1beta expression vs. WT in APP and APP-LGF treated mice, respectively). Similar results were observed when we analyzed the potential effects of LGF in Tumor Necrosis Factor-alpha (TNF-alpha) protein expression in the hippocampus (92 ± 6 (n = 6) and 88 ± 10 (n = 8) % of TNF-alpha expression vs. WT in APP and APP-LGF treated mice, respectively) and cerebral cortex (95 ± 6 (n = 5) and 107 ± 9 (n = 5) % of TNF-alpha expression vs. WT in APP and APP-LGF treated mice, respectively). This latter cytokine mediates LGF-induced neuroregeneration/neuroprotection [6,20].

LGF also modulated the expression of the transcription factor Nrf2, and the class B scavenger receptor CD36, two proteins that regulate oxidative stress and inflammatory responses in AD. As shown in Figure 5D, Nrf2 protein levels were reduced in the hippocampus and cerebral cortex of APPswe mice, and LGF treatment up-regulated Nrf2 protein expression to reach control values. LGF treatment reduced the levels of CD36 that is over-expressed in the hippocampus of APPswe mice (Figure 5C,E). Besides, LGF up-regulated CD36 protein expression in the hippocampus of WT mice (Figure 5C,E), but it lacked activity in the cerebral cortex, a brain structure where neither APP nor APP-LGF mice showed any alteration in CD36 protein levels (Figure 5C).

2.5. LGF Modulates the Expression of Proteins Involved in Cell Survival

Our previous studies showed how in an experimental model of Parkinson's disease, LGF potentiates cell survival through the regulation of Bcl2 and Bax protein expression [9]. In the hippocampus of APPswe mice the Bcl2/Bax ratio was significantly reduced, and LGF treatment increased this ratio to control values (Figure 6A). This effect was due to a reduction in the expression of the pro-apoptotic protein Bax which levels were significantly up-regulated in the hippocampus of APPswe mice (Figure 6B).

Akt is another protein involved in cell survival modulated by LGF in neurodegeneration [9]. As shown in Figure 6C, phospho-Akt/Akt ratio was up-regulated in the hippocampus of APPswe mice where phospho-Akt levels were significantly increased in comparison with WT mice (Figure 6D). The APP-LGF group of mice also showed an increased phospho-Akt/Akt ratio and higher levels of phospho-Akt than control mice (Figure 6C,D). Neither Bcl2/Bax nor phospho-Akt/Akt ratio were affected in the cerebral cortex at any of the experimental conditions used in this study (Figure 6A,B).

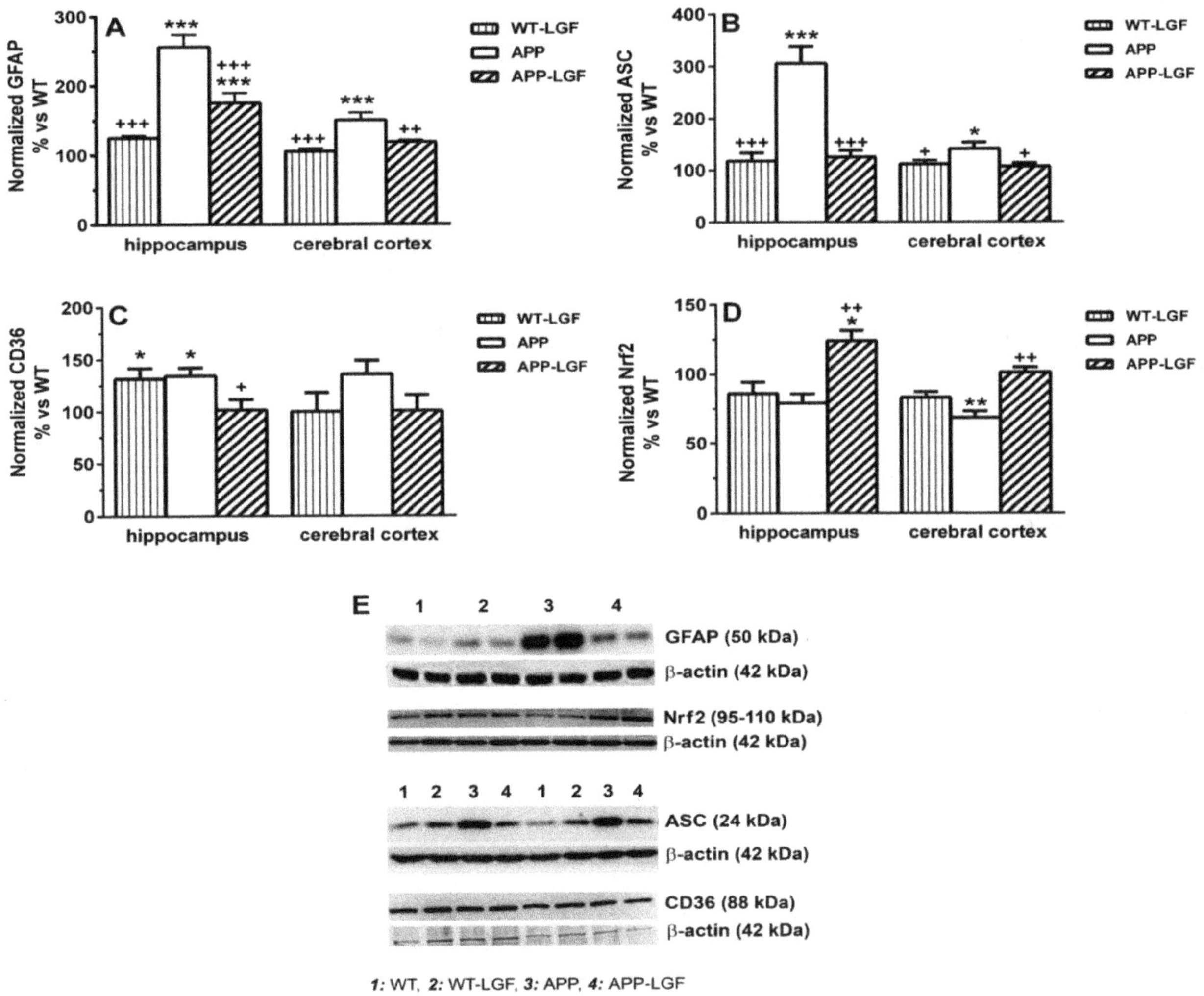

Figure 5. LGF reduces the inflammatory response in APPswe mice. Panel (**A**) shows how LGF significantly reduces GFAP protein expression in the cerebral cortex and hippocampus of APPswe. LGF administration also decreases the expression of ASC (**B**), which is a protein involved in the production of pro-inflammatory cytokines. Panel (**C**) shows quantitative Western blot analysis of the receptor scavenger CD36 that is over-expressed in the hippocampus of APP mice. Panel (**D**) represents the quantitative analysis of the transcription factor Nrf2 as an oxidative stress regulator. Representative Western blots of GFAP, Nrf2, ASC, CD36 and their respective β-actin as charge are shown in panel (**E**). Results represent the mean ± SEM of 4 to 10 independent mice. The statistical analysis was performed by one-way ANOVA followed by Newman–Keuls test. * $p \leq 0.05$, ** $p \leq 0.01$, *** $p \leq 0.001$ vs. WT. + $p \leq 0.05$, ++ $p \leq 0.01$, +++ $p \leq 0.001$ vs. APPswe mice.

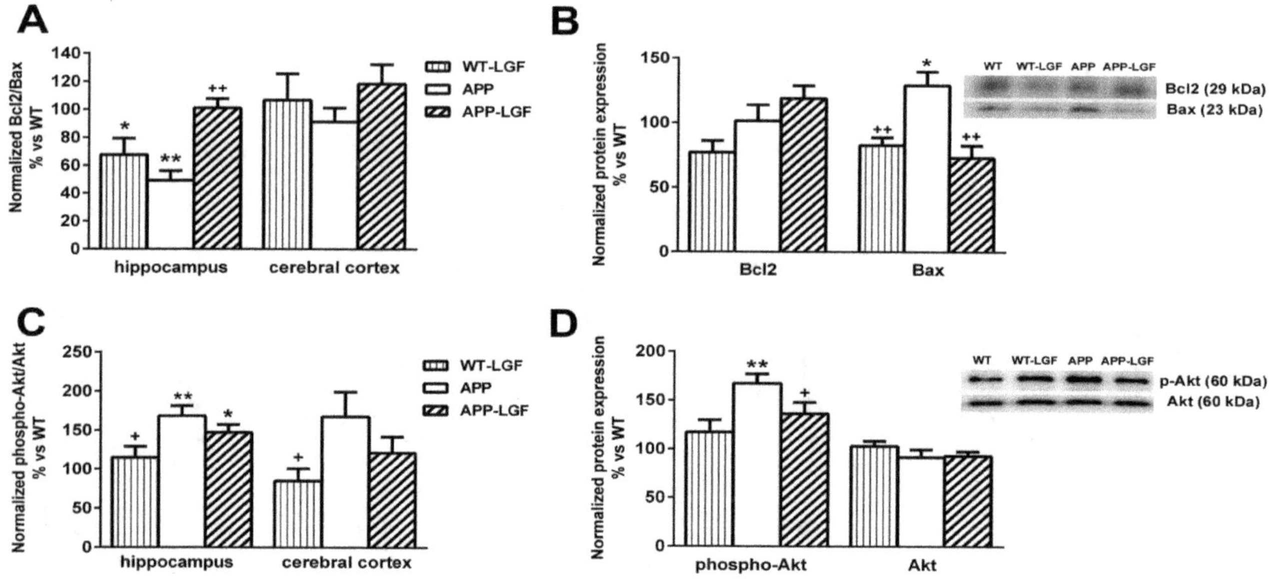

Figure 6. Effect of LGF on the expression of proteins involved in cell survival. Protein expression was analyzed by Western blot using specific antibodies against Bcl2, Bax, p-Akt and Akt. Panel (**A**), shows that LGF increases Bcl-2/Bax ratio in the hippocampus. This effect is mainly due to a reduction in Bax protein levels (**B**). Panels (**C**,**D**) show that phospho-Akt/Akt ratio (**C**) and phospho-Akt protein levels (**D**) are significantly increased in the hippocampus of APP and APP-LGF treated mice. Results represent the mean ± SEM of 4 to 8 independent mice. The statistical analysis was performed by one-way ANOVA followed by Newman–Keuls test. * $p \leq 0.05$, ** $p \leq 0.01$, vs. WT.+ $p \leq 0.05$, ++ $p \leq 0.01$ vs. APPswe mice.

3. Discussion

In the experimental model of AD used in this study (APPswe mouse), LGF treatment reduced Aβ and phospho-Tau protein levels as well as the number of Aβ plaques with a diameter higher than 25 μm. LGF administration also modulated protein ubiquitination and HSP70 protein levels, reduced glial reactivity and inflammation, and up-regulated the expression of proteins involved in cell survival. These LGF beneficial effects correlate with a better cognitive outcome in APPswe mice.

Amyloid-β aggregation and deposition of Aβ plaques are considered as causative agents in AD, so many therapies have been directed to modify Aβ levels (reviewed in [21]). Under our experimental conditions, LGF modulated Aβ by reducing its levels to WT values in the hippocampus and cerebral cortex. This reduction was observed in the expression of those Aβ peptides with a molecular weight lower than 60 kDa. This fraction includes the Aβ1-42 peptide that has been extensively studied due to its abundance in patients predisposed to AD [22] and mouse models of AD [19]. Here, we also show that LGF treatment reduced the accumulation of polyubiquitinated proteins, and up-regulated HSP70 protein expression in both structures. The high levels of ubiquitinated proteins observed in APPswe mice indicate that proteins are not correctly proteolyzed, probably due to the generation of free radicals and/or an inflammatory environment promoted by the accumulation of Aβ HSP70 is a chaperone which overexpression could suppress the progression of AD by promoting Aβ clearance (reviewed in [23]). HSP70-mediated Aβ clearance from the brain has been associated with the up-regulation of insulin-degrading enzyme (IDE) and transforming growth factor β1 (TGF-β1) [24]. This study did not evaluate IDE and TGF-β1 expression but LGF administration significantly reduced plasmatic levels of insulin in an experimental model of atherosclerosis in mice [25], and modulated the synthesis of TGF-β1 in bile duct-ligated rats [11].

Another major histopathological characteristic in AD is neurofibrillary tangles composed of aggregates of hyperphosphorylated forms of the protein associated with Tau microtubules [26,27]. As shown here, LGF treatment reduced phospho-Tau/Tau ratio in the hippocampus of APPswe mice.

Interestingly, Tau homeostasis is controlled through the action of molecular chaperones, such as HSP70 [28,29] that, as noted above, was up-regulated in this structure. In the case of the cerebral cortex, phosphoTau/Tau ratio in APP mice was not significantly different from untreated WT mice but, in this brain structure, LGF treatment reduced phospho-Tau/Tau ratio in both, WT and APP mice. At present we do not have a possible explanation for this event. We could suggest that this is a potential specific effect of LGF not associated to the accumulation of Aβ plaques and inflammation observed in APP mice. However, according to our results it does not seem the case because similar results were not observed in the hippocampus of WT mice where, as already mentioned, LGF did not reduced p-Tau/Tau ratio. Besides HSP70, which was also up-regulated in the cerebral cortex of APP-LGF mice, LGF could modulate Tau phosphorylation in this brain structure by different mechanisms not analyzed in this study. Further studies must be conducted in order to elucidate these discrepancies.

Activated microglia and reactive astrocytes are two pathological markers observed in AD [30–32]. Both cell types are considered cell targets of LGF in the CNS [6,7,9,20]. According to the present results, LGF significantly reduced proliferation (as measured by BrdU incorporation and PCNA protein expression) and Iba1 protein levels, which are two features of activated microglia. These results are in agreement with previous studies that show how chronic administration of LGF reduced microglia cell reactivity in an experimental model of Parkinson's disease in rats [9] and in ataxic rats [15]. Our immunohistochemical studies also suggest that the administration of LGF could prime microglia to acquire a phagocytic phenotype. Thus, although the number of Iba1-positive cells was not reduced in APP-LGF treated mice, this treatment increased by 3-fold the percentage of Iba1-positive cells that invaded Aβ plaques and reduced the number of Aβ large plaques while increasing the number of smaller plaques, which would explain the slight, but not significant increase observed in this parameter. How LGF modulates microglia activity in APPswe mice is unknown but, as mentioned above, LGF could stimulate TGFβ1expression that is a cytokine that stimulates Aβ clearance through activation of phagocytic microglia [33]. On the other hand, activation of phagocytic microglia has been associated with increased levels of interleukin 6 and TNF-alpha [34]. This latter cytokine seems to play an important role in the mitogenic cascade of LGF in the liver, and in LGF-induced neuroregeneration (reviewed in [6]) and neuroprotection [20].

Reactive astrogliosis is a well-known hallmark of AD that is identified, among others, by an increased expression of GFAP. We also found that LGF reduced GFAP over-expression in the hippocampus and cerebral cortex of APPswe mice, suggesting that astrocytes are potential targets of LGF in this experimental model of AD. Microglia cell reactivity to Aβ and phagocytic activity are also under the regulation of astrocytes [35] so, their stimulation with LGF could lead to the release of factors with antioxidant and/or anti-inflammatory effects that could modulate both events. In this regard, we should mention that LGF modulates the expression of TNF-alpha in cultures of mesencephalic glia [20], and significantly reduced by 36 ± 11% the expression of ASC in these cultures ($p \leq 0.05$ vs. untreated cultures).

The anti-oxidative and anti-inflammatory activities of LGF have also been observed in vivo. Thus, chronic LGF decreased oxidized glutathione concentration in ataxic mice [14], and reduced TNF-alpha protein levels in 6-OHDA-lesioned rats [9]. As presented here, LGF modulates the expression of several proteins that regulate oxidative stress and inflammatory responses in AD. ASC is an adaptor protein that participates in the production of pro-inflammatory cytokines, and contributes to the inflammatory response and cognitive impairment in AD pathology [36–39]. Chronic administration of LGF down-regulated ASC protein levels in the hippocampus and cerebral cortex of APPswe mice. In these mice, ASC is mainly expressed by microglia, which is associated with Aβ plaques (Reimers et al. manuscript in preparation). Because ASC released by microglia forms an aggregate complex with Aβ that promotes inflammation [37,39], we may argue that ASC reduction is associated with a potential anti-inflammatory effect of LGF in this experimental model of AD. Although we were unable to detect any significant change in TNF-alpha and Il-1beta protein expression at the experimental time analyzed in this study, we cannot exclude the possibility that LGF modulates the expression of these cytokines at earlier times of treatment, as observed for TNF-alpha in 6-OHDA-lesioned rats [9]. In addition, small changes in the levels of both proteins may not be detected by Western blot analysis, so that it may be necessary to use other methods with higher sensitivity as ELISA. Other studies have reported that reduced levels of ASC stimulate phagocytosis in glial cells in a mouse model of AD [40], so LGF-induced down-regulation of ASC could also mediate the increase in phagocytic activity proposed in our study.

CD36 is a class B scavenger receptor involved in phagocytosis which expression in microglia plays a key role in the Aβ-mediated activation of this cell type (reviewed in [41]). Moreover, CD36 over-expression in microglia seems to mediate the inflammatory processes associated to Aβ pathology in transgenic mice [42], and the production of ROS in response to Aβ in AD human brains [43,44]. Similarly, the increased levels of CD36 observed in the hippocampus of APPswe mice could contribute to creating an inflammatory environment in this structure. According to our results, LGF treatment could modulate inflammation and/or ROS production in the APPswe hippocampus by decreasing CD36 protein expression and, in consequence, its interaction with Aβ in this structure. In fact, the inhibition of Aβ interaction with CD36 has been proposed as a potential therapeutic strategy in AD [45]. An interesting observation of our study is that LGF up-regulated CD36 levels in the hippocampus of WT mice. These high levels of CD36 could promote the phagocytic activity of microglia to improve the clearance of debris that is accumulated in the normal brain during the processes of aging [46,47]. Although similar results were observed in the cerebral cortex of APPswe and APP-LGF treated mice, no statistically significant differences were detected. Perhaps CD36 levels are not sufficient to be detected through Western blot in this structure, or we need to study a higher number of mice, or mice at different ages. De facto, we were unable to detect CD36 up-regulation in the hippocampus of thirteen months old APPswe mice (100 ± 7 (n = 4) and 104 ± 6 (n = 4) % of CD36 expression in WT and APPswe mice, respectively).

Nrf2 is a transcription factor that regulates oxidative stress [48,49] and anti-inflammatory responses [50,51]. Nrf2 mRNA and protein deficiency have been observed in AD patients [52,53] and AD models in mice [54,55]. As shown here, LGF up-regulated Nrf2 protein levels that were reduced in the cerebral cortex and the hippocampus of APPswe mice. Nrf2 up-regulation ameliorated cognitive impairment in APP Knock-in AD mice [56], and in APPswe/PSEN1dE9 hypoxic mice, the intranasal administration of Nrf2 modulated CD36 protein expression, reduced Aβ deposition, and improved spatial memory [57]. In both studies, these beneficial effects were associated to a reduction in oxidative stress and neuroinflammation promoted by the increased levels of Nrf2. Since in our mice LGF significantly ameliorates cognitive impairment, we may consider that up-regulation of Nrf2 could underlie this behavioral improvement through the activation of anti-oxidant and anti-inflammatory responses, as has been reported in other experimental pathologies[58].

Our previous results indicate a potential neuroprotective role of LGF in the brainstem and cerebellum of ataxic rats [15], and in the substantia nigra and striatum of 6-hydroxydopamine-lesioned rats [9]. In both experimental models of neurodegeneration, LGF raised the ratio Bcl2/Bax due to the up-regulation of the anti-apoptotic protein Bcl2, which is involved in the survival of neural cells [59]. In the experimental model of AD used in this study, LGF also restored Bcl2/Bax ratio to control values, but this effect was due to the down-regulation of the pro-apoptotic protein Bax that was over-expressed in the hippocampus of APPswe mice. Up-regulation of Bax has been observed in neurons that exhibit neurofibrillary tangle pathology [60], and APP transgenic mice [61]. Besides, a neuroblastoma cell line co-transfected with Swedish mutant APP showed a higher Bax/Bcl2 ratio [62]. LGF-induced down-regulation of Bax could contribute to decreasing the excessive neuronal apoptosis reported in AD [63]. The increase in Bax levels observed in APPswe could result in neuronal death. However, APPswe mice did not show any reduction in the expression of the specific nuclear neuronal marker NeuN in the hippocampus (100 ± 8 (n = 6) and 99 ± 10 (n = 5) % of NeuN expression in WT and APP mice, respectively), and cerebral cortex (100 ± 7 (n = 6) and 99 ± 12 (n = 5) % of NeuN expression in WT and APP mice, respectively). These results agree with the lack of neuronal death previously reported in this experimental model of AD [64,65]. Akt, is a serine/threonine kinase which phosphorylated form plays a critical role in the regulation of neuronal survival [66,67] that has been involved in the pathogenesis of AD [68]. Our results showed an increased phospho-Akt/Akt ratio in the APPswe hippocampus due to the higher levels of phospho-Akt observed in this brain structure. Phospho-Akt may protect neuronal cell death through different mechanisms including the phosphorylation and inhibition of cytosolic pro-apoptotic proteins (reviewed in [69]). Because the phosphorylation of Bax by active Akt affects its translocation to the mitochondria [70], we may consider the up-regulation of phospho-Akt in the hippocampus as an intrinsic mechanism to protect neurons of Bax-mediated apoptotic cell death in the APPswe mice.

From our study, we cannot define if the observed effects of LGF are due to a direct or indirect action of the factor on the brain of APPswe mice. A potential direct action would imply that LGF could cross the blood–brain barrier by binding to specific receptors found in the endothelium known as RAGE receptors (receptors for advanced glycation end-products) [71]. In fact, LGF show some structural similarities with the advanced glycation end products (AGE) which structure is mainly based on albumins bound to glucose with the ability to change albumin conformation [72]. RAGE receptors are also expressed by astrocytes and microglia [73], and their activation elicits TNF-alpha release from these cells [73].

Present results show how LGF treatment also improves memory performance impairment in APPswe mice. The APPswe mice in comparison with the WT animals, had a reduced ambulatory behavior in the Y-maze, as shown by the total number of entrances and this pattern was unchanged by LGF treatment, so we may consider that motor activity and anxiety were affected in this experimental model of AD. However, the alternance index in the Y-maze, which is an indicator of mnemonic function, was significantly reduced in these mice. LGF treatment recovered this important parameter of working memory to similar values to those observed in WT mice. Other studies have reported a reduction in the exploratory behavior from 10 months old APPswe mice that are coincident with the presence of Aβ plaque depositions in the hippocampus and cerebral cortex (reviewed in [74]). Thus, LGF-induced reduction in Aβ plaques size and levels could contribute to the cognitive improvement observed in our study. In addition, LGF could ameliorate the exploratory behavior in these mice through the reduction of glial reactivity, and its anti-inflammatory and anti-oxidative responses referred to above.

The marble-burying test index was lower in the APPswe mice than in WT mice, and LGF rescued this behavioral parameter. Other studies have shown reduced scrabble behavior and buried marbles in mice with cortical and hippocampal lesions [75] and in Tg-APP/PS1 mice [76]. In the latter study, the behavioral deficits were attributed to the accumulation of Aβ in the brain, so we may consider that the beneficial effects observed in APP-LGF treated mice could be in part due to the reduction in Aβ levels promoted by the factor.

4. Materials and Methods

4.1. Ethics Statement

The Ethics Committee of the Hospital Ramón y Cajal, Madrid (animal facilities ES280790002001) approved on 11 May 2015 all the protocols related to the use of laboratory animals. All procedures associated with animal experiments were in accordance with Spanish legislation (RD 53/2013) and the European Union Council Directive (2010/63/EU).

4.2. LGF Purification

LGF was obtained and purified from serumof rats that were subjected to a bile duct ligation for 5 weeks, as previously described by Díaz-Gil et al. [77]. The quantitation of the purity of LGF was performed by HPLC [78] and serum samples that showed the highest concentrations of the growth factor were chosen to continue with the process. The method included three chromatographic procedures using DEAE-cellulose, Sephadex G-150, and hydroxylapatite. The absence of contaminants and other growth factors (purity) in the LGF samples was also evaluated according to the standard criteria described by Díaz-Gil et al. [5,77,79]. All LGF preparations showed a single band in SDS-PAGE electrophoresis and were lyophilized and stored at 4 °C until use. Finally, LGF aliquots were dissolved in saline prior to intraperitoneal administration.

4.3. Transgenic Animals

The Tg2576 line over-expressing human APP695 was used as a model of AD in this study. This line contains the human mutated APPswe that includes the double mutation M671L and K670N under the control of the prion protein promoter [18]. This mouse line of AD was generously donated by Dr. Carro [80]. These mice develop age-dependent AD-type neuropathology [18]. Tg2576 mice show elevated levels of the major soluble form of brain amyloid (Aβ1-40) at 1 year old. An intercross between APP Tg2576 and Wild-type (WT) C57BL6 was performed in order to obtain WT littermate controls.

Transgenic (Tg) animals were generated by breeding the mice according to the following diagram: male APPswe × female WT → APPswe (50/57.6) and WT (50/42.4)—(the numbers in brackets show the expected/found genotype frequencies of the offspring expressed in %).

Eighteen WT mice were divided into 2 experimental groups, WT control (WT, $n = 11$) and LGF treated group (WT-LGF, $n = 7$). APPswe mice were also divided in APPswe control (APP, $n = 12$) and LGF treated APPswe (APP-LGF, $n = 16$). Four mice per group were used for histological assays, and 4 to 10 mice were used for biochemical studies. All mice included in each experimental group were used for behavioral studies. The animals were studied at 21 months of age.

4.4. Genotype by PCR

The genotype of each animal was confirmed as described by Carro et al. [80]. Genomic DNA was extracted from the mouse tail using the High Pure PCR template preparation kit (Roche, Barcelona, Spain) according to the manufacturer's instructions. Briefly, 150 ng of DNA was amplified by polymerase chain reaction (PCR) using the specific primers described in [80] to detect mutant human APP sequence.

4.5. LGF and BrdU Administration

Twenty-month-old mice received 2 weekly 100 μL i.p. injections of saline used as a vehicle (WT and APP groups) or LGF (1.6 μg/100 μL) (WT-LGF and APP-LGF groups) for 3 weeks. This optimal dose of LGF has been used in different model systems using an identical or similar schedule [13,14]. Mice were sacrificed 1 week after the last treatment with vehicle or LGF (Figure 7).

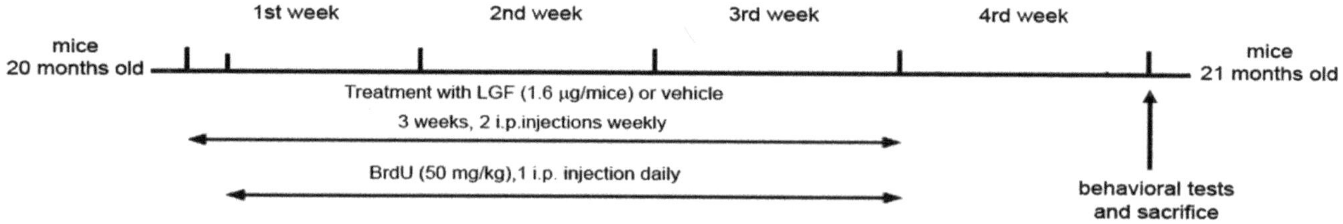

Figure 7. Representative scheme showing the methodological procedure followed for the administration of LGF or vehicle to 20 months old WT and APPswe mice.

To determine whether the i.p. administration of LGF increased cell proliferation, a group of WT and APP animals were injected daily for 3 weeks with the mitotic marker 5-bromodeoxyuridine (BrdU) (50 mg/kg i.p.), starting 24 h after the beginning of LGF/saline injections.

4.6. Behavioral Studies

Exploratory behavior and body weight were measured before treatment initiation to allocating the animals to the experimental groups (WT, WT-LGF, APP, APP-LGF). After 3 weeks of treatment with vehicle or LGF, mice were subjected to behavioral analysis. Two behavioral tests were carried out in this study: Y-maze test and marble burying test.

4.6.1. Y-Maze

Spatial working memory was measured using the Y-maze behavioral paradigm. The Y-maze test is based on the natural exploratory preference of mice to alternate arms when exploring a new environment. The spontaneous alternation behavior of mice in the Y-maze was analyzed to assess short term memory impairment in mice, following the methodology previously reported by Perucho et al. [81,82]. Testing takes place in a Y-shaped maze with three white, opaque plastic arms spaced at an angle of 120 degrees. Briefly, after acclimatizing the mice to the behavioral room (30 min), each mouse was placed at the same end of one arm of the Y-maze and allowed to move freely through the maze for 5 min. The number of arms entered, as well as the number of spontaneous alternations, defined as a sequence of entries in each of 3 consecutive arms without repetition, were recorded to determinate the alternation rate. The percentage of alternation score was calculated as follows:

$$\text{Spontaneous alternation\%} = \left(\frac{\text{number of spontaneous alternations}}{\text{total number of arm entries} - 2}\right) \times 100 \quad (1)$$

4.6.2. Marble Burying Test

Marble burying was assessed as an additional measure of exploratory digging. This test is a useful paradigm to study repetitive compulsive-like behaviors based on the observation of rodents burying objects in their bedding, a phenomenon dependent on hippocampal function [75]. Briefly, mice were individually housed in a cage filled with 5 cm of wood chip bedding for a 30 min testing period of acclimation, and continued throughout the test session. Tests were performed between 18:00 and 20:00 h, under standard laboratory conditions of temperature, 22 ± 2 °C, 12 h light:dark cycle, relative humidity 50–60% and with food and water restriction. The mice were placed individually for 30 min in plastic cages, with 9 marbles placed on top of the bedding material, in a 3 × 3 grid with 4 cm center-to-center spacing. A new cage, clean marbles and fresh bedding were used for each mouse. At the end of that time, each mouse was returned to its home cage and the number of marbles uncovered; completely buried (not visible); 2/3 covered (only top visible) and half covered, were counted. This classification was used to obtain a "buried index", as an indication of activity and interaction with their environment [83].

4.7. Antibodies and Immunochemicals for Immunohistochemistry

The primary antibodies used in this study were: rabbit polyclonal anti-Iba1 (1:100; Wako Chemicals USA, Inc., Los Angeles, CA, USA), mouse monoclonal anti-5-bromodeoxyuridine (BrdU, 1:25; DakoCytomation, Glostrup, Denmark), and mouse monoclonal anti-Aβ (6E10, 1:100; Covance, Emeryville, CA, USA). The secondary antibodies used were: Alexa Fluor-568 goat anti-mouse IgG, and Alexa Fluor-488 goat anti-rabbit IgG (1:400; both from Molecular Probes; Eugene, OR, USA), fluorescein-conjugated goat anti-mouse IgG (1:25; Jackson ImmunoResearch Laboratories Inc., West Grove, PA, USA).

4.8. Tissue Processing, Immunohistochemistry and Morphometric Analyses

Four weeks after the beginning of LGF or saline treatment transgenic mice were perfused intracardially under deep anesthesia with 10 mL of heparinized isotonic saline, followed by 40 mL of 4% paraformaldehyde. Brains were postfixed in the same solution for 24 h at 4 °C, cryoprotected and frozen, before sectioning into 20 μm-thick coronal sections in a cryostat. For quantitative measurements and immunohistochemical analysis of the dorsal hippocampus and dorsal cortex, coronal sections were obtained at the antero-posterior level of −2.5 to −3 mm from Bregma [84].

Tissue sections were mounted on coated FLEX IHC microscope slides (DakoCytomation, Glostrup, Denmark), treated with sodium acetate 10 mM, pH 6.0, at 95 °C for 4 min, and blocked with 5% normal goat serum (NGS) and 0.1% Triton-X 100 in phosphate buffer saline (PBS), pH 7.4, for 30 min. Primary antibodies diluted in 0.5% NGS in PBS, were applied for 24 h at 4 °C, and were visualized using fluorescent secondary anti-rabbit and anti-mouse antibodies diluted in 0.5% NGS in PBS. The slides were coverslipped in a medium containing p-phenylenediamine and bisbenzimide (Hoechst 33342; Sigma, St. Louis, MO, USA) for detection of nuclei. For double immunolabeling with anti-Iba1 and anti-BrdU antibodies, the former immunostaining was performed prior to the immunodetection of BrdU incorporated into nuclei. The latter detection needed pretreatment of sections with 2N HCl at 37°C for 30 min, previous to the NGS blocking step. In the case of Aβ immunodetection in plaques, sections were pretreated with 70% formic acid for 20 min at RT, followed by the blocking step.

For quantification of proliferating BrdU-positive cells, microglial Iba1-positive cells, and Aβ 6E10-positive plaques, panoramic views were obtained from one representative coronal section for each immunostaining technique and for each brain. These panoramic views, where the complete transversal surface of dorsal hippocampus and dorsal cortex of each cerebral hemisphere were visualized (3 mm^2 for each structure), were obtained by using the stitching tool of the software NIS ELEMENTS C, version BR 3.2 (Nikon Instruments Inc., Tokio, Japan), coupled to a Nikon ECLIPSE Ti-e microscope (Nikon Instruments Inc., Tokio, Japan) with a motorized stage, and the 10× objective. Four WT, 4 APP and 4 APPL-GF were analyzed for these evaluations. The data entered in the corresponding graphs were: (a) the mean ± SEM obtained from the data of both cerebral hemispheres (number of plaques/mm^2); (b) the mean of 2 different regions in the cortex and of 4 different regions in the hippocampus of one cerebral hemisphere (density of Iba1-positive cells); and (c) the sum of data from both hemispheres (density of BrdU-positive cells).

4.9. Brain Regions and Tissue Preparation for Biochemical Analysis

After decapitation the brain was extracted and the hippocampus and cortex were free-hand dissected, then the samples were frozen on dry ice for biochemical studies (Western blot). For the protein extraction, dried tissue samples were weighed and placed in six volumes (w/v) of phosphate-buffered saline (PBS) with protease inhibitor cocktail 1× (Calbiochem, Temecula, CA, USA) and 20 mM N-ethylmaleimide to inactivate deubiquitinating enzymes and subjected to two 30-s rounds of sonication. The lysates were immediately boiled for 5 min and centrifuged at 12,000× *g* at 4 °C for 30 min. The supernatant-PBS-inhibitors was defined as the soluble fraction and was used for protein analysis by Western blot. To obtain the total Aβ (soluble plus insoluble) fraction, the initial homogenate (200 μL) was extracted with 5 M guanidine in 6 mM Tris–HCl, pH 8.0 by rotating the sample at room temperature overnight. The sample obtained after guanidine extraction represented the total fraction. Soluble and total fractions were used for protein analysis by Western blot.

4.10. Protein Analysis

Aliquots of 20–30 μg of protein were added to sample loading buffer 2× (50 mM Tris pH 6.8, 10% glycerol, 2% SDS, 5% β-mercaptoethanol and 0.1% bromophenol blue). The electrophoresis was performed using SDS-polyacrylamide gels (10–15%) and then the samples were electro-blotted using nitrocellulose membranes (0.45 μm). The blots were blocked using TTBS solution (5% dry skimmed milk, 137 mM NaCl plus 0.1% Tween-20 and 20 mM Tris-HCl pH 7.6) at room temperature for 2 h. Once the blocking of non-specific binding was performed, the membranes were incubated overnight at 4 °C with specific primary antibodies diluted in blocking solution. Then, the membranes were washed twice for 10 min using blocking solution followed by another two washes with TTBS for 5 min. β-actin was used as a loading control and housekeeping protein. The membranes were developed by enhanced chemiluminescence detection using a commercial kit (Bio-Rad Laboratories Inc., Hercules, CA, USA) and quantified by computer-assisted video densitometry using the Bio-Rad *Quantity One* software (Bio-Rad Laboratories Inc, Hercules, CA, USA). The data of the proteins of interest analyzed in the study were normalized with respect to β-actin levels.

4.10.1. Primary Antibodies

The primary antibodies used in this study were: Mouse monoclonal amyloid-β antibody 6E10 (BioLegend Inc., San Diego, CA, USA), diluted 1:1000. Mouse monoclonal anti-HSP70 (1:1000) and rabbit polyclonal antibody against ASC (1:500) were from Santa Cruz (Temecula, CA, USA). Mouse monoclonal anti tau-5 (for measurement of total tau protein) antibody (Chemicon, Madrid, Spain) diluted 1:5000 and rabbit polyclonal to phospho-tau (phospho serine199 + serine202) (1:1000) were from Abcam (Cambridge, UK). Mouse monoclonal anti-glial fibrillar acid protein (GFAP) antibody diluted 1:5000 was from Chemicon (Madrid, Spain) and rabbit polyclonal antibody for anti-Iba1, 1:1000 was for WAKO (Japan). Rabbit anti-proliferating cell nuclear antigen (PCNA, 1:75; SantaCruz Biotechnology, Santa Cruz, CA, USA), and mouse monoclonal anti-ubiquitin antibody (1/500) was from Chemicon (Chemicon International Inc., Temecula, CA, USA). Mouse anti Bcl2 (1:250) and rabbit anti-Bax (1:250) were from Santa Cruz (Santa Cruz Biotechnology). Rabbit anti-phospho-Akt (Ser473P) (1:2000) and rabbit anti-Akt (1:2000) were from Cell Signaling Technology, Beverly, MA, USA. Rabbit anti Nrf2 (1:1000) and rabbit anti CD36 (1:500) were from Thermo Fisher Scientific, Rosemont, IL, USA. To correct and quantify the protein charge mouse monoclonal anti-β-actin antibody diluted 1:10,000 was used from Sigma.

4.10.2. Secondary Antibodies

Goat anti-mouse-IGg-HRP and anti-rabbit-IGg-HRP secondary antibodies diluted 1:1000 were purchased from Bio-Rad (Bio-Rad Laboratories Inc., Hercules, CA, USA).

4.11. Statistical Analysis

Results are expressed as mean ± SEM of (n) independent animals. Statistical analysis was performed with the GraphPad Prism software, version 6.01 (La Jolla, CA, USA). Before analysis, the Shapiro–Wilk test was used to test normality. One-way ANOVA followed by the Newman–Keuls multiple comparison test were performed. Differences were considered significant when $p \leq 0.05$.

5. Conclusions

Liver growth factor is an albumin–bilirubin complex that exhibits remarkable neuroprotective, anti-inflammatory, and anti-oxidant activities in several models of neurodegenerative diseases. In the experimental model of AD used in this study (APPswe mouse), chronic LGF treatment reduced Aβ and phospho-Tau protein levels which are the main neuropathological features associated to the disease. LGF also reduced microglia and astroglia cell reactivity and modulated the expression of ASC CD36 and Nrf2 which are proteins involved in the regulation of inflammatory and oxidative processes. Because these beneficial effects correlated with an improvement in the cognitive deficits observed in the APPswe mice, we may consider LGF as a potential new therapeutic factor for AD.

6. Patents

US 8,642,551 B2, 4 February 2014
CE, num. 09732019.6-1456, Ref. EP-883, April 2015
US 14/140.014, 26 May 2015

Author Contributions: Experimental Design, R.G.-G., J.P., D.R., M.J.C. and E.B.; performed the experiments, R.G.-G., J.P., M.V.-M., D.R., A.G., M.J.C., G.M.U.d.A. and E.B.; data Analysis: R.G.-G., M.J.C., D.R., A.J.E. and E.B. paper writing, R.G.-G., D.R., M.J.C. and E.B. All authors have read and agreed to the published version of the manuscript.

Acknowledgments: We are grateful to Miriam Novillo Pérez for technical help. We also thank the technical help provided by the Confocal Microscopy Unit of the Ramón y Cajal Institute for Health Research (IRYCIS). Our group also wants to thank Juan José Díaz Gil, who passed away on 4 November 2016, for the discovery of the Liver Growth Factor and for his exceptional dedication to pursuing knowledge about its effectiveness against neurodegenerative diseases. He will always be our great mentor and dear friend.

References

1. Bird, T.D. Alzheimer Disease Overview. In *GeneReviews®*; Adam, M.P., Ardinger, H.H., Pagon, R.A., Wallace, S.E., Bean, L.J.H., Stephens, K., Amemiya, A., Eds.; University of Washington, Seattle: Seattle, WA, USA; pp. 1993–2020.
2. De-Paula, V.J.; Radanovic, M.; Diniz, B.S.; Forlenza, O.V. Alzheimer's disease. *Subcell. Biochem.* **2012**, *65*, 329–352. [CrossRef] [PubMed]
3. Serrano-Pozo, A.; Frosch, M.P.; Masliah, E.; Hyman, B.T. Neuropathological alterations in Alzheimer disease. *Cold Spring Harb. Perspect. Med.* **2011**, *1*, a006189. [CrossRef] [PubMed]
4. Gandy, S.; DeKosky, S.T. Toward the treatment and prevention of Alzheimer's disease: Rational strategies and recent progress. *Annu. Rev. Med.* **2013**, *64*, 367–383. [CrossRef] [PubMed]
5. Díaz-Gil, J.J.; Escartin, P.; Garcia-Canero, R.; Trilla, C.; Veloso, J.J.; Sanchez, G.; Moreno-Caparros, A.; Enrique de Salamanca, C.; Lozano, R.; Gavilanes, J.G.; et al. Purification of a liver DNA-synthesis promoter from plasma of partially hepatectomized rats. *Biochem. J.* **1986**, *235*, 49–55. [CrossRef]
6. Gonzalo-Gobernado, R.; Calatrava-Ferreras, L.; Perucho, J.; Reimers, D.; Casarejos, M.J.; Herranz, A.S.; Jimenez-Escrig, A.; Diaz-Gil, J.J.; Bazan, E. Liver growth factor as a tissue regenerating factor in neurodegenerative diseases. *Recent Pat. CNS Drug Discov.* **2014**, *9*, 173–180. [CrossRef] [PubMed]
7. Gonzalo-Gobernado, R.; Reimers, D.; Herranz, A.S.; Diaz-Gil, J.J.; Osuna, C.; Asensio, M.J.; Baena, S.; Rodriguez-Serrano, M.; Bazan, E. Mobilization of neural stem cells and generation of new neurons in 6-OHDA-lesioned rats by intracerebroventricular infusion of liver growth factor. *J. Histochem. Cytochem.* **2009**, *57*, 491–502. [CrossRef]
8. Reimers, D.; Herranz, A.S.; Diaz-Gil, J.J.; Lobo, M.V.; Paino, C.L.; Alonso, R.; Asensio, M.J.; Gonzalo-Gobernado, R.; Bazan, E. Intrastriatal infusion of liver growth factor stimulates dopamine terminal sprouting and partially restores motor function in 6-hydroxydopamine-lesioned rats. *J. Histochem. Cytochem.* **2006**, *54*, 457–465. [CrossRef]
9. Gonzalo-Gobernado, R.; Calatrava-Ferreras, L.; Reimers, D.; Herranz, A.S.; Rodriguez-Serrano, M.; Miranda, C.; Jimenez-Escrig, A.; Diaz-Gil, J.J.; Bazan, E. Neuroprotective activity of peripherally administered liver growth factor in a rat model of Parkinson's disease. *PLoS ONE* **2013**, *8*, e67771. [CrossRef]
10. Reimers, D.; Osuna, C.; Gonzalo-Gobernado, R.; Herranz, A.S.; Diaz-Gil, J.J.; Jimenez-Escrig, A.; Asensio, M.J.; Miranda, C.; Rodriguez-Serrano, M.; Bazan, E. Liver growth factor promotes the survival of grafted neural stem cells in a rat model of Parkinson's disease. *Curr. Stem. Cell Res. Ther.* **2012**, *7*, 15–25. [CrossRef]
11. Díaz-Gil, J.J.; Garcia-Monzon, C.; Rua, C.; Martin-Sanz, P.; Cereceda, R.M.; Miquilena-Colina, M.E.; Machin, C.; Fernandez-Martinez, A.; Garcia-Canero, R. The anti-fibrotic effect of liver growth factor is associated with decreased intrahepatic levels of matrix metalloproteinases 2 and 9 and transforming growth factor beta 1 in bile duct-ligated rats. *Histol. Histopathol.* **2008**, *23*, 583–591. [CrossRef]
12. Díaz-Gil, J.J.; Munoz, J.; Albillos, A.; Rua, C.; Machin, C.; Garcia-Canero, R.; Cereceda, R.M.; Guijarro, M.C.; Trilla, C.; Escartin, P. Improvement in liver fibrosis, functionality and hemodynamics in CCI4-cirrhotic rats after injection of the Liver Growth Factor. *J. Hepatol.* **1999**, *30*, 1065–1072. [CrossRef]
13. Martinez-Galan, L.; del Puerto-Nevado, L.; Perez-Rial, S.; Diaz-Gil, J.J.; Gonzalez-Mangado, N.; Peces-Barba, G. Liver growth factor improves pulmonary fibrosis secondary to cadmium administration in mice. *Arch. Bronconeumol.* **2010**, *46*, 20–26. [CrossRef]

14. Calatrava-Ferreras, L.; Gonzalo-Gobernado, R.; Reimers, D.; Herranz, A.S.; Casarejos, M.J.; Jimenez-Escrig, A.; Regadera, J.; Velasco-Martin, J.; Vallejo-Munoz, M.; Diaz-Gil, J.J.; et al. Liver Growth Factor (LGF) Upregulates Frataxin Protein Expression and Reduces Oxidative Stress in Friedreich's Ataxia Transgenic Mice. *Int. J. Mol. Sci.* **2016**, *17*, 2066. [CrossRef] [PubMed]
15. Calatrava-Ferreras, L.; Gonzalo-Gobernado, R.; Reimers, D.; Herranz, A.S.; Jimenez-Escrig, A.; Diaz-Gil, J.J.; Casarejos, M.J.; Montero-Vega, M.T.; Bazan, E. Neuroprotective Role of Liver Growth Factor "LGF" in an Experimental Model of Cerebellar Ataxia. *Int. J. Mol. Sci.* **2014**, *15*, 19056–19073. [CrossRef]
16. Heneka, M.T.; O'Banion, M.K.; Terwel, D.; Kummer, M.P. Neuroinflammatory processes in Alzheimer's disease. *J. Neural. Transm. (Vienna)* **2010**, *117*, 919–947. [CrossRef]
17. Huang, W.J.; Zhang, X.; Chen, W.W. Role of oxidative stress in Alzheimer's disease. *Biomed. Rep.* **2016**, *4*, 519–522. [CrossRef]
18. Hsiao, K.; Chapman, P.; Nilsen, S.; Eckman, C.; Harigaya, Y.; Younkin, S.; Yang, F.; Cole, G. Correlative memory deficits, Abeta elevation, and amyloid plaques in transgenic mice. *Science* **1996**, *274*, 99–102. [CrossRef]
19. Lee, Y.W.; Kim, D.H.; Jeon, S.J.; Park, S.J.; Kim, J.M.; Jung, J.M.; Lee, H.E.; Bae, S.G.; Oh, H.K.; Son, K.H.; et al. Neuroprotective effects of salvianolic acid B on an Abeta25-35 peptide-induced mouse model of Alzheimer's disease. *Eur. J. Pharmacol.* **2013**, *704*, 70–77. [CrossRef]
20. Gonzalo-Gobernado, R.; Reimers, D.; Casarejos, M.J.; Calatrava Ferreras, L.; Vallejo-Munoz, M.; Jimenez-Escrig, A.; Diaz-Gil, J.J.; Ulzurrun de Asanza, G.M.; Bazan, E. Liver Growth Factor Induces Glia-Associated Neuroprotection in an in Vitro Model of Parkinson's Disease. *Brain Sci.* **2020**, *10*, 315. [CrossRef]
21. Arbor, S.C.; LaFontaine, M.; Cumbay, M. Amyloid-beta Alzheimer targets—Protein processing, lipid rafts, and amyloid-beta pores. *Yale J. Biol. Med.* **2016**, *89*, 5–21. [PubMed]
22. Butterfield, D.A.; Swomley, A.M.; Sultana, R. Amyloid beta-peptide (1-42)-induced oxidative stress in Alzheimer disease: Importance in disease pathogenesis and progression. *Antioxid. Redox Signal.* **2013**, *19*, 823–835. [CrossRef] [PubMed]
23. Lu, R.C.; Tan, M.S.; Wang, H.; Xie, A.M.; Yu, J.T.; Tan, L. Heat shock protein 70 in Alzheimer's disease. *Biomed. Res. Int.* **2014**, *2014*, 435203. [CrossRef] [PubMed]
24. Hoshino, T.; Murao, N.; Namba, T.; Takehara, M.; Adachi, H.; Katsuno, M.; Sobue, G.; Matsushima, T.; Suzuki, T.; Mizushima, T. Suppression of Alzheimer's disease-related phenotypes by expression of heat shock protein 70 in mice. *J. Neurosci.* **2011**, *31*, 5225–5234. [CrossRef] [PubMed]
25. Surra, J.C.; Guillen, N.; Barranquero, C.; Arbones-Mainar, J.M.; Navarro, M.A.; Gascon, S.; Arnal, C.; Godino, J.; Guzman, M.A.; Diaz-Gil, J.J.; et al. Sex-dependent effect of liver growth factor on atherosclerotic lesions and fatty liver disease in apolipoprotein E knockout mice. *Histol. Histopathol.* **2010**, *25*, 609–618. [PubMed]
26. Avila, J. Alzheimer disease: Caspases first. *Nat. Rev. Neurol.* **2010**, *6*, 587–588. [CrossRef]
27. Hernandez, F.; Avila, J. Tauopathies. *Cell Mol. Life Sci.* **2007**, *64*, 2219–2233. [CrossRef] [PubMed]
28. Dou, F.; Netzer, W.J.; Tanemura, K.; Li, F.; Hartl, F.U.; Takashima, A.; Gouras, G.K.; Greengard, P.; Xu, H. Chaperones increase association of tau protein with microtubules. *Proc. Natl. Acad. Sci. USA* **2003**, *100*, 721–726. [CrossRef]
29. Miyata, Y.; Koren, J.; Kiray, J.; Dickey, C.A.; Gestwicki, J.E. Molecular chaperones and regulation of tau quality control: Strategies for drug discovery in tauopathies. *Future Med. Chem.* **2011**, *3*, 1523–1537. [CrossRef]
30. Dossi, E.; Vasile, F.; Rouach, N. Human astrocytes in the diseased brain. *Brain Res. Bull.* **2018**, *136*, 139–156. [CrossRef]
31. Sarlus, H.; Heneka, M.T. Microglia in Alzheimer's disease. *J. Clin. Investig.* **2017**, *127*, 3240–3249. [CrossRef]
32. Taipa, R.; Ferreira, V.; Brochado, P.; Robinson, A.; Reis, I.; Marques, F.; Mann, D.M.; Melo-Pires, M.; Sousa, N. Inflammatory pathology markers (activated microglia and reactive astrocytes) in early and late onset Alzheimer disease: A post mortem study. *Neuropathol. Appl. Neurobiol.* **2018**, *44*, 298–313. [CrossRef] [PubMed]
33. von Bernhardi, R.; Eugenin-von Bernhardi, L.; Eugenin, J. Microglial cell dysregulation in brain aging and neurodegeneration. *Front. Aging Neurosci.* **2015**, *7*, 124. [CrossRef] [PubMed]
34. Kakimura, J.; Kitamura, Y.; Takata, K.; Umeki, M.; Suzuki, S.; Shibagaki, K.; Taniguchi, T.; Nomura, Y.; Gebicke-Haerter, P.J.; Smith, M.A.; et al. Microglial activation and amyloid-beta clearance induced by exogenous heat-shock proteins. *FASEB J.* **2002**, *16*, 601–603. [CrossRef] [PubMed]
35. Von Bernhardi, R.; Ramirez, G. Microglia-astrocyte interaction in Alzheimer's disease: Friends or foes for the nervous system? *Biol. Res.* **2001**, *34*, 123–128. [CrossRef] [PubMed]

36. Franklin, B.S.; Bossaller, L.; de Nardo, D.; Ratter, J.M.; Stutz, A.; Engels, G.; Brenker, C.; Nordhoff, M.; Mirandola, S.R.; Al-Amoudi, A.; et al. The adaptor ASC has extracellular and 'prionoid' activities that propagate inflammation. *Nat. Immunol.* **2014**, *15*, 727–737. [CrossRef] [PubMed]
37. Friker, L.L.; Scheiblich, H.; Hochheiser, I.V.; Brinkschulte, R.; Riedel, D.; Latz, E.; Geyer, M.; Heneka, M.T. beta-Amyloid Clustering around ASC Fibrils Boosts Its Toxicity in Microglia. *Cell Rep.* **2020**, *30*, 3743–3754. [CrossRef]
38. Scott, X.O.; Stephens, M.E.; Desir, M.C.; Dietrich, W.D.; Keane, R.W.; de Rivero Vaccari, J.P. The Inflammasome Adaptor Protein ASC in Mild Cognitive Impairment and Alzheimer's Disease. *Int. J. Mol. Sci.* **2020**, *21*, 4674. [CrossRef]
39. Venegas, C.; Kumar, S.; Franklin, B.S.; Dierkes, T.; Brinkschulte, R.; Tejera, D.; Vieira-Saecker, A.; Schwartz, S.; Santarelli, F.; Kummer, M.P.; et al. Microglia-derived ASC specks cross-seed amyloid-beta in Alzheimer's disease. *Nature* **2017**, *552*, 355–361. [CrossRef]
40. Couturier, J.; Stancu, I.C.; Schakman, O.; Pierrot, N.; Huaux, F.; Kienlen-Campard, P.; Dewachter, I.; Octave, J.N. Activation of phagocytic activity in astrocytes by reduced expression of the inflammasome component ASC and its implication in a mouse model of Alzheimer disease. *J. Neuroinflamm.* **2016**, *13*, 20. [CrossRef]
41. Doens, D.; Fernandez, P.L. Microglia receptors and their implications in the response to amyloid beta for Alzheimer's disease pathogenesis. *J. Neuroinflamm.* **2014**, *11*, 48. [CrossRef]
42. Martin, E.; Boucher, C.; Fontaine, B.; Delarasse, C. Distinct inflammatory phenotypes of microglia and monocyte-derived macrophages in Alzheimer's disease models: Effects of aging and amyloid pathology. *Aging Cell* **2017**, *16*, 27–38. [CrossRef] [PubMed]
43. Coraci, I.S.; Husemann, J.; Berman, J.W.; Hulette, C.; Dufour, J.H.; Campanella, G.K.; Luster, A.D.; Silverstein, S.C.; El-Khoury, J.B. CD36, a class B scavenger receptor, is expressed on microglia in Alzheimer's disease brains and can mediate production of reactive oxygen species in response to beta-amyloid fibrils. *Am. J. Pathol.* **2002**, *160*, 101–112. [CrossRef]
44. Ricciarelli, R.; D'Abramo, C.; Zingg, J.M.; Giliberto, L.; Markesbery, W.; Azzi, A.; Marinari, U.M.; Pronzato, M.A.; Tabaton, M. CD36 overexpression in human brain correlates with beta-amyloid deposition but not with Alzheimer's disease. *Free Radic. Biol. Med.* **2004**, *36*, 1018–1024. [CrossRef] [PubMed]
45. Wilkinson, K.; Boyd, J.D.; Glicksman, M.; Moore, K.J.; El Khoury, J. A high content drug screen identifies ursolic acid as an inhibitor of amyloid beta protein interactions with its receptor CD36. *J. Biol. Chem.* **2011**, *286*, 34914–34922. [CrossRef] [PubMed]
46. Conde, J.R.; Streit, W.J. Microglia in the aging brain. *J. Neuropathol. Exp. Neurol.* **2006**, *65*, 199–203. [CrossRef] [PubMed]
47. Mosher, K.I.; Wyss-Coray, T. Microglial dysfunction in brain aging and Alzheimer's disease. *Biochem. Pharmacol.* **2014**, *88*, 594–604. [CrossRef]
48. Itoh, K.; Chiba, T.; Takahashi, S.; Ishii, T.; Igarashi, K.; Katoh, Y.; Oyake, T.; Hayashi, N.; Satoh, K.; Hatayama, I.; et al. An Nrf2/small Maf heterodimer mediates the induction of phase II detoxifying enzyme genes through antioxidant response elements. *Biochem. Biophys. Res. Commun.* **1997**, *236*, 313–322. [CrossRef]
49. Suzuki, T.; Muramatsu, A.; Saito, R.; Iso, T.; Shibata, T.; Kuwata, K.; Kawaguchi, S.I.; Iwawaki, T.; Adachi, S.; Suda, H.; et al. Molecular Mechanism of Cellular Oxidative Stress Sensing by Keap1. *Cell Rep.* **2019**, *28*, 746–758. [CrossRef]
50. Itoh, K.; Mochizuki, M.; Ishii, Y.; Ishii, T.; Shibata, T.; Kawamoto, Y.; Kelly, V.; Sekizawa, K.; Uchida, K.; Yamamoto, M. Transcription factor Nrf2 regulates inflammation by mediating the effect of 15-deoxy-Delta(12,14)-prostaglandin j(2). *Mol. Cell Biol.* **2004**, *24*, 36–45. [CrossRef]
51. Kobayashi, E.H.; Suzuki, T.; Funayama, R.; Nagashima, T.; Hayashi, M.; Sekine, H.; Tanaka, N.; Moriguchi, T.; Motohashi, H.; Nakayama, K.; et al. Nrf2 suppresses macrophage inflammatory response by blocking proinflammatory cytokine transcription. *Nat. Commun.* **2016**, *7*, 11624. [CrossRef]
52. Kerr, F.; Sofola-Adesakin, O.; Ivanov, D.K.; Gatliff, J.; Gomez Perez-Nievas, B.; Bertrand, H.C.; Martinez, P.; Callard, R.; Snoeren, I.; Cocheme, H.M.; et al. Direct Keap1-Nrf2 disruption as a potential therapeutic target for Alzheimer's disease. *PLoS Genet* **2017**, *13*, e1006593. [CrossRef] [PubMed]
53. Youssef, P.; Chami, B.; Lim, J.; Middleton, T.; Sutherland, G.T.; Witting, P.K. Evidence supporting oxidative stress in a moderately affected area of the brain in Alzheimer's disease. *Sci. Rep.* **2018**, *8*, 11553. [CrossRef] [PubMed]

54. Joshi, G.; Gan, K.A.; Johnson, D.A.; Johnson, J.A. Increased Alzheimer's disease-like pathology in the APP/PS1DeltaE9 mouse model lacking Nrf2 through modulation of autophagy. *Neurobiol. Aging.* **2015**, *36*, 664–679. [CrossRef] [PubMed]
55. Rojo, A.I.; Pajares, M.; Garcia-Yague, A.J.; Buendia, I.; van Leuven, F.; Yamamoto, M.; Lopez, M.G.; Cuadrado, A. Deficiency in the transcription factor NRF2 worsens inflammatory parameters in a mouse model with combined tauopathy and amyloidopathy. *Redox. Biol.* **2018**, *18*, 173–180. [CrossRef]
56. Uruno, A.; Matsumaru, D.; Ryoke, R.; Saito, R.; Kadoguchi, S.; Saigusa, D.; Saito, T.; Saido, T.C.; Kawashima, R.; Yamamoto, M. Nrf2 Suppresses Oxidative Stress and Inflammation in App Knock-In Alzheimer's Disease Model Mice. *Mol. Cell Biol.* **2020**, *40*. [CrossRef]
57. Wang, C.Y.; Wang, Z.Y.; Xie, J.W.; Cai, J.H.; Wang, T.; Xu, Y.; Wang, X.; An, L. CD36 upregulation mediated by intranasal LV-NRF2 treatment mitigates hypoxia-induced progression of Alzheimer's-like pathogenesis. *Antioxid. Redox Signal.* **2014**, *21*, 2208–2230. [CrossRef] [PubMed]
58. Giron-Martinez, A.; Perez-Rial, S.; Terron-Exposito, R.; Diaz-Gil, J.J.; Gonzalez-Mangado, N.; Peces-Barba, G. Proliferative Activity of Liver Growth Factor is Associated with an Improvement of Cigarette Smoke-Induced Emphysema in Mice. *PLoS ONE* **2014**, *9*, e112995. [CrossRef]
59. Frebel, K.; Wiese, S. Signalling molecules essential for neuronal survival and differentiation. *Biochem. Soc. Trans.* **2006**, *34*, 1287–1290. [CrossRef]
60. Eckert, A.; Marques, C.A.; Keil, U.; Schussel, K.; Muller, W.E. Increased apoptotic cell death in sporadic and genetic Alzheimer's disease. *Ann. N. Y. Acad. Sci.* **2003**, *1010*, 604–609. [CrossRef]
61. Feng, Z.; Qin, C.; Chang, Y.; Zhang, J.T. Early melatonin supplementation alleviates oxidative stress in a transgenic mouse model of Alzheimer's disease. *Free Radic. Biol. Med.* **2006**, *40*, 101–109. [CrossRef]
62. Yan, Y.; Gong, K.; Ma, T.; Zhang, L.; Zhao, N.; Zhang, X.; Tang, P.; Gong, Y. Protective effect of edaravone against Alzheimer's disease-relevant insults in neuroblastoma N2a cells. *Neurosci. Lett.* **2012**, *531*, 160–165. [CrossRef] [PubMed]
63. Obulesu, M.; Lakshmi, M.J. Apoptosis in Alzheimer's disease: An understanding of the physiology, pathology and therapeutic avenues. *Neurochem. Res.* **2014**, *39*, 2301–2312. [CrossRef] [PubMed]
64. King, D.L.; Arendash, G.W. Behavioral characterization of the Tg2576 transgenic model of Alzheimer's disease through 19 months. *Physiol. Behav.* **2002**, *75*, 627–642. [CrossRef]
65. Takeuchi, A.; Irizarry, M.C.; Duff, K.; Saido, T.C.; Hsiao Ashe, K.; Hasegawa, M.; Mann, D.M.; Hyman, B.T.; Iwatsubo, T. Age-related amyloid beta deposition in transgenic mice overexpressing both Alzheimer mutant presenilin 1 and amyloid beta precursor protein Swedish mutant is not associated with global neuronal loss. *Am. J. Pathol.* **2000**, *157*, 331–339. [CrossRef]
66. Noshita, N.; Lewen, A.; Sugawara, T.; Chan, P.H. Evidence of phosphorylation of Akt and neuronal survival after transient focal cerebral ischemia in mice. *J. Cereb. Blood Flow Metab.* **2001**, *21*, 1442–1450. [CrossRef] [PubMed]
67. Zhao, H.; Sapolsky, R.M.; Steinberg, G.K. Phosphoinositide-3-kinase/akt survival signal pathways are implicated in neuronal survival after stroke. *Mol. Neurobiol.* **2006**, *34*, 249–270. [CrossRef]
68. Matsuda, S.; Nakagawa, Y.; Tsuji, A.; Kitagishi, Y.; Nakanishi, A.; Murai, T. Implications of PI3K/AKT/PTEN Signaling on Superoxide Dismutases Expression and in the Pathogenesis of Alzheimer's Disease. *Diseases* **2018**, *6*, 28. [CrossRef]
69. Chong, Z.Z.; Li, F.; Maiese, K. Activating Akt and the brain's resources to drive cellular survival and prevent inflammatory injury. *Histol. Histopathol.* **2005**, *20*, 299–315. [CrossRef]
70. Gardai, S.J.; Hildeman, D.A.; Frankel, S.K.; Whitlock, B.B.; Frasch, S.C.; Borregaard, N.; Marrack, P.; Bratton, D.L.; Henson, P.M. Phosphorylation of Bax Ser184 by Akt regulates its activity and apoptosis in neutrophils. *J. Biol. Chem.* **2004**, *279*, 21085–21095. [CrossRef]
71. Sagare, A.P.; Winkler, E.A.; Bell, R.D.; Deane, R.; Zlokovic, B.V. From the liver to the blood-brain barrier: An interconnected system regulating brain amyloid-beta levels. *J. Neurosci. Res.* **2011**, *89*, 967–968. [CrossRef]
72. Thornalley, P.J. Cell activation by glycated proteins. AGE receptors, receptor recognition factors and functional classification of AGEs. *Cell Mol. Biol. (Noisy-Le-Grand)* **1998**, *44*, 1013–1023. [PubMed]
73. Park, I.H.; Yeon, S.I.; Youn, J.H.; Choi, J.E.; Sasaki, N.; Choi, I.H.; Shin, J.S. Expression of a novel secreted splice variant of the receptor for advanced glycation end products (RAGE) in human brain astrocytes and peripheral blood mononuclear cells. *Mol. Immunol.* **2004**, *40*, 1203–1211. [CrossRef] [PubMed]

74. Ameen-Ali, K.E.; Wharton, S.B.; Simpson, J.E.; Heath, P.R.; Sharp, P.; Berwick, J. Review: Neuropathology and behavioural features of transgenic murine models of Alzheimer's disease. *Neuropathol. Appl. Neurobiol.* **2017**, *43*, 553–570. [CrossRef] [PubMed]
75. Deacon, R.M. Digging and marble burying in mice: Simple methods for in vivo identification of biological impacts. *Nat. Protoc.* **2006**, *1*, 122–124. [CrossRef] [PubMed]
76. Kim, T.K.; Han, H.E.; Kim, H.; Lee, J.E.; Choi, D.; Park, W.J.; Han, P.L. Expression of the plant viral protease NIa in the brain of a mouse model of Alzheimer's disease mitigates Abeta pathology and improves cognitive function. *Exp. Mol. Med.* **2012**, *44*, 740–748. [CrossRef] [PubMed]
77. Díaz-Gil, J.J.; Rua, C.; Machin, C.; Cereceda, R.M.; Garcia-Canero, R.; de Foronda, M.; Perez de Diego, J.; Trilla, C.; Escartin, P. Hepatic growth induced by injection of the liver growth factor into normal rats. *Growth Regul.* **1994**, *4*, 113–122. [PubMed]
78. Singh, J.; Bowers, L.D. Quantitative fractionation of serum bilirubin species by reversed-phase high-performance liquid chromatography. *J. Chromatogr.* **1986**, *380*, 321–330. [CrossRef]
79. Díaz-Gil, J.J.; Sanchez, G.; Trilla, C.; Escartin, P. Identification of biliprotein as a liver growth factor. *Hepatology* **1988**, *8*, 484–486. [CrossRef]
80. Carro, E.; Trejo, J.L.; Gomez-Isla, T.; LeRoith, D.; Torres-Aleman, I. Serum insulin-like growth factor I regulates brain amyloid-beta levels. *Nat. Med.* **2002**, *8*, 1390–1397. [CrossRef]
81. Perucho, J.; Casarejos, M.J.; Gomez, A.; Solano, R.M.; de Yebenes, J.G.; Mena, M.A. Trehalose protects from aggravation of amyloid pathology induced by isoflurane anesthesia in APP(swe) mutant mice. *Curr. Alzheimer Res.* **2012**, *9*, 334–343. [CrossRef]
82. Perucho, J.; Casarejos, M.J.; Rubio, I.; Rodriguez-Navarro, J.A.; Gomez, A.; Ampuero, I.; Rodal, I.; Solano, R.M.; Carro, E.; Garcia de Yebenes, J.; et al. The effects of parkin suppression on the behaviour, amyloid processing, and cell survival in APP mutant transgenic mice. *Exp. Neurol.* **2010**, *221*, 54–67. [CrossRef] [PubMed]
83. Casarejos, M.J.; Perucho, J.; Gomez, A.; Munoz, M.P.; Fernandez-Estevez, M.; Sagredo, O.; Fernandez Ruiz, J.; Guzman, M.; de Yebenes, J.G.; Mena, M.A. Natural cannabinoids improve dopamine neurotransmission and tau and amyloid pathology in a mouse model of tauopathy. *J. Alzheimers Dis.* **2013**, *35*, 525–539. [CrossRef] [PubMed]
84. Franklin, K.; Paxinos, G. *The Mouse Brain in Stereotaxic Coordinates*, 3rd ed.; Academic Press: San Diego, CA, USA, 2007.

Permissions

All chapters in this book were first published by MDPI; hereby published with permission under the Creative Commons Attribution License or equivalent. Every chapter published in this book has been scrutinized by our experts. Their significance has been extensively debated. The topics covered herein carry significant findings which will fuel the growth of the discipline. They may even be implemented as practical applications or may be referred to as a beginning point for another development.

The contributors of this book come from diverse backgrounds, making this book a truly international effort. This book will bring forth new frontiers with its revolutionizing research information and detailed analysis of the nascent developments around the world.

We would like to thank all the contributing authors for lending their expertise to make the book truly unique. They have played a crucial role in the development of this book. Without their invaluable contributions this book wouldn't have been possible. They have made vital efforts to compile up to date information on the varied aspects of this subject to make this book a valuable addition to the collection of many professionals and students.

This book was conceptualized with the vision of imparting up-to-date information and advanced data in this field. To ensure the same, a matchless editorial board was set up. Every individual on the board went through rigorous rounds of assessment to prove their worth. After which they invested a large part of their time researching and compiling the most relevant data for our readers.

The editorial board has been involved in producing this book since its inception. They have spent rigorous hours researching and exploring the diverse topics which have resulted in the successful publishing of this book. They have passed on their knowledge of decades through this book. To expedite this challenging task, the publisher supported the team at every step. A small team of assistant editors was also appointed to further simplify the editing procedure and attain best results for the readers.

Apart from the editorial board, the designing team has also invested a significant amount of their time in understanding the subject and creating the most relevant covers. They scrutinized every image to scout for the most suitable representation of the subject and create an appropriate cover for the book.

The publishing team has been an ardent support to the editorial, designing and production team. Their endless efforts to recruit the best for this project, has resulted in the accomplishment of this book. They are a veteran in the field of academics and their pool of knowledge is as vast as their experience in printing. Their expertise and guidance has proved useful at every step. Their uncompromising quality standards have made this book an exceptional effort. Their encouragement from time to time has been an inspiration for everyone.

The publisher and the editorial board hope that this book will prove to be a valuable piece of knowledge for researchers, students, practitioners and scholars across the globe.

List of Contributors

Kyung Hee Lee
Department of Dental Hygiene, Division of Health Science, Dongseo University, Busan 47011, Korea

Myeounghoon Cha
Department of Physiology, Yonsei University College of Medicine, Seoul 03722, Korea

Bae Hwan Lee
Department of Physiology, Yonsei University College of Medicine, Seoul 03722, Korea
Brain Korea 21 PLUS Project for Medical Science, Yonsei University College of Medicine, Seoul 03722, Korea

Vage Markosyan, Zufar Safiullov, Andrei Izmailov, Filip Fadeev, Mikhail Sokolov, Maksim Kuznetsov, Dmitry Trofimov, Evgeny Kim, Airat Gibadullin, Farid Bashirov and Rustem Islamov
Department of Medical Biology and Genetics, Kazan State Medical University, 420012 Kazan, Russia

Grayr Kundakchyan and Ilnur Salafutdinov
Institute of Fundamental Medicine and Biology, Kazan [Volga Region] Federal University, 420008 Kazan, Russia

Leniz Nurullin
Kazan Institute of Biochemistry and Biophysics, Federal Research Center of Kazan Scientific Center of Russian Academy of Sciences, 119991 Kazan, Russia

Beom Seok Kang, Bo Young Choi, A Ra Kho, Song Hee Lee, Dae Ki Hong, Jeong Hyun Jeong, Min Kyu Park and Sang Won Suh
Department of Physiology, College of Medicine, Hallym University, Chuncheon 24252, Korea

Dong Hyeon Kang
Department of Medical Science, College of Medicine, Hallym University, Chuncheon 24252, Korea

Xinyue Dong, Jin Gao, Yujie Su and Zhenjia Wang
Department of Pharmaceutical Sciences, College of Pharmacy and Pharmaceutical Sciences, Washington State University, Spokane, WA 99202, USA

Motomasa Tanioka
Department of Physiology, Yonsei University College of Medicine, Seoul 03722, Korea
Brain Korea 21 PLUS Project for Medical Science, Yonsei University College of Medicine, Seoul 03722, Korea

Wyun Kon Park
Department of Anesthesiology and Pain Medicine, Anesthesia and Pain Research Institute, Yonsei University College of Medicine, Seoul 03722, Korea

Joohyun Park
Brain Korea 21 PLUS Project for Medical Science, Yonsei University College of Medicine, Seoul 03722, Korea
Department of Anatomy, Yonsei University College of Medicine, Seoul 03722, Korea

Jong Youl Kim, Sumit Barua and Ye Jun Jeong
Department of Anatomy, Yonsei University College of Medicine, Seoul 120-752, Korea

Jong Eun Lee
Department of Anatomy, Yonsei University College of Medicine, Seoul 120-752, Korea
BK21 Plus Project for Medical Sciences, and Brain Research Institute, Yonsei University College of Medicine, Seoul 120-752, Korea

Kyoung-Ha Park
Division of Cardiovascular Diseases, Hallym University Medical Center, Anyang 14068, Korea

Man-Sup Lim
Department of Medical Education, College of Medicine, Hallym University, Chuncheon 24252, Korea

Jonas Ort, Benedikt Kremer, Hans Clusmann, Anke Höllig and Ute Lindauer
Department of Neurosurgery, Medical Faculty, RWTH Aachen University, 52074 Aachen, Germany

Linda Grüßer and Romy Blaumeiser-Debarry
Department of Anaesthesiology, Medical Faculty, RWTH Aachen University, 52074 Aachen, Germany

Mark Coburn
Department of Anaesthesiology and Intensive Care Medicine, University Hospital Bonn, 53127 Bonn, Germany

Luca Colucci-D'Amato
Department of Environmental, Biological and Pharmaceutical Sciences and Technologies, University of Campania "Luigi Vanvitelli", 81100 Caserta, Italy
Inter University Center for Research in Neurosciences (CIRN), University of Campania "Luigi Vanvitelli", 80131 Naples, Italy

Luisa Speranza
Department of Neuroscience, Albert Einstein College of Medicine, New York, NY 10461, USA

Floriana Volpicelli
Department of Pharmacy, School of Medicine and Surgery, University of Naples Federico II, 80131 Naples, Italy

Md Ezazul Haque, Mahbuba Akther and Shofiul Azam
Department of Applied Life Science, Graduate School, Konkuk University, Chungju 27478, Korea

In-Su Kim
Department of Biotechnology, Research Institute of Inflammatory Disease (RID), College of Biomedical and Health Science, Konkuk University, Chungju 27478, Korea

Dong-Kug Choi
Department of Applied Life Science, Graduate School, Konkuk University, Chungju 27478, Korea
Department of Biotechnology, Research Institute of Inflammatory Disease (RID), College of Biomedical and Health Science, Konkuk University, Chungju 27478, Korea

Juan Perucho, Manuela Vallejo-Muñoz, Maria José Casarejos, Diana Reimers, Ana Gómez, Gonzalo M. Ulzurrun de Asanza and Eulalia Bazán
Servicio de Neurobiología, Instituto Ramón y Cajal de Investigación Sanitaria (IRYCIS), 28034 Madrid, Spain

Rafael Gonzalo-Gobernado
Servicio de Neurobiología, Instituto Ramón y Cajal de Investigación Sanitaria (IRYCIS), 28034 Madrid, Spain
National Centre for Biotechnology (CNB), CSIC, 28049 Madrid, Spain

Adriano Jiménez-Escrig
Servicio de Neurobiología, Instituto Ramón y Cajal de Investigación Sanitaria (IRYCIS), 28034 Madrid, Spain
Servicio de Neurología, Hospital Ramón y Cajal, 28034 Madrid, Spain

Index

www.ingramcontent.com/pod-product-compliance
Lightning Source LLC
LaVergne TN
LVHW081018210926
848485LV00004B/891